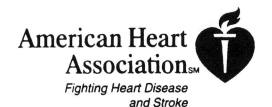

American Heart Association℠

Fighting Heart Disease
and Stroke

Monograph Series

DISCONTINUOUS CONDUCTION IN THE HEART

Previously published:

Cardiovascular Applications of Magnetic Resonance
Edited by Gerald M. Pohost, MD

Cardiovascular Response to Exercise
Edited by Gerald F. Fletcher, MD

Congestive Heart Failure: Current Clinical Issues
Edited by Gemma T. Kennedy, RN, PhD, and Michael H. Crawford, MD

Atrial Arrhythmias: State of the Art
Edited by John P. DiMarco, MD, PhD, and Eric N. Prystowsky, MD

Invasive Cardiology: Current Diagnostic and Therapeutic Issues
Edited by George W. Vetrovec, MD, and Blase Carabello, MD

Syndromes of Atherosclerosis: Correlations of Clinical Imaging and Pathology
Edited by Valentin Fuster, MD, PhD

Exercise and Heart Failure
Edited by Gary J. Balady, MD, and Ileana L. Piña, MD

Sudden Cardiac Death: Past, Present, and Future
Edited by Sandra B. Dunbar, RN, DSN, Kenneth A. Ellenbogen, MD, and Andrew E. Epstein, MD

Hormonal, Metabolic, and Cellular Influences on Cardiovascular Disease in Women
Edited by Trudy M. Forte, PhD

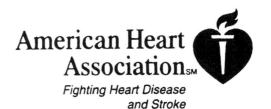

American Heart
Associationsm
*Fighting Heart Disease
and Stroke*

Monograph Series

DISCONTINUOUS CONDUCTION
IN THE HEART

Edited By

Peter M. Spooner, PhD

*Director, Arrhythmia Research Program,
Division of Heart and Vascular Diseases,
National Heart, Lung, and Blood Institute,
National Institutes of Health,
Bethesda, Maryland*

Ronald W. Joyner, MD, PhD

*Professor, Pediatrics and Physiology,
Emory University School of Medicine,
Atlanta, Georgia*

José Jalife, MD

*Professor and Chairman,
Department of Pharmacology,
Professor of Pediatrics and Medicine, SUNY Health Science Center,
Syracuse, New York*

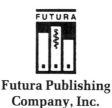

**Futura Publishing
Company, Inc.**
Armonk, NY

Library of Congress Cataloging-in-Publication Data

Discontinuous conduction in the heart / edited by Peter M. Spooner,
    Ronald W. Joyner, Jose Jalife.
        p.   cm. — (American Heart Association monograph series)
    Summaries of presentations from a 1995 research workshop
sponsored by the Basic Science Council of the American Heart
Association and the National Heart, Lung, and Blood Institute in
Hilton Head, S.C.
    Includes bibliographical references and index.
    ISBN 0-87993-669-X
    1. Arrhythmia—Pathophysiology—Congresses. 2. Heart conduc-
tion system—Congresses.   I. Spooner, Peter M. II.   Joyner,
Ronald W.   III. Jalife, Jose.   IV. American Heart Association. Basic
Science Council.   V. National Heart, Lung, and Blood Institue.
VI. Series.
    [DNLM: 1. Heart Conduction System—physiopathology—
congresses.
2. Arrhythmia—physiopathology—congresses.
WG 202 D611 1997]
RC685.A65D55 1997
616.1'2807—dc21
DNLM/DLC
for Library of Congress   97-23561
                                                                   CIP

Copyright © 1997
Futura Publishing Company, Inc.

Published by
Futura Publishing Company
135 Bedford Road
Armonk, New York 10504

LC #: 97-6841
ISBN #: 0-87993-669x

Preface

Discontinuity in cardiac conduction—multidimensional divergence and anisotropy in intertissue and intercellular communication between cardiocytes—is an important feature of the mechanisms determining the coordination and spread of electrical activation throughout the heart. In ischemic, scarred, or hemodynamically compromised hearts, it also represents the source of arrhythmic disturbances that claim the lives of thousands of patients each year.

Understanding the nature and structural and functional origin of cardiac discontinuities, and determining their effects on pathways of depolarizing and repolarizing potentials across the myocardium, are also an effort that, over the past two decades, has provided a fascinating new view of cardiac physiology.

Structural disorganization and block within macroscopic pathways of conduction have long been recognized as part of the "anatomic substrate" of many life-threatening arrhythmias. Development of corrective surgical and ablative strategies that address such macroscopic discontinuities represents an important and ongoing contribution of interventional cardiology. Recognition that microscopic discontinuities between cells of the contracting myocardium also modulate conductivity on a beat-by-beat/day-by-day basis and can result in aberrant macroscopic conduction is a more recent concept whose significance is just beginning to be appreciated.

Development of an improved understanding of arrhythmias that incorporates perception of both microscopic and macroscopic discontinuities has been hindered by a lack of fundamental information on their role in vivo. It is an area that has only recently begun to be explored. To paraphrase Dr Madison Spach, one of the field's pioneers:

> A major problem in cardiac electrophysiology is our lack of knowledge about inter-cellular current flow and cell-to-cell conduction. The increasing need to understand normal and abnormal conduction events at a cellular and sub-cellular level is related to mounting evidence that cardiac conduction is essentially discontinuous in nature, owing to recurrent resistive discontinuities created by cellular interconnections, or gap junction channels between adjacent cells. Discontinuous propagation at a microscopic level contrasts

with our longstanding (views) of cardiac conduction at a macroscopic scale, an understanding (focused on) . . . current mechanisms . . . in a continuous syncytium. The consequences (of the differences) are considerable . . . .[1]

The consequences are indeed . . . "considerable," and as supported by the information presented here, they indicate that our views at both levels require revision. Once considered largely within the realm of cardiac esoterica, new discoveries on the nature of membrane function and on the dynamic, nonlinear basis of excitation in arrhythmic hearts[2] present new prospects for understanding arrhythmogenesis and for its potential control.

The purpose of this volume is to present a series of views on discontinuous conduction, each encompassing a different dimension of cellular biological, molecular, or electrophysiological diversity, at different structural levels within the heart. Our goal was to review not only laboratory results but also implications for antiarrhythmic intervention. Thus, for example, the role of ventricular gap junctions is considered not just in terms of connexin molecular diversity and three-dimensional structure but also with the view that changes in their distribution, gating, or regulation could underlie changes in conduction velocity in ischemic zones and, like other ion channels, present new targets for drug therapy.

Each chapter presents the work of a leading group of experts drawn from across the United States and Europe to discuss views on discontinuities at multiple levels of propagation with, in many cases, dissimilar perspectives on similar phenomena. The chapters, which have been especially written for this publication, are based on presentations given in a workshop that was jointly sponsored by the Basic Science Council of the American Heart Assocation (AHA) and the National Heart, Lung, and Blood Institute (NHLBI).

The contributions published in the text represent the first collective attempt to integrate understanding of the molecular and cellular basis of discontinuities with new knowledge of global patterns of activation. Particular progress is reported in several important areas: new information on the diversity, structure, and function of different gap junction proteins; the availability of new theoretical and cellular models to predict the effects of changes in discontinuities and ion flux on conduction;

---

[1] Spach MS. Microscopic basis of anisotropic propagation in the heart. In: Zipes DP, Jalife J, eds. *Cardiac Electrophysiology.* New York, NY: WB Saunders Co; 1995:204–216.
[2] Jalife J, Davidenko JM, Michaels DC. A new perspective in the mechanisms of arrhythmias and sudden cardiac death: spiral waves of excitation in heart muscle. *J Cardiovasc Electrophysiol.* 1991;2:S133–S152.

and new gene targeting strategies with the potential to alter currents and discontinuities in vivo. The importance of these developments in our understanding of reentrant and other conduction arrhythmias in situ and in guiding future research is a major focus of the chapters that follow.

Kathryn A. Taubert, PhD
Peter M. Spooner, PhD

Acknowledgment

The ideas presented in this text were developed from initial discussions on an NHLBI workshop with two confirmed proponents of the importance of discontinuities in cardiology, Drs David Spray, Albert Einstein Colege of Medicine, and Ronald Joyner, Emory College of Medicine. In addition, an outstanding committee consisting of Drs Penny Boyden, Columbia University, Augustus Grant, Duke University, and José Jalife, Syracuse University, assisted with the selection and organization of topics and authors. Each also provided essential assistance in ensuring the quality and timeliness of the papers subsequent to the workshop.

All of those involved believe that publication of the work here will facilitate sharing of new perspectives in the search for safer, more effective ways to deal with arrhythmic disease. On behalf of the AHA, its Basic Science Council, and the Division of Heart and Vascular Diseases, the NHLBI, each of use would like to add our personal and professional thanks to the organizing committee and to each of the participants whose work is represented. All of us are also very much indebted to the leadership and staff of both organizations who provided the generous and essential support that made the effort possible.

Contributors

Michael A. Beardslee, MD   Cardiology Fellow, Cardiovascular Division, Washington University Medical School, St Louis, MO

Viviana M. Berthoud, PhD   Postdoctoral Fellow and Research Associate, Department of Pediatrics, Washington University School of Medicine, St Louis, MO

Eric C. Beyer, MD, PhD   Associate Professor of Pediatrics and Cell Biology and Physiology, Division of Pediatric Hematology/Oncology, Washington University School of Medicine, St Louis, MO

Penelope A. Boyden, PhD   Professor, Department of Pharmacology, College of Physicians and Surgeons of Columbia University, New York, NY

Candido Cabo, PhD   Post Doctoral Fellow, SUNY Health Science Center, Syracuse, NY

Wayne E. Cascio, MD   Associate Professor of Medicine, Division of Cardiology, Department of Medicine, University of North Carolina School of Medicine, Chapel Hill, NC

Bruce J. Darrow, MD, PhD   Resident Physician, Department of Internal Medicine, Columbia-Presbyterian Hospital, New York, NY

Jorge M. Davidenko, MD   Associate Professor, Department of Pharmacology, SUNY Health Science Center, Syracuse, NY

Lloyd M. Davis, MBBS, PhD   Staff Specialist Cardiologist, Westmead Hospital, Westmead, Australia

Jacques M. T. de Bakker, PhD   Department of Experimental Cardiology, University of Amsterdam Academic Medical Center, Amsterdam, The Netherlands

Mario Delmar, MD, PhD   Associate Professor, Department of Pharmacology, SUNY Health Science Center, Syracuse, NY

Stephen M. Dodge, MD   Resident Physician, Internal Medicine, Washington University School of Medicine, St Louis, MO

Williard S. Ellis, PhD   Department of Medicine and the Cardiovascular Research Institute, University of California, San Francisco, CA

Vladimir G. Fast, MD   Department of Physiology, University of Bern, Bern, Switzerland

Glenn I. Fishman, MD   Associate Professor, Department of Medicine, Section of Molecular Cardiology, Albert Einstein College of Medicine, Bronx, NY

Leonard S. Gettes, MD   Henry A. Foscue Distinguished Professor of Cardiology, University of North Carolina School of Medicine, Chapel Hill, NC

Augustus O. Grant, MB, ChB, PhD   Associate Professor, Cardiovascular Division, Department of Medicine, Duke University Medical Center, Durham, NC

Patricia A. Guerrero, MD   Cardiology Fellow, Cardiovascular Division, Washington University School of Medicine, St Louis, MO

Jose Jalife, MD   Professor and Chairman, Department of Pharmacology, Professor of Pediatrics and Medicine, SUNY Health Science Center, Syracuse NY

Michiel J. Janse, MD   Department of Experimental Cardiology, University of Amsterdam Academic Medical Center, Amsterdam, The Netherlands

Timothy A. Johnson, PhD   Research Associate Professor, Division of Cardiology, Department of Medicine, University of North Carolina School of Medicine, Chapel Hill, NC

Habo J. Jongsma, PhD   Professor of Medical Physiology, Chair, Department of Medical Physiology and Sports Medicine, Universiteit Utrecht, Utrecht, The Netherlands

Mark E. Josephson, MD   Director, Harvard Thorndike Electrophysiology Institute, Cardiovascular Division, Beth Israel Hospital, Boston, MA

Ronald W. Joyner, MD, PhD   Professor, Pediatrics and Physiology, Emory University School of Medicine, Atlanta, GA

Jonathan M. Kalman, MBBS, PhD   Department of Medicine and the Cardiovascular Research Institute, University of California, San Francisco, CA

Charles J. H. J. Kirchhoff, MD, PhD   Fellow, Harvard Thorndike Electrophysiology Institute, Cardiovascular Division, Beth Israel Hospital, Boston, MA

André G. Kléber, MD   Professor, Department of Physiology, University of Bern, Bern, Switzerland

James G. Laing, PhD   Postdoctoral Fellow, Department of Pediatrics, Washington University School of Medicine, St. Louis, MO

Michael D. Lesh, MD   Associate Professor, Cardiac Electrophysiology, Department of Medicine and the Cardiovascular Research Institute, University of California, San Francisco, CA

Eduardo Marban, MD, PhD   Professor of Medicine, Section of Molecular and Cellular Cardiology, Johns Hopkins University, Baltimore, MD

Gregory E. Morley, PhD   Postdoctoral Associate, Department of Pharmacology, SUNY Health Science Center, Syracuse, NY

Barbara Muller-Borer, PhD   Post Doctoral Fellow, Division of Cardiology, Department of Medicine, University of North Carolina School of Medicine, Chapel Hill, NC

Jeffrey E. Olgin, MD   Department of Medicine and the Cardiovascular Research Institute, University of California, San Francisco, CA

Brian O'Rourke, PhD   Assistant Professor of Medicine, Section of Molecular and Cellular Cardiology, Johns Hopkins University, Baltimore, MD

Arkady Pertsov, PhD   Associate Professor, Department of Pharmacology, SUNY Health Science Center, Syracuse, NY

Brian Ramza, MD, PhD   Postdoctoral Fellow in Cardiology, Johns Hopkins University, Baltimore, MD

Stephan Fohr, MD   Department of Physiology, University of Bern, Bern, Switzerland

Dmitry Romashko, PhD   Postdoctoral Research Fellow, Section of Molecular and Cellular Cardiology, Johns Hopkins University, Baltimore, MD

Michael R. Rosen, MD   Gustavus A. Pfeiffer Professor of Pharmacy, Professor of Pediatrics, College of Physicians and Surgeons of Columbia University, New York, NY

Yoram Rudy, PhD   Professor, Department of Biomedical Engineering, Case Western Reserve University, Cleveland, OH

Jeffrey E. Saffitz, MD, PhD   Professor of Pathology and Medicine, Washington University School of Medicine, St. Louis, MO

Robin M. Shaw, BS Sc   Research Assistant, Cardiac Bioelectricity Research and Training Center, Department of Biomedical Engineering, Case Western Reserve University, Cleveland, OH

Madison S. Spach, MD   Professor of Pediatrics and Cell Biology, Duke University Medical Center, Durham, NC

Peter M. Spooner, PhD   Director of Arrhythmia Research Program, Division of Heart and Vascular Diseases, National Heart, Lung, and Blood Institute, National Institutes of Health, Bethesda, MD

David C. Spray, PhD   Professor of Neuroscience and Medicine, Departments of Neuroscience and Medicine, Albert Einstein College of Medicine, Bronx, NY

C. Frank Starmer, PhD   Professor of Computer Science and Medicine, Duke University Medical Center, Durham, NC

Josef Starobin, PhD   Research Associate, Departments of Medicine (Cardiology) and Computer Science, Duke University Medical Center, Durham, NC

Harold C. Strauss, MD   Professor of Medicine and Pharmacology, Duke University Medical Center, Durham, NC

Peter N. Tadros, MD   Research Fellow, Cardiovascular Division, Washington University School of Medicine, St Louis, MO

Steven M. Taffet, PhD   Associate Professor, Department of Microbiology and Immunology, SUNY Health Science Center, Syracuse, NY

Kathryn A. Taubert, PHD   Senior Science Consultant, American Heart Association, Dallas, TX

Henk E. D. J. ter Keurs, MD, PhD   Professor of Medicine and Medical Physiology, University of Calgary Health Science Centre, Calgary, Alberta, Canada

Richard D. Veenstra, PhD   Associate Professor, Department of Pharmacology, SUNY Health Science Center, Syracuse, NY

Monique J. Vink, MD   Research Fellow, Department of Neuroscience, Albert Einstein College of Medicine, Bronx, NY

Andrew L. Wit, PhD   Professor, Columbia University College of Physicians and Surgeons, New York, NY

Mark Yeager, MD, PhD   Director, Research and Staff Cardiologist, Division of Cardiovascular Diseases, Scripps Research Institute, La Jolla, CA

Ying Ming Zhang, MSc   Department of Medicine, University of Calgary Health Science Center, Calgary, Alberta, Canada

Contents

Normal Cardiac Conduction
Introduction

Harold C. Strauss, MD

In the past, the heart was treated as an anatomic and electrical syncytium, because early electrophysiological studies[1-3] suggested that cardiac cells were connected by low-resistance pathways. Measurements of passive membrane properties in isolated cardiac Purkinje strands were well described by a one-dimensional cable equation.[1,3] As a result, analysis of propagation focused on measurements of the magnitude of the peak of the sodium current (phase O $\dot{V}_{max}$), conduction velocity and safety factor for propagation. Such measurements were used to elucidate the mechanism of conduction slowing under conditions designed to simulate different pathological conditions. In addition, studies were also designed to elucidate the mechanism of antiarrhythmic drug action which coincided with the introduction of numerous sodium channel blockers (Class I antiarrhythmic drugs) into the field. Unfortunately, the assumptions of one-dimensional cable theory are rarely met in cardiac muscle,[3] and the development of mathematical and analytical theories appropriate for treatment of experimental results obtained with two or three dimensions has been an enormous problem.

Advances in instrumentation and experimental approaches permitted cardiac investigators to characterize sarcolemmal ionic and gap junction currents and identify the proteins that formed the basis of those currents. In addition, a series of intriguing observations indicated that conduction in the heart is more appropriately described as being discontinuous rather than continuous. The initial three chapters that comprise the first section of the book provide an appreciation for how advances in our study of sarcolemmal ion channels, molecular biology of gap junction proteins, and the experimental and theoretical basis of discontinuous conduction have increased our understanding of scientific issues underlying cardiac conduction, cardiac arrhythmias, and sudden cardiac death.

The first chapter, by Dr. Spach, provides an elegant review of how our treatment of propagation evolved from consideration of conduction in the heart as being continuous to one in which conduction is viewed as being discontinuous at the microscopic level. The conduction discontinuity was due to the discrete microscopic resistances produced by the intercellular connections. These in turn produce electrical loading effects on the sarcolemmal ionic current. The significance of Spach's hypothesis is underscored by his demonstration that major conduction disturbances known to produce reentry can occur solely on the basis of variations in geometric arrangement of the gap junctions in the direction of propagation. The critical observations were that propagation velocity and rate of depolarization of the transmembrane potential were dependent on the direction of propagation in ventricular and atrial muscle. This finding poses new challenges in identifying therapeutic targets for arrhythmias. It suggests that the anatomic details of the arrangement of individual myocytes, their irregular shapes, and the nonuniform distribution of gap junctions are important in the structural analysis of conduction. Subsequent studies have demonstrated that gap junctional currents vary greatly and that different gap junction orientations may be used for current flow in different directions.

How does excitation spread occur in individual cells as a function of propagation direction on a subcellular level? It then becomes important to consider that the greatest load inside each cell occurs in membrane patches next to the intercalated disks at the end of cells. Hence, the safety factor for propagation would be enhanced by increasing Na current density in the area of the cell membrane near the gap junction and would provide some rationale for the initially puzzling observations by Cohen,[4] who noted an increased density of Na^+ channel protein near the gap junction. Finally, Dr. Spach suggests that the long-term changes in cellular connectivity during aging, ie, loss of a diffuse distribution and lateral connections between cells and their effects on conductivity are unexplored. In addition, loss of side-to-side coupling between groups of cells appears to be a major mechanism for unidirectional block and reentry by producing spatial differences in the effective refractory period. This chapter places in much better perspective the importance of each topic dealt with in greater detail in the remaining chapters in the text and in this way represents a most elegant introduction to the field from one of its leading proponents.

Chapter 2, by Dr. Jongsma, underscores the importance of gap junction channels in forming the low-resistance pathways between cells. Gap junction size (ie, the number of parallel conducting intercellular channels), gap junction distribution, and properties of the intracellular channels contribute importantly to passive current spread and, as a result, propagation. This chapter reviews the morphology and distribution of gap junctions, the structure and distribution of gap junction channels, their modulation, and the consequences for conduction of the cardiac impulse. In the heart, messenger RNAs for six connexin (Cx) species have been detected, although only three have been shown to be expressed. There are considerable differences in the tissue distribution of these three. Gating kinetics of Cx43 are influenced by phosphorylation state and intracellular pH, suggesting that changes in cell signaling and intracellular acidification during myocardia ischemia for example, may explain the substantial changes in passive membrane properties and conduction that have been observed experimentally. As yet, however, there are few definitive functional data indicating that conduction properties are modified by phosphorylation.

Although we tend to think of connexins as being of importance only in the mature heart, studies in which the Cx43 gene is genetically knocked out in mice identified a potentially extremely important role for connexins in development.[5] Cx43 is abundant in many parts of the heart but is probably not necessary for conduction in the embryonal and early neonatal heart. However, the Cx43 knockout mice die of developmental defects in the right ventricular outflow tract. Similarly, some pediatric patients with visceroatrial heterotaxia have point mutations at putative phosphorylation sites in the Cx43 carboxy-terminus[6] These observations, in concert with other data discussed by Dr. Jongsma, suggest that Cx43 not only plays an essential role in creating an electrical syncytium in the heart but also may provide a communication pathway for signaling molecules to move between cells during development, thereby playing a critical role in normal cardiac development.

Dr. Marban and colleagues remind us in Chapter 3 that sarcolemmal ion channels not only are necessary for transmitting the impulse but also are capable of modifying excitation on a beat-to-beat basis. Although much attention has been devoted to the study of voltage-gated ion channels, this chapter emphasizes the importance of a ligand-gated K^+ channel, namely the ATP-sensitive K^+ channel ($I_{K,ATP}$). Its role in the adaptive response to myocardial ischemia and ATP depletion is widely appreciated. However, the recent discovery of an intrinsic metabolic oscillator in individual heart cells strongly suggests that glycolytic oscillation can occur during substrate deprivation and/or anoxia-reoxygenation and drive $I_{K,ATP}$, resulting in large oscillations in membrane K^+ conductance. Such cyclical changes in membrane current could form the basis of inhomogeneities and perhaps arrhythmogenesis.

References

1. Weidman S. The electrical constants of Purkinje fibres. *J Physiol (Lond)*. 1952; 118:348–360.
2. Weidman S. The diffusion of radiopotassium across intercalated disks of mammalian cardiac muscle. *J Physiol (Lond)*. 1966;187:323–342.
3. Fozzard HA, Arnsdorf MF. Cardiac electrophysiology. In: Fozzard HA, Haber E, Jennings RB, Katz AM, Morgan HE, eds. *The Heart and Cardiovascular System: Scientific Foundations*. New York, NY: Raven Press; 1992:63–98.
4. Cohen SA. Immunocytochemistry of rat cardiac sodium channels. *Circulation*. 1991;84(suppl II):II–182. Abstract.
5. Reaume AG, deSousa PA, Kulkarni S, Langille BL, Zhu D, Davies TC, Juneja SG, Kidder GM, Rossant J. Cardiac malformation in neonatal mice lacking connexin43. *Science*. 1995;267:1831–1834.
6. Britz-Cunningham SH, Maithili MS, Craig WZ, Fletcher WH. Mutations of the connexin43 gap-junction gene in patients with heart malformations and defects of laterality. *N Engl J Med*. 1995;332:1323–1329.

Chapter 1

Discontinuous Cardiac Conduction:
Its Origin in Cellular Connectivity With Long-Term Adaptive Changes That Cause Arrhythmias

Madison S. Spach, MD

The object of this chapter is to describe how emergent new conduction behavior occurs as a result of microscopic changes in the discrete nature of cellular connectivity of the myocardium. These relatively new conduction phenomena are discontinuous in nature, and they provide important theoretical and experimental challenges to synthesize a complete theory linking discontinuous conduction at a microscopic scale with continuous conduction at the larger, macroscopic level. In this endeavor, it will be important to distinguish differences in wave-front movement and conduction block caused by intrinsic variations in membrane ionic properties of continuous media versus wave-front movement from block due to conduction abnormalities caused by differences in electrical loading secondary to variations in the distribution of the electrical connections between cells.

A Major Missing Factor

Although it has long been appreciated that cardiac muscle is composed of discrete cells connected together by "low-resistance" connections, the electrical effects produced by the irregular distribution of

This work was supported by U.S. Public Health Service Grant HL 50537 and the North Carolina Supercomputing Center.

From: Spooner PM, Joyner RW, Jalife J (eds). *Discontinuous Conduction in the Heart.* Armonk, NY: Futura Publishing Company, Inc.; © 1997.

these connections between cells and between bundles have been considered of minor importance. It has been assumed, therefore, that the myocardial architecture has electrical properties equivalent to those of continuously uniform geometry and resistance in the direction of propagation. In such structures, there is a positive correlation between the peak magnitude of the membrane sodium current (as expressed by $\dot{V}_{max}$), the conduction velocity, and the safety factor of conduction.[1-3] Thus, $\dot{V}_{max}$ and the safety factor of propagation have long been closely associated in the analysis of action potentials that propagate in a continuous medium. These considerations have been reinforced by the success achieved in the application of continuous cable theory to the analysis of impulse conduction in nerve axons.[4,5] In a continuous medium, spatial variations in membrane ionic currents are necessary to produce conduction disturbances. The mechanisms of arrhythmias, therefore, have been considered to be limited to the intrinsic ionic properties of the sarcolemma, eg, inhomogeneities of action potential duration in the widely used "leading-circle" concept.[6]

Consequently, basic research has focused on the measurement of the sarcolemmal ionic currents in isolated single cells, and the greatest successes of modern cardiac electrophysiology have been the "molecular dissection" of the sarcolemmal ionic current channels. A profound effect of these achievements has been the development of a framework for the mechanisms of cardiac conduction disturbances as well as for the associated pharmacological therapy of reentrant arrhythmias that focuses on the intrinsic kinetics of the sarcolemmal ionic currents.[7] In contrast to the remarkable advances in basic science, however, the management of clinical arrhythmias, and especially of atrial fibrillation, the most commonly encountered chronic arrhythmia in patients, remains far from satisfactory.[8,9] In addition, the clinical application of antiarrhythmic pharmacological agents targeted to block the sarcolemmal ionic channels recently encountered a major setback. Clinical trials, such as the CAST study,[10] have shown that the chronic administration of these pharmacological agents produces serious proarrhythmic effects in adults with structural heart disease, even though the drugs may suppress the appearance of conducted premature impulses. Although the serious proarrhythmic effects of drugs designed to block the sarcolemmal ionic channels have created difficult clinical problems, they also have generated a perplexing problem for basic scientists: most available information focuses on electrophysiological changes that occur when the activity of sarcolemmal ionic current channels is altered, yet clinical evidence now suggests that there is a "major missing factor" that is important in reentrant arrhythmias.

Concomitant with the foregoing developments, the picture of a different type of mechanism producing cardiac conduction disturbances began to be developed in 1981. At that time, our experimental results led us to propose the hypothesis that cardiac conduction was discontinuous in nature at a microscopic level because of the presence of resistive discontinuities produced by the cellular connections that, in turn, produce electrical loading effects on the sarcolemmal ionic currents.[11] In retrospect, this concept represents a major departure from the long-held idea that cardiac muscle behaves like a continuous syncytium, and it provides a new field to determine the mechanisms underlying the widely known but poorly understood link between "structural heart disease" and cardiac arrhythmias. Thereupon, we were able to accumulate considerable experimental evidence to support a theory of discontinuous conduction and to suggest its importance by demonstrating that all of the major conduction disturbances known to produce reentry can occur solely on the basis of variations in the geometric arrangement (topology) of the gap junctions in the direction of propagation, especially in tissues with sparse side-to-side coupling between cells, which occurs in association with microfibrosis.[12,13] In addition, we found that "anisotropic reentry" occurred in adult canine atrial bundles in the absence of spatial differences in action potential duration (Figure 1).[11] Subsequently, considerable information has been presented from numerous laboratories, including our own, that discontinuities of conduction due to the discrete nature of cellular connectivity in cardiac muscle play an important role in arrhythmias.[14–18]

On the basis of the foregoing, the primary candidate for the currently "major missing factor" is discontinuous conduction in cardiac bundles that undergo changes in the distribution of the gap junctions. That is, small changes in the distribution of the gap junctions at a microscopic level produce large changes in conduction behavior at a global anatomic level.[11–13] Accordingly, the central question for cardiac electrophysiology now becomes, How do microscopic variations in the geometric arrangement of the gap junctions that couple the nonlinear membranes of individual cells produce marked changes in the electrical behavior of the entire heart?

This chapter addresses that question by developing a picture of how the distribution of the gap junctions of mature normal ventricular myocardium produces the events of discontinuous conduction at a microscopic level. The major feature is the presence of increases in electrical load and the magnitude of the sodium current localized to the cell membrane adjacent to the gap junctions. This picture is then expanded to incorporate the observation that the normal myocardium undergoes adaptive changes in the arrangement of the gap junctions throughout life.[12,19] With these changes, there is a concomitant loss of side-to-side cellular coupling, which is arrhythmogenic. The major premise of this chapter is the following syllogism: changes in the electrical behavior

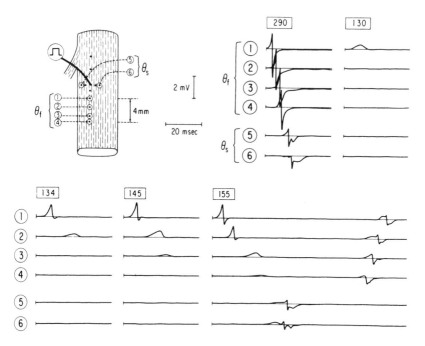

Figure 1. Abnormal conduction events leading to anisotropic reentry. Drawing (upper left) shows locations of stimulating and recording electrodes on a crista terminalis atrial preparation from an adult dog. Waveforms in rest of figure were recorded from extracellular electrodes at numbered sites. Numbers in boxes represent delay time (in milliseconds) between prior normal stimulus and a premature stimulus. If premature stimulus was started in absolute refractory period and its delay was increased, earliest distant extracellular potential occurred at delay of 130 ms. Activity being recorded was clearly decremental, because it was recorded only by closest electrode along long axis of fibers. As premature stimulus interval was increased from 134 to 145 ms, decremental propagation in longitudinal direction increased in strength and was observed at greater distances. At 155 ms, stable but very slow propagation (0.05 m/s) occurred in transverse direction, while longitudinally, there was decremental conduction to block. Lower panel, at 155 ms, second group of waveforms at electrodes 1 through 4 represents reentry with reentrant excitation propagating back toward stimulus electrode. Reprinted with permission from Reference 11.

of normal myocardium occur primarily as a result of adaptive changes in the geometric arrangement of the gap junctions,[18] a process that begins at birth and continues through the aging process. Consequently, superimposed abnormal states, such as hypertrophy[15] and healing after infarction,[14] induce marked acceleration, abnormal enhancement, or recapitulation of the long-term adaptive changes in the spatial arrangement of gap junctions that evolve in normal hearts.

Major Advances Produced by the Application of Continuous Cable Theory to Cardiac Muscle

The development of a complete theory of discontinuous conduction for normal and abnormal conduction phenomena will require the step-by-step development of an approximate electrical description of the microarchitecture of a variety of cardiac structures, beginning with normal myocardium.[20,21] The continuous cable theory[22] used by Hodgkin and Huxley[5] to create a quantitative description of impulse conduction in nerve axons provides the foundation for development of any concept or model of discontinuous conduction based on an electrical description of the myocardial architecture. Before going on to discontinuous propagation, therefore, it is important first to establish how ideas about conduction disturbances developed as they evolved on the basis of the assumption that cardiac impulse conduction occurred in a continuous syncytium.

The initial application of a structural theory to the conduction of impulses in excitable tissues was based on a theory developed outside the realm of biology. In 1855, Lord Kelvin (Sir William Thomson) had published a solution to a similar problem from engineering, that of a leaky one-dimensional cable, for application to the transatlantic telegraph cable.[22] Kelvin derived the now-classic continuous cable equation

$$1/(r_i + r_o) \, (\partial^2 V/\partial x^2) = i_m \tag{1}$$

where r_i and r_o are the resistances per unit length of the inside and outside conductors, respectively; V is the transmembrane potential; ∂x measures the distance along one spatial dimension; and i_m is the net current through the membrane per unit length.

By the early 1920s, a clear picture had developed of the general electrical characteristics of living cells.[23] It was known that a conductive cell interior is surrounded by a thin, poorly conducting membrane that, in turn, is surrounded by conductive extracellular fluid. It was soon realized that Lord Kelvin's cable equation might apply to excitative structures, such as elongated nerves.[24,25] In 1946, Hodgkin and Rushton[4] produced a quantitative demonstration of the accuracy of this analogy by combining an analytic solution of the cable equation for a passive linear membrane (membrane resistance r_m of a unit length and capacitance c_m per unit length),

$$1/(r_i + r_o) \, (\partial^2 V/\partial x^2) = i_m = (V_m/r_m) + c_m(\partial V_m/\partial t), \tag{2}$$

with extracellular potential measurements in a thin film of solution surrounding a lobster axon immersed in oil.

The application of continuous one-dimensional cable theory to cardiac muscle began with Weidmann[26] in the 1950s. Based on the assumption then prevalent that cardiac cells formed a literal syncytium with cytoplasmic continuity (continuous medium), he duplicated the Hodgkin-Rushton experiment[4] on a Purkinje fiber. Weidmann obtained a satisfactory fit at a macroscopic level with the solutions of Equation 2 and extracted passive parameters for the preparation from his fit: ie, current injected within a single cell altered the potential in cells that were multiple cell lengths distant from the cell in which current was injected.

With the introduction of electron microscopy, however, it became clear that cytoplasmic continuity did not exist between cardiac cells.[27-29] Woodbury and Crill[30] noted the apparent paradox this caused because of the high resistance of the sarcolemmal membrane. To obtain an answer to the question of how the local circuit gets from cell to cell, as observed by Weidmann,[26] Woodbury and Crill measured changes in the transmembrane potential induced by intracellular current injection. They found that the length constant of voltage decay was longer than the cell length in the longitudinal direction and longer than the cell width in the transverse direction. Consequently, they concluded that there must be "low-resistance" connections between cells at the intercalated disk to get the current from one cell to another. Subsequently, Barr et al[31] were able to localize this continuity to the gap junction (nexus). By the late 1960s, the paradox seemed to be resolved: although the heart consists of individual cells entirely surrounded by high-resistance membrane, there are pathways between cells of sufficiently high conductance to cause the tissue to behave functionally like a continuous syncytium. Continuous cable theory, therefore, was assumed to apply to small bundles of cardiac cells. This theory was then used in numerous experiments at a macroscopic scale to extract passive parameters and to explain differences in propagation from region to region on the basis of a difference in membrane properties, ie, a difference in the characteristics or density of the membrane channels for the excitatory ionic currents.

Ionic currents, however, by themselves do not determine propagation, so their characteristics must be combined with a theory of the appropriate structure, including its geometry and linear electrical properties. Because of the variable shapes of cardiac myocytes, their nonuniform arrangement, and the irregular distribution of the gap junctions, it has not been possible to achieve analytical solutions of equations that electrically describe cardiac tissue at a microscopic level. Numerical computer simulations have therefore become invaluable in identifying the kinds of propagation phenomena that might be produced by the architecture of the myocardium. Until recently, however, because of the complexity of the microarchitecture, computer models of multidimensional propagation have represented cellular connectivity as the averaged effect of many cells at the much larger macroscopic level, a scale at which propagating excitation waves appear to be continuous, even if anisotropic.[32,33]

The first clear experimental correlations between propagation velocity and the angle between the wave front and the long fiber axis were published in 1959 by Draper and Mya-Tu[34] and Sano et al.[35] Although they did not verify the wave-front orientation, both concluded that the propagation velocity in ventricular muscle is approximately three to four times larger in the direction of the long axis of the fibers than in the transverse direction. Clerc[36] subsequently postulated that the directional difference in propagation velocity in relation to the orientation of the fibers is due to the directional difference in axial resistivity. To obtain the relative values of axial resistivity along and perpendicular to the long axis of the fibers, he measured the peak values of intracellular and extracellular potential gradients during propagation in young calf ventricular muscle. He related the velocity and the resistance measurements by assuming a continuous but anisotropic two-dimensional (2D) sheet model and a constant shape of the action potential at all sites for all directions of conduction. He concluded that the resistance values he measured accounted for the velocity differences according the classic inverse-square relationship that had been shown by Hodgkin[37] in a continuous cable:

$$\theta = k(1/(\sqrt{r_i}), \tag{3}$$

where θ is the conduction velocity, k is a constant depending on the membrane properties, and r_i is the internal resistance per unit length. For the case of a continuous cable, Hodgkin[37] concluded that changes in velocity (θ) secondary to changes in internal resistance (r_i) would occur according to the reciprocal relationship shown in Equation 3 without altering the temporal shape of the action potential.

Initial Evidence That Conduction Is Discontinuous in Cardiac Muscle

In 1981, we encountered serious difficulty in applying the above ideas to the analysis of propagation of depolarization at a microscopic level.[11] The problem is most clearly illustrated by recapitulating the events as they occurred at that time. We were conducting experiments on the origin of extracellular potential waveforms in anisotropic cardiac bundles,[38] using the assumption that such bundles have continuous passive electrical properties. This assumption was consistent with the then-recent experimental analysis by Clerc[36] of anisotropic velocity differences in young calf ventricular muscle, in which he found no directional differences in the shape of the upstroke of the action potential. However, we observed variations in the rate of depolarization of the transmembrane potential that were dependent on the direction of propagation in normal adult atrial and ventricular canine muscle.[11] Greater values of $\dot{V}_{max}$ occurred during slow transverse conduction across the fibers (TP) in the direction of high axial resistance, and lower $\dot{V}_{max}$ values occurred with fast conduction along the long axis of the fibers (LP) in the direction of low axial resistance. The reproducible directional differences in $\dot{V}_{max}$ clearly were not due to changes in the membrane ionic properties, because each microelectrode impalement site served as its own control when the direction of conduction was altered.

Defining Discontinuous Conduction

We were unable to find any mechanism known at that time to account for this result. The directional variations in the rate of depolarization of the transmembrane potential could not occur in a continuous medium because in such structures, differences in velocity due to differences in axial resistance do not alter the time course of the action potential.[37] Having eliminated all known factors as a possible explanation, we hypothesized that cardiac conduction is discontinuous in nature at a microscopic level because of recurrent discontinuities of intracellular resistance produced by the cellular connections, which, in turn, alter the membrane ionic currents by means of electrical loading.[11] At a microscopic level, propagation of the excitatory process occurs with recurrent delays and hesitations at localized sites of elevated intracellular resistance that correspond to the cell boundaries and gap junctions. As illustrated schematically in Figure 2, depending on the direction of conduction, the propagation of excitation within cells stops at the boundaries produced by the nonjunctional (sarcolemmal) membrane, creating incremental or "boundary" block ($\rightarrow$|). However, the process does not actually stop at the connections between cells, ie, at the gap junctions. Rather, variable delays and hesitations in propagation occur at the gap junctions dependent on the time required for sufficient current to flow across each gap junction to discharge the capacitance of the sarcolemmal membrane on the other side to initiate excitation in the downstream cells.

Significance of Discontinuous Conduction

The major question about the above phenomenon is whether it represents merely second-order conduction events at a microscopic

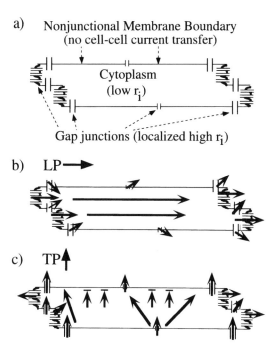

a) Nonjunctional Membrane Boundary
(no cell-cell current transfer)

Cytoplasm
(low r_i)

Gap junctions (localized high r_i)

b) LP→

c) TP↑

Figure 2. Schematic representation of discontinuous propagation events of a single cardiac myocyte within a multicellular network. a, In intracellular space, gap junctions represent local areas of increased resistance relative to that of cytoplasm, and there is no transfer of cell-to-cell current via nonjunctional (sarcolemmal) membrane. b, c, Arrows indicate direction of current flow in direction of conduction. During longitudinal propagation (LP), conduction delays occur primarily at cellular connections at ends of elongated cell. During transverse propagation (TP), total time required to excite all the sarcolemmal membrane of the cell is much less than during LP, and conduction stops at lateral border of cell (→|). This delay permits sufficient current transfer to occur across gap junctions to discharge capacitance of sarcolemmal membrane on other side gap junctions and turn on excitatory mechanism of adjacent laterally connected cells.

scale or whether it indicates that the distribution of gap junctions in different conduction pathways may be important in producing the conduction disturbances that initiate reentrant arrhythmias. To answer that question, we used the preceding ideas about discontinuous conduction to perform experiments demonstrating that changes in the distribution of the gap junctions in the path of propagating excitation waves independently produce all of the major conduction abnormalities that initiate reentry.[11–13,15] The conduction disturbances in this category are (1) decremental conduction, (2) unidirectional block, and (3) very slow conduction (<0.1 m/s). All of these conduction disturbances played a major role in producing the events leading to anisotropic reentry in the muscle bundle illustrated in Figure 1.

How can we be sure that the patterns of propagation with decremental conduction and reentry illustrated in Figure 1 were not due to spatial differences in action potential duration? To ensure that this mechanism was not the cause of the events, we made the following checks. (1) The time of return of local excitability (as an index of action potential duration) was measured at multiple sites within the entire area of the reentry circuit. The measured premature intervals were 151 ms at the stimulus site and 144 ms at electrode 4 (the site at which LP decremental block occurred), a variation in the opposite direction required to explain the decremental conduction on the basis of action potential differences. (2) The stimulus electrode and a few of the recording electrodes were moved to other sites within the initial measurement area, and a portion of the sequence of premature stimuli was repeated. For all sites tested in similar preparations, the pattern of simultaneous decremental conduction (longitudinal, LP) and nondecremental (transverse, TP) propagation was observed for some range of delay of the premature stimulus, and these events produced anisotropic microreentry in atrial bundles from elderly individuals.[15] Thus, the unusual conduction patterns were not due to spatial differences in the action potential; rather, they were related to the direction of the fiber orientation, with different arrangements of the cellular connections in the longitudinal and transverse pathways.

The significance of discontinuous conduction, therefore, is that it introduces a major class of new mechanisms that cause cardiac arrhythmias. These new mechanisms are based on variations in the topology of the gap junctions that, in turn, create nonuniform loading effects on the sarcolemmal membrane that alter the ionic currents. Consequently, discontinuous conduction poses a new challenge in terms of the long-term goal of identifying therapeutic targets for cardiac arrhythmias. The framework of therapeutic targets aimed at correcting the underlying conduction disturbances must now be expanded to include not only the long-known effects of regional variations in the sarcolemmal membrane ionic channel properties but also the recently found effects of variations in electrical loading due to different geometric arrangements of the gap junctions.[39]

Approaching Discontinuous Conduction at a Microscopic Level

Significant problems become apparent, however, when one attempts to study the mechanisms of conduction events related to discontinuous conduction at a microscopic level. Foremost is the fact that electrical loading, like the effective coupling conductance between cells,[40] is strongly dependent on the nonuniform topology of the gap junctions in multicellular networks and thus cannot be measured directly. Nor can the problem be reduced to isolated cell pairs, which removes the nonuniform loading effects produced by the irregular distribution of the gap junctions in naturally occurring tissues. These features most likely account for the lack of available information about the most fundamental features of cardiac conduction—the events of excitation spread inside individual cells and the events that occur when the excitatory impulse is transferred from one cell to its neighbors in multidimensional cardiac muscle.

We therefore hypothesized that variations in electrical load associated with different directions of conduction alter $\dot{V}_{max}$ because of changes in the spatial relationships between the impalement site of a microelectrode and the surrounding microscopic electrical boundaries encountered by different excitation waves.[41] These boundaries correspond to the different sizes and shapes of the impaled and contiguous cells and the distribution of their associated electrical connections. If this hypothesis is correct, these boundary relationships would also be different for small patches of sarcolemmal membrane located at different sites within a cell, thus implying that there are intracellular spatial variations in electrical load, which would produce variations of $\dot{V}_{max}$ inside individual cells. Examining $\dot{V}_{max}$ therefore becomes important because it is the only experimental measurement that provides a sensitive index of changes in the electrical load on the membrane as "seen" at a highly localized membrane patch (ie, the microelectrode impalement site). Furthermore, under conditions during which the intrinsic properties of the membrane ionic channels do not change, variations in $\dot{V}_{max}$ due to loading (boundary) effects produce associated changes in the sodium current. For example, decreases in $\dot{V}_{max}$ due to an increase in electrical load are associated with increases in I_{Na},[42,43] which is opposite to the classic relationship in which increases in I_{Na} are associated with increases in $\dot{V}_{max}$.

In view of the above, one experimental approach to evaluate spatial differences in electrical load at a microscopic level is to measure $\dot{V}_{max}$ at multiple sites and, at each site, to introduce a simple intervention that changes the complex geometric relationships between the impalement site, the boundaries of the impaled and contiguous cells, and the associated cellular interconnections. This intervention is a change in the direction of propagation from along the longitudinal to the transverse axis of the fibers and a reversal of the direction of conduction along each of these axes, ie, "four-way conduction," which does not alter the intrinsic properties of the membrane ionic currents. Figure 3

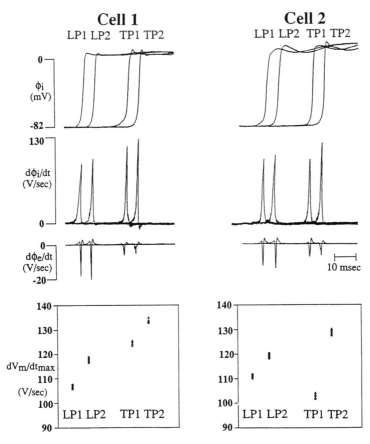

Figure 3. Upstrokes of intracellular action potential ϕ_i (top), derivatives of ϕ_i and extracellular potential ϕ_e (middle), and values of maximum rate of change of transmembrane potentials dV_m/dt_{max} (bottom) for five beats during propagation in each of four directions. In vitro measurements were performed in epicardium of normal adult canine left ventricular muscle with uniform anisotropic electrical properties. Reversal of plane-wave conduction was introduced along longitudinal axis of fibers (LP1 and LP2) and along an axis across fibers (TP1 and TP2) to produce "four-way conduction" at each impalement site. Cell 1 (left) represents typical result obtained in 35 cells, and cell 2 (right) represents atypical result obtained in 5 cells. Waveforms of intracellular potential (ϕ_i) are shown, as are their first derivatives (dϕ_i/dt) and first derivatives of extracellular potential (dϕ_e/dt), which illustrate calculation of dV_m/dt_{max} as dϕ_i/dt minus dϕ_e/dt. Multiple values of dV_m/dt_{max} for each direction (bottom) demonstrate that differences in dV_m/dt_{max} produced by four directions of conduction considerably exceeded slight beat-to-beat variations in values obtained during propagation in a given direction. Reprinted with permission from Reference 41.

shows the considerable variability of electrical loading effects within individual cells that became manifest from microelectrode measurements of transmembrane potentials by this method within small areas of well-coupled uniform anisotropic tissue[21,41]: (1) with any given direction of plane-wave conduction at a macroscopic level, $\dot{V}_{max}$ varied from site to site (not shown); (2) $\dot{V}_{max}$ at a single impalement site could be forced to have many values by causing a macroscopic planar wave front to propagate in multiple directions (Figure 3) and (3) at most impalement sites, TP $\dot{V}_{max}$ was greater than LP $\dot{V}_{max}$ (Figure 3, cell 1), but at a few sites (12.5%), one of the directions of transverse conduction produced the smallest $\dot{V}_{max}$ value of all four directions (Figure 3, cell 2). These results show that at each impalement site there is a unique relationship between LP $\dot{V}_{max}$ and TP $\dot{V}_{max}$ and also with 180° shifts in conduction direction along each axis.

Implications of the Variability of $\dot{V}_{max}$ at a Cellular Level

We asked the question as to whether the experimental variations in $\dot{V}_{max}$, along with the anisotropic differences in extracellular potential waveforms and their derivatives,[41] could be accounted for by a model with continuous internal resistance and "discontinuities" of the plasma membrane ionic current properties. A continuous 2D media model was used with "discontinuities" of the membrane ionic properties represented by periodic abrupt spatial changes in the maximum sodium conductance from 20 to 35 mS/cm^2 and vice versa (Spach MS, Heidlage JF, unpublished observations). The computer simulation results demonstrated that "membrane discontinuity" sites produced gradual spatial changes in the conduction events (eg, local velocity change and change in $\dot{V}_{max}$) that occurred over distances of several hundred micrometers. These changes could not account for the experimentally measured changes in $\dot{V}_{max}$, and none of the computed extracellular waveforms or their derivatives fit the experimental results. Only when an associated resistive discontinuity in intracellular space was added did the computed results begin to show a resemblance to those recorded experimentally. Thus, we concluded that the events of discontinuous propagation require recurrent discontinuities of axial resistance rather than abrupt spatial differences in membrane ionic properties in an otherwise continuous syncytium. Furthermore, we were also unable to find a satisfactory explanation for the measured variability of $\dot{V}_{max}$ based on curvature of the wave fronts[44,45] or on currently available models with resistive discontinuities at regularly spaced intervals.[46–49]

At this point, it is necessary to have some information about how cell-to-cell current flow (charge transfer) occurs across the nonuniformly distributed gap junctions during propagation in different directions in cardiac muscle. Such information is necessary in order to know whether the gap junctional "feedback" effects through electrical loading produce changes in the excitatory ionic currents in association with $\dot{V}_{max}$ changes within individual cells. To begin to make experimental measurements of the changes in the currents across a single gap junction plaque during conduction of the action potential, however, one must first locate the cellular connection and then measure the potential difference across the gap junctional plaque by monitoring the potential at sites very close to both sides of the gap junctional membrane (within a few micrometers). Such measurements have not been achieved and, at this point, the technical requirements are far beyond the resolution capabilities of available experimental techniques.

Thus, an important challenge for the future will be to develop new technology that provides high spatial-temporal resolution of simultaneously measured events at many sites, with each site identified with respect to the geometry of individual cells in the multicellular network. To design experiments that will use such to-be-developed techniques and to know how to interpret the results obtained therefrom, an associated theoretical basis will have to be developed for conduction at a microscopic level. From a practical standpoint, such a theoretical basis will require numerical computer models that approximate the complexities of the microstructure of the myocardium.

Electrical Description of the Architecture of Normal Mature Ventricular Myocardium and Its Application to Discontinuous Conduction

Details of the arrangement of cardiomyocytes, their irregular shapes, and the nonuniform distribution of their gap junctions have not entered into analyses of cardiac conduction up to this point. Without a realistic electrical model of cardiac architecture, there are insurmountable experimental problems in evaluating electrical loading effects within a given cell of a multicellular network. Thus, the only way we knew to address the problem of load variations within individual cells was to develop a 2D multicellular model that approximates the associated discrete myocardial architecture and mimics the "four-way conduction" experiments in the cellular model to determine whether the $\dot{V}_{max}$ behavior in the model is similar to that of real tissue.

We therefore developed a 2D cellular model to explore whether the $\dot{V}_{max}$ variability observed at random sites reflected variable patterns of excitation events within individual cells of normal adult left ventricular muscle.[20,21] We chose to approximate the architecture of adult left ventricular epicardium because it has the greatest variety of cell shapes and sizes, along with the highest degree of anisotropic coupling of cells, that we have encountered.[11,13,41] The distribution of cell shapes and the gap junctional arrangement chosen for any one model, however, represents only one of an infinite number of possible arrangements. Thus, rather than focus on a specific structure, we examined the concept that the variable sizes and shapes of cardiomyocytes, along with the nonuniform arrangement of their interconnections, have a major effect on conduction at a microscopic size scale.

We adhered to the constraint that all of the gap junctional channels (connexins) of mature myocytes were in the immediate region of the intercalated disks, as demonstrated for normal mature mammalian ventricular myocytes.[50–52] The Hodgkin-Huxley model[5] with Ebihara-Johnson kinetics[53] was used to approximate the fast sodium current. Construction of the model based on the measured geometry of myocytes from normal adult canine left ventricles, as well as the manner in which the cells were electrically coupled together to form a 2D multicellular network, is illustrated in Figure 4. The distribution of three types of gap junctions (Figure 4B) was approximated by use of available data from Saffitz's laboratory.[50] Detailed results are presented in recent publications, along with a description of the model, the assignment of conductance values to the gap junctions, the numerical analysis techniques, and verification of the model.[20,21]

Are Gap Junctional Delays and Intracellular Depolarization Events Influenced by Loading Effects of the Cellular Network?

To establish whether differences in electrical load alter junctional delays between normally coupled cells, we first created a minimal load by isolating a pair of myocytes that had a normal effective coupling conductance [$g_j(eff)$] value of 1.2 μS (Figure 5, top). When one of the cells was excited with a threshold stimulus of 0.5-ms duration, there was prolonged latency of V_m at -44 to -45 mV before simultaneous activation of both cells occurred (not shown). Throughout the myocytes, $\dot{V}_{max}$ varied between 268 and 275 V/s, the high values reflecting a minimal electrical load. The absence of a junctional delay was similar to the experimental result of Weingart and Maurer,[54] who used a threshold stimulus. When the stimulus was increased to two times threshold, however, a junctional delay of 55 μs occurred (Figure 5A) and $\dot{V}_{max}$ increased to a range of 289 to 321 V/s.

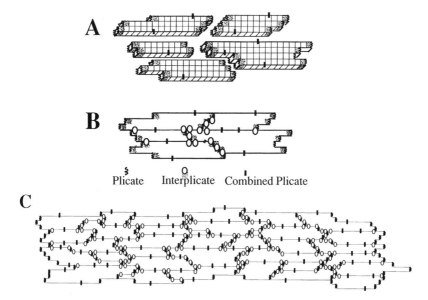

Figure 4. Formation of a 33-myocyte basic unit of 2D cellular model. A, Outlines of five myocytes and manner in which they were fitted together to form a group of cells. Stippled areas next to intercalated disks represent locations of interplicate gap junctional membrane. Grids show 10×10-μm segments that represent sarcolemmal membrane patches and interior of each cell (depth$=11.3$ μm). B, Arrangement of three types of gap junctions (symbols) that electrically interconnect myocytes. C, Arrangement of 33 myocytes and distribution of their intercellular connections (symbols). The 33-cell unit was replicated longitudinally and vertically by fitting ends and sides together to form cellular arrays of different sizes and shapes. Modified with permission from Reference 21.

When the same cell pair was incorporated into the 2D cellular network, cell "x" was connected to 7 cells and cell "y" to 6 cells. During transverse propagation, $\dot{V}_{max}$ in both cells decreased to values between 165 and 179 V/s, and the junctional delay increased to 165 μs (Figure 5B). Despite the significant intercellular conduction delay, the action potential upstrokes maintained a smooth contour (Figure 5B), as occurs experimentally during TP.[11] The effects of loading on the sodium current and the kinetics of the sodium channels were demonstrated by the following changes in the patches of membrane (darkened segments) on each side of the gap junction shown at the top of Figure 5: (1) In the isolated cell pair, total I_{Na} averaged 46 μC/cm^2 (Figure 5D). (2) In the isolated cell pair, total g_{Na} averaged 2.4 mS-ms/cm^2, and it increased to 3.05 mS-ms/cm^2 (27% increase) in the cellular network (not shown).

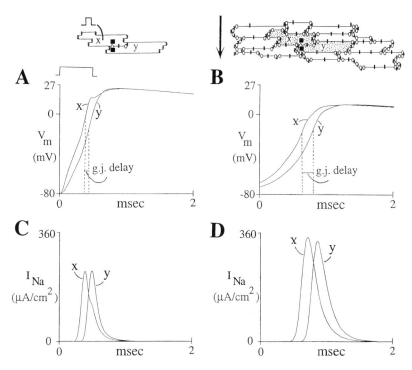

Figure 5. Loading effects of cellular network on impulse transfer between two well-coupled myocytes. Two cells are shown in isolation (top left) and within cellular network (top right); solid squares mark membrane segments, one on each side of an interplicate junction, where V_m and I_{Na} were recorded. Two myocytes were coupled by 1 plicate, 2 interplicate, and 1 combined plicate gap junction, which produced an effective gap junctional conductance [$g_j(eff)$] value of 1.2 μS. Gap junctional (g.j.) delay was determined as time difference in $\dot{V}_{max}$ of two segments. A, Gap junction delay of 55 μs following a two-times-threshold stimulus to cell "x" with cell pair in isolation. Stimulus symbol shows shape and duration (0.5 ms) of current pulse. B, Gap junction delay of 165 μs with cell pair incorporated into 2D cellular array. Macroscopic plane-wave transverse propagation (arrow) was initiated along a line located more than three resting space constants from group of cells shown. C, Time course of I_{Na} in isolated cell pair. D, Time course of I_{Na} during transverse propagation with cell pair incorporated into cellular network. Reprinted with permission from Reference 21.

Effects of Myocardial Architecture on the Spatial Distribution of Depolarization

The effects of the discrete nature of myocardial architecture on the spatial distribution of the depolarization phase of the action potential are shown in Figure 6. Depolarization extended approximately one resting space constant (λ) during both LP and TP ($\lambda_L = 1.3$ mm, $\lambda_T = 0.4$ mm[20]). The macroscopic conduction velocities produced a TP/LP velocity ratio of 0.31, with a TP velocity of 0.15 m/s and an LP velocity of 0.48 m/s, values that agree with experimental data in uniform anisotropic ventricular muscle.[11,38] The LP spatial pattern of depolarization approximated a smooth curve with large changes of the transmembrane potential (V_m) inside each cell and small V_m discontinuities at the connections between cells (Figure 6, LP). The LP pattern was similar to the spatial potential wavefront demonstrated by Rudy and Quan[55] in a 1D cable with intercalated disks at 100-μm intervals. During TP, however, the pattern was just the opposite: large discontinuities of V_m occurred between cells, and V_m showed little change across the interior of each cell (Figure 6, TP). The overall effect of the irregularities of V_m as a function of distance was well described as a single exponential process ($r = .99$) over many cells in the foot of the spatial action potential, as shown by the solid line for TP in Figure 6. Thus, at the macroscopic level, the discrete cellular changes in V_m become averaged and appear consistent with the continuous (exponential) approximation of the passive spread of currents in cardiac bundles.[20,56]

What Is the Nature of Excitation Spread Through the Cellular Network?

The sensitivity of propagating depolarization to the boundaries and gap junctions of the individual myocytes was best revealed by perspective plots that provided a microscopic view of the multidimensional spatial distribution of the activation times. Figure 7 presents a representative result for five interconnected myocytes. The group of cells analyzed (Figure 7, top) was located 3 λ from the stimulus site.

During longitudinal propagation, step increases of activation time (discontinuities) occurred in the region of the end-to-end connections between cells (Figure 7A). During LP, however, the major increases in activation time occurred along the sarcolemmal membrane within each myocyte. A major feature of LP was that the locations of the propagation discontinuities along the longitudinal axis corresponded to the irregular distribution of the plicate junctions. These irregular longitudi-

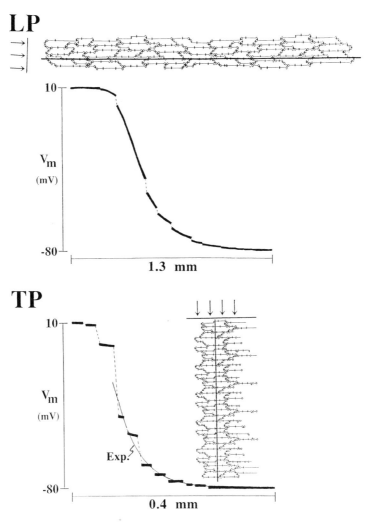

Figure 6. Spatial distribution of depolarization within 2D cellular network during longitudinal (LP) and transverse (TP) propagation. Spatial depolarization curve during LP (arrows) is a plot of V_m values at each consecutive segment along horizontal solid line overlying cellular network. Values of V_m were obtained at same instant of time. Spatial depolarization curve during TP (arrows) is a similar plot of V_m values at each consecutive segment along vertical solid line overlying network of cells. In each spatial depolarization curve, bold solid portion represents change of V_m within cells, and dashed lines represent step changes in V_m at gap junctions and cell borders. Solid line superimposed on foot of TP spatial depolarization curve (Exp.) is best fit of a single exponential to V_m values between -80 and -20 mV ($r = .99$). Reprinted with permission from Reference 21.

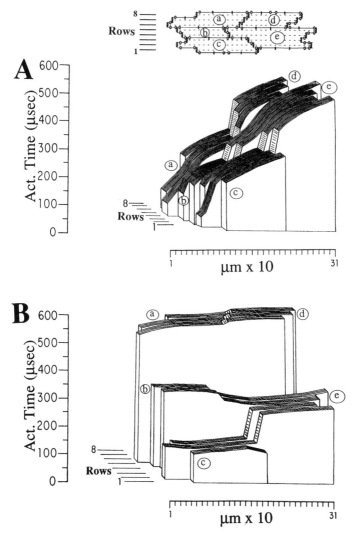

Figure 7. Perspective plots of activation times depicting propagating depolarization through a network of five myocytes at center of 2D cellular model. During LP and TP, time of $\dot{V}_{max}$ was determined at each segment (8 rows of longitudinal marks) within five myocytes (top). A, Longitudinal propagation in a left-to-right direction. B, Transverse propagation in a bottom-to-top direction. In each perspective plot, activation times along each of eight rows of 10×10-μm segments are plotted as function of distance along longitudinal axis of cells. Hatched steps in each perspective plot denote delays across plicate gap junctions. In both panels, letters a through e are included to identify each myocyte with activation times along corresponding rows depicted in five myocytes (top). Reprinted with permission from Reference 21.

nal local delays at the end-to-end connections of myocytes produced asynchrony of excitation in different portions of myocytes located side by side. Thus, superimposed on the overall smooth process of LP, the nonuniformly distributed longitudinal and lateral discontinuities of propagating depolarization reflected the irregular shapes of the cells (Figure 7A).

With TP, there were large lateral "jumps" in activation time between cells, whereas within each myocyte there was almost simultaneous activation of the sarcolemma (Figure 7B). The lateral "jumps" in activation time coincided with the lateral borders of the underlying cells. A few sites displayed prominent longitudinal discontinuities of activation time that were due to the asynchrony of activation of two irregularly shaped cells connected end to end (Figure 7B, cells c and e). This asynchrony occurred because the lateral border of the earliest-activated cell extended further in the direction of the approaching wave front than did the lateral border of the adjoining cell, which was activated later. During TP, however, only small differences in activation time occurred across the end-to-end connections of most cells, eg, the small activation time discontinuity between cells a and d. The pattern of transverse excitation spread, therefore, was quite different from that of LP. TP occurred as large "jumps" in activation time between the lateral borders of juxtaposed cells, and within individual myocytes there was almost simultaneous activation of the entire sarcolemmal membrane.

A general conclusion of the results shown in Figure 7 is that conduction is indeed discontinuous at a microscopic scale, and the discontinuities of propagation are more prominent during transverse than longitudinal conduction. Moreover, plane waves do not occur at a microscopic level because of the disruption of the excitation wave by the irregular cell boundaries and the associated nonuniformly distributed gap junctions.

How Does Cell-to-Cell Current Flow Occur During Propagation in Different Directions?

To answer this question, we assessed the corresponding transfer of charge across each gap junction of the same five-cell group (cf Figure 7, top) during LP and TP. We calculated the net charge transferred across each gap junction by (1) obtaining the voltage-difference curve of the upstrokes of the transmembrane action potentials of the two segments on either side of each gap junction and (2) multiplying the area of the voltage-difference curve by the associated value of the gap junctional conductance. The average net charge transferred across the

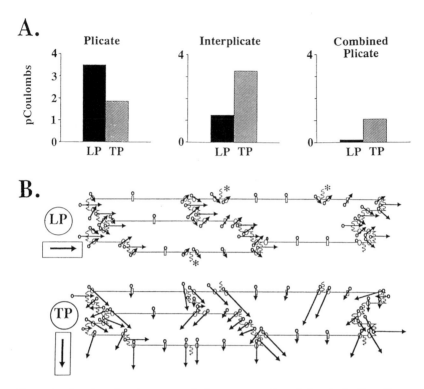

Figure 8. Gap junctional currents during propagation of depolarization. Group of five cells analyzed was same as those shown at top of Figure 7. A, Mean values of net charge (picocoulombs) transferred across each gap junction during propagation of upstroke of action potential in longitudinal (LP) and transverse (TP) directions. Number of gap junctions was 23 plicate, 49 interplicate, and 15 combined plicate. (Types of gap junctions are illustrated in Figure 4B.) B, Magnitude and direction of net charge transfer across each gap junction during upstroke of action potential are represented by length and direction of each arrow. Length of arrows within boxes represents 0.33 pC.

plicate, interplicate, and combined plicate junctions for the five cells during longitudinal and transverse propagation is shown in Figure 8A. As can be seen, each type of gap junction demonstrated a considerably different mean value of net transfer of charge during propagation in the longitudinal versus the transverse direction ($P<.001$).

To view the gap junctional currents during the propagation of depolarization in greater detail, we analyzed each cell of the group to compare the specific differences in charge transfer across each gap junction during LP and TP. A typical result is shown in Figure 8B for three of the interconnected cells. The magnitude and direction of total charge transfer during the propagation of depolarization across each gap junction are represented by the length and direction of each arrow. The considerable differences in the amount of charge transferred across each junction, as well as differences in the direction of current flow, can be seen for LP and TP. During LP, the asterisks at the top of Figure 8B mark two intercalated disks that separated myocytes located above the cell shown. The associated arrows illustrate that during LP, part of the charge transfer between two directly connected cells occurred by current flow around the intercalated disk via another cell.[20]

The results therefore demonstrate that the magnitude of the gap junctional currents varies greatly and that different gap junctions are used for cell-to-cell current flow (charge transfer) for different directions of propagation. We found the differences in gap junctional current during LP and TP to be associated with similar differences in the mean gap junctional time delay and mean peak voltage across the gap junctions ($P<.001$).[21] Consequently, the longer the delay in transfer of the depolarization phase of the action potential across a gap junction, the greater the cell-to-cell charge transferred via the gap junction. Furthermore, because of the complex arrangement of the gap junctions at the intercalated disks, during LP part of the current flow between cells directly coupled end-on-end occurs around the intercalated disk via a laterally juxtaposed cell.

How Does Excitation Spread Occur Within Individual Cells During Different Directions of Conduction?

Representative intracellular excitation sequences during longitudinal propagation are presented in Figure 9A, which shows isochrones within each of the same five interconnected myocytes used in the foregoing analysis of gap junctional currents. During LP, the mean time to excite all of the membrane within each cell was 226 ± 78 μs (range, 68 to 348 μs; n = 11). Except for slight bending at intercalated disks near the ends of the irregularly shaped cells, the isochrones maintained a vertical orientation throughout each cell. Within each cell, however, the isochrones shifted farther apart as excitation moved from the area where the action potential entered the cell to the area where it exited the cell. Consequently, the major intracellular feature of LP was that conduction was slower in the proximal part and faster in the distal part of each cell. These subcellular events produced an alternating sequence of slower and faster conduction along the path of longitudinal conduction throughout the cellular network. Reversing the direction of longitudinal conduction showed that the subcellular differences in the speed of conduction were not caused by variations in cross-sectional area within the cells. When the direction of longitudinal conduction was

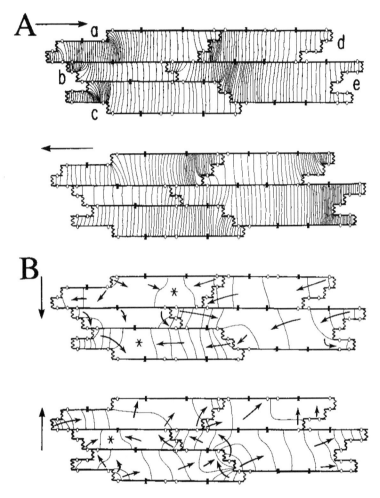

Figure 9. Intracellular excitation sequences during "four-way" conduction along longitudinal and transverse axes of myocytes. A, Isochrones within each of five myocytes (a through e) during propagation in both directions (arrows) along longitudinal axis of cells. Isochrones are separated by 4 μs. B, Intracellular isochrones during propagation in both directions (arrows) along transverse axis of cells. Isochrones are separated by 3 μs. Asterisks represent sites of intracellular collisions during transverse propagation. Cells a through e are same five myocytes as at top of Figure 7. Reprinted with permission from Reference 21.

reversed, the proximal part of each cell (with respect to the direction of LP) remained the region of slowest conduction and the distal part of each cell remained the region of fastest conduction.

The major subcellular feature of transverse conduction was the rapidity with which excitation spread throughout each cell (Figure 9B). During TP, the mean intracellular conduction time was 21 ± 10 μs (range, 8 to 39 μs) for the same cells in which the mean intracellular conduction time during LP was 226 μs ($P<.001$). Another major difference was that during TP, the pattern of intracellular excitation spread was different in each cell (Figure 9B). Within the same cell, the isochrones were oriented in different directions, and the pattern within each myocyte changed drastically when the direction of conduction was reversed along the transverse axis of the cells. For example, collisions occurred in cells a and c when the direction of TP was from top to bottom (Figure 9B, ↓, asterisks). However, when the direction of TP was reversed (Figure 9B, ↑), a collision occurred only in cell b. We did not find a myocyte that demonstrated an intracellular collision during both directions of TP.

Does $\dot{V}_{max}$ Have the Same Value Throughout a Cell for Each Direction of Conduction?

We found $\dot{V}_{max}$ to vary within all cells of the 2D network for all directions of conduction. Representative results of "four-way conduction" are shown for two cells in Figure 10. During LP (Figure 10A), $\dot{V}_{max}$ was lowest in the proximal part ("input" region) of each myocyte, where intracellular conduction was slowest. $\dot{V}_{max}$ increased to its maximal value between the middle and distal fourth of each cell. In the distal part ("output region") of each myocyte, $\dot{V}_{max}$ decreased, although conduction was fastest in this region. During LP, the $\dot{V}_{max}$ minima at the distal output region of the myocytes had higher values than did the minima at the proximal input region ($P<.001$). The fluctuating values of $\dot{V}_{max}$ within each myocyte resulted in an alternating sequence of lower and higher $\dot{V}_{max}$ values along the longitudinal axis of the network of cells.

When we compare the model results to the experimentally observed variations in $\dot{V}_{max}$ at different locations along the axis of conduction, it is reasonable to assume that in the experiments, the tip of the microelectrode varied randomly in its intracellular location relative to the ends of each impaled cell. Consequently, at different subcellular locations within different cells, the values of $\dot{V}_{max}$ would be different because of the fluctuations of $\dot{V}_{max}$ within the individual cells. Therefore, the cellular model results were consistent with the experimental

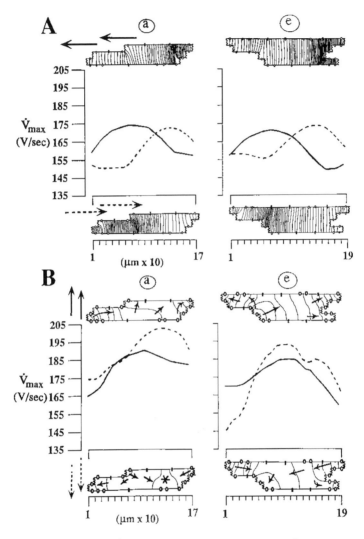

Figure 10. Distribution of $\dot{V}_{max}$ within two myocytes during "four-way conduction." In each graph, values of $\dot{V}_{max}$ are plotted as a function of distance (μm) along a line of consecutive segments extending between ends of each myocyte. A, Longitudinal propagation in both directions along long axis of cells. A cellular outline with accompanying intracellular excitation sequence for each direction of longitudinal propagation (isochrones separated by 4 μs) is presented for each direction of LP. B, Transverse propagation in both directions along an axis transverse to long axis of cells. An outline of each myocyte with accompanying intracellular excitation sequence is presented for each direction of TP (isochrones separated by 3 μs). Myocytes a and e are those of previous figures.

variety of $\dot{V}_{max}$ values observed at different impalement sites during LP.[21,41]

During TP, there was considerable cell-to-cell variation, although the intracellular pattern of a $\dot{V}_{max}$ maximum with two minima was maintained, as occurred during LP (Figure 10B). The mean $\dot{V}_{max}$ value within almost every cell was greater during TP than during LP. However, the TP $\dot{V}_{max}$ minima near the ends of each cell were often lower than the LP $\dot{V}_{max}$ maximum located near the center of each cell. Consequently, there was considerable overlap of TP $\dot{V}_{max}$ and LP $\dot{V}_{max}$ when values from different subcellular areas of the same or different myocytes were compared. When the paired values of $\dot{V}_{max}$ were compared at each segment, however, TP $\dot{V}_{max}$ was greater than LP $\dot{V}_{max}$ throughout most cells. Near the ends of a few myocytes, however, there was a reversal of the usual TP>LP $\dot{V}_{max}$ relationship. For example, in Figure 10B ($\Downarrow$), at the left end of cell e, the value of $\dot{V}_{max}$ during TP in a top-to-bottom direction was less than the value of $\dot{V}_{max}$ at that site during LP in either direction along the axis of the cells. These areas near the ends of a few myocytes probably provide a subcellular basis for the experimental result that at a few implement sites, TP $\dot{V}_{max}$ was less than LP $\dot{V}_{max}$.[21,41]

Nonuniformity of Electrical Load Inside Cells Indicated by $\dot{V}_{max}$ Intracellular Variations

Because the ionic properties of the surface membranes of all of the cells of the 2D cellular model were identical, we concluded that the variations of $\dot{V}_{max}$ could be accounted for only by associated variations of electrical load within individual cells. In the presence of constant membrane ionic channel properties, there is an inverse relationship between electrical load and $\dot{V}_{max}$.[42,43] It follows that for all directions of conduction, therefore, the greatest load inside each cell occurred in membrane patches next to the intercalated disks at the ends of the cells (areas of the $\dot{V}_{max}$ minima), and the intracellular area of least load (highest value of $\dot{V}_{max}$) was located toward or near the center of each cell. Thus, the membrane areas of greatest electrical load within each cell were concentrated at the intercalated disks where currents were received from and transferred to adjacent cells via the associated gap junctions. This subcellular distribution of electrical load can be accounted for by the following. (1) The small portion of the cell surface membrane that is adjacent to the input gap junctions is the first area of the cell to be excited. Consequently, $\dot{V}_{max}$ in this area is decreased by the loading effects of most of the membrane of the cell, which is yet to be depolarized. (2) The area of membrane just proximal to the output intercalated disks is influenced by the loading effects of the gap junctional current needed to initiate excitation of the membrane on the other side of the output gap junction, which is membrane constituting the input area of the next cell, an area of maximal load because of the yet-to-be-depolarized major portion of that cell.

An additional feature in most cells was that the $\dot{V}_{max}$ minimum adjacent to the input intercalated disks had a lower value than that of the $\dot{V}_{max}$ minimum located just proximal to the output intercalated disks. This relative difference in the values of the two $\dot{V}_{max}$ minima indicates that the electrical load is less in the output region than in the input area of most cells. The relatively lower load on the membrane in the output area can be accounted for by the "boundary effect" of the discontinuity in the path of conduction caused by the discrete increase in resistance of the adjacent output gap junctions (cf Figure 2). That is, the elevated resistance of the output gap junctions produces a discontinuity that, in turn, has a boundary effect[42] that diminishes the load and tends to elevate $\dot{V}_{max}$ in the area just proximal to the discontinuity. As a result, discontinuous propagation is characterized by the gap junctions producing interactive loading effects on the same area of membrane. For example, loading produced by the transfer of current across the output gap junctions tends to decrease $\dot{V}_{max}$ (local increase in electrical load) in the output region of each cell, whereas the concomitant boundary effect of the discontinuity produced by the output gap junctions tends to increase $\dot{V}_{max}$ (local decrease in electrical load) in the same area of the cell.

Variations in the Magnitude of I_{Na} Within Individual Cells

To evaluate the associated effects of loading on the sodium current inside cells, we analyzed the total amount of I_{Na} generated by each 10×10-μm patch of the surface membrane within 16 myocytes of the 2D model.[21] The subcellular spatial variation in the magnitude of I_{Na} was the same as that of $\dot{V}_{max}$, with an inverse relationship between the two (LP: $r = -.78$, $P<0.001$; TP: $r = -.87$, $P<.001$; n=564 segments). A typical relationship between excitation spread, $\dot{V}_{max}$, and I_{Na} within a single myocyte is shown in Figures 11 and 12 for LP and TP, respectively. During LP, the magnitude of I_{Na} was greatest in the proximal part of the myocyte, less in the distal part, and least in a region located between the middle and distal fourth of the cell (Figure 11C). During TP, the magnitude of I_{Na} was greatest near the ends of the myocyte and lowest in the central area of the cell (Figure 12C). The subcellular variations in the magnitude of I_{Na} were also linked to variations in the

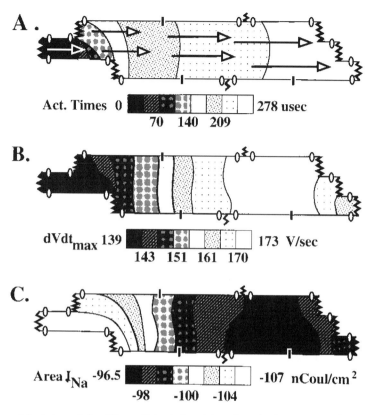

Figure 11. Intracellular 2D spatial relationships of excitation spread, $\dot{V}_{max}$, and magnitude of I_{Na} within a single myocyte during longitudinal propagation. A, Map of intracellular excitation sequence. B, Map of distribution of dV/dt_{max}. C, Map of total charge (nC/cm²) carried by sodium current. Isovalue map of distribution of sodium current (Area I_{Na}) was constructed from values of total depolarizing sodium current of each 10×10-μm segment (nC/cm²) within myocyte. Opposite patterns of B and C are due to inverse relation between $\dot{V}_{max}$ and magnitude of I_{Na} in each membrane segment. Relationships are shown for myocyte c of Figure 9.

kinetics of the sodium channels; the total sodium conductance was proportional to total I_{Na} in each segment ($r=.99$, $P<.001$, n$=564$).

Significance of Subcellular Variation of I_{Na} Due to Discontinuous Conduction

These microscopic spatial variations in the magnitude of I_{Na} are the hallmark of discontinuous conduction, a feature quite different

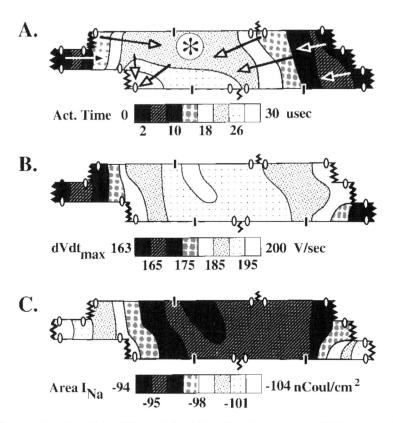

Figure 12. Intracellular 2D spatial relationships between excitation spread, $\dot{V}_{max}$, and I_{Na} within a single myocyte during transverse propagation. Relationships are shown for same myocyte as in Figure 11. A, Map of intracellular excitation sequence. Asterisk denotes an intracellular collision. B, Map of distribution of dV/dt_{max}. C, Map of total charge (nC/cm^2) carried by sodium current.

from that which occurs in a continuous syncytium. Localization of increased I_{Na} to surface membrane regions adjacent to the input and output gap junctions of each cell provides a striking similarity to the same regions in which Cohen[57] demonstrated an increased density of the sodium channel protein in rat cardiac myocytes. He showed that antibodies against portions of the amino-terminus and carboxy-terminus and I-II interdomain region of the rat cardiac sodium channel labeled the surface membrane adjacent to the intercalated disks at the ends of cardiac myocytes more intensely than the remainder of the surface membrane. Subcellular variations in the density of the Na^+ channels also have been demonstrated by voltage clamp measurements in Purkinje cells by Makielski et al[58] and with the loose-patch-clamp technique in ventricular cells by Antoni et al.[59]

The specific locations of increased I_{Na} due to enhanced electrical loading at the ends of the cells (Figures 11C and 12C) provide an important consideration as to why it would be advantageous to increase the density of functional sodium channels in these areas of the surface membrane. The safety factor of conduction would be improved by the following. (1) Increasing I_{Na} in the input area would augment current flow throughout the cytoplasm to discharge the capacitance and enhance activation of the Na^+ channels of the remainder of the membrane of each cell. (2) Increasing I_{Na} in the output area would augment cell-to-cell conduction by increased transfer of charge across the output gap junctions. The results therefore suggest that there is a close spatial relationship between the input and output gap junctions, increased electrical load on the juxtaposed cell membrane that increases the magnitude of I_{Na}, and the associated increased density of Na^+ channel protein demonstrated by Cohen.[57] The significance of these relationships is that the distribution of the gap junctions creates the patterns of subcellular loading that increase the magnitude of I_{Na} near the input and output gap junctions in the path of the propagating excitation wave. Consequently, subcellular variations in both electrical load and the expression of the Na^+ channel protein in the surface membrane appear to be linked to the topology of the gap junctions.

An important challenge is the clarification of these relationships to answer the question, Does the enhanced subcellular loading that produces an increased magnitude of I_{Na} near the gap junctions serve as a supramolecular mechanism that affects second messengers to enhance expression of ion-channel proteins in these specific areas of the cell membrane? If so, it is possible that the direction of conduction may influence the density of Na^+ channels in specific subcellular areas because the maximal intracellular load is at the input and output gap junctions of each cell.

Long-Term Changes in Cellular Connectivity From Birth Through Aging

Changes in the Distribution of Gap Junctions Within Individual Myocytes

In contrast to the foregoing picture of mature ventricular cells, the distribution of the electrical and mechanical connections within neonatal cardiac myocytes is quite different.[60–63] In human ventricular muscle, Peters et al[63] demonstrated in neonatal myocytes that the gap junctions (connexin [Cx] 43) and fascia adherens junctions (N-cadherin) are distributed in a punctate manner over the entire surface of each cell. Although the gap junctions and fascia adherens junctions generally have a close spatial association, the two types of junctions frequently are not closely adjacent in infants but become increasingly so with maturation of the intercalated disk. Furthermore, during early childhood the gap junctions and fascia adherens junctions lose their diffuse distribution as lateral connections between adjacent cells, and both types of junctions become progressively confined to the large transverse terminals characteristic of the intercalated disks of adult ventricular myocytes.[50–52] The adult pattern of the distribution of gap junctions at the intercalated disks is achieved at about 6 years of age in humans.[63]

For comparative purposes, Figure 13 shows a drawing of a typical result obtained by immunolabeling of Cx43 in neonatal and adult canine ventricular myocardium in our recent studies (Spach MS, Dolber PC, unpublished observations), using methods previously described by Dolber et al.[52] The neonatal myocyte is small and has a smooth spindle shape, and the surface membrane of the entire cell is covered by punctate labeling of Cx43. The adult ventricular myocyte is much larger and has an irregular shape because of the staggered arrangement of the transverse-oriented intercalated disks, and there are large areas along the cell surface that have no gap junctions (Cx43). These age differences in single myocytes illustrate that during the long interval of normal physiological hypertrophy and growth after birth there is a loss of gap junctions (Cx43) along the sides of individual cardiac myocytes. Concomitantly, gap junctions (Cx43) become concentrated in large transverse-oriented disks toward the ends of mature cells as well as in a few disks scattered along the length of the adult myocyte.

A. Neonate

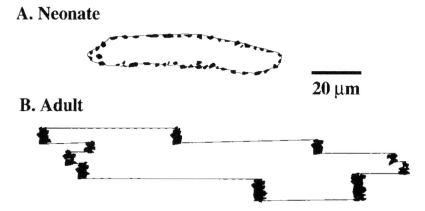

20 μm

B. Adult

Figure 13. Drawing of a typical neonatal (A) and adult (B) canine ventricular myocyte to illustrate characteristic differences in size and shape of cells and associated differences in distribution of immunolabeled gap junctions (connexin43).

The effects on microscopic conduction of these changes in cellular geometry and cellular connectivity are unexplored, and they present an important area for future study. As noted earlier, new techniques and/or approaches will be needed, especially in this case because of the small size of neonatal myocytes. Consequently, at this point a major need is the development of numerical multidimensional models that include the details of cellular geometry and connectivity at different ages after birth. We have only preliminary experimental and model data in newborn ventricular preparations. With the caveat that the data are quite preliminary, the variability of microscopic conduction events appears to be less in neonatal than in adult ventricular myocardium, eg, less variation of $\dot{V}_{max}$ inside individual myocytes, with smaller differences in $\dot{V}_{max}$ for different directions of conduction. These preliminary results suggest that cellular loading is different in well-coupled networks of small, young cells than in well-coupled networks of large, mature cells. Whether these differences play a role clinically in the increase of arrhythmias with increasing age (and size) from birth remains to be determined. However, it can be said at this point that changes in the size and shape of individual myocytes, along with changes in the distribution of the gap junctions, alter the effects of electrical loading on conduction within cells and on cell-to-cell conduction.

Loss of Side-to-Side Coupling Between Groups of Normal Cells With Development of Microfibrosis

In the preceding paragraphs, both neonatal and adult myocytes have been considered to be located in networks in which each cell is connected to numerous surrounding cells,[50–52] thus producing tight electrical coupling (relatively low resistance) in all directions. In such tissues, smooth extracellular waveforms occur during conduction in all directions, as shown for transverse conduction in Figure 14A. We have designated such tissues as being characterized by uniform anisotropy. Bundles of this type have been shown to encompass large areas of the normal canine ventricle[13] and pectinate atrial bundles from children.[19] It quickly became apparent, however, that with the progression of time, some bundles change their passive properties from uniform anisotropy to those of nonuniform anisotropy,[12,13] as indicated by the development of multiphasic extracellular waveforms during transverse conduction (Figure 14B, middle).

The appearance of multiphasic extracellular waveforms during TP indicates asynchronous excitation of small groups of cells due to loss of side-to-side coupling,[12] which produces a zigzag course of propagating

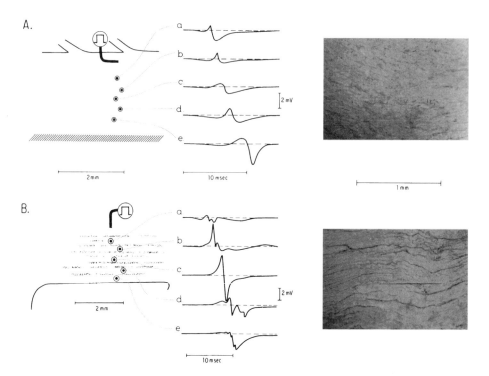

Figure 14. Transverse propagation in uniform (A) and nonuniform (B) aniso-tropic canine atrial muscle bundles. A, Crista terminalis; B, limbus of fossa ovalis. The two preparations were from same atrium of a puppy 1 week after birth. Extracellular waveforms recorded during transverse propagation are shown on left. Smooth single deflections occurred with uniform anisotropy (A), and irregular multiphasic waveforms occurred with nonuniform anisotropy (B). Associated microscopic structure of uniform versus nonuniform anisotropy is shown on right. In newborn crista with uniform anisotropy, collagenous tissue is distributed among myocytes in a scattered and irregular manner (A). In limbus with nonuniform anisotropy, collagenous tissue is organized into fine connective tissue septa (microfibrosis), which appear as wavy horizontal lines that separate individual myocytes and groups of myocytes along long axis of fibers (B). By adulthood in dogs, many areas of atrium, including crista, demonstrate nonuniform anisotropic properties with connective tissue septa and multiphasic extracellular waveforms similar to those shown in B. Reprinted with permission from Reference 12.

depolarization through the poorly coupled but juxtaposed groups of cells.[19] These waveforms have consistently been associated with the appearance of fine, longitudinally oriented collagenous septa (microfi-brosis) that surround individual cells and small groups of cells (Figure 14B, right). We have found that the development of microfibrosis with loss of side-to-side connections between groups of cells (nonuniform anisotropy) occurs normally in atrial bundles at two greatly separated time intervals: (1) in the crista terminalis and limbus of fossa ovalis of the dog during the first several months of life (Figure 14)[12] and (2) in adult human atrial pectinate bundles during the aging process.[19] These changes also occur in adult patients with atrial hypertrophy.[19] Furthermore, similar changes develop between birth and adulthood in selected areas of normal canine ventricles, ie, at the apex of the left ventricle (an area of tortuous movement) and in areas adjacent to coronary blood vessels. These regions in normal ventricular muscle are associated with development of connective tissue septa, and they produce local ventricular areas that have multiphasic waveforms during transverse conduction.[64]

Long-Term Loss of Side-to-Side Fiber Coupling Produces Very Slow Conduction of Normal Action Potentials

Although the membrane depolarization properties remain the same, several changes occur in the propagation of normal action potentials in bundles that undergo loss of side-to-side coupling between groups of cells (microfibrosis).[19] These changes are illustrated by the conduction differences in a mature atrial pectinate muscle with uniform anisotropic properties from a 12-year-old child (Figure 15A, left) and in a pectinate muscle with nonuniform anisotropic properties from a 64-year-old adult (Figure 15B, left). In the child's bundle (uniform anisotropy), normal action potentials propagate from a single stimulus site with a gradual transition from longitudinal to transverse conduction to produce teardrop-shaped isochrones. The associated extracellular waveforms are smooth in contour, with a large biphasic deflection during fast LP and a small deflection with slower TP. Such bundles in both atrial and ventricular muscle produce an LP/TP velocity ratio between 2.5 and 4.

In the adult nonuniform anisotropic bundle (Figure 15B, left), the spread of normal action potentials from a single stimulus site produces a very narrow zone (in this case 100 μm wide) of fast longitudinal conduction and the transition to TP is abrupt, so there are no teardrop-shaped isochrones. Also, microscopic conduction is quite irregular during TP, as indicated by the multiphasic deflections in the low-amplitude extracellular waveforms (Figure 15B, left). Bundles with these conduction characteristics have a high LP/TP velocity ratio, ranging from 7 to 15. Histologically, these bundles demonstrate small collagenous septa marking areas in which there is an absence of side-to-side coupling

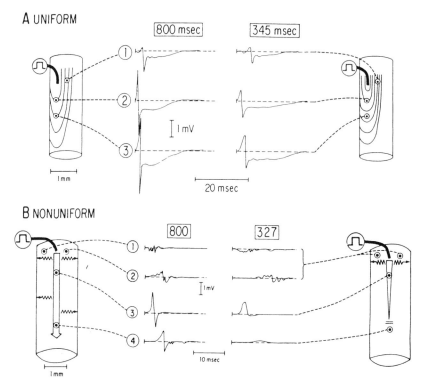

Figure 15. Difference in propagation responses of normal and premature action potentials in uniform (A) and nonuniform (B) anisotropic human atrial muscle bundles. In each panel, normal excitation sequence and a few measured extracellular waveforms are shown on left and those of an early premature impulse on right. Time intervals between stimuli are shown within boxes above each group of extracellular waveforms. A, Isochrones are drawn at 1-ms intervals. Atrial bundle was from a 12-year-old boy. B, Excitation sequence is represented by symbols because excitation sequence at a microscopic level was so complex that it was not possible to construct isochrone maps with a reasonable degree of accuracy. In drawing of normal conduction (left), elongated open arrow denotes narrow region of fast longitudinal conduction; on right, elongated triangle represents decremental conduction to block along long axis of fibers. Atrial bundle was from a 64-year-old woman. Reprinted with permission from Reference 15.

between small groups of cells for 2 to 10 cell lengths.[15,19] This feature is noted because mature atrial myocytes have quite importantly been shown to have fewer lateral gap junctions between their ends than do ventricular myocytes.[65] However, these differences in individual myocytes have been put forth as the cause of the high LP/TP velocity ratio in some atrial bundles (eg, crista terminalis) compared with the low LP/TP ratio in ventricular muscle.[65] In mature atrial and ventricular bundles that have uniform anisotropic properties, we have consistently found low LP/TP velocity ratios, <4. Furthermore, only when multiphasic shapes of the extracellular waveforms occur in atrial or ventricular bundles does a high LP/TP velocity ratio (nonuniform anisotropy) develop.[19] These features therefore suggest a different explanation. Rather than arising because the lateral connections are limited to the ends of each atrial myocyte, the development of a high LP/TP velocity ratio (>7) in atrial muscle occurs when individual myocytes are formed into elongated groups of cells without coupling to juxtaposed lateral fibers for multiple cell lengths.[12,15,19]

It is now clear that a major effect of the loss of side-to-side connections between elongated groups of cells is a significant decrease in the effective velocity of conduction across fibers. This decrease largely accounts for the high LP/TP ratio exhibited by nonuniform anisotropic bundles with microfibrosis. For example, in atrial pectinate bundles from children (uniform anisotropy), we found the mean effective transverse conduction velocity to be 0.12 m/s.[15] In larger pectinate muscle bundles from adults >50 years old (nonuniform anisotropy), however, the mean effective transverse velocity was only 0.085 m/s ($P<.01$),[15] a value similar to very slow conduction of the AV node. Very slow conduction (<0.07 m/s) was previously considered to require modification of the membrane depolarization currents to produce "depressed" membrane properties with "slow upstroke" action potentials, as occurs within the AV node. In the bundle from a 64-year-old subject in Figure 15B, however, normal action potentials propagated across the fibers with an effective velocity of 0.05m/s. In numerous nonuniform anisotropic human atrial bundles from subjects >60 years old, we found effective conduction velocities as low as 0.03 m/s in the presence of normal, fast upstroke action potentials.[15] This type of slow conduction of fast upstroke action potentials due to nonuniform anisotropy most likely will become increasingly important in the future identification of the cause of low conduction velocities that must be present within some areas of reentrant circuits for the circuit to be small enough to be maintained within the size of a specific chamber of the heart.

We have considered the collagenous septa within nonuniform anisotropic bundles to mark areas in which there could not be side-to-side electrical coupling between cells. That is, there are no sarcolemmal apposition sites between cells at which collagenous septa separate the fibers, and consequently, current cannot flow in a side-to-side direction between the cytoplasmic domains of adjacent cells at these sites. The use of collagenous septa as "markers" of "insulated" side-to-side electrical barriers is noted here to emphasize that from an electrophysiological viewpoint, the principal feature is the distribution of the gap junctions rather than the connective tissue per se. The connective tissue does not produce a barrier to current flow in extracellular space because of its porous structure produced by the fibrillar nature of types I and III collagen in the heart.[66]

Loss of Side-to-Side Fiber Coupling Generates a Major Mechanism for Unidirectional Block and Reentry

When the effective refractory period of one pathway is longer than that of another, impulses can continue to propagate in the pathway with the shorter refractory period when a premature impulse is initiated at an interval that is less than that of the effective refractory period of another pathway. These differences are the generic cause of any type of unidirectional block, whether multidimensional in nature[11,13,15] or of the "antegrade-retrograde" type with 180° differences in a 1D structure.[67,68] The importance of unidirectional block is that it must occur in order for the remaining propagating excitation wave to circulate back and reexcite the initial stimulus area (circus movement), a process that is integral to initiating a reentrant arrhythmia.

In the past, any spatial difference in the effective refractory period that produces unidirectional block has been considered to be due to intrinsic ionic current differences of the sarcolemmal membrane, eg, spatial inhomogeneities of repolarization.[6] In contrast to this long-held idea, however, the representative results of Figure 15 demonstrate that the underlying cause of differences in the effective refractory period of two pathways is more complex. Figure 15A (right) shows the effects of reducing the premature stimulus interval in the uniform anisotropic bundle of the 12-year-old child. When the premature interval was decreased to the earliest stimulus that would produce a propagated response (345 ms), all waveforms remained smooth in contour as they decreased in amplitude. Earlier premature stimuli failed to produce conduction in any direction in these preparations; ie, propagation stopped in all directions simultaneously in uniform anisotropic preparations. This result was typical of bundles from subjects <20 years old: directional differences in the effective refractory period and reentry could not be induced in bundles with tight electrical coupling in all directions and no histological evidence of microfibrosis. In the nonuniform anisotropic atrial bundle from the 64-year-old subject, however, when the premature interval was reduced to 327 ms, decremental longitudinal conduction to block occurred while stable slow transverse conduction persisted (Figure 15B, right). Additional slight changes in the premature interval resulted in anisotropic reentry within the muscle bundle.[15] The same response occurred when the stimulus site was shifted to different locations throughout the bundle.

Mechanisms of Unidirectional Block

Several features of the unidirectional block in nonuniform anisotropic cardiac bundles are noteworthy with regard to changing concepts. First, the differences in the effective refractory period within the pathways of LP and TP occurred in the absence of spatial differences in the action potential duration.[11,15] Second, the pattern of unidirectional block depended on the presence of discontinuities. If the medium of propagation were continuous, propagation would have to fail in both directions simultaneously. Thus, there are two factors that produce spatial differences in the effective refractory period: (1) spatial differences in the intrinsic ionic current properties of the cellular membranes of different areas and (2) differences in the pattern of cellular connectivity, which produce loading differences for each direction of propagation with respect to the orientation of the fibers.

In the past, unidirectional block usually has been thought of in terms of one-dimensional propagation: antegrade or retrograde propagation.[67,68] As shown in Figure 15, the angular dependence is more general and can be related to cell orientation, with differences in the distribution of the gap junctions encountered with different directions of conduction. This feature is significant because a theory or rule that applies to conduction in 1D structures can break down during multidimensional conduction at a microscopic level. For example, we found that the irregular distribution of the gap junctions (discontinuities) in two dimensions produces propagation events qualitatively different from those that occur with similar discontinuities in a 1D structure (cf Appendix of Reference 21).

Conclusions

The results presented here demonstrate not only that the discrete nature of cardiac muscle produces discontinuous conduction but also that propagation is stochastic in nature at a microscopic level. Instead of being orderly, stable, and continuous as the averaged events appear to be at the larger macroscopic (tissue) size, propagation at a microscopic level is seething with change and disorder by virtue of varying excitatory events and delays between cells. An integral component of the stochastic nature of cardiac propagation is that the irregular distribution of the cellular connections create inhomogeneities of electrical load that affect conduction inside individual cells and influence conduction delays across gap junctions. This process produces discontinuous propagation as a primary reflection of the nonuniformities of electrical load produced by the nonuniform distribution of the cellular interconnections.

A major feature of the stochastic nature of conduction at a microscopic level is that it provides a highly protective effect against cardiac conduction disturbances, which lead to global arrhythmias. For example, changing the direction of conduction markedly alters the intracellular excitatory events and the gap junctional delays, and the excitatory events feed back on one another from cell to cell. By means of intracellular variations of electrical load, the stochastic nature of normal propagation provides a way to reestablish the general trend of wavefront movement after variations in excitation events occur. However, when the great variety of events throughout the medium at this small scale is overridden by the development of separated groups of cells, the electrical load is distributed over a larger area. The myocardial architecture may then fail to reestablish a smoothed wave front, and the microarchitecture become proarrhythmic. As shown in Figure 15, when cell group regularization occurs as a result of the loss of side-to-side connections, unidirectional block, slow conduction, and reentry occur in the absence of repolarization inhomogeneities. Thus, the normal maintenance of an adequate number of side-to-side electrical connections between fibers throughout the myocardium provides protection against the initiation of reentrant arrhythmias. Conversely, the loss of side-to-side electrical connections between fibers (nonuniform anisotropic properties) is associated with an enhanced propensity for the initiation of reentrant arrhythmias.

It is not surprising that as one explores cardiac conduction on a smaller and smaller scale, the events that occur are not consistent with continuous cable theory, as they are at the larger macroscopic level. The cellular conduction events were found to be considerably more variable and complicated than can be discerned at a macroscopic level where the discrete cellular effects are averaged. That the stochastic behavior of conduction events at a microscopic level leads to deterministic or statistically predictable behavior as a large multicellular network is also not surprising. This relationship is similar to the stochastic behavior of individual sodium ion channel currents that produce highly predictable macroscopic currents when many channels are involved.

This analysis shows that there is an increase in electrical loading of the cell membrane localized to the input and output gap junctions. The increased electrical load, in turn, produces an increase in I_{Na} in these subcellular areas, which are the same subcellular regions in which an increase in the density of Na^+-channel protein has been demonstrated by Cohen.[57] Thus, the gap junctions and density distribution of Na^+-channel proteins are linked topologically to areas of increased electrical loading, a feature that should enhance the safety factor of discontinuous conduction. Recently, increased density of Kv1.5 K^+-channel proteins also has been demonstrated in the same subcellular regions adjacent to the gap junctions at the ends of cardiac myocytes.[69,70] The effects on conduction of an increase in the density of functional ionic channels that augment the depolarizing and repolarizing currents in these subcellular areas provide an important area for future study. Changes in the expression and in the kinetics of specific ionic channels that occur in disease states have recently been reviewed by Boyden and Jeck.[71] An intriguing question is whether there are disease-induced changes in the density distribution of ionic channels that are linked to topological changes in the gap junctions by the subcellular distribution of intracellular loading that increases I_{Na} near the input and output gap junctions of individual cells (Figures 11C and 12C).

Changes in the Topology of Gap Junctions as a Major Adaptive Mechanism and Therapeutic Target

The effective coupling conductance between cells within a network can be altered in two ways: by changing the conductance, g_j, of the individual gap junctions (ie, the number of unitary channels or their conductance) or by altering the spatial arrangement of the gap junctions. Changes in g_j are known to involve several factors, eg, intracellular pH,[72] second messengers (cAMP),[73] and steady-state voltage gradients (≈ 100 mV) across gap junctions.[74] Immunohistochemical labeling studies also have shown that there are different isoforms of the connexins in different cardiac structures,[75] and the connexin differences are associated with different unitary conductances of the gap junction channels.[76] At this point, it is not clear how to integrate information about the different isoforms of cardiac gap junction proteins and their different unitary conductances into a detailed conduction model for different cardiac structures. For example, the effects on g_j of differences in the conductance of the unitary channels can be offset by varying the number of channels within each gap junctional plaque. Furthermore, Vink et al[77] recently presented evidence that in genetically ablated Cx43 mice, the absence of Cx43 (the major gap junction protein of the mammalian ventricle) is associated with compensatory expression of other connexins. A general effect of the various isoforms is variation of the intercellular diffusion of substances, such as anionic morphogens,[77] which is related to variations in pore size of the individual channels.

The second general mechanism of altering cellular connectivity, changing the topology of the gap junctions, is relatively unexplored. The results presented here show that there is a long-term tendency for regularization of the stochastic arrangement of the cellular connections to occur by formation of small groups of cells secondary to the loss of side-to-side fiber coupling. The following statement summarizes the general process:

> Adaptive cardiac structural mechanisms elicit changes in the pattern of cellular connectivity during growth, development, and aging and with disease. A general feature is the loss of side-to-side connections in association with the development of small collagenous septa. This process produces small elongated groups of cells of variable lengths (3 to 10 cells long) and of variable widths (1 to 5 cells wide). An important feature of the normal stochastic distribution of the gap junctions is that at a given age, it provides the initial condition from which time-dependent adaptive mechanisms alter the spatial pattern of the cellular interconnections to produce a variety of spatial patterns that result in emergent new electrical behavior of the heart.

The foregoing generates a major question: What are the factors that control the loss of side-to-side electrical coupling between fibers in different cardiac structures? At this point, little is known about the biological factors that produce these time-dependent changes in the topology of gap junctions in otherwise normal cardiac muscle. The close association between an increase in fine collagenous septa and a progressive decrease in side-to-side electrical coupling between cardiac fibers has been impressive in data accumulated thus far.[12,13,15,19] Terracio et al[78] demonstrated in vitro that fibroblasts become oriented perpendicular to the direction of stretch, which is remarkably similar to the orientation of the fibroblasts of the connective tissue in the nonuniform anisotropic cardiac preparations we have studied. With regard to collagen, Weber et al[79] recently reviewed the interrelationships between function, structural remodeling, and regulatory mechanisms of collagen in preserving tissue architecture of the myocardium.

On the basis of the close association between collagenous septa and the distribution of side-to-side electrical connections between cardiac fibers, we suggest the following hypothesis for future investigation: genetic expression of the systems that regulate the distribution of collagenous septa and the side-to-side electrical connections between cardiac fibers are under similar developmental and regional control.[18] The significance of this hypothesis should be enhanced and sustained by the challenge to find a way to alter the topology of the cellular interconnections as a therapeutic target for life-threatening cardiac arrhythmias.[39]

Acknowledgments   I wish to express my appreciation to Roger C. Barr, Paul C. Dolber, J. Francis Heidlage, and C. Frank Starmer for their continuing collaboration in the work presented here.

References

1. Hodgkin AL, Katz B. The effect of sodium ions on the electrical activity of the giant axon of the squid. *J Physiol (Lond).* 1949;108:37–77.
2. Weidmann S. The effect of the cardiac membrane potential on the rapid availability of the sodium-carrying system. *J Physiol (Lond).* 1955;127: 213–224.
3. Hunter PJ, McNaughton PA, Noble D. Analytical models of propagation in excitable cells. *Prog Biophys Mol Biol.* 1975;30:99–144.
4. Hodgkin AL, Rushton WAH. The electrical constants of a crustacean nerve fibre. *Proc R Soc London B.* 1946;133:444–479.
5. Hodgkin AL, Huxley AF. A quantitative description of membrane current and its application to conduction and excitation in nerve. *J Physiol (Lond).* 1952;117:500–544.
6. Allessie MA, Bonke FIM, Schopman FJG. Circus movement in rabbit atrial muscle as a mechanism of tachycardia, III: the "leading circle" concept: a new model of circus movement in cardiac tissue without the involvement of an anatomical obstacle. *Circ Res.* 1977;41:9–18.
7. Task Force of the Working Group on Arrhythmias of the European Society of Cardiology. The Sicilian gambit: a new approach to the classification of antiarrhythmic drugs based on their actions on arrhythmogenic mechanisms. *Circulation.* 1991;84:1831–1851.
8. Werkö L. Atrial fibrillation. In: Olsson SB, Allessie MA, Campbell RWF, eds. *Atrial Fibrillation: Mechanisms and Therapeutic Strategies.* Armonk, NY: Futura Publishing Co; 1994:1–13.
9. Campbell RWF. Atrial fibrillation: management with class 1c drugs. In: Olsson SB, Allessie MA, Campbell RWF, eds. *Atrial Fibrillation: Mechanisms and Therapeutic Strategies.* Armonk, NY: Futura Publishing Co; 1994: 273–286.
10. Cardiac Arrhythmia Suppression Trial (CAST) Investigators. Preliminary report: effect of encainide and flecainide on mortality in a randomized trial of arrhythmia suppression after myocardial infarction. *N Engl J Med.* 1989; 321:406–412.
11. Spach MS, Miller WT III, Geselowitz DB, et al. The discontinuous nature of propagation in normal canine cardiac muscle: evidence for recurrent discontinuities of intracellular resistance that affect the membrane currents. *Circ Res.* 1981;48:39–45.
12. Spach MS, Miller WT III, Dolber PC, et al. The functional role of structural complexities in the propagation of depolarization in the atrium of the dog: cardiac conduction disturbances due to discontinuities of effective axial resistivity. *Circ Res.* 1982;50:175–191.
13. Spach MS, Dolber PC. The relation between discontinuous propagation in anisotropic cardiac muscle and the "vulnerable period" of reentry. In: Zipes

DP, Jalife J, eds. *Cardiac Arrhythmias: Mechanisms and Management.* New York, NY: Grune & Stratton; 1985:241–252.

14. Ursell PC, Gardner PI, Albala A, et al. Structural and electrophysiological changes in the epicardial border zone of canine myocardial infarcts during infarct healing. *Circ Res.* 1985;56:436–451.

15. Spach MS, Dolber PC, Heidlage JF. Influence of the passive anisotropic properties on directional differences in propagation following modification of the sodium conductance in human atrial muscle: a model of reentry based on anisotropic discontinuous propagation. *Circ Res.* 1988;62:811–832.

16. Luke RA, Saffitz JE. Remodeling of ventricular conduction pathways in healed canine infarct border zones. *J Clin Invest.* 1991;87:1594–1602.

17. Smith JH, Green CR, Peters NS, et al. Altered patterns of gap junction distribution in ischemic heart disease: an immunohistochemical study of human myocardium using laser scanning confocal microscopy. *Am J Pathol.* 1991;139:801–821.

18. Spach MS. Changes in the topology of gap junctions as an adaptive structural response of the myocardium. *Circulation.* 1994;90:1103–1106.

19. Spach MS, Dolber PC. Relating extracellular potentials and their derivatives to anisotropic propagation at a microscopic level in human cardiac muscle: evidence for electrical uncoupling of side-to-side fiber connections with increasing age. *Circ Res.* 1986;58:356–371.

20. Spach S, Heidlage JF. A multidimensional model of cellular effects on the spread of electrotonic currents and on propagating action potentials. *Crit Rev Biomed Eng.* 1992;20:141–169.

21. Spach MS, Heidlage JF. The stochastic nature of cardiac propagation at a microscopic level: an electrical description of myocardial architecture and its application to conduction. *Circ Res.* 1995;76:366–380.

22. Thomson W. On the theory of the electric telegraph. [From *Proc Royal Soc,* May 1855.] In: Sir William Thomson [Lord Kelvin]. *Mathematical and Physical Papers.* Vol 2. Cambridge, UK: Cambridge University Press; 1884:61–76.

23. Cole KS. *Membranes, Ions, and Impulses.* Berkeley, Calif: University of California Press; 1968:1–59.

24. Hermann L. Allgemeine Nervenphysiologie. In: Hermann L, ed. *Handbuch der Physiologie.* Vol 2. Leipzig, Germany: Vogel; 1879:1–196.

25. Rushton WAH. A physical analysis of the relation between threshold and interpolar length in the electrical excitation of medulated nerve. *J Physiol (Lond).* 1934;82:332–352.

26. Weidmann S. The electrical constants of Purkinje fibres. *J Physiol (Lond).* 1952;127:348–360.

27. Söstrand FS, Andersson E. Electron microscopy of the intercalated disc of cardiac muscle tissue. *Experientia.* 1954;10:369–370.

28. Van Breemen VL. Intercalated discs in heart muscle studied with the electron microscope. *Anat Rec.* 1953;117:49–63.

29. Muir AR. An electron microscope study of the embryology of the intercalated disc in the heart of the rabbit. *J Biophys Biochem Cytol.* 1957;3:193–202.

30. Woodbury JW, Crill WE. On the problem of impulse conduction in the atrium. In: Florey E, ed. *Nervous Inhibition.* New York, NY: Pergamon Press; 1961:124–135.

31. Barr L, Dewey MM, Berger W. Propagation of action potentials and the structure of the nexus in cardiac muscle. *J Gen Physiol.* 1965;48:797–823.

32. Joyner RWF, Ramón F, Moore JW. Simulation of action potential propagation in an inhomogeneous sheet of coupled excitable cells. *Circ Res.* 1975; 36:654–661.

33. Henriquez CS. Simulating the electrical behavior of cardiac tissue using the bidomain model. *Crit Rev Biomed Eng.* 1993;21:1–77.
34. Draper MH, Mya-Tu M. A comparison of the conduction velocity in cardiac tissues of various mammals. *Q J Exp Physiol.* 1959;44:91–109.
35. Sano T, Takayama N, Shimamoto T. Directional difference of conduction velocity in cardiac ventricular syncytium studied by microelectrodes. *Circ Res.* 1959;7:262–267.
36. Clerc L. Directional differences of impulse spread in trabecular muscle from mammalian heart. *J Physiol (Lond).* 1976;255:335–346.
37. Hodgkin AL. A note on conduction velocity. *J Physiol (Lond).* 1954;125:221–224.
38. Spach MS, Miller WT, Miller-Jones E, et al. Extracellular potentials related to intracellular action potentials during impulse conduction in anisotropic canine cardiac muscle. *Circ Res.* 1979;45:188–204.
39. Spach MS, Starmer CF. Altering the topology of gap junctions in nonuniform anisotropy: a major therapeutic target for atrial fibrillation. *Cardiovasc Res.* 1995;30:336–344.
40. Socolar SJ. The coupling coefficient as an index of junctional conductance. *J Membr Biol.* 1977;34:29–37.
41. Spach MS, Heidlage JF, Darken ER, et al. Cellular $\dot{V}_{max}$ reflects both membrane properties and the load presented by adjoining cells. *Am J Physiol.* 1992;263:H1855–H1863.
42. Spach MS, Kootsey JM. Relating the sodium current and conductance to the shape of transmembrane and extracellular potentials by simulation: effects of propagation boundaries. *IEEE Trans Biomed Eng.* 1985;BME-32:743–755.
43. Spach MS, Dolber PC, Heidlage JF, et al. Propagating depolarization in anisotropic human and canine cardiac muscle: apparent directional differences in membrane capacitance. *Circ Res.* 1987;60:206–219.
44. Suenson M. Interaction between ventricular cells during the early part of excitation in the ferret heart. *Acta Physiol Scand.* 1985;125:81–90.
45. Cabo C, Pertsov AM, Baxter WT, et al. Wave-front curvature as a cause of slow conduction and block in isolated cardiac muscle. *Circ Res.* 1994;75:1014–1028.
46. Joyner RW. Effects of the discrete pattern of electrical coupling on propagation through an electrical syncytium. *Circ Res.* 1982;50:192–200.
47. Rudy Y, Quan W. A model study of the effects of the discrete cellular structure on electrical propagation in cardiac tissue. *Circ Res.* 1987;61:815–823.
48. Leon LJ, Roberge FA. Directional characteristics of action potential propagation in cardiac muscle: a model study. *Circ Res.* 1991;69:378–395.
49. Fast VG, Kléber AG. Microscopic conduction in cultured strands of neonatal rat heart cells measured with voltage-sensitive dyes. *Circ Res.* 1993;73:914–925.
50. Hoyt RH, Cohen ML, Saffitz JE. Distribution and three-dimensional structure of intercellular junctions in canine myocardium. *Circ Res.* 1989;64:563–574.
51. Gourdie G, Green CR, Severs NJ. Gap junction distribution in adult mammalian myocardium revealed by anti-peptide antibody and laser scanning confocal microscopy. *J Cell Sci.* 1991;99:41–55.
52. Dolber PC, Beyer EC, Junker JL, et al. Distribution of gap junctions in dog and rat ventricle studied with a double-label technique. *J Mol Cell Cardiol.* 1992;24:1443–1457.

53. Ebihara L, Johnson EA. Fast sodium current in cardiac muscle: a quantitative description. *Biophys J.* 1980;32:779–790.
54. Weingart R, Maurer P. Action potential transfer in cell pairs isolated from adult rat and guinea pig ventricles. *Circ Res.* 1988;63:72–80.
55. Rudy Y, Quan W. A model study of the effects of the discrete cellular structure on electrical propagation in cardiac tissue. *Circ Res.* 1987;61: 815–823.
56. Weidmann S. Electrical constants of trabecular muscle from mammalian heart. *J Physiol (Lond).* 1970;210:1041–1054.
57. Cohen SA. Immunocytochemistry of rat cardiac sodium channels. *Circulation.* 1991;84(suppl II):II-182. Abstract.
58. Makielski JC, Sheets MF, Hanck DA, et al. Sodium current in voltage clamped internally perfused canine cardiac Purkinje cells. *Biophys J.* 1987; 52:1–11.
59. Antoni H, Böcker D, Eickhorn R. Sodium current kinetics in intact rat papillary muscle: measurements with the loose-patch-clamp technique. *J Physiol (Lond).* 1988;406:199–213.
60. van Kempen MJA, Fromaget C, Gros D, et al. Spatial distribution of connexin-43, the major cardiac gap junction protein in the developing and adult rat heart. *Circ Res.* 1991;68:1638–1651.
61. Fromaget C, El Aoumari A, Gros D. Distribution pattern of connexin43, a gap-junctional protein, during the differentiation of mouse heart myocytes. *Differentiation.* 1992;51:9–20.
62. Gourdie RG, Green CR, Severs NJ, et al. Immunolabeling patterns of gap junction connexins in the developing and mature rat heart. *Anat Embryol.* 1992;185:363–378.
63. Peters NS, Severs NJ, Rothery SM, et al. Spatiotemporal relationship between gap junctions and fascia adherens junctions during postnatal development of human ventricular myocardium. *Circulation.* 1994;90:713–725.
64. Spach MS, Dolber PC. Abnormalities in depolarization mediating arrhythmogenic mechanisms: focus on anisotropy and reentry. In: Singh BN, Wellens HJJ, Hiraoka M, eds. *Electropharmacological Control of Cardiac Arrhythmias.* Armonk, NY: Futura Publishing Co; 1994:83–99.
65. Saffitz JE, Kanter HL, Green KG, et al. Tissue-specific determinants of anisotropic conduction velocity in canine atrial and ventricular myocardium. *Circ Res.* 1994;74:1065–1070.
66. Weber KT, Sun Y, Tyagi SC, et al. Collagen network of the myocardium: function, structural remodeling and regulatory mechanisms. *J Mol Cell Cardiol.* 1994;26:279–292.
67. Starmer CF, Lastra AA, Nesterenko VV, et al. Proarrhythmic response to sodium channel blockage: theoretical model and numerical experiments. *Circulation.* 1991;84:1364–1377.
68. Shaw RM, Rudy Y. The vulnerable window for unidirectional block in cardiac tissue: characterization and dependence on membrane excitability and intercellular coupling. *J Cardiovasc Electrophysiol.* 1995;6:115–131.
69. Barry DM, Trimmer JS, Merlie JP, et al. Differential expression of voltage-gated K^+ channel subunits in adult rat heart: relation to functional K^+ channels? *Circ Res.* 1995;77:361–369.
70. Mays DJ, Foose JM, Philipson LH, et al. Localization of the Kv1.5 K^+ channel in explanted cardiac tissue. *J Clin Invest.* 1995;96:282–292.
71. Boyden PA, Jeck CD. Ion channel function in disease. *Cardiovasc Res.* 1995; 29:312–318.

72. Spray DC, Stern JH, Harris AL, et al. Gap junctional conductance: comparison of sensitivities to H and Ca ions. *Proc Natl Acad Sci U S A.* 1982;79: 441–445.

73. Saez JC, Spray DC, Nairn AC, et al. cAMP increases junctional conductance and stimulates phosphorylation of the 27-kDa principal gap junction polypeptide. *Proc Natl Acad Sci U S A.* 1986;83:2473–2477.

74. Veenstra RD. Voltage-dependent gating of gap junction channels in embryonic chick ventricular cell pairs. *Am J Physiol.* 1990;258:C662–C672.

75. Davis LM, Rodefeld ME, Green K, et al. Gap junction protein phenotypes of the human heart and conduction system. *J Cardiovasc Electrophysiol.* 1995; 6:813–822.

76. Veenstra RD, Wang HZ, Westphale EM, et al. Multiple connexins confer distinct regulatory and conductance properties of gap junctions in developing heart. *Circ Res.* 1992;71:1277–1283.

77. Vink MJ, Fishman GI, Vieira D, et al. Properties of gap junction channels in neonatal cardiac myocytes from wild type and connexin43 (Cx43) knockout (KO) mice. *Circulation.* 1995;92(suppl I):I-41. Abstract.

78. Terracio L, Miller B, Borg TK. Effects of cyclic mechanical stimulation of the cellular components of the heart: in vitro. *In Vitro.* 1988;24:53–58.

79. Weber KT, Sun Y, Tyagi SC, et al. Collagen network of the myocardium: function, structural remodeling and regulatory mechanisms. *J Mol Cell Cardiol.* 1994;26:279–292.

Chapter 2

Gap Junction Channels and Cardiac Conduction

Habo J. Jongsma

Conduction of the cardiac impulse depends on a number of morphological and functional parameters. One the one hand, conduction velocity is determined by the ability of individual myocytes to generate fast-rising, large-amplitude action potentials, which is dependent on the resting membrane potential, ie, the number and density of I_{K1} channels and the extracellular potassium concentration, and the number and density of voltage-activated sodium and calcium channels. On the other hand, the geometry and the cellular composition of the myocardium are critically important for the spread of electrical activation from the sinoatrial node toward the atria and ventricles. The size, shape, and orientation of myocytes, the presence and distribution of nonexcitable connective tissue, including fibroblasts, the size and shape of the extracellular space, and the organization of the muscular tissue in specialized structures like the sinoatrial node, the atrioventricular node, and the ventricular conduction system all influence conduction velocity at both the macroscopic and microscopic scale. Conduction of action potentials throughout the heart occurs by way of local circuit currents that flow from each cell to its neighbors via specialized membrane structures called gap junctions containing intercellular channels. The density of local circuit current determines the speed with which a particular cell excites its neighbors to generate an action potential and thus the velocity of spread of electrical activation. Therefore, apart from the factors mentioned above, gap junction size (ie, number of parallel conducting intercellular channels), gap junction distribution, and properties of the intercellular channels contribute importantly to conduction

Supported in part by: NWO grant 900–516–093; NHS grant M93-002

From: Spooner PM, Joyner RW, Jalife J (eds). *Discontinuous Conduction in the Heart.* Armonk, NY: Futura Publishing Company, Inc.; © 1997.

velocity and activation patterns in the myocardium. As a result of the rapid progress of molecular and cell biological techniques in the past decade, it has become clear that gap junction channels are far more complicated entities than the simple passive holes between cells they were previously considered to be. The new insights have been summarized in several reviews.[1-4] In the following, I will briefly discuss those aspects of gap junction function that relate to (discontinuous) conduction of the cardiac action potential.

Morphology and Distribution of Cardiac Gap Junctions

Gap junctions are aggregates of intercellular channels commonly organized into plaques of various sizes. They are recognized in transmission electron micrographs as regions in which the membranes of neighboring cells come very close together, leaving a gap of ~2 to 4 nm. In freeze-fracture replicas and in x-ray diffraction studies, gap junctions are seen as densely packed arrays of particles ~9 nm in diameter, which are commonly thought to represent gap junction channels.[6] In many species, groups of particles are arranged in specific patterns (see Reference 6 for a review) apparently designed to isolate small groups of particles by particle-free membrane domains. Although not definitively proven, the physiological relevance for this arrangement can be explained along two lines of reasoning. On the one hand, for intercellular channels to form, two apposing membranes must come fairly close together. It has been argued by Abney et al[7] that energetically, the optimal arrangement is obtained by packing many channels as close together as possible. On the other hand, it has been shown by Wilders and Jongsma[8] that gap junction channels in large arrays have a much higher cytosolic access resistance than those in isolation or in small arrays. Gap junction channels in large contiguous arrays are therefore less effective conductors of electrical current. As suggested by Hall and Gourdie,[6] arrangement of channels in small groups separated by particle-free aisles might overcome the access resistance effect while retaining the energetically favorable close packing. Support for this notion comes from the observation that gap junctions in nonexitable tissues like liver often consist of very large arrays of channels[5] not separated by particle-free membrane domains. Using antibodies against gap junction proteins (see below) and confocal microscopy, Gourdie et al[9] reconstructed en face views of intercalated disks between mammalian (including human) ventricular cells. They demonstrated a peculiar arrangement of gap junctions in the disk, with relatively large plaques lining the perimeter and numerous much smaller ones in the central region. Whether such an arrangement improves electrical interaction between neighboring cells is at present not known.

Electrical interaction between cardiac myocytes is determined not only by the arrangement of channels in a gap junction but of course also by the total number of channels between them. The more channels between cells (preferably in not too large contiguous arrays, because of the acess resistance problem), the more current can flow between cells at a given potential difference between them; the excitation threshold is reached more quickly, and conduction velocity is higher. When considering the relation between conduction velocity and number of gap junction channels between cells, one should also take into account the size of the cells. Small cells need less current to reach threshold than large cells because of the smaller membrance capacitance to be discharged[10] and the resistivity of the extracellular spaces that form the return path of the local circuit current.[11] Attempts have been made to estimate the number of gap junction channels needed between cells to obtain action potential propagation with physiologically meaningful delay.[12] The actual conductance values found are generally much higher than predicted.[13,14] This may mean that gap junctional conductance has a large safety factor or that the extracellular resistance, which was not taken into account in the above-mentioned calculation, necessitates a substantially larger junctional conductance.

An important factor determining the pattern of impulse conduction is the distribution of gap junctions along the myocyte perimeter. In canine ventricular cells, with width-to-length ratios of 1 to 6, approximately equal numbers of gap junctions are found all around the cells. This should give rise to considerable anisotropy in the sense that longitudinal conduction should be much faster than transverse conduction. Because of the complicated packing arrangement of the cells, however, impulses traveling in the transverse direction have to cross on average only 3.5 cell borders for every single crossing of a cell boundary in the longitudinal direction,[15] giving rise to less anisotropy of conduction than surmised from tissue geometry only. In contrast, in the crista terminalis, where gap junctions occur in the intercalated disks only,[15] conduction velocity is much more anisotropic and also faster in the longitudinal direction.

Nodal tissue conducts impulses very slowly[16] because its gap junctions are small and sparse,[17–19] and Purkinje fibers conduct impulses very fast because they are abundantly connected by large gap junctions.[20,21]

The overall conductance of a gap junction is determined by the conductance of each of the channels that compose it. In the following, recent data will be reviewed which suggest that this remark is not as trivial as it may appear.

Structure and Distribution of Gap Junction Channels

Gap junction channels span the membranes between two neighboring cells. They are formed by the head-to-head alignment of two hemichannels—connexons—contributed by each of the apposed cells. Each connexon in turn is composed of six protein molecules belonging to the gene family of the connexins, of which in mammals at least 14 members have been cloned.[4] The amino acid sequences deduced from connexin cDNAs combined with hydropathy plots indicate that all connexins have four membrane-spanning regions.[1] Labeling studies with antibodies directed against C-terminal and N-terminal amino acid sequences suggest that both the N-terminus and C-terminus are located intracellularly. This arrangement causes the molecules to have two extracellular loops and one intracellular loop. In the N-terminus, both extracellular loops and the four membrane-spanning segment amino acid sequences are well conserved between connexins. Important differences between different connexins are found in the sequence and number of amino acid residues in the intracellular loop and C-terminus. The extracellular loops of all connexins thus far examined are stabilized by intramolecular disulfide bridges, there being one bridge within each of the two loops and one between them. The extracellular loops are responsible for the docking of two apposed connexons to form a gap junction channel. This docking by noncovalent linking is very tight, as evidenced by the resistance of gap junctions against splitting along the gap by denaturing salt concentrations or by mechanical forces.

Connexin molecules are named according to the species they are derived from and their putative molecular weight as calculated from their cDNAs (eg, rCx43 is rat connexin with a molecular weight of 43 kD). In heart, the message for Cx37, Cx40, Cx43, Cx45, Cx46, and Cx50 has been detected. Between cardiac myocytes, Cx40, Cx43, and Cx45 proteins have been shown to be expressed. There are considerable differences in the tissue distribution of these three connexins not only within hearts of one species but also between comparable parts of hearts of different species.[22] Cx43 appears to be the most abundant and most ubiquitous of the three myocardial connexins; it is detected immunocytochemically in all parts of the heart of all mammalian species studied, with the notable exception of the sinoatrial node of most species, including humans, and proximal parts of the conduction system of rat and mouse. In rabbit and hamster sinoatrial node, Cx43 has been reported to be present,[18,23] but the resolution of the immunofluorescence data did not allow assessment of whether the distribution of Cx43 in these species is the same as in guinea pig and cow, in which

Cx43 immunolabeling is confined to strands of atrial cells interdigitating with strands of nodal cells.[19,24] In dog sinoatrial node,[25] a distribution comparable to the one in guinea pig and cow has been reported. In other species, the sinoatrial node has not been studied in sufficient detail to warrant a conclusion. Preliminary experiments in our laboratory suggest that in mouse, very little if any Cx43 is detectable in the nodal area. In rat and mouse, no Cx43 can be detected in the proximal part of the ventricular conduction system[26,27]; instead, Cx40 is detected here. Cx40 is also present abundantly in the atria of guinea pig, mouse, rabbit, cow, and human.[22,28] In dog, Cx40 appears to be present in all parts of the heart,[25] albeit in low amounts. Saffitz's group has reported Cx45 protein to be present in low amounts in all parts of dog and human heart, colocalized with Cx43.[29] To appreciate the significance of these findings for conduction of the cardiac impulse, it is necessary to briefly review the properties of gap junction channels made of the different cardiac connexins.

Properties and Modulation of Gap Junction Channels

On the basis of the dimensions of the pore in gap junction channels as inferred from electron image analysis and x-ray scattering[30,31] and the specific conductivity of the intracellular fluid filling the pore, the conductance of these channels has classically been estimated to be ~100 pS.[32] Simple calculations using this number and numbers of channels taken from freeze-fracture replicas resulted in the widely held belief that gap junctional conductance could never be a limiting factor for impulse propagation. At present, the conductance of gap junction channels made from the different cardiac connexins and the biophysical properties of the channels and their direct surroundings are known. This knowledge has changed our ideas considerably. Cx43 channels have a main single channel conductance of 45 to 50 pS (the value is dependent on the solution filling the pipettes used for recording; in this chapter, all values mentioned are for ±120 mmol/L potassium glutamate or potassium gluconate; these values are almost identical to those measured with the perforated-patch technique[33] and can thus be considered to be close to the in vivo values). Two minor states of ±20 and ±70 pS have been reported as well. The preponderance of these three states is influenced by (de)phosphorylating treatments[34–36]: activation of protein kinase C (PKC) and, in some species, of protein kinase G (PKG) increases the relative proportion of low-conductance states, whereas addition of phosphatase to the pipette-filling solution increases the proportion of high-conductance states. As may be expected,

PKG activation decreases total junctional conductance in neonatal rat heart cells, whereas PKC activation increases it.[35] Apparently, PKC activation not only increases the number of low-conductance events but also increases the probability of their being open. Dye coupling experiments, which are generally used to assess gap junction channel permeability, showed a decrease in number of stained cells after treatment with both PKC and PKG, suggesting that low-conductance states have lower permeability than higher-conductance states. Cx43 channels in myocytes and in transfected cells are not sensitive to protein kinase A (PKA) activation[36,37] (but see Reference 38). Long-term incubation of neonatal myocytes with dibutyryl-cAMP, however, increases Cx43 expression significantly.[39]

Cx43 channels are rather ion-unselective. Veenstra et al[40] reported that the selectivity of anions over cations is only 1.17 and that cation selectivity follows the Eisenman series I (see Reference 41), meaning that cation permeability is determined primarily by the hydration energies of the ions and not by the radius of the pore. The channels are weakly sensitive to transjunctional voltage differences[42,43] and to changes in membrane potential.[44] When transjunctional voltage is increased, Cx43 channels tend to close with a time constant of >50 ms.[45] Macroscopically, a residual conductance of 30% to 40% of the initial value remains when a transjunctional voltage of ≥100 mV is applied to Cx43 gap junctions; whether this implies that the lower-conductance state is less voltage-sensitive than higher-conductance states[45] or that gap junction channels, once opened, never can close completely[46] is still a matter of debate.

Cx43 gap junction conductance is decreased by intracellular acidification due to a decrease in the probability of the channels' being open. The mechanism of action of H^+ ions on Cx43 is not completely elucidated. Ek et al[47] and Hermans et al[48] have shown that histidines in the intracellular loop are involved: replacement of His^{95} by an acid or polar residue decreases pH sensitivity, as does replacement of His^{126} by the neutral residue glutamine. Replacement of His^{142} by glutamine, however, increased pH sensitivity.[48] Truncation of the C-terminus of Cx43 by 125-amino-acid residues decreases pH sensitivity, which could be restored by coinjecting the message for both the truncated Cx43 and the truncated part together in *Xenopus* oocytes.[47] These findings have led Delmar and coworkers to postulate a kind of ball-and-chain mechanism for pH-induced closure of gap junction channels comparable to the membrane voltage–induced inactivation of potassium channels.[49] It was recently shown[50] that substitution of Asp^{379} in the C-terminal of Cx43 has the same effect on pH sensitivity as truncation. It is a matter of debate whether pH sensitivity is a direct effect or is mediated through changes in cytosolic calcium, as has been suggested by Peracchia et al[51] on the basis of experiments with calcium chelators. We (Rook and Jongsma, unpublished observations) found that even working with well-calcium-buffered pipette-filling solutions, when measuring gap junctional conductance, it is difficult to keep intracellular pCa constant when intracellular pH is changed in the voltage-clamped cells. Some caution in the interpretation of pH experiments in which cystosolic calcium is not monitored, therefore, would appear to be necessary. It seems safe to conclude at this moment that Ca^{2+} and H^+ ions influence Cx43 junctional conductance synergistically, as has also been proposed by Burt.[52] Although the very first experiment demonstrating modulation of junctional conductance, the "healing-over" phenomenon described by Délèze,[53] involved calcium, the modulation of gap junction conductance by this ion per se is still controversial. Spray[54] maintains that cardiac gap junction channels close only when intracellular calcium concentrations reach unphysiologically high values, whereas others[55,56] presented evidence that Cx43 gap junctions close by increase of calcium concentrations within the physiological range, possibly by a calmodulin-mediated mechanism.[51] This matter can only be settled by simultaneous measurement of junctional conductance and intracellular calcium concentration.

Cx40 gap junction channels have a main single-channel conductance of 157 pS (172 pS with KCl in the pipette) when measured in transfected N2A cells.[57] Sometimes minor conductance states at 32 and 80 pS were observed. In adult rabbit atria, which express a substantial amount of Cx40, a conductance state of 180 pS (with CsCl in the pipette) was found next to one of 100 pS attributable to Cx43.[14] The cation-over-anion selectivity of Cx40 channels is five times higher than that of Cx43 channels, which may partly explain the low permeability to anionic dyes of Cx40 channels compared with Cx43 channels.[40] Like Cx43, Cx40 has been shown to be a phosphoprotein,[4] but the functional response of Cx40 channels to (de)phosphorylating treatments is as yet unknown.

Gap junctions composed of Cx45 channels are steeply voltage-sensitive: they are half inactivated at transjunctional voltages of 15 to 20 mV and reach maximal steady-state inactivation (92%) at 40 to 50 mV.[58] Cx45 channels have single-channel conductances of 36 and 22 pS, with the lower conductance being more abundant at higher transjunctional voltages, which may mean that the 36-pS conductance state is more voltage-sensitive than the 22-pS state.[37] Cx45 is also a phosphoprotein,[4] and stimulation of PKC opens an additional conductance of 16 pS, but whether this causes a reduction of overall Cx45 gap junctional conductance has not been investigated.[37] Cx45 channels are not influenced by either PKG or PKA stimulation. Hermans et al[59] recently demonstrated that Cx45 gap junctions are more pH_i-sensitive than Cx43 gap junctions: reducing pH_i from 7.0 to 6.3 decreased Cx43 conductance to 40% of control values, while Cx45 channels completely closed. All information about Cx45 channels has been gathered in mammalian cell lines or in oocytes injected with Cx45 mRNA. Properties of Cx45 channels in cardiac myocytes have not yet been investigated.

The description above serves to illustrate that gap junction channel behavior is much more complicated than previously thought, yet no attention has been paid to transcriptional regulation. Of the three cardiac connexins, only the promoter region of Cx43 has been identified,[60] and some regulatory protein-binding sequences have been found. Links with conduction remain to be established. The above-mentioned upregulation of Cx43 expression, concomitant with an increase in conduction velocity in neonatal rat cardiac myocytes[39] by long-term incubation of cultures with cAMP, might be a first step in that direction.

A further complication arises when it is appreciated that cardiac myocytes often express more than one connexin type. Because the extracellular loops of all connexins are very conserved, the possibility exists that heterotypic junctional channels may be formed between cells, with one cell contributing a connexon made of, eg, Cx43 molecules and another cell contributing a connexon made of, eg, Cx45 molecules. Several older studies indicate that cells from different organs or different cells from the same organ can become coupled by gap junctions.[61,62] Using the oocyte and coupling-deficient mammalian cell expression systems, this issue was systematically studied (for a review see Reference 4). In these systems, it has been established that of the cardiac connexins, Cx45 can form functional channels with Cx40 and Cx43. Interestingly, Cx40 and Cx43 are not able to form functional channels.[63,64] The behavior of heterotypic channels is complicated. Open-channel resistance seems to be the sum of the resistances of the two different connexons,[62,65] whereas permeability of heterotypic channels, as assessed with dyes, seems to be governed by that of the connexon that in the homotypic configuration forms a channel with the lower permeability of the two. Voltage sensitivity of heterotypic channels is dependent on the polarity of the voltage on which the channel closes.[65,66] This behavior is not seen in homotypic channels, which have two identical gates in series. It causes heterotypic channels to exhibit rectifying behavior.[62,66] In addition to heterotypic channels, it is theoretically possible to have gap junction channels consisting of heteromeric connexons in tissues expressing more than one type of connexin. Heteromeric connexons are built from different connexin molecules. Jiang et al[67] presented evidence for the existence of such heteromeric connexons in the lens, and Sosinsky[68] argued that in liver, Cx32 and Cx26, coexpressed in the same gap junction, preferentially formed homomeric connexons, which, however, are able to form heterotypic channels.

Consequences for Conduction of the Cardiac Impulse

The far from complete review of experimental results concerning the distribution and properties of gap junction channels presented above makes clear that intercellular communication in the myocardium is quite complex. What are the consequences of this complexity for electrical communication? It seems clear that all parts of the heart contain amply sufficient gap junctions to guarantee fast impulse conduction, with the possible exception of the nodal areas. In the latter areas, small gap junctions have been detected ultrastructurally but not beyond doubt immunocytochemically, possibly because their small size prevents detection. Cx43 is detected abundantly in many parts of the heart but seems not to be absolutely necessary for conduction at least in the embryonic and early neonatal stages. Reaume et al[69] showed that mice in which the Cx43 gene was deleted were born viable but died subsequently because of a developmental defect in the right outflow tract. The developmental importance of Cx43 is underscored by the finding[70] that patients with visceroatrial heterotaxia, showing various cardiac malformations, may exhibit Cx43 point mutations. When tested in transfected cells, the mutated Cx43 forms channels with reduced dye permeability. In adult ventricular myocardium, Cx43 is almost the only connexin expressed and thus seems to be essential for impulse conduction. It has been shown that in embryonic heart, Cx40 is widely expressed in both atrium and ventricle.[22,26] This raises the possibility that Cx40 can serve impulse conduction as well as Cx43 and that it does so when no Cx43 is present. In this respect, it is interesting that Vink et al[71] recorded single gap junctional channel conductances of 90 to 220 pS in pairs of neonatal myocytes from Cx43 knockout mice, possibly due to Cx40 channels. In adult normal ventricle of many species, no Cx43 is detected in the proximal parts of the conduction system. Instead, Cx40 is expressed. On the one hand, this may be advantageous for speed of impulse conduction, because Cx40 gap junctions have lower resistance than Cx43 gap junctions of the same size. On the other hand, current leakage from cells of the conduction system to surrounding septal myocytes might be prevented because Cx40 cannot form functional heterotypic channels with Cx43,[63] which would speed up impulse propagation also. In atrium, Cx40 and Cx43 are generally coexpressed. Although it cannot be excluded that Cx40 expression here is a remnant of development, it might improve conduction velocity in a tissue in which no specialized conduction pathways are present.

Bastide et al[72] found enhanced Cx40 expression in hypertrophic rat hearts, and they suggested that this may help to maintain proper conduction velocity in these enlarged hearts. All in all, the picture arises that regulation of Cx40 expression is an important means for the heart to ensure adequate conduction velocity of the cardiac impulse in various regions of the heart under various conditions. More definitive conclusions await the creation of Cx40 knockout mice.

There is abundant evidence that gap junction channel conductance can be modified by a wide variety of environmental factors, such as activity of the autonomous cardiac nerves, metabolic status of the cells, and intracellular ion concentrations. Although most of the published data concern Cx43 gap junction channels, there is no reason to doubt that Cx40 and Cx45 channel conductances can be modified also. It is well established that the occurrence of cardiac arrhythmias under a variety of conditions is governed by changes in refractory period and changes in conduction velocity. In particular, an increase in dispersion of refractoriness has been implicated as arrhythmogenic. In the same way, local changes in gap junctional conductance induced by local changes in autonomic nervous activity or local changes in cellular metabolism under pathological circumstances might increase dispersion in conduction velocity and thus the incidence of cardiac arrhythmias.

References

1. Bennett MV, Barrio LC, Bargiello TA, Spray DC, Hertzberg E, Saez JC. Gap junctions: new tools, new answers, new questions. *Neuron.* 1991;6:305–320.
2. Beyer EC. Gap junctions. *Int Rev Cytol.* 1993;137C:1–37.
3. Jongsma HJ, Rook MB. Morphology and electrophysiology of cardiac gap junction channels. In: Zipes DP, Jalife J, eds. *Cardiac Electrophysiology: From Cell to Bedside.* 2nd ed. Philadelphia, Pa: WB Saunders; 1995:115–126.
4. Bruzzone R, White TW, Paul DL. Connections with connexins: the molecular basis of direct intercellular signaling. *Eur J Biochem.* 1996;238:1–27.
5. Makowski L. X-ray diffraction studies of gap junction structure. *Adv Cell Biol.* 1988;2:119–158.
6. Hall JE, Gourdie RG. Spatial organization of cardiac gap junctions can affect access resistance. *Microsc Res Tech.* 1995;31:446–451.
7. Abney JR, Braun J, Owicki JC. Lateral interactions among membrane proteins: implications for the organization of gap junctions. *Biophys J.* 1987;52:441–454.
8. Wilders R, Jongsma HJ. Limitations of the dual voltage clamp method in assaying conductance and kinetics of gap junction channels. *Biophys J.* 1992;63:942–953.
9. Gourdie RG, Green CR, Severs NJ. Gap junction distribution in adult mammalian myocardium revealed by an anti-peptide antibody and laser scanning confocal microscopy. *J Cell Sci.* 1991;99:41–55.
10. Wilders R, Kumar R, Joyner RW, et al. Action potential conduction between a ventricular cell model and an isolated ventricular cell. *Biophys J.* 1996;70:281–295.
11. Kleber AG, Riegger CB, Janse MJ. Electrical uncoupling and increase of

extracellular resistance after induction of ischemia in isolated arterially perfused rabbit papillary muscle. *Circ Res.* 1987;61:271–279.

12. Wilders R, Jongsma HJ. Beating irregularity of single pacemaker cells isolated from the rabbit sinoatrial node. *Biophys J.* 1993;65:2601–2613.

13. Metzger P, Weingart R. Electric current flow in cell pairs isolated from adult rat hearts. *J Physiol (Lond).* 1985;366:177–195.

14. Verheule S, Hermans MMP, Kwak BR, Jongsma HJ. Properties of gap junction channels in adult rabbit atrium and ventricle. *Pflugers Arch.* 1995;430: R143.

15. Saffitz JE, Kanter HL, Green KG, Tolley TK, Beyer EC. Tissue-specific determinants of anisotropic conduction velocity in canine atrial and ventricular myocardium. *Circ Res.* 1994;74:1065–1070.

16. Bleeker WK, Mackaay AJ, Masson-Pevet M, Bouman LN, Becker AE. Functional and morphological organization of the rabbit sinus node. *Circ Res.* 1980;46:11–22.

17. Masson-Pévet M, Bleeker WK, Gros D. The plasma membrane of leading pacemaker cells in the rabbit sinus node. *Circ Res.* 1979;45:621–629.

18. Trabka Janik E, Coombs W, Lemanski LF, Delmar M, Jalife J. Immunohistochemical localization of gap junction protein channels in hamster sinoatrial node in correlation with electrophysiologic mapping of the pacemaker region. *J Cardiovasc Electrophysiol.* 1994;5:125–137.

19. Ten Velde I, De Jonge B, Verheijck EE, et al. Spatial distribution of connexin 43, the major cardiac gap junction protein, visualizes the cellular network for impulse propagation from sinoatrial node to atrium. *Circ Res.* 1995;76: 802–811.

20. Pressler ML, Munster PN, Huang X. Gap junction distribution in the heart: functional relevance. In: Zipes DP, Jalife J, eds. *Cardiac Electrophysiology: From Cell to Bedside.* 2nd ed. Philadelphia, Pa: WB Saunders; 1996:144–151.

21. Oosthoek PW, Virágh S, Lamers WH, Moorman AFM. Immunohistochemical delineation of the conduction system, II: the atrioventricular node and Purkinje fibers. *Circ Res.* 1993;73:482–491.

22. Van Kempen MJA, Ten Velde I, Wessels A, et al. Differential connexin distribution accommodates cardiac function in different species. *Microsc Res Tech.* 1995;31:420–436.

23. Anumonwo JM, Wang HZ, Trabka Janik E, et al. Gap junctional channels in adult mammalian sinus nodal cells: immunolocalization and electrophysiology. *Circ Res.* 1992;71:229–239.

24. Oosthoek PW, Virágh S, Mayen AEM, Van Kempen MJA, Lamers WH, Moorman AFM. Immunohistochemical delineation of the conduction system, I: the sinoatrial node. *Circ Res.* 1993;73:473–48.

25. Kanter HL, Laing JG, Beyer EC, Green KG, Saffitz JE. Multiple connexins colocalize in canine ventricular gap junctions. *Circ Res.* 1993;73:344–350.

26. Delorme B, Dahl E, Jarry-Guichard T, et al. Developmental regulation of connexin 40 gene expression in mouse heart correlates with the differentiation of the conduction system. *Dev Dyn.* 1995;204:358–371.

27. van Kempen MJ, Fromaget C, Gros D, Moorman AF, Lamers WH. Spatial distribution of connexin43, the major cardiac gap junction protein, in the developing and adult rat heart. *Circ Res.* 1991;68:1638–1651.

28. Gros A, Jarry-Guichard T, Ten Velde I, et al. Restricted distribution of connexin40, a gap junctional protein, in mammalian heart. *Circ Res.* 1994; 74:839–851.

29. Chen SC, Davis LM, Westphale EM, Beyer EC, Saffitz JE. Expression of

multiple gap junction proteins in human fetal and infant hearts. *Pediatr Res.* 1994;36:561–566.

30. Unwin PNT, Zampighi G. Structure of the junction between communicating cells. *Nature.* 1980;283:545–549.
31. Caspar DLD, Goodenough DA, Makowski L, Philips WC. Gap junction structures, I: correlated electron microscopy and x-ray diffraction. *J Cell Biol.* 1977;74:605–628.
32. Simpson I, Rose B, Loewenstein WR. Size limit of molecules permeating the junctional membrane channels. *Science.* 1977;197:294–296.
33. Takens-Kwak BR, Jongsma HJ. Cardiac gap junctions: three distinct single channel conductances and their modulation by phosphorylating treatments. *Pflugers Arch.* 1992;422:198–200.
34. Moreno AP, Saez JC, Fishman GI, Spray DC. Human connexin43 gap junction channels: regulation of unitary conductances by phosphorylation. *Circ Res.* 1994;74:1050–1057.
35. Kwak BR, van Veen TAB, Analbers LJS, Jongsma HJ. TPA increases conductance but decreases permeability in neonatal rat cardiomyocyte gap junction channels. *Exp Cell Res.* 1995;220:456–463.
36. Kwak BR, Saez JC, Wilders R, et al. Effects of cGMP-dependent phosphorylation on rat and human connexin43 gap junction channels. *Pflugers Arch.* 1995;430:770–778.
37. Kwak BR, Hermans MMP, De Jonge HR, Lohmann SM, Jongsma HJ, Chanson M. Differential regulation of distinct types of gap junction channels by similar phosphorylating conditions. *Mol Biol Cell.* 1995;6:1707–1719.
38. Burt JM, Spray DC. Inotropic agents modulate gap junctional conductance between cardiac myocytes. *Am J Physiol.* 1988;254:H1206–H1210.
39. Darrow BJ, Fast VG, Kleber AG, Beyer EC, Saffitz JE. Direct link between gap junction remodeling and changes in conduction in cultured myocytes. *Circulation.* 1995;92(suppl I):1–40. Abstract.
40. Veenstra RD, Wang HZ, Beblo DA, et al. Selectivity of connexin-specific gap junctions does not correlate with channel conductance. *Circ Res.* 1995;77:1156–1165.
41. Hille B. *Ionic Channels of Excitable Membranes.* 2nd ed. Sunderland, Mass: Sinauer; 1992.
42. Rook MB, Jongsma HJ, van Ginneken AC. Properties of single gap junctional channels between isolated neonatal rat heart cells. *Am J Physiol.* 1988;255:H770–H782.
43. Veenstra RD. Voltage-dependent gating of gap junction channels in embryonic chick ventricular cell pairs. *Am J Physiol.* 1990;258:C662–C672.
44. White TW, Bruzzone R, Wolfram S, Paul DL, Goodenough DA. Selective interactions among the multiple connexin proteins expressed in the vertebrate lens: the second extracellular domain is a determinant of compatibility between connexins. *J Cell Biol.* 1994;125:879–892.
45. Moreno AP, Rook MB, Fishman GI, Spray DC. Gap junction channels: distinct voltage-sensitive and -insensitive conductance states. *Biophys J.* 1994;67:113–119.
46. Bukauskas FF, Weingart R. Voltage-dependent gating of single gap junction channels in an insect cell line. *Biophys J.* 1994;67:613–625.
47. Ek JF, Delmar M, Perzova R, Taffet SM. Role of histidine 95 on pH gating of the cardiac gap junction protein connexin43. *Circ Res.* 1994;74:1058–1064.
48. Hermans MMP, Kortekaas P, Jongsma HJ, Rook MB. The role of histidines on pH sensitivity of connexins 43 and 45. *Pflugers Arch.* 1995;430:R144.

49. Catterall WA. Structure and function of voltage-gated ion channels. *Annu Rev Biochem.* 1995;64:493–531.
50. Calero GA, Ek-Vitorin JF, Taffet JM, Delmar M. Mutation of a single amino acid (asp379) prevents pH regulation of connexin43. *Biophys J.* 1996;70: A208.
51. Peracchia C, Wang X, Li L, Peracchia LL. Inhibition of calmodulin expression prevents low-pH-induced gap junction uncoupling in Xenopus oocytes. *Pflugers Arch.* 1996;431:379–387.
52. Burt JM. Block of intercellular communication: interaction of intracellular H^+ and Ca^{2+}. *Am J Physiol.* 1987;253:C607–C612.
53. Délèze J. The recovery of resting potential and input resistance in sheep heart injured by knife or laser. *J Physiol (Lond).* 1970;208:547–562.
54. Spray DC, Bennett MVL. Physiology and pharmacology of gap junctions. *Annu Rev Physiol.* 1985;47:281–303.
55. Lazrak A, Peracchia C. Gap junction gating sensitivity to physiological internal calcium regardless of pH in Novikoff hepatoma cells. *Biophys J.* 1993;65:2002–2012.
56. Dahl G, Isenberg G. Decoupling of heart muscle cells: correlation with increased cytoplasmic calcium activity and with changes in nexal ultrastructure. *J Membr Biol.* 1980;53:63–75.
57. Beblo DA, Wang HZ, Beyer EC, Westphale EM, Veenstra RD. Unique conductance, gating, and selective permeability properties of gap junction channels formed by connexin40. *Circ Res.* 1995;77:813–822.
58. Moreno AP, Laing JG, Beyer EC, Spray DC. Properties of gap junction channels formed of connexin 45 endogenously expressed in human hepatoma (SKHep1) cells. *Am J Physiol.* 1995;268:C356–C365.
59. Hermans MMP, Kortekaas P, Jongsma HJ, Rook MB. pH sensitivity of the cardiac gap junction proteins, connexin 45 and 43. *Pflugers Arch.* 1995;431: 138–140.
60. De Leon JR, Buttrick PM, Fishman GI. Functional analysis of the connexin43 gene promoter in vivo and in vitro. *J Mol Cell Cardiol.* 1994;26:379–389.
61. Epstein ML, Gilula NB. A study of communication specificity between cells in culture. *J Cell Biol.* 1977;75:769–787.
62. Rook MB, van Ginneken AC, de Jonge B, el Aoumari A, Gros D, Jongsma HJ. Differences in gap junction channels between cardiac myocytes, fibroblasts, and heterologous pairs. *Am J Physiol.* 1992;263:C959–C977.
63. Bruzzone R, Haefliger JA, Gimlich R, Paul D. Connexin40, a component of gap junctions in vascular endothelium, is restricted in its ability to interact with other connexins. *Mol Biol Cell.* 1993;4:7–20.
64. Elfgang C, Eckert R, Lichtenberg Frate H, et al. Specific permeability and selective formation of gap junction channels in connexin-transfected HeLa cells. *J Cell Biol.* 1995;129:805–817.
65. Moreno AP, Fishman GI, Beyer EC, Spray DC. Human Cx43 and human Cx45 expressed in a mammalian cell line: heterotypic channels conserve the electrophysiological properties of hemichannels. In: Kanno Y, ed. *1993 International Meeting on Gap Junctions.* Hiroshima 734: Department of Physiology and Oral Physiology; 1993:69.
66. Verselis VK, Ginter CS, Bargiello TA. Opposite voltage gating polarities of two closely related connexins. *Nature.* 1994;368:348.
67. Jiang JX, White TW, Goodenough DA. Changes in connexin expression and distribution during chick lens development. *Dev Biol.* 1995;168:649–661.
68. Sosinsky G. Mixing of connexins in gap junction membrane channels. *Proc Natl Acad Sci U S A.* 1995;92:9210–9214.

69. Reaume AG, De Sousa PA, Kulkarni S, et al. Cardiac malformation in neonatal mice lacking connexin43 [see comments]. *Science.* 1995;267:1831–1834.
70. Britz Cunningham SH, Shah MM, Zuppan CW, Fletcher WH. Mutations of the connexin43 gap-junction gene in patients with heart malformations and defects of laterality. *N Engl J Med.* 1995;332:1323–1329.
71. Vink MJ, Fishman GI, Vieira D, Spray DC. Properties of gap junction channels in neonatal cardiac myocytes from wild type and connexin43 (Cx43) knockout (KO) mice. *Circulation.* 1995;92(suppl I):1–41. Abstract.
72. Bastide B, Neysse L, Ganten D, Paul M, Willecke K, Traub O. Gap junction protein connexin40 is preferentially expressed in vascular endothelium and conductive bundles of rat myocardium and is increased under hypertensive conditions. *Circ Res.* 1993;73:1138–1149.

Chapter 3

Nonjunctional Channels of Cardiac Cells and Metabolic Oscillations as Contributors to Discontinuous Conduction

Eduardo Marban, MD, PhD,
Brian Ramza, MD, PhD,
Dmitry Romashko, PhD, and
Brian O'Rourke, PhD

Although one reflexively thinks of gap junctions when the topic of conduction is raised, it is important to remember that ionic channels in the surface membrane not only are necessary for transmitting the impulse but also are capable of modifying excitation on a beat-to-beat basis. Cooley et al[1] simulated the changes in conduction that would occur in a simple Hodgkin-Huxley cable when the surface membrane conductance is scaled by a factor η. If $\eta < 0.26$, only decremental waves were possible. At values of η just above 0.26, the distinction between decremental and regenerative conduction became blurred; the concept of "threshold" became meaningless, along with the built-in safety of refractoriness.

Modern physiological approaches have yielded important insights into the mechanisms that underlie cellular excitability. Mechanisms that can reduce excitability are particularly relevant for this monograph. One such mechanism, based on work from our laboratory, will be discussed. We[2] have demonstrated that energy metabolism becomes unstable when cells are stressed by substrate deprivation or by anoxia/reoxygenation. The oscillations of cellular energy charge drive huge fluctuations in membrane potassium conductance due to activa-

From: Spooner PM, Joyner RW, Jalife J (eds). *Discontinuous Conduction in the Heart.* Armonk, NY: Futura Publishing Company, Inc.; © 1997.

tion of ATP-dependent potassium channels. Individual cells become cyclically inexcitable when such oscillations are present. In an electrical network, entire regions of the heart may become cyclically inexcitable, even if gap junctional conductance were to remain unaffected. By producing cyclical changes in excitability, such oscillations of membrane current may form the basis for a new arrhythmogenic principle.

Metabolic Control of Ion Homeostasis

Maintenance of the ionic gradients that support biological excitability and signal transduction ultimately depends on active transport. Thus, it is not surprising that cells have evolved a rich variety of mechanisms whereby changes in cellular energy state regulate ion channels, pumps, and transporters. Most examples of metabolic regulation are straightforwardly adaptive, enabling cells that are energetically robust to function to their fullest while energetically compromised cells can shut off processes that demand energy. In at least a few instances (eg, the pancreatic β-cell, as discussed below), the regulatory mechanisms not only provide a safety net but are also used physiologically for signal transduction. The level of regulation ranges from transcriptional activation (eg, increased expression of a Na^+/H^+ exchanger gene in rabbit hearts during ischemia[3]) to direct modification of ion channel gating by energy metabolites such as ATP.

The best-known example is the ATP-dependent potassium channel ($I_{K,ATP}$), which turns on when intracellular [ATP] falls to submillimolar levels. $I_{K,ATP}$ was first discovered in heart,[4,5] where the channel is plentiful.[6] $I_{K,ATP}$ renders inexcitable myocardial cells that are energetically depleted.[6] During coronary arterial occlusion (a common clinical situation that accounts for $\approx$300 000 cases of sudden death annually[7]), [ATP] falls to submillimolar levels within minutes and $I_{K,ATP}$ is turned on.[8] The adaptive value of $I_{K,ATP}$ in ischemic stress is much debated. While clearly an energy-sparing mechanism, the activation of $I_{K,ATP}$ during coronary occlusion may also contribute to arrhythmias by producing inhomogeneity of excitability in the heart and by facilitating extracellular K^+ accumulation.[9]

Metabolic Oscillations

Oscillatory behavior has come to be recognized as central to a number of key biological systems.[10] One of the first biochemical oscillators to be characterized was the glycolytic oscillator,[11] which appears to underlie the oscillations of membrane current and excitation-contraction (E-C) coupling.

In cytosolic extracts of yeast,[12] mammalian heart,[13] or skeletal muscle,[14] direct measurements of the metabolic intermediates of glycolysis reveal large periodic oscillations. These generally occur spontaneously, but they can be amplified by critically timed additions of certain metabolic intermediates, as discussed below. In bovine heart cytosolic extracts studied at 15.5°C, the concentrations of glycolytic intermediates clearly oscillate, and do so with a period of ≈20 minutes.[13] In yeast extracts, in which temperature sensitivity has been studied most extensively, the period of the oscillations varies from several hours at 0°C to ≈13 seconds at 37°C[12]; most studies find periods of 1 to 10 minutes at room temperature. Such oscillations have also been observed in intact yeast,[15] blowfly larvae,[16] and ascites tumor cells.[17]

To understand how this phenomenon arises, it is useful to recognize that oscillations can be readily established whenever a rate-limiting enzyme in a cascade responds to small changes in metabolites with large changes in activity. Phosphofructokinase, which catalyzes the phosphorylation by ATP of fructose 6-phosphate to fructose 1,6-diphosphate, fulfills these criteria.[18] The rate of glycolysis is controlled primarily by the activity of phosphofructokinase. This enzyme is allosterically stimulated by ADP and AMP and is inhibited by ATP and citrate. Various lines of evidence support the idea that phosphofructokinase drives the glycolytic oscillator. In cardiac cytosolic extracts,[13] metabolites upstream from phosphofructokinase (eg, glucose 6-phosphate and fructose 6-phosphate) oscillate 180° out of phase with respect to downstream reaction products. The sudden addition of ADP to yeast extracts resets the phase of the oscillations[12] in a manner consistent with the known allosteric modulation of phosphofructokinase by ADP. Finally, quantitative modeling based primarily on metabolite feedback on phosphofructokinase activity has successfully reproduced all the major features of the glycolytic oscillator.[18,19]

Glycolytic oscillations are so ubiquitous that there is reason to wonder how they evolved and whether they impart a selective advantage to cells. In general terms, the most responsive control systems are those that operate far from equilibrium; only under nonequilibrium conditions can feedback control effectively fine-tune the activity of biological enzymes. Such control is particularly important for enzymes that determine net energy flux, since energy supply must be rapidly responsive to changes in energy demand. Thus, the glycolytic oscillator represents a prototypical biological control system operating under nonequilibrium conditions.[20] In addition to such theoretical considerations, the pancreatic β-cell, which is specialized to sense glucose and to release insulin, constitutes one clear-cut example of a physiological role for glycolytic oscillations. Glucose leads to β-cell depolarization and to Ca^{2+} influx via L-type calcium channels. Depolarization does not continue indefinitely, nor is it graded; it occurs in bursts. The rate of bursting is governed by the level of extracellular glucose, with high glucose leading to summation of the bursts and greater insulin release. Glycolytic oscillations have been proposed to drive $I_{K,ATP}$ cyclically, producing a bias current that underlies the overall bursting pattern.[21,22] A key role for the glycolytic oscillator is supported by evidence that $I_{K,ATP}$ is much more sensitive to glycolytically derived ATP than to ATP generated by oxidative phosphorylation.[23] Similar lines of evidence indicate a preferential role for glycolysis in supplying ATP to ion-motive ATPases in the surface membrane of vascular smooth muscle cells.[24] Such functional compartmentation may reflect the fact that up to 50% of phosphofructokinase is bound to the surface membrane, at least in erythrocytes and in brain cells.[25] When so bound, the activity of phosphofructokinase increases over that of the free cytosolic form, providing yet another rationale for local effects of this enzyme and its metabolites on ion channels.

Metabolic Oscillations in Heart Cells

Ventricular myocytes subjected to mild metabolic stress, such as the withdrawal of fuel substrates from the medium, suffer no obvious ill effects as judged by visual inspection: cells remain rod-shaped with crisp striations for at least several hours. This is presumably due to the low metabolic demand of quiescent cells, coupled with the fact that heart cells contain abundant glycogen and free fatty acids that can serve, at least temporarily, as endogenous sources of energy. Nevertheless, myocytes studied under glucose-free conditions gave us the first indication that primary metabolic oscillations can be manifested in intact mammalian cells. Figure 1 shows membrane currents and the fluorescence of Calcium Green (a long-wavelength Ca^{2+} indicator; Molecular Probes) from two guinea pig ventricular cells studied with whole-cell patch clamp using the following solutions (in mmol/L): intracellular: potassium glutamate 120, KCl 25, NaCl 10, $MgCl_2$ 0.5, MgATP 0.2 to 5, HEPES 10 (pH 7.2), and Calcium Green 0.03; extracellular: NaCl 140, KCl 5, $MgCl_2$ 1, $CaCl_2$ 2, HEPES 10 (pH 7.4), and glucose 0 to 10. Patch pipettes had resistances of 1 to 3 MΩ. The voltage protocol, repeated every 6 seconds, consisted of steps from -80 to -40 mV for 100 ms, followed by a 200-ms pulse to $+10$ mV. The left portion of Figure 1A shows six consecutive responses to such stimuli from a cell under glucose-free conditions. The first pulse is entirely unremarkable: the step to -40 mV elicits a very large sodium current that activates

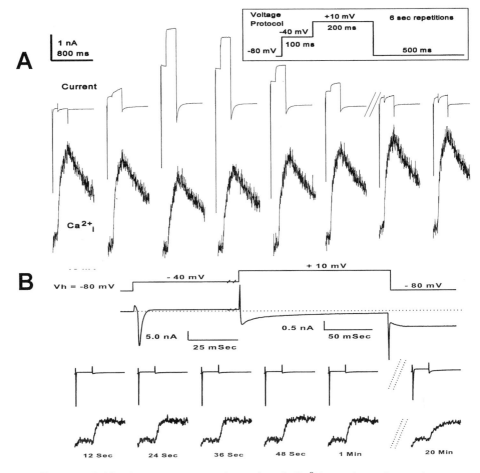

Figure 1. A, Membrane currents and cytoplasmic Ca^{2+} in a guinea pig ventricular myocyte during a metabolic oscillation. Voltage protocol illustrated in inset was applied repetitively every 6 seconds. B, Stability of membrane currents and Ca^{2+} transients in a cell studied in glucose-containing solution. Panel A and subsequent figures reprinted, with permission, from reference 2. Copyright 1994 American Association for the Advancement of Science.

and inactivates rapidly; subsequent depolarization to 0 mV turns on I_{Ca} and evokes a sizable Ca^{2+} transient. Normally this type of response can be obtained over and over during the course of an experiment; Figure 1B illustrates the stability of the membrane currents and Ca^{2+} signals in a "sister" cell studied for 20 minutes under control conditions (same solutions, except for 10 mmol/L glucose extracellularly). In contrast, the cell studied under glucose-free conditions developed a background current over the next 6 to 12 seconds (Figure 1A). This background current, which dominates the third and fourth membrane

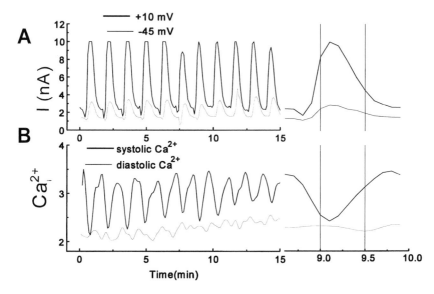

Figure 2. Phase and period of oscillations in membrane current (top) and in [Ca^{2+}]$_i$ (bottom). Values of membrane current from an experiment like that in Figure 1 are plotted at the ends of the prepulse and the test pulse. The systolic and diastolic [Ca^{2+}]$_i$ are the maxima and minima, respectively, of Calcium Green fluorescence. On the right are shown traces during one cycle at an expanded time base.

current records, is small at the holding potential but large and outward at −40 mV and even more so at 10 mV. As the background current became larger and larger, the amplitude of the Ca^{2+} transients declined progressively. After peaking at 12 to 18 seconds, membrane currents spontaneously returned toward normal. The last two records in Figure 1A, obtained just 72 and 78 seconds after the initial one, show virtually complete disappearance of the background current and restoration of normal Ca^{2+} transients.

Figure 2 shows a time course plot of the oscillations in current (A) and intracellular Ca^{2+} (B) in another cell studied under glucose-free conditions. From the onset of the experiment, a large background current (A) was cyclically activated with a period of 1 to 2 minutes. The average period of the oscillations in eight cells equaled 1.66 minutes (±0.21 minutes, SD). A general finding that is again exemplified here is the outward direction of the current at potentials positive to E$_K$ (−86 mV in this experiment). In perfect synchrony with the peaks of the membrane current oscillations, panel B reveals cyclical dips in Ca^{2+} transient amplitude (primarily due to changes in systolic Ca^{2+}). This inverse phase relationship is readily apparent by the expanded traces on the right.

With simple removal of external glucose, such oscillations were observed in 55 of 109 cells (51%). If these oscillations are related to the glycolytic oscillator, their variability can be readily understood. Quantitative modeling of the glycolytic oscillator has revealed that metabolic oscillations can only be sustained over a certain range of substrate influx rates.[18] Isolated cells are known to contain variable amounts of endogenous glycogen[26]; since the amount of glycogen limits the rate of substrate influx into glycolysis under glucose-free conditions,[27] it is not surprising that some cells do not oscillate with simple withdrawal of external substrate. We now recognize that cells that are not oscillating spontaneously can generally be induced to do so by transient perturbations of intracellular metabolite concentrations. Figure 3A shows an example in which oscillations were initiated by photolysis of internal caged ADP in a cell that was not oscillating spontaneously in glucose-free solution. This finding can be readily rationalized: the sudden rise in internal [ADP] feeds back upon and alters the activity of phosphofructokinase, perturbing the system such that oscillations are triggered. This finding has been confirmed in 11 other cells. Sudden changes of intracellular [ATP] (by flash photolysis of caged ATP) can also initiate oscillations (n = 4 cells, not shown) or reset their phase (n = 3). Thus, our data support the notion that the oscillatory response is latent within every cell.

The absence of substrates is not required to initiate the oscillations. Figure 3B shows an example in which they were triggered after a brief exposure to the mitochondrial uncoupler 2,4-dinitrophenol. As described previously during severe metabolic inhibition,[28] exposure to dinitrophenol suppresses and eventually eliminates Ca^{2+} transients (Figure 3B) in association with the development of a large outward current (Figure 3A), presumably $I_{K,ATP}$. Dinitrophenol was then washed out with normal solution containing 10 mmol/L glucose. Ca^{2+} transients quickly recovered as the outward current disappeared. About 7 minutes after washout of dinitrophenol, membrane currents and $[Ca^{2+}]_i$ spontaneously and unexpectedly began to oscillate. The oscillations were similar in amplitude, period, and phase to those in Figures 1 and 2; however, they were damped and disappeared over the next 10 minutes. It is noteworthy that these oscillations began and ended while the cell was bathed in normal Tyrode's solution. The fact that the oscillations were initiated during recovery from severe metabolic inhibition hints that the key factor may not be substrate availability but rather the relative balance of various energy metabolites within the cell. This interpretation is bolstered by the new findings that photo-

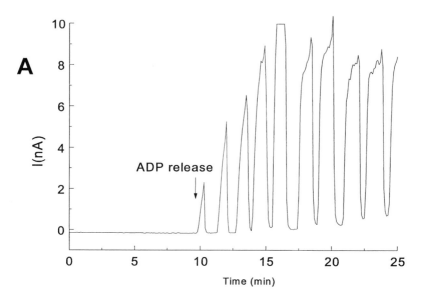

A

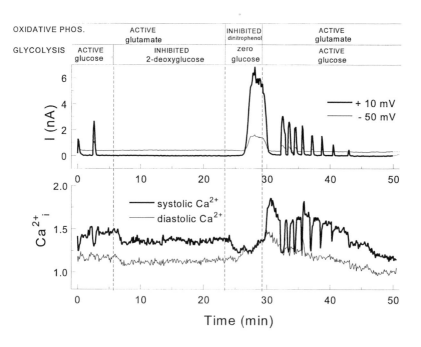

B

release of caged ADP or ATP can initiate oscillations or reset their phase.

Because the cyclical background currents appear to be K^+-selective and resemble the current induced by dinitrophenol (Figure 3), we hypothesize that the oscillations reflect cyclical activation of $I_{K,ATP}$. The preliminary experiment in Figure 4A supports this interpretation. The application of 200 μmol/L glibenclamide, a known blocker of $I_{K,ATP}$, quickly suppressed the background current oscillations. In other cells, concentrations of glibenclamide as low as 10 μmol/L were found to suffice to block the current oscillations. Another preliminary experiment further implicates $I_{K,ATP}$ while shedding additional light on the potential metabolic trigger. $I_{K,ATP}$ is believed to be particularly sensitive to glycolytically derived ATP,[23] so we tested the effect of restoring glucose to a cell that was oscillating in its absence. The addition of 10 mmol/L glucose to the external solution suppressed both the current oscillations and those in $[Ca^{2+}]_i$. We have found that concentrations of glucose as low as 1 mmol/L can suffice to inhibit the oscillations (O'Rourke et al, 1994[2]).

To begin to probe the physiological impact of the oscillations, we switched to current clamp to measure the membrane potential in a cell that was first noted to be oscillating under voltage-clamp conditions. Figure 5A shows the results. Action potentials stimulated by brief depolarizing currents applied every 6 seconds started out long (typical for a guinea pig myocyte at room temperature; see representative records at the top and time course of action potential duration below), periodically shortened to nothing more than a stimulus artifact, and later re-lengthened.

The metabolic challenges presented to these cells do not even come close to being lethal. All cells in which we have observed metabolic oscillations have been entirely unselected and "normal" in appearance. Indeed, cells that exhibit oscillations in substrate-free external medium resume behaving unexceptionally within seconds of substrate reintroduction (eg, Figure 4A). When maintained in physiological solutions, cells isolated from the same hearts remain conventional in their behavior, contain the usual complement of ionic currents, and exhibit robust

---

Figure 3. Initiation of oscillations by photolysis of internal caged ADP (A) or during recovery from severe metabolic inhibition (B). A, A cell containing 1 mmol/L caged ADP was illuminated with a 1-ms flash of UV light at the time indicated by the arrow, initiating oscillations of membrane current (values plotted were at the end of pulses to 0 mV). B, Top, Timing of application of metabolic inhibitors; middle, membrane current values at ends of pulses to -50 mV (dashed line) and 10 mV (solid line); bottom, systolic (solid) and diastolic (dashed) Calcium Green fluorescence.

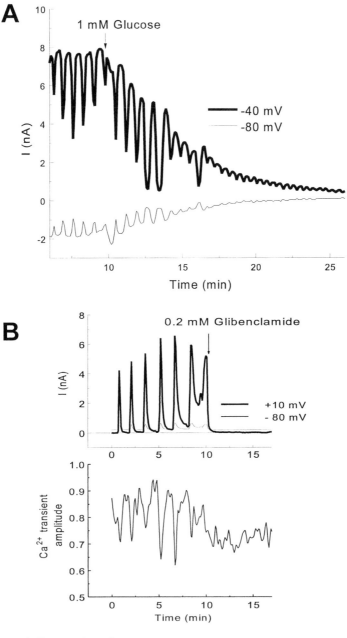

Figure 4. A, Termination of oscillations by exposure to 10 mmol/L glucose. B, Suppression of the oscillating currents by the $I_{K,ATP}$ blocker glibenclamide. Top panels, Membrane currents; bottom panels, Ca^{2+} transient amplitude (systolic minus diastolic Calcium Green fluorescence).

E-C coupling (Figure 1B). If the excitability of otherwise normal heart cells can indeed oscillate when they are subjected to modest metabolic stress (as suggested by Figure 5A), it is difficult to overstate the potential implications for arrhythmogenesis (and for the regulation of contraction). Our thinking about arrhythmogenesis has been heavily influenced by models in which there is a fixed structural basis for arrhythmias.[29] While much has been learned about arrhythmias that propagate around a healed myocardial infarct, little is known about the basis of sudden cardiac death during ischemia (a much more common problem). If groups of metabolically stressed cells in an ischemic region (or in the border zone) can turn on and off in response to an intrinsic metabolic oscillator, excitability may become sufficiently inhomogeneous to induce reentry on a microscopic scale, which in turn could initiate ventricular fibrillation. It is also easy to imagine circumstances in which electrically coupled cells in the heart may undergo metabolic oscillations, but these oscillations are out of phase with each other. Although excitability may be maintained in the tissue as a whole due to electrotonic interactions, Ca^{2+} transients would presumably remain inhomogeneous due to the metabolic oscillations in individual cells. Such inhomogeneity of Ca^{2+} transients would be expected to produce gross contractile dysfunction, because fully activated cells dissipate some of their mechanical energy in pulling their more compliant neighbors.[30]

It is worth highlighting the fact that the oscillations described here are unlike any oscillatory responses described previously in heart cells. Oscillations of intracellular $[Ca^{2+}]$ mediated by the sarcoplasmic reticulum (SR) in the heart are well known (see Reference 32 and the references cited therein), but the present phenomenon is not triggered by SR Ca^{2+} release: background current oscillates even when the membrane is held at a fixed potential, during which $[Ca^{2+}]_i$ remains constant (see Figure 5B). The effect of glucose, as well as many other features of the oscillations, are entirely consistent with the following hypothesis: The glycolytic oscillator is latent in every cell but is suppressed when cellular energy charge is high. The oscillator can be unmasked by relatively minor metabolic perturbations that suffice to trigger broad swings in the activity of phosphofructokinase. The resultant oscillations in ATP and ADP produce cyclical activation of $I_{K,ATP}$.

In the intact tissue, heart cells are coupled to each other by gap junctions. Thus, oscillations must be synchronized in order for regions of the heart to become cyclically inexcitable. Such synchronization could occur because of the timing of a shared external stimulus (eg, ischemia and reperfusion); alternatively, diffusion of metabolites from one cell to its neighbors through gap junctions may suffice to synchronize metabolic oscillations. It is even possible that synchronization may

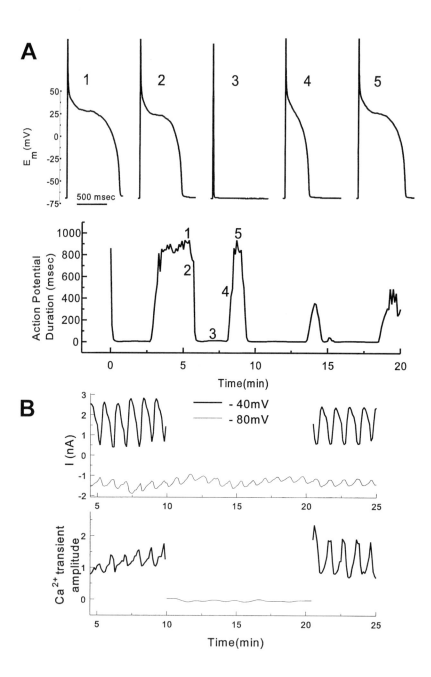

occur via a diffusible extracellular messenger. Evidence for the latter has been obtained in multicellular yeast suspensions, which can oscillate synchronously despite the absence of cell-cell connections.[15]

Summary

The presence of an intrinsic metabolic oscillator in individual heart cells is a startling finding. Modest, reversible perturbations of cellular metabolism can cause otherwise normal cells to become temporarily inexcitable. The results strongly indicate that glycolytic oscillations are primary and that these drive $I_{K,ATP}$. The mechanism of the associated defect in E-C coupling remains to be determined but may well involve cyclical suppression of Ca^{2+} entry due to direct MgATP-dependent modulation of calcium channels.[32] Although electrophysiological inhomogeneities have long been suspected to cause arrhythmias, the inhomogeneities have usually been attributed to fixed structural lesions or to progressive metabolic deterioration.[29] The idea that an inherent metabolic rhythm can be unmasked in stressed but viable cells adds a new level of complexity (and many new opportunities) to our thinking about arrhythmogenesis and ischemic dysfunction. Recent evidence suggesting that pharmacological manipulation of ATP-sensitive K^+ channel activity alters the functional consequences of ischemic insult highlights the importance of the proposed line of inquiry.[33] The ultimate significance of the phenomenon in cardiac disease states will be determined only after detailed characterization of the oscillatory response in single cells, in cell pairs, in tissue, and in mathematical network models.

References

1. Cooley JW, Dodge FA, Cohen H. Digital computer solutions for excitable membrane models. *J Cell Comp Physiol.* 1965;66:S99–S109.

◄──

Figure 5. A, Oscillations in action potential duration. Top row shows representative responses elicited by brief depolarizing current pulses applied every 6 seconds; bottom row shows action potential duration at 90% repolarization as a function of time. B, Persistence of oscillations in membrane current at a fixed membrane potential (-80 mV) in the absence of evoked Ca^{2+} transient. The membrane currents (top) and systolic/diastolic Ca^{2+} signals (bottom) during our conventional voltage protocol (until the 10-minute time point) and when the same cell was held at a constant potential of -80 mV (between the 10- and 20-minute time points).

2. O'Rourke B, Ramza BM, Marban E. Oscillations of membrane current and excitability driven by metabolic oscillations in heart cells. *Science.* 1994;265: 962–966.
3. Dyck JR, Lopaschuk GD. Identification of a small Na^+/H^+ exchanger-like message in the rabbit myocardium. *FEBS Lett.* 1992;310:255–299.
4. Trube G, Hescheler J. Inward-rectifying channels in isolated patches of the heart cell membrane: ATP-dependence and comparison with cell-attached patches. *Pflugers Arch.* 1984;401:178–184.
5. Noma A. ATP-regulated K^+ channels in cardiac muscle. *Nature.* 1983;305: 147–148.
6. Nichols CG, Ripol C, Lederer WJ. ATP-sensitive potassium channel modulation of the guinea pig ventricular action potential and contraction. *Circ Res.* 1991;68:280–287.
7. Shen W-K, Hammil SC. Survivors of acute myocardial infarction: who is at risk for sudden cardiac death? *Mayo Clin Proc.* 1991;66:950–962.
8. Weiss JN, Venkatesh N, Lamp ST. ATP-sensitive K^+ channels and cellular K^+ loss in hypoxic and ischaemic mammalian ventricle. *J Physiol (Lond).* 1992;447:649–673.
9. Wilde AAM, Escande D, Schumacher CA et al. Potassium accumulation in the globally ischemic mammalian heart: a role for the ATP-sensitive potassium channel. *Circ Res.* 1990;67:835–843.
10. Tsien RW, Tsien RY. Calcium channels, stores, and oscillations. *Annu Rev Cell Biol.* 1990;6:715–760.
11. Berridge MJ, Rapp PE. A comparative survey of the function, mechanism and control of cellular oscillators. *J Exp Biol.* 1979;81:217–279.
12. Chance B, Schoener B, Elsaesser S. Control of the waveform of oscillations of the reduced pyridine nucleotide level in a cell-free extract. *Proc Nat Acad Sci U S A.* 1964;52:337–341.
13. Frenkel R. Control of reduced diphosphopyridine nucleotide oscillations in beef heart extracts, II: oscillations of glycolytic intermediates and adenine nucleotides. *Arch Biochem Biophys* 1968;125:157–165.
14. Tornheim K, Lowenstein JM. The purine nucleotide cycle, IV: interactions with oscillations of the glycolytic pathway in muscle extracts. *J Biol Chem.* 1974;249:3241–3247.
15. Hess B, Boiteux A. Mechanism of glycolytic oscillation in yeast, I: aerobic and anaerobic growth conditions for obtaining glycolytic oscillation. *Hoppe Seylers Z Physiol Chem.* 1968;349:1567–1574.
16. Collatz K-G, Horning M. Age dependent changes of a biochemical rhythm: the glycolytic oscillator of the blowfly *Phormia terraenovae. Comp Biochem Physiol.* 1990;96:771–774.
17. Ibsen KH, Schiller KW. Oscillations of nucleotides and glycolytic intermediates in aerobic suspension of Ehrlich ascites tumor cells. *Biochim Biophys Acta.* 1967;131:405–407.
18. Tornheim K. Oscillations of the glycolytic pathway and the purine nucleotide cycle. *J Theor Biol.* 1979;79:491–541.
19. Markus M, Kuschmitz D, Hess B. Chaotic dynamics in yeast glycolysis under periodic substrate input flux. *FEBS Lett.* 1984;172:235–238.
20. Prigogine I. *Order Out of Chaos; Man's New Dialogue With Nature.* New York, NY: Random House; 1984.
21. Cook DL, Satin LS, Hopkins WF. Pancreatic cells are bursting, but how? *Trends Neurosci.* 1991;14:411–414.
22. Corkey BE, Tornheim K, Deeney JT et al. Linked oscillations of free Ca^{2+}

and the ATP/ADP ratio in permeabilized RINm5F insulinoma cells supplemented with a glycolyzing cell-free muscle extract. *J Biol Chem.* 1988;263: 4254–4258.

23. Weiss JN, Lamp ST. Glycolysis preferentially inhibits ATP-sensitive K⁺ channels in isolated guinea pig cardiac myocytes. *Science.* 1987;238:67–69.

24. Hardin CD, Raeymaekers L, Paul RJ. Comparison of endogenous and exogenous sources of ATP in fueling Ca^{2+} uptake in smooth muscle plasma membrane vesicles. *J Gen Physiol.* 1992;99:21–40.

25. Uyeda K. Interactions of glycolytic enzymes with cellular membranes. In: Stadtman ER, Chock PB, eds. *Current Topics in Cellular Regulation.* New York, NY: Academic Press; 1992:31–48.

26. Chen V, McDonough KH, Spitzer JJ. Effects of insulin on glucose metabolism in isolated heart myocytes from adult rats. *Biochim Biophys Acta.* 1985; 846:398–404.

27. Kusuoka H, Marban E. Mechanism of the diastolic dysfunction induced by glycolytic inhibition: does ATP derived from glycolysis play a favored role in cellular Ca^{2+} homeostasis in ferret myocardium? *J Clin Invest.* 1994; 93:1216–1223.

28. Goldhaber JI, Parker JM, Weiss JN. Mechanisms of excitation-contraction coupling failure during metabolic inhibition in guinea-pig ventricular myocytes. *J Physiol (Lond).* 1991;443:371–386.

29. Wit AL, Janse MJ. *The Ventricular Arrhythmias of Ischemia and Infarction: Electrophysiological Mechanisms.* Mount Kisco, NY: Futura Publishing Co, Inc; 1993.

30. Kort AA, Lakatta EG, Marban E, Stern MD, Wier WG. Fluctuations in intracellular $[Ca^{2+}]$ and their effect on tonic tension in canine cardiac Purkinje fibres. *J Physiol.* 1985;367:291–308.

31. Marban E, Robinson SW, Wier WG. Mechanisms of arrhythmogenic delayed and early afterdepolarizations in ferret ventricular muscle. *J Clin Invest.* 1986;78:1185–1192.

32. O'Rourke B, Backx PH, Marban E. Phosphorylation-independent modulation of L-type calcium channels by magnesium-nucleotide complexes. *Science.* 1992;257:245–248.

33. Lynch JJ Jr., Sanguinetti MC, Kimura S, Bassett AL. Therapeutic potential of modulating potassium currents in the diseased myocardium. *FASEB J.* 1992;6:2952–2960.

Discontinuous Conduction and Arrhythmias
Introduction

Augustus O. Grant, MB, ChB, PhD

For decades, the conceptual basis for the origin of cardiac arrhythmias was dominated by the "membrane hypothesis." Slow conduction and block, the critical bases for reentry, were postulated to be the result of a decrease in the excitatory current carried by sodium or calcium ions or of heterogeneities in repolarization. The therapeutic effects of commonly used drugs were interpreted as resulting from the block of these currents. Two events provided an impetus for reevaluation of the membrane hypothesis. In 1981, Spach et al[1] demonstrated nonuniform anisotrophy and discontinuous propagation in myocardial bundles. Slow transverse conduction with normal upstroke velocities were observed; conversely, rapid longitudinal conduction was observed with slow upstroke velocities. These relationships were the opposite of those predicted for conduction in a continuous medium. The directional differences in conduction were the result of structural anisotropy. At both the microscopic and macroscopic levels, effective internal resistance is lower in the longitudinal direction. The safety of conduction is determined by the relationship between current sources and sinks. The lower longitudinal resistance forms a larger current sink, making conduction failure in this direction more likely. A differential failure in conduction may therefore occur entirely on the basis of structure and result in reentry. Extension of these studies by Spach and other investigators emphasized the role of abnormal structure as a basis for cardiac arrhythmias. The results of the CAST study[2] are consistent with a critical role of structure. Drugs that were relatively safe in patients with structurally normal hearts proved lethal in the scarred postinfarction heart.

The three contributions in this section by Kirchhof and Josephson,[3]

Lesh et al,[4] and Saffitz et al[5] examine the clinical and structural evidence for discontinuous propagation as a basis for cardiac arrhythmias. The clinical studies do not permit the direct demonstration of discontinuous propagation possible with detailed mapping studies in vitro. Few data have been provided by intraoperative mapping. A majority of the data depend on the interpretation of intracardiac electrograms obtained during endocardial mapping of arrhythmias. Split or fractionated electrograms have been interpreted as markers of discontinuous propagation. The asynchronous activation of closely spaced bundles results in a decrease in the amplitude, prolongation of the duration, and multiple phases in the electrogram. Although the question of motion artifact has been raised about the form of these electrograms, substantial data now link fractionated electrograms to the occurrence of discontinuities of propagation and anisotropic reentry. This and some unquestionable markers of discontinuous propagation in clinical arrhythmias are reviewed by Kirchhof and Josephson[3] and Lesh et al.[4]

The Naturally Occurring Experiment: AV Node Reentry

Atrioventricular (AV) node reentry is a "clue" disease. In retrospect, clinical evidence that discontinuous propagation is the cause of most AV nodal reentrant tachycardias (AVNRTs) preceded many of the detailed in vitro studies of discontinuous propagation and anisotropic reentry.[6] The reproducible initiation and termination of AVNRT and the demonstration of an excitable gap support the occurrence of reentry. The most compelling evidence for discontinuous propagation is provided by the stimulus-response curve of the AV node during premature stimulation. The discontinuous response curves suggested the presence of dual AV nodal pathways. Distinct fast (β) and slow (α) pathways within the AV node having different refractory periods were proposed (reviewed in Reference 6). Kirchhof and Josephson[3] review the evidence that the dual pathways are functional rather than structural. In this particular arrhythmia, for which there is strong evidence for discontinuous propagation, fractionated extracellular electrograms were recorded in vitro during directional changes in propagation, supporting the interpretation of the fractionated waveforms.

The pathways for reentry may not be confined to the anatomic node.[7,8] This is emphasized by the high success rate of radiofrequency "modification of the AV node" for the cure of AV nodal reentrant tachycardia with ablation site(s) in the posteroinferior right atrium.[9] Why is the AV node a likely site for the occurrence of discontinuous propagation? Saffitz et al[5] point out that AV nodal myocytes are connected by a "very small and sparsely distributed (gap) junction." The result is a low safety factor for conduction over the AV node. The orientation of fibers in the approaches to the AV node also favors directional differences in the safety factor of conduction.

The importance of membrane properties of the AV node cannot be overlooked. The nodal cells have low resting membrane potentials and slow upstroke velocities, dependent on the calcium current.[10] Because of the reduced membrane potential, recovery of the calcium current from inactivation is slow. Refractoriness persists for a significant time beyond complete repolarization. These characteristics make the AV node a site of decremental conduction and block. The efficacy of the calcium channel blocking drugs and adenosine in terminating AVNRT support an important role of the membrane properties of the nodal cells in reentry.

A simple unanswered question is hidden in the discussion of AVNRT by Kirchhof and Josephson.[3] They point out that 10% to 15% of patients have discontinuous stimulus-response curves, yet only a minority of patients develop AVNRT. Presumably, conditioning and initiating factors such as autonomic tone and the occurrence of spontaneous atrial or ventricular premature beats are important in the transition to clinical arrhythmia.

Atrial Flutter/Fibrillation

Lesh et al[4] review the evidence for discontinuous propagation during typical atrial flutter. The arrhythmia results from macroscopic reentry. The smooth-walled atrial structures are activated in a inferior-to-superior direction. The circuit is completed by conduction in a counterclockwise direction over the crista terminalis and the eustachian ridge. Lesh et al combine intracardiac ultrasound with electrode catheter mapping to assess conduction during typical atrial flutter. In their hands, intracardiac ultrasound proved very useful in the identification of intraatrial structures such as the crista terminalis. They were particularly concerned about the basis for the isolation of the reentrant circuit. Split potentials were recorded in the electrograms, suggesting that discontinuous propagation was originating from the crista terminalis. They suggest that the discontinuous propagation across the crista terminalis may provide a mechanism for isolation. Saffitz et al[5] point out a directional distribution of gap junctions in the crista terminalis, with these low-resistance connections occurring primarily at the ends of cells. Radiofrequency ablation applied to the low right atrium has been very effective in terminating this arrhythmia.[11] This is consistent with a reentrant mechanism but does not address the basis for reentry.

Although atrial fibrillation is more common than atrial flutter, fewer data on its mechanisms exist. Spach and Starmer[12] examined conduction in human atrial bundles in vitro. They found nonuniform isotropic properties in the bundles removed from older subjects but not in those from children and young adults. The data are consistent with the known age distribution of atrial fibrillation: it is rare in childhood even in the presence of marked atrial enlargement, and its prevalence increases with advancing age.

Lesh et al[4] discuss two possible mechanisms of clinical atrial fibrillation: (1) a rapid ectopic focus with exit block and (2) reentry resulting from one or more wavelets in the atria. They suggest that the ectopic focus may be protected from the rest of the atrium by discontinuous propagation. A delicate balance must be involved, because the focus has to excite the atrium, yet its activity should not be loaded by a low resistance (large sink) to the atrium. Their success in ablating atrial fibrillation with lesions in the region of the proposed ectopic focus would support the occurrence of the first mechanism. However, it is likely that this mechanism accounts for a minority of cases of clinical atrial fibrillation. In general, both the surgical and catheter ablation of atrial fibrillation usually require more extensive lesions that also involve the left atrium.[13] This is more consistent with reentry occurring over a large area of the atria.

Ventricular Tachycardia

Ventricular tachycardia has multiple causes, including coronary artery disease, hypertensive cardiovascular disease, hypertrophic cardiomyopathy, and congenital and acquired QT-interval prolongation. Kirchhof and Josephson[3] provide a very comprehensive review of the role of discontinuous propagation in ventricular tachycardia, focusing primarily on arrhythmias occurring in the setting of coronary artery disease. Even in this single entity, the mechanisms of arrhythmia are likely to differ in acute ischemia compared with the chronic healed infarction. Changes in structure and the associated discontinuous propagation are probably more important in the chronic healed infarction. The evidence for a role of discontinuous propagation in the genesis of ventricular tachycardia is indirect but no less compelling. Endocardial electrograms showing fractionated potentials of low amplitude and long duration have provided the major clue. De Bakker et al[14] showed that such electrograms could be recorded from endocardial resection of patients with ventricular tachycardia. They showed that relatively normal action potentials could be recorded from several cells. This observation diminishes the significance of changes in membrane properties as a possible mechanism of ventricular tachycardia in healed myocardial infarction. In contrast, hyperkalemia, low pH, and increased intracellular calcium activity produce definite changes in the action potential in the acutely ischemic heart.

Studies from Josephson's laboratory clearly show a relationship between ventricular tachycardia and fractionated potentials recorded with electrode catheters. Quantitative and qualitative changes in the fractionated electrograms occur after initiation of ventricular tachycardia. The most significant change is in the duration; electrical activity may become continuous and thus span diastole. Termination of ventricular tachycardia by pacing may result in disappearance of the diastolic activity.

What is the structural basis for discontinuous propagation in chronic ischemic heart disease? At a gross level, the replacement fibrosis forms a basis for separation of fiber bundles. In their contribution, however, Saffitz et al[5] point out that more subtle changes in cell coupling may occur. "Peri-infarct myocytes are connected by fewer and shorter gap junctions than are normal cells." However, to emphasize the role of multiple contributing factors, they point out that the healed infarcts of patients with arrhythmias do not appear to be structurally different from those without arrhythmias. The difference in arrhythmia experience may depend on triggering events.

Conclusions

The available data suggest that discontinuous propagation plays a central role in the common clinical arrhythmias. This has major implications in our therapy for cardiac arrhythmias. Treatments that affect properties of the sarcolemma are doomed to have limited success. In myocardial infarction, treatment to prevent arrhythmias should begin immediately. Angiotension-converting enzyme inhibitors limit fibrosis after coronary artery occlusion.[15] This may be a basis for their benefit in postinfarction patients. Our drug development strategies should shift from membrane-active drugs to therapies that can regulate the expression of gap junctions or that provide exogenous replacement of junctions. Many hurdles will have to be overcome to bring these strategies to the clinic. However, the low efficacy of many of our current therapies and the magnitude of the problem should encourage us to make a commitment to develop newer and more appropriate therapeutic strategies.

References

1. Spach MS, Miller WT III, Geselowitz DG. The discontinuous nature of propagation in normal canine cardiac muscle. *Circ Res.* 1981;48:39–54.

2. CAST Investigators. Preliminary report: effect of encainide and flecainide on mortality in a randomized trial of arrhythmia suppression after myocardial infarction. *N Engl J Med.* 1989;321:406–421.
3. Kirchhof CJHJ, Josephson ME. The role of discontinuous conduction/nonuniform anisotropy in clinical arrhythmias. In Spooner PM, Joyner RW, Jalife J, eds. *Discontinuous Conduction in the Heart.* Armonk, NY: Futura Publishing Co., Inc.; 1997.
4. Lesh MD, Kalman JM, Olgin JE, Ellis WS. The role of discontinuous electrical propagation in clinical atrial arrhythmias-current evidence and future directions. In Spooner PM, Joyner RW, Jalife J, eds. *Discontinuous Conduction in the Heart.* Armonk, NY: Futura Publishing Co., Inc.; 1997.
5. Saffitz JE, Beyer EC, Darrow BJ, Guerrero PA, Beardslee MA, Dodge SM. Gap junction structure, conduction and arrhythmogenesis directions for future research. In Spooner PM, Joyner RW, Jalife J, eds. *Discontinuous Conduction in the Heart.* Armonk, NY: Futura Publishing Co., Inc.; 1997.
6. Zeng W, Mazgalev T, Munk AA, Shrier A, Jalife J. Dual atrioventricular pathways revisited: on the cellular mechanisms of discontinuous atrioventricular nodal recovery and the gap phenomenon. In Zipes DP, Jalife J, eds. Cardiac Electrophysiology: From Cell to Bedside. Philadelphia: WB Saunders Co. 1995;31:325.
7. Janse MJ, Anderson RH, McGuire MA, Ho Sy. "A-V nodal" re-entry, I: "A-V nodal" re-entry revisited. *J Cardiovasc Electrophysiol.* 1993;5:561–572.
8. McGuire MA, Janse MJ, Ross DL. "A-V nodal" re-entry, II: A-V nodal, A-V junctional or atrionodal re-entry? *J Cardiovasc Electrophysiol.* 1993;5: 573–586.
9. Jackman WM, Beckman KJ, McClelland JH, et al. Treatment of supraventricular tachycardia due to atrioventricular nodal re-entry by radiofrequency catheter ablation of slow pathway conduction. *N Engl J Med.* 1992; 327:313–318.
10. Meijler FL, Janse MJ. Morphology and electrophysiology of the mammalian atrioventricular node. *Physiol Rev.* 1988;68:608–647.
11. Feld G, Fleck P, Chen PS, et al. Radio-frequency catheter ablation for the treatment of human type 1 atrial flutter: identification of a critical zone in the re-entrant circuit by endocardial mapping techniques. *Circulation.* 1992; 86:1233–1240.
12. Spach MS, Starmer CF. Altering the topology of gap junctions: a major therapeutic target for atrial fibrillation. *Cardiovasc Res.* 1995;30:336–344.
13. Cox JL, Boineau JP, Schuessler RB, Jaquiss RDB, Lappas DG. Modification of the maze procedure for atrial flutter and atrial fibrillation. *J Thorac Cardiovasc Surg.* 1995;110:473–484.
14. De Bakker JMT, van Capella FJL, Janse MJ, et al. Re-entry as a cause of ventricular tachycardia in patients with chronic ischemic heart disease: electrophysiologic and anatomic correlation. *Circulation.* 1988;77:581–606.
15. Linz W, Wiemer G, Gohlke P, Unger T, Scholkens BA. Contributions of kinins to the cardiovascular actions of angiotensin-converting enzyme inhibitors. *Pharmacol Rev.* 1995;47:25–49.

Chapter 4

Gap Junction Structure, Conduction, and Arrhythmogenesis:
Directions for Future Research

Jeffrey E. Saffitz, MD, PhD,
Eric C. Beyer, MD, PhD,
Bruce J. Darrow, MD, PhD,
Patricia A. Guerrero, MD,
Michael A. Beardslee, MD,
and Stephen M. Dodge, MD

Recent progress in elucidating the role of gap junctions in cardiac conduction has been substantial, but these advances have been largely descriptive rather than mechanistic. A great deal is now known about the molecular features of cardiac connexins, their distributions in the heart, and the functional properties of the channels they form in experimental expression systems. Discoveries in the past 5 years indicate that (1) individual cardiac myocytes express at least three different connexins, each of which forms channels with distinct biophysical properties, including unitary conductances, voltage dependencies, and ionic permeabilities; (2) the cardiac connexins are phosphoproteins, and their posttranslational modification may exert a wide range of effects, includ-

Work in the authors' laboratories was supported by National Institutes of Health Grants HL50598 and HL45466. Bruce J. Darrow was supported by NIH Training Grant T32 NS07129; Patricia A. Guerrero and Michael A. Beardslee were supported by NIH Training Grant T32 HL0708; Patricia A. Guerrero was also supported by an NRSA Grant from the National Institutes of Health. Dr. Beyer is an Established Investigator of the American Heart Association.

From: Spooner PM, Joyner RW, Jalife J (eds). *Discontinuous Conduction in the Heart.* Armonk, NY: Futura Publishing Company, Inc.; © 1997.

ing alterations in single-channel conductance, gating, channel assembly and intracellular transport, and connexin protein turnover; (3) cardiac tissues characterized by distinct anisotropic conduction properties (eg, nodes and bundles in the conduction system and atrial and ventricular myocardium) express different combinations of the connexins; (4) myocytes in functionally disparate cardiac tissues are interconnected by distinct tissue-specific spatial arrangements of gap junctions; (5) the number, size, and three-dimensional distribution of gap junctions change rapidly in response to physiological or pathophysiological processes; and (6) the half-lives of connexins in cultured neonatal rat ventricular myocytes are very short ($t_{1/2} = 1.5$ to 3 hours).

These observations broadly summarize the state of current knowledge of the role of gap junctions in cardiac conduction and arrhythmogenesis and form the basis for two major hypotheses: (1) the conduction properties of specific cardiac tissues are specified, in part, by multiple factors, including the types of connexins expressed; the number, size, and spatial distribution of gap junctions interconnecting myocytes in each tissue; the biophysical properties of the channels formed by each connexin; and other factors, including posttranslational modifications such as phosphorylation; and (2) changes in type of connexin expressed, gap junction number, and spatial distribution directly alter conduction and may thereby contribute to arrhythmogenesis. Although these hypotheses are supported by a large body of indirect or circumstantial evidence, there has been no direct test of the functional roles of multiple connexins expressed in individual cardiac myocytes, nor has the role of structural features of intercellular junctions as determinants of cardiac conduction and as potential determinants of arrhythmogenesis been critically evaluated.

The purpose of this chapter is to highlight specific questions that, in the authors' opinions, are important targets for future research. The current state of knowledge pertaining to each question is briefly summarized, and specific experimental approaches are proposed.

Why Does the Heart Express Multiple Connexins?

Connexins are members of a multigene family of proteins, each encoded by a single gene at different chromosomal loci.[1] More than a dozen members have been cloned and sequenced, and their tissue distributions have been characterized. A major milestone in gap junction research was the recent realization that individual differentiated cells express multiple connexins. This was first shown in hepatocytes.[2] In the heart, at least three individual connexin proteins, Cx43, Cx40, and Cx45, have been shown unequivocally to be expressed in cardiac myocytes.[3,4] Other connexins, including Cx37,[5] Cx46,[6] and the connexin-related protein MP70,[7] have been identified in cardiac tissues by use of nucleic acid or antibody probes, but it is uncertain whether these proteins are expressed by cardiac myocytes or other cells in the heart, such as vascular endothelium, smooth muscle, valvular tissues, stromal elements, etc.

The absolute amounts of the cardiac connexins expressed by individual myocytes have not been rigorously quantified, partly because of differences in concentrations and affinities of monospecific antibodies used to identify them. However, although information on the absolute amounts of Cx43, Cx40, and Cx45 in the heart is lacking, there is no doubt that functionally distinct cardiac tissues express these three proteins in different patterns. For example, Cx40 is expressed in the nodes and bundles of the cardiac conduction system[8–13] and is readily identified in atrial myocardium,[10–12] but its expression by the ventricle is highly limited and may be absent. Detection of Cx40 mRNA in ventricular homogenates must be interpreted with caution because the protein has been clearly localized to intramural coronary vessels.[13,14] Immunohistochemical identification of Cx40 expression by ventricular endocardial and subendocardial myocyte bundles[13] could reflect some ventricular myocyte expression of Cx40 in these sites or may be attributable to fibers of the Purkinje system, which express abundant Cx40. In any event, a highly consistent tissue distribution of Cx40 has been observed in the hearts of many mammals, including humans. In contrast, Cx43, which appears to be the most abundant cardiac connexin, is widely expressed in both atrial and ventricular muscle and in most but not all components of the conduction system.[8–10,15–17] Many investigators have failed to identify Cx43 in at least some specialized myocytes of the sinoatrial and atrioventricular nodes.[10,16,17] Cx45 has been detected in all cardiac tissues, but it appears to be present in lower abundance[3,4,10,14] than other connexins in myocytes that coexpress Cx45 with Cx43 and/or Cx40. It should be emphasized, however, that this conclusion is based on comparisons of immunochemical signal intensity by immunohistochemistry and Western blotting, and concentrations and affinities of monospecific antibodies are largely unknown.

Electrophysiological analysis of single-channel events in communication-deficient cells transfected with known connexin DNA sequences has revealed a wide range of biophysical properties of channels formed by different connexins.[18–28] These include unitary conductances, voltage dependencies, and ionic permeabilities. The fact that different connexins form channels with unique properties, combined with the distinct patterns of multiple connexin expression in different conductive tissues of the heart, strongly suggests that the conduction properties of cardiac tissue are influenced by connexin expression phenotypes. At present, however, there has been no direct test of this hypothesis.

Recognition that individual cardiac myocytes express at least three different connexins and that functionally distinct cardiac tissues express these proteins in different amounts raises fundamental questions. What biological purposes other than current transfer are served by expression of multiple connexins in individual cardiac myocytes? What are the individual contributions of specific connexin gene products to the conduction properties of functionally distinct cardiac tissues in the normal heart? Does expression of specific combinations of connexins confer specific conduction properties on a cardiac tissue? Answering these questions will be challenging, because many factors ultimately contribute to the conduction properties of cardiac tissues, and it may be difficult to experimentally isolate the effects of just one. An approach that overcomes this difficulty is theoretical analysis using computer simulations of cardiac conduction in models that incorporate molecular and structural features of real tissue. Highly sophisticated models of the cardiac action potential have proved helpful in gaining insights into mechanisms underlying the generation of normal and abnormal intracellular currents.[29–32] A challenge for the future will be to incorporate the complexities of intercellular current transfer into models that include other important structural complexities of myocardial intercellular connections. Gaining insight into the biological and physiological roles of individual connexins by this approach will require greater understanding than currently exists about the relative amounts and subcellular distributions of individual connexins within myocyte gap junctions and about the regulation of individual channel function. It may be anticipated, however, that as information is gained from experimental studies of connexin expression and function, parallel advances will occur in the theoretical analysis of the individual roles of connexins in cardiac conduction.

Another important strategy that is already being widely implemented involves genetic manipulation of expression of specific genes in transgenic or knockout mice.[33,34] In the case of genes important in cardiac electrophysiology, this approach has only recently been applied. For example, a Cx43 knockout mouse has been produced[35] in which null mutants develop to term but die shortly after birth, apparently as a result of a poorly defined cardiac abnormality involving right ventricular outflow tract obstruction. At present, only limited, preliminary electrophysiological studies have been performed in the Cx43 knockout mouse.[36] Future detailed studies should shed light on the role of this protein in cardiac conduction. It can be anticipated that all of the cardiac connexins, as well as many other genes encoding proteins important in cardiac electrophysiology, will be manipulated by either knockout or transgenic strategies to alter their expression in cardiac tissues. This approach will undoubtedly be informative. But whereas the technology for producing transgenic and knockout mice is becoming widely available, advances in murine cardiac electrophysiology are also necessary to achieve its full potential. Because of its small size and rapid heart rate, the mouse heart has not been widely used in experimental cardiac electrophysiology. Until large-animal transgenic strategies are better developed, it seems imperative that cardiac electrophysiologists develop the means to analyze conduction in the mouse heart to take advantage of these advances. Functional analysis of gene products expressed in simple systems such as the *Xenopus* oocyte is of value, but eventually it will be necessary to return to the animal to elucidate the contributions of individual genes.

Another approach that combines advantages of both analyses in noncardiac expression systems and genetically manipulated animals is the use of primary cultures of cardiac myocytes to help define the role of individual genes in conduction and arrhythmogenesis. Recent reports have described sarcolemmal and junctional currents in individual cells or cell pairs derived from disaggregated fetal, neonatal, or adult mouse hearts.[37,38] This approach will also be useful in determining the functions of individual connexins from genetically altered mice. Moreover, genetic manipulation of connexin expression can be performed directly in more conventional neonatal rat ventricular myocytes in vitro by means of adenoviral or other gene transfer approaches. Adenoviral gene transfer in primary myocyte cultures is attractive because of its high efficiency, the lack of dependence of gene transfer on cell division, and the absence of the immune system activation that complicates adenoviral gene transfer in vivo. Another advantage of in vitro systems is exemplified by recent studies in which neonatal rat ventricular myocytes have been grown in patterned arrays that exhibit many of the anisotropic structural complexities of myocardium in vivo.[39–41] These patterned growth cultures, combined with optical mapping to assess conduction with great temporal and spatial resolution and the potential for genetic or pharmacological manipulation of expression, dramatically illustrate the potential to elucidate the electrophysiological consequences in primary culture systems.

What Are the Physiological Regulators of Gap Junctional Channel Conductance?

The original concept of gap junction channels as indiscriminate pores that close only in response to profound pathophysiological stimuli associated with the death of one member of a coupled cell pair (eg, acidosis and marked increases in intracellular calcium) has given way to recognition of a far more complex regulation. It has been known for several years that multiple signal transduction pathways can affect gap junction channel function, but the molecular mechanisms and the role of these pathways in physiological and pathophysiological processes are barely understood. Many connexins (including Cx43, Cx45, and Cx40) are phosphoproteins. Recent evidence has implicated connexin phosphorylation in multiple biological processes, including changes in single-channel conductance states, protein assembly into functional channels and their incorporation into channel arrays in gap junctions, and possibly connexin degradation as well.[18,19,21–24,42,43] Indeed, phosphorylation of different amino acids in individual connexins may alter different biological functions. At present, knowledge about the sites of phosphorylation within individual connexin sequences, the kinases and phosphatases that regulate it, and the biological and electrophysiological consequences remains fragmentary. Sorting out the complexities of connexin regulation will be arduous, but potential insights into the basic biology as well as development of efficacious therapeutics to modulate junctional conductance in patients with heart disease will be great. In this regard, a recent report identifying a peptide that appears to interact specifically with gap junction channels[44] may provide a tantalizing new direction for such research.

To What Extent Do Specific Spatial Arrangements Determine Anisotropic Conduction Properties of Normal Tissues?

A striking feature of the normal heart is the diversity of structural "blueprints" on how myocytes are interconnected in three-dimensional tissues. Knowledge in this area is incomplete, but an interesting picture has emerged relating the structure and distribution of intercellular connections at gap junctions to electrophysiological properties of specific conductive tissues of the heart. An example of functionally relevant, tissue-specific three-dimensional packing geometries that we have studied is the comparison of the left ventricle with the crista terminalis in the canine heart.[11] We have found that a typical myocyte in the canine left ventricle is connected on average to 11 or 12 other myocytes. Roughly equivalent numbers of junctions occur between neighboring cells oriented in side-to-side and end-to-end apposition. Although concentrated at the ends of ventricular myocytes, gap junctions also occur at many other points along the cell body, leading to complex patterns of overlapping cells in ventricular muscle. Whereas the ratio of cell length to width of isolated canine ventricular myocytes is ≈6:1, the overlapping pattern of cells in ventricular tissue results in an "effective" length-to-width ratio of only 3.4:1. This geometry is consistent with the moderate degree of anisotropy observed in conduction velocities in ventricular muscle compared with other tissues, such as the atrial bundles known as the crista terminalis.[45] Because activation wave fronts moving through a uniform sheet of ventricular myocardium readily cross intercellular junctions and propagate in both longitudinal and transverse directions, the elongated shape of ventricular myocytes becomes a principal determinant of conduction velocity anisotropy, because wave fronts must traverse more intercellular junctions and encounter greater resistance in the transverse than the longitudinal direction.

In contrast to the ventricle, nonuniformity or anisotropy of conduction velocity in the crista terminalis depends not only on cell shape, but also on anisotropic distribution of intercellular junctions.[11] Crista terminalis myocytes are smaller than ventricular myocytes but have an identical length to-width-ratio. Longitudinal conduction velocity in the crista is greater than in the ventricle, but transverse propagation is considerably slower. This leads to a ratio of longitudinal to transverse velocity of ≈10:1 in the crista compared with a directional ratio of only ≈3:1 in ventricular muscle.[45,46] Because differences in membrane ionic currents in the crista and ventricle cannot fully account for their disparate degrees of conduction velocity anisotropy, structural features appear to play a major role. For example, in contrast to the distribution of junctions in ventricular myocytes, gap junctions in crista terminalis myocytes are located mainly at the true ends of the cells.[11] Thus, whereas a single ventricular myocyte is connected in three-dimensional tissue to 11 or 12 neighbors, with numerous intercellular connections occurring between cells in end-to-end and side-to-side juxtaposition, myocytes of the crista terminalis are connected to only six or seven neighbors, but on average, four or five of these are connected in predominantly end-to-end apposition.[11] Accordingly, longitudinal propagation in the crista is facilitated by numerous intercellular junctions, whereas transverse intercellular current transfer can occur at far fewer locations. Thus, wavefronts may have to zigzag, traveling a longer conduction pathway than in tissue composed of myocytes more extensively interconnected side-to-side.

Detailed three-dimensional reconstructions of cellular packing geometries have not been described for all cardiac tissues, but qualitative morphological studies have revealed vastly different structural features of intercellular coupling that undoubtedly contribute importantly to the anistropic properties of nodes and bundles in the conduction system. For example, sinoatrial and atrioventricular node myocytes are interconnected by very small, sparsely distributed junctions, a structural pattern that is consistent with the slow conduction in these specialized conductive tissues.[10,47,48] At the other end of the spectrum, cells of the His-Purkinje network form fiber bundles containing numerous very large lateral and end-to-end junctions.[10,16,46] This arrangement apparently converts a parallel array of myocytes into a larger, more homogeneous conductive cable that facilitate rapid conduction.

Another recently recognized feature of cardiac intercellular junctions concerns changes in size and spatial distribution of gap junctions during cardiac growth and development. Ventricular myocytes of the late fetal, neonatal, and infant heart are characterized by numerous, small gap junctions distributed uniformly throughout the cell surface. In contrast, adult ventricular myocytes express larger gap junctions that are concentrated mainly at the ends of the cells or at discrete points along the cell body with an intervening sarcolemma devoid of junctions.[49] Mechanisms responsible for the establishment of these two distinct patterns of gap junction distribution are unknown. One clue may be that surviving myocytes at the borders of healing myocardial infarcts exhibit a gap junction pattern reminiscent of the "fetal" pattern,[50] consistent with the notion that remodeling of conduction pathways in response to injury may mirror developmental processes during establishment of the adult pattern.

The presence of different spatial patterns of intercellular junctions in cardiac tissues that have different conduction properties strongly implicates the number, size, and spatial distribution of gap junctions as independent determinants of conduction properties. However, structural determinants of tissue electrophysiology remain poorly understood. Moreover, the mechanisms underlying the development of specific packing geometries in the heart are unknown. How are tissue-specific arrangements of end-to-end and side-to-side connections established? Are these inherent features of the tissue arising as a consequence of morphogenesis? To what extent are spatial arrangements of gap junctions determined by mechanical forces? Are the distributions of gap junctions mainly a consequence of the locations of intercalated disks, such that junctions form at sites where mechanical stabilization of neighboring cells is provided by adjacent disks?

Identification of molecular mechanisms responsible for spatial arrangements of gap junctions in distinct cardiac tissues will depend on fundamental advances in cardiac morphogenesis. However, some aspects can be studied today. One approach involves application of defined mechanical stresses to cardiac myocytes in vitro to determine alterations in structure and distribution of intercellular junctions. This strategy has been used to identify mechanisms whereby stretch activates expression of early response and contractile protein genes during the hypertrophic response.[51,52]

Do Hybrid Connexin Channels Form Between Cardiac Myocytes?

The fact that gap junctions between cardiac myocytes contain multiple connexins, each of which forms channels with specific biophysical properties, provides enormous potential for the fine control of intercellular communication. One intriguing aspect is the possibility that cardiac myocytes express heterotypic channels composed of hemichannels made of different connexins as well as heteromeric channels in which each hemichannel contains multiple connexin. At present, however, little is known about the presence of heterotypic or heteromeric channels in complex organs such as the heart.

Immunohistochemical analysis has shown that different connexins colocalize in individual gap junctions in cardiac myocytes,[4] but even with confocal techniques, the resolution of light microscopy is insufficient to reveal how individual proteins are distributed within the large arrays in gap junctions. Recent scanning-transmission electron microscopic studies of freeze-fractured hepatic gap junctions identified microdomains in which two hepatic connexins, Cx26 and Cx32, appear to be segregated.[53] Whether separation of connexins into such microdomains occurs in cardiac junctions is unknown.

Molecular properties of heterotypic gap junction channels have been characterized in several studies using *Xenopus* oocyte expression systems. Of relevance is one study of heterotypic channels expressing the cardiac connexins Cx40, Cx43, and Cx37.[54] Oocytes expressing Cx40 formed functional heterotypic channels with oocytes expressing Cx37, but cells expressing Cx40 did not form functional channels with those expressing Cx43, even though these proteins formed characteristic homotypic channels. These observations may have implications for current flow in intact heart. Atrial myocytes which express both Cx43 and Cx40 within individual gap junctions, may be able to form only homotypic channels with defined but limited functions. In addition, there may be some situations in which intercellular connections exhibit a considerable degree of connexin "mismatch." For example, sinus node cells in most species express little or no Cx43 but appear to connect with atrial myocytes that express Cx43. Similarly, distal Purkinje fibers, which express Cx40 abundantly, appear to form junctions with ventricular myocytes, which express little or no Cx40. Thus, disparate connexin phenotypes at critical "junctions" within the cardiac conduction system might play a role in the functional specialization of these regions.

Insights into the role of heterotypic channels in the heart may come from studies in which the expression of connexins is altered genetically and the functional consequences are analyzed in isolated cell pairs. As more information becomes available on the biophysical properties of heterotypic channels in heterologous expression systems, computer simulations may also provide insight into their potential biological roles.

What Mechanisms Underlie Remodeling of Intercellular Connections in Response to Myocardial Injury and What Are Their Implications for Arrhythmogenesis?

Increasing evidence implicates alterations in gap junctions in the pathogenesis of heart disease, either as a result of acquired changes in the amount or distribution of connexins or through mutations in individual connexin genes. Mutations in amino acid residues that are putative targets for phosphorylation in Cx43 have been associated with congenital cardiac malformations in patients exhibiting visceroatrial heterotaxia.[55] The causal link between Cx43 gene mutations and the expression of these malformations has not yet been established, but advances in this area can be anticipated.

Myocardial responses to injury are associated with alterations in cell-to-cell communication implicated in arrhythmogenesis and possibly other forms of heart disease. However, the range of potential pathophysiological change in intercellular communication is broad, and the responsible mechanisms and functional consequences are highly complex and poorly understood. Rapid alterations in junctional conductance probably contribute importantly to the development of conduction abnormalities in acute myocardial ischemia. Ischemic myocytes rapidly accumulate Ca^{2+} and H^+ in amounts sufficient to decrease junctional coupling.[56,57] Long-chain acylcarnitines and other potent arrhythmogenic lipid metabolites accumulate rapidly within the sarcolemma of ischemic myocytes and may decrease junctional conductance and also impair ion currents, leading to alterations in excitability, automaticity, and conduction.[58] It is plausible to speculate that different connexins may form channels with differential responses to acidosis, Ca^{2+}, and other mediators of ischemia, such that effects on conduction depend on the connexin phenotype in a given cardiac tissue. This question could be studied by characterizing responses of defined channels to pathophysiological stimuli in expression systems. It may also be possible to evaluate the effects of ischemia on channel function and myocardial conduction in cultured myocytes or intact animals in which the expression of specific connexins has been manipulated genetically.

Alterations in the number or distribution of myocyte gap junctions probably plays an important role in the development of arrhythmia substrates that accompany chronic myocardial responses to injury, for example, healing after acute myocardial infarction or remodeling in response to pressure or volume overload.[59–62] Reentrant ventricular tachyarrhythmias in patients who have survived previous myocardial infarction are often dependent on regions of slow, heterogeneous propagation leading to conduction delay or block in viable but structurally altered myocardium bordering the healed infarct.[63,64] Despite the distinctly abnormal propagation of wave fronts through the border zone, intracellular recordings of resting membrane potential and action potential upstroke velocities in these regions are typically normal or near normal.[65] Thus, slow conduction leading to reentry in regions bordering healed infarcts may be attributable primarily to alterations in current transfer between myocytes at gap junctions.

Morphometric analysis of intercellular connections in healed canine infarct border zones has shown that peri-infarct myocytes are connected by fewer and shorter gap junctions than are normal cells.[59] The number of cells connected to each individual ventricular myocyte is reduced by nearly half in border zone regions, primarily as the result of selective loss side-to-side junctions.[59] Thus, wave fronts activating these regions in a transverse direction would propagate more slowly, and wave fronts might be forced to zigzag through the tissue until they reenter postrefractory tissue and initiate the next beat of the tachycardia. Indeed, a zigzag course of activation has been documented in scarred human papillary muscles in which transverse propagation was impaired by collagenase barriers.[64]

Because of the enormous diversity in the number and spatial distribution of intercellular connections at gap junctions in the heart, critical structural determinants of "anatomic substrates" of cardiac arrhythmias have not been defined in detail. In fact, all patients who survive myocardial infarction are left with infarct scars. However, the pathological anatomy of "anatomic substrates" that have been surgically excised from patients with reentrant ventricular tachycardias is not different in obvious ways from the variable admixtures of surviving myocytes and scar tissue in healed infarcts of patients with no apparent history of ventricular tachycardia. Perhaps the location of myocardial scars in relation to "triggers" is the major determinant of whether the common, stereotypical pathological change in injured myocardium actually becomes an "anatomic substrate." Alternatively, there may be more subtle patterns of surviving myocytes and scar tissue that create specific conduction abnormalities that increase the risk of arrhythmogenesis independent of location relative to triggers. Elucidation of the structural determinants of lethal arrhythmias will probably require detailed analysis of microconduction and identification of the electrophysiological consequences of different event patterns of injury and scarring.

Little is known about mechanisms leading to the remodeling of gap junction distribution in diseased myocardium. It seems probable, however, that remodeling of conduction pathways in infarct border zones is a complex process involving perturbations of connexin gene expression and changes in rates of connexin protein synthesis and degradation. Detailed understanding of regulatory sequences in cardiac connexin genes will be critical in dissecting transcriptional mechanisms of connexin expression. Identification of specific response elements in the promoters of connexin genes will provide further insights into signal transduction pathways and mechanisms that link changes in connexin expression to the full repertoire of responses to myocyte injury. Future identification of nuclear binding factors that interact with connexin gene promoters might also shed light on systems regulating tissue-specific expression of connexins in functionally distinct tissues of the mammalian heart.

Beyond the transcriptional level, multiple potential translational and posttranslational mechanisms may be important in controlling communication at gap junctions. For example, regulation of connexin turnover is largely unexplored but could represent an important aspect of the development of arrhythmia substrates in response to injury. The morphological spectrum of myocyte responses to diverse forms of injury is nonspecific and consists of degenerative changes, including partial or nearly complete loss of sarcomeres, accumulation of glycogen, and disorganization and loss of sarcoplasmic reticulum.[66,67] These changes, often referred to as "myocytolysis," are typically observed in myocytes in "chronic ischemic" states (eg, "hibernating myocardium"), in cardiomyopathies, and in congestive heart failure. Not much is known about the intracellular mechanisms that cause myocytolysis, but the morphological manifestations appear to be reversible and correlate with the degree of ventricular dysfunction. The loss of myofibrils in response to diverse forms of injury suggests that activation of cellular proteolytic systems is involved.

We and others have shown that Cx43 and Cx45 turn over rapidly ($t_{1/2} = 1.5$ to 3 hours) in cultured neonatal rat ventricular myocytes.[22,43] Recent work in our laboratory has implicated ubiquitin-dependent proteosomal degradation in Cx43 proteolysis.[68] However, in the context of the response to injury, there have been no studies of Cx43 turnover dynamics in the adult heart. Other proteins involved in intercellular adhesion have been found to turn over rapidly in subconfluent cell cultures but to turn over much more slowly once stable junctions form between confluent, contact-inhibited cells.[69] Regulated degradation of gap junction channel proteins could therefore be important in maintaining steady-state distributions intercellular connections in the normal adult heart under basal conditions, and activation of connexin proteolysis in response to injury might mediate remodeling of conduction pathways in the pathogenesis of arrhythmias.

Conclusions

Great progress has been achieved recently in understanding the biology of cardiac gap junctions. With respect to understanding their role in cardiac conduction, this progress appears to be limited mainly to a more detailed description of cardiac connexins and their distributions throughout the heart. The challenge for the future will be to determine how molecular, biophysical, and structural features of cell-to-cell communication via gap junctions contributes to the conduction properties of cardiac tissues and to elucidate the pathophysiological consequences of changes in connexin expression and gap junction number and spatial distribution in diseased myocardium. Meeting this challenge will require new approaches that combine contemporary tools of cellular and molecular biology with electrophysiology. It will also be important to develop new experimental systems that encompass the complexity of the heart but that are also amenable to genetic manipulation and electrophysiological analysis.

References

1. Beyer EC, Goodenough DA, Paul DL. Connexin family of gap junction proteins. *J Membr Biol.* 1990;116:187–194.
2. Traub O, Look J, Dermietzel R, et al. Comparative characterization of the 21-kD and 26-kD gap junction proteins in murine liver and cultured hepatocytes. *J Cell Biol.* 1989;108:1039–1051.
3. Kanter HL, Saffitz JE, Beyer EC. Cardiac myocytes express multiple gap junction proteins. *Circ Res.* 1992;70:438–444.
4. Kanter HL, Laing JG, Beyer EC, et al. Multiple connexins colocalize in canine ventricular myocyte gap junctions. *Circ Res.* 1993;73:344–350.
5. Reed KE, Westphale EM, Larson DM, et al. Molecular cloning and functional expression of human connexin37, an endothelial cell gap junction protein. *J Clin Invest.* 1993;91:997–1004.
6. Paul DL, Ebihara L, Takemoto LJ, et al. Connexin46, a novel lens gap junction protein, induces voltage-gated currents in nonjunctional plasma membrane of Xenopus oocytes. *J Cell Biol.* 1991;115:1077–1089.
7. Harfst E, Severs NJ, Green CR. Cardiac myocyte gap junctions: evidence

for a major connexon protein with an apparent relative molecular mass of 70,000. *J Cell Sci.* 1990;96:591–604.

8. Kanter HL, Laing JG, Beau SL, et al. Distinct patterns of connexin expression in canine Purkinje fibers and ventricular muscle. *Circ Res.* 1993;72: 1124–1131.

9. Gourdie RG, Severs NJ, Green CR, et al. The spatial distribution and relative abundance of gap-junctional connexin40 and connexin43 correlate to functional properties of components of the cardiac atrioventricular conduction system. *J Cell Sci.* 1993;105:985–991.

10. Davis LM, Kanter HL, Beyer EC, et al. Distinct gap junction protein phenotypes in cardiac tissues with disparate conduction properties. *J Am Coll Cardiol.* 1994;24:1124–1132.

11. Saffitz JE, Kanter HL, Green KG, et al. Tissue-specific determinants of anisotropic conduction velocity in canine atrial and ventricular myocardium. *Circ Res.* 1994;74:1065–1070.

12. Gros D, Jarry-Guichard T, Ten Velde I, et al. Restricted distribution of connexin40, a gap junctional protein, in mammalian heart. *Circ Res.* 1994; 74:839–851.

13. Bastide B, Neyses L, Ganten D, et al. Gap junction protein connexin40 is preferentially expressed in vascular endothelium and conductive bundles of rat myocardium and is increased under hypertensive conditions. *Circ Res.* 1993;73:1138–1149.

14. Chen S, Davis LM, Westphale EM, et al. Expression of multiple gap junction proteins in human fetal and infant hearts. *Pediatr Res.* 1994;36:561–566.

15. van Kempen MJ, Fromaget C, Gros D, et al. Spatial distribution of connexin43, the major cardiac gap junction protein, in the developing and adult rat heart. *Circ Res.* 1991;68:1638–1651.

16. Oosthoek PW, Viragh S, Lamers WH, et al. Immunohistochemical delineation of the conduction system, II: the atrioventricular node and the Purkinje fibers. *Circ Res.* 1993;73:482–491.

17. Oosthoek PW, Viragh S, Mayen AEM, et al. Immunohistochemical delineation of the conduction system, I: the sinoatrial node. *Circ Res.* 1993;73: 473–481.

18. Musil LS, Beyer EC, Goodenough DA. Expression of gap junction protein connexin43 in embryonic chick lens: molecular cloning, ultrastructural localization, and post-translational phosphorylation. *J Membr Biol.* 1990;116: 163–175.

19. Lau AF, Hatch Pigott V, Crow DS. Evidence that heart connexin43 is a phosphoprotein. *J Mol Cell Cardiol.* 1991;23:659–663.

20. Veenstra RD, Wang H-Z, Westphale EM, et al. Multiple properties of gap junctions in developing heart. *Circ Res.* 1992;71:1277–1283.

21. Moreno AP, Sáez JC, Fishman GI, et al. Human connexin43 gap junction channels: Regulation of unitary conductances by phosphorylation. *Circ Res.* 1994;74:1050–1057.

22. Laird DW, Puranam KL, Revel JP. Turnover and phosphorylation dynamics of connexin43 gap junction protein in cultured cardiac myocytes. *Biochem J.* 1993;273:67–72.

23. Takens Kwak BR, Jongsma HJ. Cardiac gap junctions: three distinct single channel conductances and their modulation by phosphorylating treatments. *Pflugers Arch.* 1992;422:198–200.

24. Moreno AP, Fishman GI, Spray DC. Phosphorylation shifts unitary conductance and modifies voltage dependent kinetics of human connexin43 gap junction channels. *Biophys J.* 1992;62:51–53.

25. Veenstra RD, Wang H-Z, Beblo DA, et al. Selectivity of connexin-specific gap junctions does not correlate with channel conductance. *Circ Res.* 1995; 77:1156–1165.
26. Beblo DA, Wang H-Z, Beyer EC, et al. Unique conductance, gating, and selective permeability properties of gap junction channels formed by connexin40. *Circ Res.* 1995;77:813–822.
27. Traub O, Eckert R, Lichtenberg-Fraté H, et al. Immunochemical and electrophysiological characterization of murine connexin40 and -43 in mouse tissues and transfected human cells. *Eur J Cell Biol.* 1994;64:101–112.
28. Veenstra RD, Wang H-Z, Beyer EC, et al. Selective dye and ionic permeability of gap junction channels formed by connexin45. *Circ Res.* 1994;75: 483–490.
29. Luo C, Rudy Y. A dynamic model of the cardiac ventricular action potential, I: simulations of ionic currents and concentration changes. *Circ Res.* 1994; 74:1071–1096.
30. Luo C, Rudy Y. A dynamic model of the cardiac ventricular action potential, II: afterdepolarizations, triggered activity, and potentiation. *Circ Res.* 1994; 74:1097–1113.
31. Rudy Y. Reentry: insights from theoretical simulations in a fixed pathway. *J Cardiovasc Electrophysiol.* 1995;6:115–131.
32. Zeng J, Laurita KR, Rosenbaum DS, et al. Two components of the delayed rectifier K^+ current in ventricular myocytes of the guinea pig type: theoretical formation and their role in repolarization. *Circ Res.* 1995;77:1–13.
33. Chien KR. Molecular advances in cardiovascular biology. *Science.* 1993;269: 916–917.
34. Field LJ. Transgenic mice in cardiovascular research. *Annu Rev Physiol.* 1993;55:97–114.
35. Reaume AG, de Sousa PA, Kulkarni S, et al. Cardiac malformation in neonatal mice lacking connexin43. *Science.* 1995;267:1831–1834.
36. Vink M, Fishman GI, Vieira D, et al. Properties of gap junction channels in neonatal cardiac myocytes from wild type and connexin43 knockout mice. *Circulation.* 1995;92(suppl I):I-41. Abstract.
37. Nuss HB, Marban E. Electrophysiological properties of neonatal mouse cardiac myocytes in primary culture. *J Physiol (Lond).* 1994;479:265–279.
38. Davies MP, An RH, Doevendans P, et al. Developmental changes in ionic channel activity in the embryonic murine heart. *Circ Res.* 1996;78:15–25.
39. Fast V, Kléber AG. Microscopic pattern of electrical excitation in strands of cultured rat heart cells. *Circ Res.* 1993;73:914–925.
40. Fast V, Kléber AG. Anisotropic conduction in monolayers of neonatal rat heart cells cultured on collagen substrates. *Circ Res.* 1994;75:591–595.
41. Fast V, Kléber AG. Cardiac tissue geometry as a determinant of unidirectional conduction block: assessment of microscopic excitation spread by optical mapping in patterned cell cultures and in a computer model. *Cardiovasc Res.* 1995;29:694–707.
42. Laing JG, Westphale EM, Engelmann GL, et al. Characterization of the gap junction protein connexin45. *J Membr Biol.* 1994;139:31–40.
43. Darrow BJ, Laing JG, Lampe PD, et al. Expression of multiple connexins in cultured neonatal rat ventricular myocytes. *Circ Res.* 1995;76:381–387.
44. Dhein S, Tudyka T, Schott M, et al. A new antiarrhythmic peptide improves cellular coupling: a possible new antiarrhythmic mechanism. *Circulation.* 1995;92(suppl I):I-641. Abstract.
45. Spach MS, Miller WT III, Geselowitz DB, et al. The discontinuous nature

of propagation in normal canine cardiac muscle: evidence for recurrent discontinuities of intracellular resistance that affect the membrane currents. *Circ Res.* 1981;48:39–54.

46. Pressler ML, Münster PN, Huang X. Gap junction distribution in the heart: functional relevance. In: Zipes DP, Jalife J, eds. *Cardiac Electrophysiology: From Cell to Bedside.* 2nd ed. Philadelphia, Pa: WB Saunders; 1995:144–151.

47. Trabka-Janik E, Coombs W, Lemanski LF, et al. Immunohistochemical localization of gap junction protein channels in hamster sinoatrial node in correlation with electrophysiologic mapping of the pacemaker region. *J Cardiovasc Electrophysiol.* 1994;5:125–137.

48. Opthof T. Gap junctions in the sinoatrial node: immunohistochemical localization and correlation with activation pattern. *J Cardiovasc Electrophysiol.* 1994;5:138–143.

49. Peters NS, Severs NJ, et al. Spatiotemporal relation between gap junctions and fascia adherens junctions during postnatal development of human ventricular myocardium. *Circulation.* 1994;90:713–725.

50. Smith JH, Green CR, Peters NS, et al. Altered patterns of gap junction distribution in ischemic heart disease. *Am J Pathol.* 1991;139:801–821.

51. Komuro I, Kaida T, Shibazaki Y, et al. Stretching cardiac myocytes stimulates protooncogene expression. *J Biol Chem.* 1990;265:3595–3598.

52. Komuro I, Katoh Y, Kaida T, et al. Mechanical loading stimulates cell hypertrophy and specific gene expression in cultured rat cardiac myocytes. *J Biol Chem.* 1991;266:1265–1268.

53. Sosinsky G. Mixing of connexins in gap junction membrane channels. *Proc Natl Acad Sci U S A.* 1995;92:9210–9214.

54. Bruzzone R, Haefliger JA, Gimlich RL, et al. Connexin40, a component of gap junctions in vascular endothelium, is restricted in its ability to interact with other connexins. *Mol Biol Cell.* 1993;4:7–20.

55. Britz-Cunningham SH, Shah MM, Zuppan CW, et al. Mutations of the connexin43 gap junction gene in patients with heart malformations and defects of laterality. *N Engl J Med.* 1995;332:1323–1329.

56. Kléber AG, Fleischauer J, Cascio WE. Ischemia-induced propagation failure in the heart. In: Zipes DP, Jalife J, eds. *Cardiac Electrophysiology: From Cell to Bedside.* 2nd ed. Philadelphia, Pa: WB Saunders; 1995:174–182.

57. Noma A, Tsuboi N. Dependence of junctional conductance on proton, calcium and magnesium ions in cardiac paired cells of guinea pigs. *J Physiol (Lond).* 1987;282:193–211.

58. Wu J, McHowat J, Saffitz JE, et al. Inhibition of gap junctional conductance by long-chain acylcarnitines and their preferential accumulation in junctional sarcolemma during hypoxia. *Circ Res.* 1993;72:879–889.

59. Luke RA, Saffitz JE. Remodeling of ventricular conduction pathways in healed canine infarct border zones. *J Clin Invest.* 1991;87:1594–1602.

60. Severs NJ. Pathophysiology of gap junctions in heart diseases. *J Cardiovasc Electrophysiol.* 1994;5:462–475.

61. Peters NS, Green CR, Poole-Wilson PA, et al. Reduced content of connexin43 gap junctions in ventricular myocardium from hypertrophied and ischemic hearts. *Circulation.* 1993;88:864–875.

62. Campos De Carvalho AC, Tanowitz HB, Wittner M, et al. Trypanasoma infection decreases intercellular communication between cardiac myocytes. *Prog Cell Res.* 1993;3:193–197.

63. Janse MJ, Wit AL. Electrophysiological mechanisms of ventricular arrhythmias resulting from myocardial ischemia and infarction. *Physiol Rev.* 1989; 69:1049–1069.

64. de Bakker MJT, van Capelle FJL, Janse MJ, et al. Slow conduction in the infarcted human heart: "zigzag" course of activation. *Circulation.* 1993;88: 915–926.
65. Dillon SM, Allessie MA, Ursell PC, et al. Influences of anisotropic tissue structure on reentrant circuits in the epicardial border zone of subacute canine infarcts. *Circ Res.* 1988;63:182–206.
66. Maes A, Flameng W, Nuyts J, et al. Histological alterations in chronically hypoperfused myocardium: correlation with PET findings. *Circulation.* 1994;90:735–745.
67. Ausma J, Schaart G, Thoné F, et al. Chronic ischemic viable myocardium in man: aspects of dedifferentiation. *Cardiovasc Pathol.* 1995;4:29–37.
68. Laing JG, Beyer EC. The gap junction protein connexin43 is degraded via the ubiquitin proteasome pathway. *J Biol Chem.* 1995;270:26399–26403.
69. Pasdar M, Nelson WJ. Kinetics of desmosome assembly in Madin-Darby canine kidney epithelial cells: temporal and spatial regulation of desmoplakin organization and stabilization upon cell-cell contact. *J Cell Biol.* 1988;106:687–695.

Role of Discontinuous Electrical Propagation in Clinical Atrial Arrhythmias:
Current Evidence and Future Directions

Michael D. Lesh, MD,
Jonathan M. Kalman, MBBS, PhD,
Jeffrey E. Olgin, MD,
and Willard S. Ellis, PhD

A substantial body of basic electrophysiological research supports the notion that discontinuous propagation due to nonuniform anisotropic coupling is an essential aspect of cardiac impulse propagation and plays an important role in arrhythmogenesis. Such evidence derives from a variety of sources, including electrographic measurements from isolated myocardium studied in baths with intracellular and extracellular microelectrodes[1,2]; multielement electrode mapping arrays of various sizes and densities[3-5]; optical mapping techniques[6,7]; histological analysis of normal and diseased myocardium, with or without direct electrophysiological correlates, including the recent capability of characterizing the structural and molecular features of intercellular coupling[2,8-11]; and corroborative theoretical work in computer models.[12-19]

Despite this extensive basic scientific foundation, only recently have we begun to apply this knowledge base to search for the "footprints" of discontinuous propagation in clinical tachyarrhythmias. Such "footprints" might include the recording of fractionated elec-

From: Spooner PM, Joyner RW, Jalife J (eds). *Discontinuous Conduction in the Heart.* Armonk, NY: Futura Publishing Company, Inc.; © 1997.

trograms indicating conduction through nonuniformly anisotropic myocardium.[13,20] Split potentials indicating conduction around a line of block also may indicate the presence of discontinuous propagation. In this chapter, we focus on the role of discontinuous propagation in a variety of clinical atrial tachycardias and review some of the evidence that can be derived from the clinical electrophysiological laboratory that discontinuous propagation is an essential feature in most, if not all, atrial tachyarrhythmias in humans. In particular, we discuss the role of the crista terminalis (CT) in the genesis of right atrial focal and reentrant tachyarrhythmias.

Our hypothesis is that much of what would appear to be functional electrophysiological properties of the atrium actually derives from anatomic structure. That is, the issue of whether atrial arrhythmias arise from alterations in functional electrical properties or from fixed anatomic abnormalities ("fixed versus functional" origin of atrial arrhythmias) represents a false dichotomy: spatial dispersion of functional properties such as conduction and refractoriness most likely derives from and is linked to fixed anatomic structure, either one normally present or an acquired abnormality.

Tools From Assessing Discontinuous Propagation in the Clinical Setting

Many of the tools readily available to the basic electrophysiologist (correlation of high-density and microelectrode recordings with histology, etc) have been unavailable to the clinician-scientist during transvascular catheter-based clinical electrophysiological testing. Although operative mapping in patients undergoing open-chest surgery has been useful, its application to the large number of patients with disparate arrhythmia mechanisms is obviously quite limited. However, several factors and techniques are converging that encourage a greater understanding of atrial arrhythmia mechanisms and the role of discontinuous propagation therein. For example, improved capabilities of digital clinical mapping systems has allowed many more recording electrodes in patients undergoing testing in the clinical electrophysiology laboratory. Also, the fact that transcatheter radiofrequency ablation is in many cases curative[21–25] has brought an increasing number of patients who would not previously have undergone electrophysiology testing to the laboratory for invasive mapping. Finally, in our laboratory we have explored the novel use of intracardiac echocardiography (ICE) as an adjunct to standard fluoroscopy to relate endocardial anatomic structures to electrophysiological properties of the atrium.[26–28]

As generally practiced, electrode catheter positioning during clinical electrophysiological studies is guided by fluoroscopy, and target sites for ablation are based on an analysis of intracardiac electrograms. However, there are limitations to the use of fluoroscopy, especially if one desires to relate anatomic structure to electrophysiological function, including failure to identify detailed features of the endocardium and the relationship between a recording catheter and specific endocardial features. Also, contact between the ablation electrode and the endocardium and lesion formation cannot be directly assessed with fluoroscopy.

The imaging system in use in our laboratory is composed of a 10-MHz ultrasound transducer mounted on the tip of a 10F, 120-cm-long, over-the-wire catheter (CVIS, Cardiovascular Imaging Systems). The original purpose of this catheter was for intravascular imaging, but we have adapted it for use in the heart. The outer diameter of the catheter is 0.333 cm, and it is passed through a 10F intravascular sheath with an internal diameter of 0.345 cm. At a focal depth of 4 cm, the axial resolution of the system is 450 μm and the lateral resolution is 750 μm. The imaging plane is orthogonal to the catheter, with a radial field of view of ≈4 cm. Images are acquired at 28 frames per second and recorded on a super VHS videotape for review. The type of imaging we can obtain is demonstrated in Figure 1. There are a number of limitations to current ICE technology, such as limited penetration to the left side of the heart and the lack of steerability and tip deflection, which limits what can be seen. It is hoped that future improved generations of this technology will allow greater resolution of anatomic detail over a larger portion of the heart.

Role of the Crista Terminalis in Atrial Tachycardias

One structure easily visualized via ICE is the CT. Because of its unique electrophysiological properties, we hypothesized that the CT plays a pivotal role in many arrhythmias arising from the right atrium. The CT can be thought of as the "AV node of the atrium." For example, just as the AV node contains relatively poor cell-to-cell coupling,[29,30] Saffitz et al[9] demonstrated the markedly anisotropic cell-to-cell coupling that occurs across the CT. In addition, the CT contains cells with a propensity for spontaneous automaticity, just as the AV node does. The CT is the site of the sinus node complex,[31] which is a distributed group of cells running a variable length along the CT. It is likely, in fact, that both the CT and the AV node have the same embryological origin. Indeed, it is probably not coincidental that the site of the sinus pacemaker complex is also a region of poor cell-to-cell coupling. As

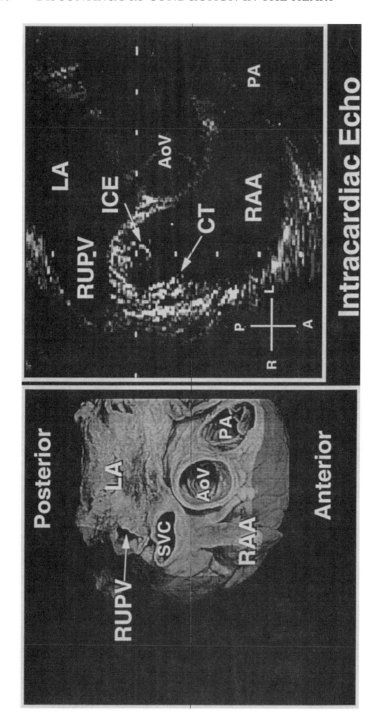

Joyner and van Capelle[32] showed, using numerical simulations of electrically coupled cells, for the relatively small sinoatrial node to be spontaneously automatic and yet be sufficiently electrically coupled to the surrounding quiescent atrial cells to initiate action potential propagation requires some degree of electrical uncoupling of the cells within the normal sinoatrial-atrial system. It follows that such uncoupling is likely to be important for the firing of cells with abnormal automaticity (ectopic atrial tachycardia foci) as well.

Role of Discontinuous Propagation in Human Atrial Flutter

Atrial flutter is an arrhythmia that has interested electrophysiologists for much of this century. A reentrant mechanism was postulated from the careful studies of Lewis et al[33] in the 1920s. Studies in animal models implicated the critical role of macroscopic barriers to delineate the circuit boundaries. For example, Rosenblueth and Garcia-Ramos[34] developed a canine model of atrial flutter by creating a crush lesion between the orifices of the venae cavae. When the lesion was extended over the free wall to the tricuspid annulus, the tachycardia terminated. Although these data suggest that the tachycardia was due to reentry set up by these artificial obstacles, careful mapping was not performed, and the precise barriers around which the circus movement occurred were not defined. Frame et al[35,36] used a similar model of atrial flutter with a Y-shaped lesion in the right atrium between the venae cavae and a connecting lesion extending toward the appendage. Interestingly, careful mapping revealed that reentry occurred around the tricuspid annulus and not around the lesion itself. The Y-shaped lesion served as a posterior discontinuity, protecting the tissue between the lesion and the tricuspid annulus from being excited, or "short circuited," from an inferiorly spreading wave front. These studies demonstrate the im-

Figure 1. Example of transcatheter intracardiac ultrasound imaging. Left, Anatomic specimen of heart viewed from above. Right, Intracardiac echo (ICE) image, a two-dimensional transaxial plane perpendicular to shaft of imaging catheter, which runs along intercaval axis in this case. Structures seen at this level include right upper pulmonary vein (RUPV) entering left atrium (LA); right atrial appendage (RAA) separated from posterior smooth-walled right atrium by crista terminalis (CT), noted as a prominent ridge extending from endocardial surface; aortic valve (AoV); and pulmonary artery (PA). In most patients, CT can be seen along length of right atrium, from superomedial to inferolateral, allowing placement of mapping catheters directly on or near CT for assessment of its electrophysiological properties in patients in electrophysiology laboratory.

portance of not one but two barriers for reentry to occur, with a second barrier to "protect" atrial tissue from short-circuit excitation by the reentrant wave front traveling around the first, as reviewed by Boyden.[37]

Initial studies using multisite endocardial mapping in patients with atrial flutter confirmed macroreentry in the right atrium, with the septal wall activated in the inferior-to-superior direction, while the free wall is activated superior-to-inferior.[38–42] Although in these studies an area of "slow conduction" was identified between the triscuspid annulus and the coronary sinus ostium and inferior vena cava, which encouraged the subsequent development of a curative ablative technique by creating a lesion across the floor of the right atrium,[22,23,42] the barrier (or barriers) accounting for the disparate activation patterns of the septum and free wall were not addressed. In addition, these mapping studies did not relate the circuit to right atrial endocardial anatomy, which was difficult because, as noted above, fluoroscopy does not allow resolution of endocardial detail.

Recently, using carefully targeted multisite endocardial activation mapping guided to 1-mm accuracy by ICE, we tested the hypothesis that the posterior barrier in human atrial flutter is formed by the crista terminalis and its inferior continuation as the eustachian ridge. Thus, the trabeculated right atrium in typical human flutter is activated in the superior-to-inferior direction, while the smooth-walled right atrium (septum) posterior to these structures is activated inferior-to-superior.[28] Evidence for discontinuous propagation at the CT and eustachian ridge included (1) disparate activation times on either side of the CT and eustachian ridge during flutter; (2) entrainment techniques showing sites just anterior to these structures to be within the critical reentrant path (the first postpacing interval at the site from which entrainment pacing was tested nearly equal to the tachycardia cycle length) and sites just posterior to be out of the circuit (the first postpacing interval at the site of entrainment pacing much longer than the tachycardia cycle length); and (3) the fact that ICE, with a multipolar catheter placed directly on the CT, recorded split potentials along the entire length of the CT and eustachian ridge as wave fronts traveled in opposite directions. A set of recordings showing the split potentials along the CT and eustachian ridge is demonstrated in Figure 2.

One might ask whether the observed split potentials are the result of fixed block versus block that develops as a functional consequence of the rapid rates during flutter. On recordings made during sinus rhythm in which activation originates at the superior aspect of the CT and propagates inferiorly, split potentials on the CT are not seen. However, if one paces from the low septum, even at slow rates, in patients with clinical atrial flutter the split potentials clearly emerge, as illus-

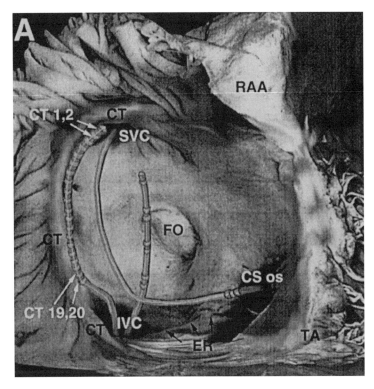

Figure 2. A, Diagram showing catheter placement in relation to right atrial anatomic structures. Idealized depiction of right atrial endocardium is viewed anterior to posterior through a reflected anterior wall. A 20-pole catheter inserted through femoral vein lies along length of crista terminalis (CT). Poles 1 and 2 are at superior margin of CT (CT 1,2), and poles 19 and 20 at inferior margin (CT 19,20) for reference to subsequent intracardiac recordings. Also shown are an octapolar catheter along interatrial septum and decapolar catheter inserted through internal jugular vein, which lies inside coronary sinus. Intracardiac echo catheter and roving catheter are not shown. RAA indicates right atrial appendage; SVC, superior vena cava; IVC, inferior vena cava; FO, fossa ovalis; ER, eustachian ridge along floor of right atrium (arrows); TA, tricuspid annulus; and CS os, coronary sinus ostium.

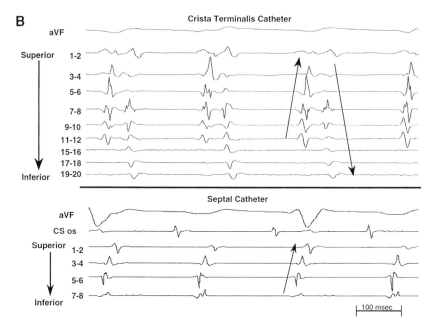

Figure 2. *(continued)* B, Electrograms from catheter lying along CT (top) and along septum (bottom). Poles 1–2 are most distal (superior) electrode pairs. Split potentials, indicative of discontinuous propagation, are recorded along length of CT, a finding characteristic of all patients with typical atrial flutter. Early component has a characteristic proximal-to-distal (low-to-high) activation sequence, and the late component has a distal-to-proximal (high-to-low) sequence. Bottom, Septal catheter is activated with a proximal-to-distal (low-to-high) sequence, and no split components are in evidence.

trated in Figure 3. This suggests that the transverse uncoupling across the CT indeed represents fixed conduction block, with the demonstration of split electrograms over the CT simply dependent on the direction in which a propagating wave front interacts with the CT.

Thus, split potentials are one type of "footprint" of discontinuous propagation that can be sought in clinical studies. The concept that the direction of wave-front propagation with respect to a zone or line of anatomic weakness (the CT or eustachian ridge in this case) determines whether split potentials will be manifest on extracellular electrogram recordings is illustrated in Figure 4. Note that the line of absent transverse coupling, such as might represent the CT or other analogous cardiac structure, causes the footprint of discontinuous conduction to be manifest only under specific circumstances, propagation perpendicular to the anatomic obstacle in this case. But this is not to say that the line of block is in any way "functional," though it is this sort of

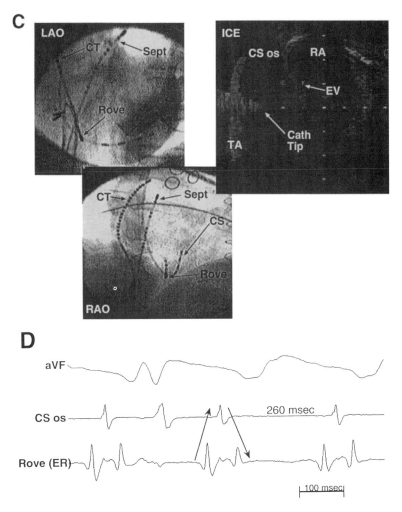

Figure 2. *(continued)* C, LAO and RAO fluoroscopic and intracardiac echo (ICE) images demonstrating position of catheters during a typical study in which ICE was used to correlate anatomy with electrophysiological function during atrial flutter. ICE images are single freeze frames. Catheters along CT, septum (Sept), and in CS are labeled in fluoroscopic images. Position of the rove catheter, which casts a characteristic fan-shaped artifact on ICE, is seen adjacent to eustachian ridge, between it and TA. LAO indicates left anterior oblique; RAO, right anterior oblique; Rove, roving/mapping catheter; LA, left atrium; RA, right atrium; and EV, eustachian valve. D, Electrograms recorded from CS os and roving catheter just anterior to eustachian ridge in a patient with atrial flutter. Split potentials indicative of discontinuous conduction are present at eustachian ridge, which, along with CT, is a continuous line of block during typical atrial flutter in humans. Modified with permission from Reference 28.

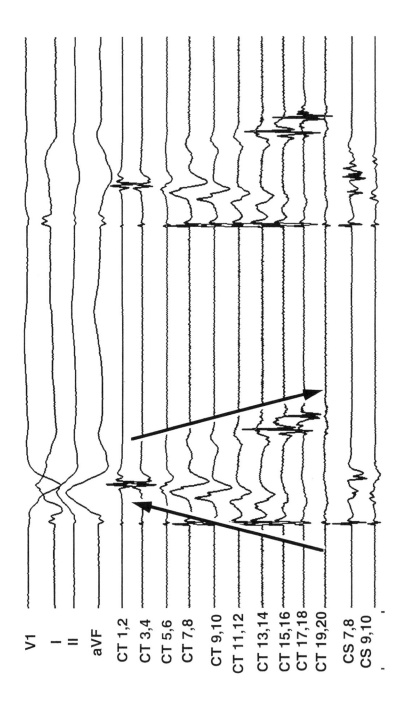

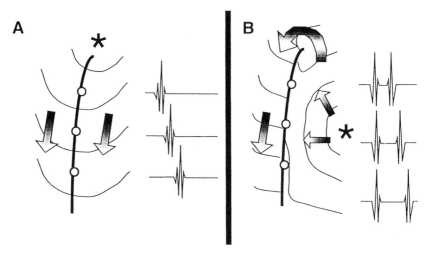

Figure 4. Given a zone or line of "anatomic weakness" (such as transverse uncoupling along crista), whether split potentials will be recorded depends on direction of wave-front propagation relative to that anatomic line. A drawing of atrium with such a line and isochronal activation contours is shown. Three simulated recording sites are shown directly along line of transverse uncoupling (open circles) along with corresponding electrograms on right of each panel. A, Propagation is parallel to line of transverse uncoupling (broad arrows), so split electrograms are not observed. B, Propagation is perpendicular to line of transverse uncoupling and split potentials are recorded because of disparate activation on either side of line of block. This paradigm explains why split potentials are not usually recorded during normal sinus rhythm in patients with a propensity for atrial flutter but are in evidence during flutter itself or pacing from low septum.

Figure 3. Surface leads and intracardiac electrograms from a 20-pole catheter on crista terminalis (CT) in a patient with atrial flutter, but during pacing from low septum at a slow rate. Note that split potentials, indicative of discontinuous propagation, are present along CT in same fashion as during atrial flutter (Figure 2B). This provides evidence that block (or very slow conduction) for wave fronts propagating transverse to CT is fixed and does not require rapid rates for its development. Fixed CT (and eustachian ridge) block may be what distinguishes those with substrate for atrial flutter from those without it, whether that block is congenital or acquired due to atrial disease and stretch.

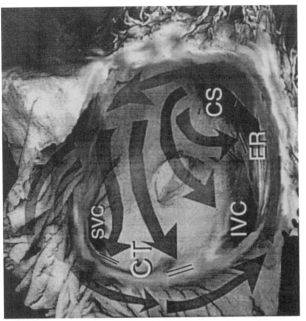

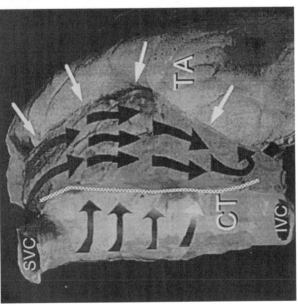

Figure 5. Diagram showing proposed circuit in human type I atrial flutter. Right, View of right atrial epicardial surface in a right posterior oblique view; left, idealized depiction of right atrial endocardium viewed anterior to posterior through a reflected anterior wall. Arrows represent atrial activation sequence during counterclockwise atrial flutter. Lines of block are marked with double lines. Two barriers are required to define a reentrant loop. Anterior barrier consists of the tricuspid annulus (TA), and posterior border is crista terminalis (CT) (sulcus terminalis, shown as a dotted line, on epicardial surface) and its extension beyond inferior vena cava (IVC) as eustachian ridge (ER). Thus, wave front is quite broad in anterior and lateral extent, comprising entire width of trabeculated right atrial free wall. It then becomes constrained to a relatively narrow isthmus in low right atrium bounded anteriorly by tricuspid valve and posteriorly by IVC, eustachian ridge, and coronary sinus ostium (CS). After emerging from low right atrium, wave front ascends septum.

circumstance that has in the past, perhaps, given rise to the false dichotomy of "fixed" versus "functional" discontinuous propagation. Fixed cell-to-cell uncoupling can be linked to an anatomic structure, yet its manifestation on recorded electrophysiological data is present only under a restricted set of circumstances.

It is our belief that what separates patients with atrial flutter—a third to a half of whom have no overt evidence of structural heart disease—from those without atrial flutter is either congenital or acquired complete transverse uncoupling along the entire length of the CT and the eustachian ridge. In other words, even in normal individuals, the CT has poor transverse coupling. It is most likely an exaggeration of this normal anisotropy that provides the structural substrate for typical atrial flutter. The precise location of the region of the CT at which this uncoupling exists cannot be resolved by our current catheter-based technology, but we suspect that it occurs at the junction where the thin-walled posterior atrium (sinus venosus descendent) joins the thicker CT such that the impedance mismatch resulting from discontinuity in the source-sink relationship at the thin-thick interface adds to the poor transverse coupling of the CT itself.

With the role of the CT and eustachian ridge now elucidated, we can express the geometry of the flutter reentrant wave front on the basis of the barriers that define it, as illustrated in Figure 5. As Boyden noted, two barriers are required to define a reentrant loop. In the case of typical atrial flutter, the anterior barrier consists of the tricuspid annulus[43] (exactly as in the canine model of Frame et al[35,36]), and the posterior border is the CT and its extension beyond the inferior vena cava as the eustachian ridge. Thus, the wave front is quite broad in its anterior and lateral extent, comprising the entire width of the trabeculated right atrial free wall. It then becomes constrained to a relatively narrow isthmus in the low right atrium bounded anteriorly by the tricuspid valve and posteriorly by the inferior vena cava, eustachian ridge, and coronary sinus ostium. After emerging from the low right atrium, the wave front emerges to ascend the septum. It is the block along the length of the CT that prevents this wave front from prematurely invading the trabeculated right atrium and "short-circuiting" the reentrant wave. Although any lesion that transsected the circuit from one fixed barrier to another would be curative, it is the relative narrowness of the low right atrial isthmus that allows atrial flutter to be cured by a transcatheter radiofrequency ablative lesion that severs the isthmus from annulus to inferior vena cava.

Although classic, typical atrial flutter rotates in a counterclockwise direction in the frontal plane, there is nothing sacrosanct about this direction of rotation, and most patients with typical atrial flutter can have atrial flutter induced in the electrophysiology laboratory that rotates in the clockwise direction.[44] Interestingly, the clockwise and counterclockwise flutters in a given patient have cycle lengths generally within 10 ms of each other and split potentials along the length of the CT and eustachian ridge in both. Thus, the role of discontinuous propagation is the same in both the counterclockwise and clockwise forms of "typical" atrial flutter.

Patients may also have a more rapid "atrial flutter," which we call "true atypical" flutter. This atypical form of atrial flutter does not use

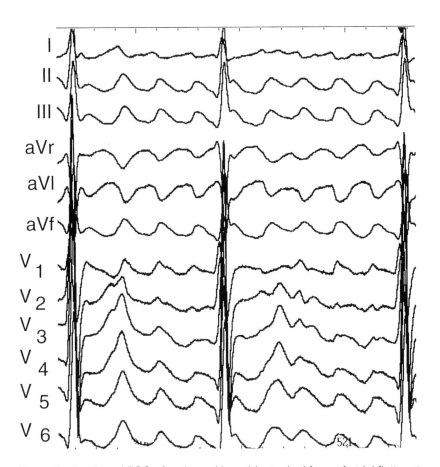

Figure 6. A, 12-lead ECG of patient with rapid, atypical form of atrial flutter at cycle length of 200 ms. B, Surface and intracardiac recordings of same patient with atypical atrial flutter. Split potentials are recorded over only approximately top half of crista terminalis (CT). While entire circuit in these rapid atypical flutters has not been delineated, a reasonable hypothesis is that discontinuous conduction over only a portion of CT might result in a rapid "circum-cristal" reentry.

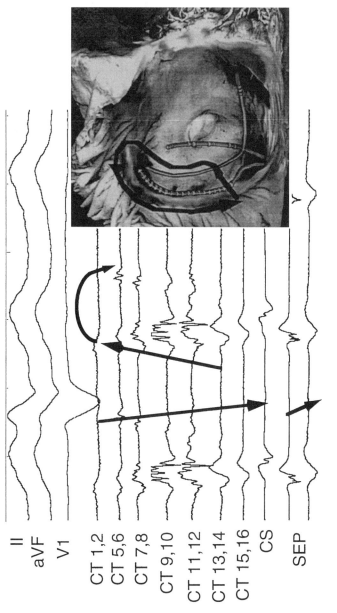

Figure 6. *(continued)*

the low right atrial isthmus. Figure 6 illustrates a patient with atypical flutter at a cycle length of 200 ms. Activation and entrainment mapping excluded a typical form of flutter. In this case, however, it appeared that only a portion of the anisotropic CT served as a pivotal line of block, as evidenced by the presence of split potentials extending only along the top several poles of a catheter placed along the CT under ICE guidance (Figure 6B). These true atypical flutters require better characterization in larger cohorts of patients, but it seems logical that discontinuous propagation, probably linked to anatomic structure but with lines of block that may be partly functional and developing only at rapid rates, helps to establish the substrate for these rapid reentrant waves, which in turn may have implications for therapy with radiofre-quency ablation. Other likely sites of discontinuous propagation that may have a role as the substrate for these types of unusual flutters include the fossa ovalis, the pulmonary vein ostia, and the coronary sinus ostium. These rapid, atypical atrial flutters may be a transitional rhythm between typical flutter and atrial fibrillation.

Role of Discontinuous Propagation in Focal Atrial Tachycardias

Another class of atrial arrhythmias have a focal origin. Although one can debate whether these "focal tachycardias" are initiated by trig-gering or phase 4 automaticity or even microreentry,[45] this debate has not addressed how the large bulk of surrounding myocardium would be prevented from electrotonically inhibiting the firing of this small focus of automaticity. We hypothesized that the relatively poor coup-ling of the CT would serve as the required substrate because not only does it contain cells with automatic properties, but the CT would also prevent electrotonic extinction of those foci. This concept is illustrated in Figure 7. A cell or small cluster of cells with a tendency toward abnormal automaticity (or triggering or microreentry) well coupled to surrounding normal atrium (Figure 7, left panel) will not be able to manifest that tendency because of electrotonic interactions. However, if the region of abnormal automaticity is in a region of poor cell-to-cell coupling (Figure 7, right panel), discontinuous propagation may allow these cells to manifest their abnormal firing. As long as the coupling is not so poor that no impulse may exit, a tachycardia can be initiated. In this case, the "footprint" of discontinuous propagation during clinical electrophysiological mapping will be fractionated electrograms, repre-senting slow conduction through poorly coupled tissue, recorded from the site of origin of the tachycardia and preceding the onset of the surface P wave, when the bulk of the normal surrounding atrium is

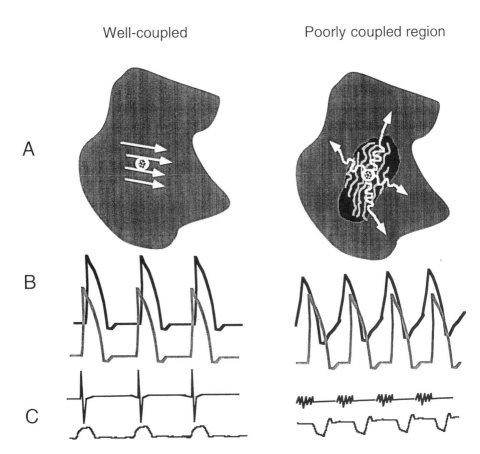

Figure 7. A-C, Illustration of concept that regardless of cellular mechanism of focal tachycardia (automaticity, triggering, microreentry), relatively poor coupling of that focus to surrounding atrium is required to prevent electrotonic extinction of such a focus. A, Drawings of atrial tissue containing a focus with a tendency toward abnormal firing. B, Simulated action potential recordings, with black tracing from abnormal focus and gray tracing from normal surrounding atrium. C, Bipolar electrogram that might be recorded from a catheter straddling central focus and surrounding atrium and corresponding simulated surface ECG P wave. A cell or small cluster of cells with a tendency toward abnormal automaticity well coupled to surrounding normal atrium (gray, A, left) will not be able to manifest that tendency due to electrotonic interactions. However, if region of abnormal automaticity is in a region of poor cell-to-cell coupling (right, black region of drawing in A), discontinuous propagation may allow these cells to manifest abnormal firing. As long as coupling is not so poor that no impulse may exit, a tachycardia can be initiated. In this case, "footprint" of discontinuous propagation during clinical electrophysiological mapping will be fractionated electrograms (C, right) representing slow conduction through poorly coupled tissue, recorded from site of origin of tachycardia and preceding onset of surface P wave, when bulk of normal surrounding atrium is finally activated, by a substantial period of time.

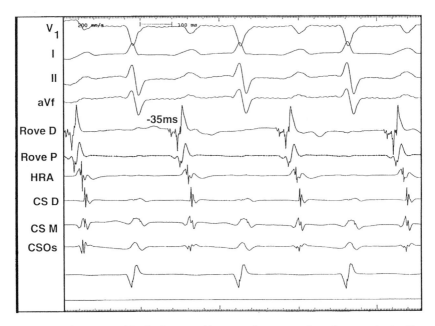

Figure 7. *(continued)* D, Surface and intracardiac recordings from patient with focal atrial tachycardia confirmed by intracardiac echo to be arising from superolateral crista terminalis. Recording from site of origin (and successful ablation) (Rove) shows a fractionated electrogram preceding onset of surface P wave by 35 ms, indicative of slow, discontinuous propagation through a region of poor coupling.

finally activated, by a substantial period of time. Indeed, using ICE-guided mapping, we have found that 14 of 18 focal right atrial tachycardias studied arose directly from the some part of the CT.[46] In addition, markedly fractionated electrograms, indicative of conduction through poorly coupled tissue, were recorded in almost all cases and preceded the onset of the surface P wave by ≥50 ms. Thus, regardless of the initiating factor, discontinuous propagation plays an essential role in focal atrial tachycardias.

Role of Discontinuous Propagation in Atrial Fibrillation

The most common atrial arrhythmia is atrial fibrillation. It is also the least well-characterized atrial arrhythmia, despite many years of elegant studies in animal models and in humans undergoing open-chest surgery. It is likely that with further study in the electrophysiology laboratory of patients with atrial fibrillation, we will come to recognize atrial fibrillation as not one disease but rather a common manifestation of several different tachycardia mechanisms. For example, given that atrial tachycardias may have a focal origin along the CT, it would not be surprising if some patients, particularly those who are young and without significant structural heart disease, may have a rapidly firing focal tachycardia that the rest of the atrium cannot track in a one-to-one ratio, thus giving the appearance of atrial fibrillation. We have seen several such patients in our laboratory, who have had their atrial fibrillation cured with a focal radiofrequency ablative lesion. In the same way that nonuniform anisotropic cell-to-cell coupling "allows" ectopic atrial tachycardia to fire without electrotonic extinction from surrounding atrium, so too might a very rapid atrial focus require uncoupling to prevent its inhibition. Indeed, poor coupling surrounding a focus of rapid automaticity may cause "fibrillatory" exit from this focus. Furthermore, even if atrial fibrillation occurs by multiple wavelets of reentry, which is thought to be the more common mechanism for "steady-state" fibrillation,[47–49] the premature beats that initiate tachycardia might well derive from foci of automaticity in regions of poor cell-to-cell coupling. The mode of initiation of atrial fibrillation requires much further study.

The incidence of focal automaticity leading to atrial fibrillation in the total population of patients with atrial fibrillation is unknown. Another potential mechanism of atrial fibrillation is rapid reentry around regions of relatively poor coupling. That is, lines of block (discontinuous propagation) may well develop at regions of relative anatomic weakness, again discounting the notion that fixed anatomic structure and functional electrophysiological properties are mutually exclusive. However, unlike atrial flutter, in which the reentrant circuit remains constant, atrial fibrillation might develop if these reentrant waves wandered to some extent around the atrium or if a "mother wavelet" remained stable but the rest of the atrium were not able to follow in a one-to-one ratio. Because of its poor transverse coupling, the CT again becomes a candidate for the pivot line around which a rapid reentrant wave (stable or unstable) might circulate. If the CT acted as the anatomic substrate for a line of functional block, then the "footprint" of decremental discontinuous propagation might appear as hypothesized in Figure 8. During pacing perpendicular to the CT, long coupled beats would pass without much delay past the CT, giving rise to relatively normal electrograms (Figure 8A). However, one might expect that premature beats would exhibit delay as they encountered the CT because of its poor transverse coupling, and split potentials would develop dynamically (Figure 8B). If the CT exhibits decremental conduction (analogous to the decremental conduction seen in the AV

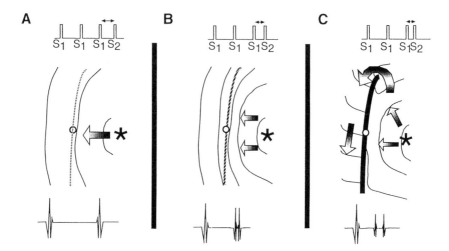

Figure 8. See Figure 4 for nomenclature. Illustration here of an anatomically based line of functional discontinuous propagation, such as might occur along crista terminalis in some cases. During pacing perpendicular to line of anatomic weakness, long coupled beats (S_1S_2, top) would pass without much delay across crista, giving rise to relatively normal electrograms (A). However, one might expect that premature beats would exhibit delay as they encountered line of anatomic weakness if it possessed poor transverse coupling, and split potentials would develop dynamically (B). More tightly coupled premature beats would result in split potentials with greater separation of two components (C) and even development of true conduction block.

node), then more tightly coupled premature beats would result in split potentials with greater separation of the two components (Figure 8C). Finally, if an early enough premature beat arrives at the CT, then micro-reentry could occur around the resulting line of block, and the split components would be even more widely separated.

We have found this situation in some patients, undergoing study in the electrophysiology laboratory, as illustrated in Figure 9. In the example shown, there appeared to be decremental conduction across the CT in response to premature beats, with the degree of decrement, and hence the separation of the two components of the split potentials recorded from the CT, inversely proportional to the coupling interval of the premature beat (Figure 9A and 9B). Finally, at the shortest coupling interval (Figure 9C), sustained atrial fibrillation results. This is perhaps a direct in vivo example of the phenomenon documented by Spach et al[50] using in vitro, fine-scale mapping in human atrial trabeculae. In young, uniformly anisotropic atrial bundles, Spach found that propagation of progressively earlier premature beats continued as a smooth process until propagation ceased simultaneously in all directions. In older, nonuniformly anisotropic bundles, premature beats produced either unidirectional block or a zigzag of longitudinal conduction with induction of microreentry.

The example shown in Figure 9 is not to say that the CT is the only structure around which a microreentrant wave might develop, leading to atrial fibrillation. Rather, it is an example of the type of anatomic structure that could give rise to an adequate degree of discontinuous propagation to support such microreentry, and it is likely that other regions of normal or diseased atria would exhibit the requisite discontinuous propagation as well. Future research will need to focus on other atrial regions, such as the ostia of the pulmonary veins or the fossa ovalis and tendon of Todaro, which might provide the substrate of discontinuous propagation leading to the initiating substrate for atrial fibrillation.

A

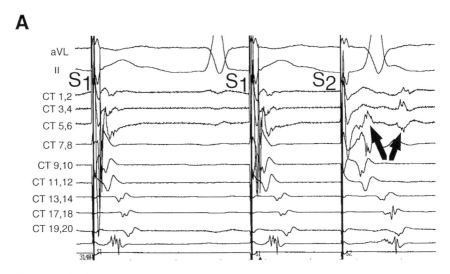

Figure 9. Surface leads I and aVL, along with intracardiac electrograms from a 20-pole catheter positioned precisely along crista terminalis (CT) under intra-cardiac echo guidance from patient with paroxysmal atrial fibrillation. Pacing from high right atrium is present (S_1), with premature beats (S_2) introduced at progressively shorter coupling intervals (numbers labeled in ms). B, Just S_2 beat is shown; C, last beat of an eight-beat basic drive (S_1) and the premature beat (S_2) is shown. There appears to be decremental conduction across crista in response to premature beats, with degree of decrement, and hence separation of two components of split potentials (arrows in A) recorded from crista, inversely proportional to coupling interval of premature beat (A and B). Finally, at shortest coupling interval (C), sustained atrial fibrillation results.

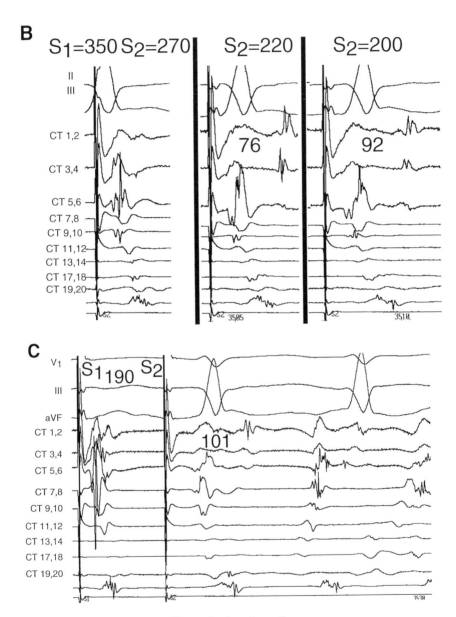

Figure 9. *(continued)*

Summary

Ultimately, one might theorize (see Figure 10) that all atrial arrhythmias require discontinuous propagation and that it is the "size
scale" of the heterogeneity of cell-to-cell coupling that varies among
arrhythmia types. Thus, discontinuous propagation on the size scale
of the entire CT and eustachian valve is the substrate for typical macroreentrant atrial flutter, and a smaller macroreentrant circuit using only
a portion of the CT yields rapid, atypical atrial flutter. When the size
of the region of discontinuous propagation becomes small enough, the
single macroreentrant circuit becomes somewhat unstable and coarse
"fib/flutter" results, often with brief paroxysms that self-terminate. As
the size scale of discontinuous propagation becomes smaller still, and
perhaps more diffuse,[51] coarse and ultimately fine (chronic) atrial fibrillation would result. A similar paradigm has been elegantly proposed
by Spach and Josephson[29] to explain how reentry due to nonuniform
anisotropy can occur in a structure as small as the AV node.

In summary, data such as split potentials and fractionated electrograms from carefully positioned intracardiac electrode catheters
combined with the use of ICE to correlate anatomy with electrophysiology have revealed considerable direct and indirect evidence for the
critical role of discontinuous propagation in patients with clinical atrial
arrhythmias.

Future studies will benefit from the development of even more
advanced technologies for correlating functional anatomy with electrophysiology. Such tools might include in vivo use of fluorescent dyes
that label connexons to assess, via transvascular catheters, the actual
distribution of cell-to-cell connections. Advances in electrographic tech-

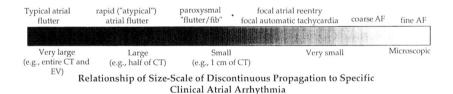

**Relationship of Size-Scale of Discontinuous Propagation to Specific
Clinical Atrial Arrhythmia**

Figure 10. Illustration of unifying paradigm through which size scale, or degree, of discontinuous propagation is matched to arrhythmia that results. At a
very large size scale, typical atrial flutter results when uncoupling extends along
entire crista terminalis (CT) and eustachian ridge. Atypical flutter might result
when discontinuous propagation occurs over only a portion of CT. Ultimately,
very fine atrial fibrillation (AF) results at end stage of atrial disease when size
scale of cell-to-cell uncoupling is at a cellular level and occurs diffusely throughout atrium. EV, eustachian valve.

niques such as statistical signal processing will be needed to identify the role of nonuniform anisotropy in atrial fibrillation in which wandering wavelets are likely to be "anchored" or to "stream" on the basis of structural anisotropy and barriers. Perhaps some of what we will learn can be done noninvasively by use of positron emission tomography, high-resolution magnetic resonance imaging, multichannel magneto-cardiography, etc. Ultimately, therapy may be based on altering the properties of discontinuous propagation in a way that "normalizes" conduction to abolish the substrate for these bothersome arrhythmias. For example, direct endomyocardial transcatheter injection of con-nexon genes might cure atrial arrhythmias by improving discontinuous propagation, representing a true "bench to bedside" achievement.

References

1. Spach MS, Miller WT, Geselowitz DB, Barr RC, Kootsey JM, Johnson EA. The discontinuous nature of propagation in normal canine cardiac muscle. Evidence for recurrent discontinuities of intracellular resistance that affect the membrane currents. *Circ Res.* 1981;48:39–54.
2. Dolber PC, Spach MS. Structure of canine Bachmann's bundle related to propagation of excitation. *Am J Physiol.* 1989;257(5 pt 2):H1446–H1457.
3. Ursell P, Gardner P, Albala A, Fenoglio J, Wit A. Structural and electrophys-iological changes in the epicardial border zone of chronic myocardial in-farcts during infarct healing. *Circ Res.* 1985;56:436–451.
4. Dillon S, Allessie M, Ursell P, Wit A. Influences of anisotropic tissue struc-ture on reentrant circuits in the epicardial border zone of subacute canine infarcts. *Circ Res.* 1988;63:182–206.
5. Hofer E, Urban G, Spach MS, Schafferhofer I, Mohr G, Platzer D. Measuring activation patterns of the heart at a microscopic size scale with thin-film sensors. *Am J Physiol.* 1994;266(5 pt 2):H2136–H2145.
6. Hill B, Courtney K. Design of a multipoint laser scanned optical monitor of cardiac action potential propagation: application to microreentry in guinea pig atrium. *Ann Biomed Eng.* 1987;15:567–577.
7. Rosenbaum D, Kaplan D, Kanai A, Ruskin J, Cohen R, Salama G. Optical maps reveal decreased spatial coupling of repolarization during arrhyth-mogenic insults. *Circulation.* 1988;78(suppl II):II-613. Abstract.
8. Gardner P, Ursell P, Fenoglio J, Wit A. Electrophysiologic and anatomic basis for fractionated electrograms recorded from healed myocardial in-farcts. *Circulation.* 1985;72:596–611.
9. Saffitz JE, Kanter HL, Green KG, Tolley TK, Beyer EC. Tissue-specific deter-minants of anisotropic conduction velocity in canine atrial and ventricular myocardium. *Circ Res.* 1994;74:1065–1070.
10. Sommer J, Scherer B. Geometry of cell and bundle appositions in cardiac muscle: light microscopy. *Am J Physiol.* 1985;248(*Heart Circ Physiol*): H792–H803.
11. Richards DA, Blake GJ, Spear JF, Moore EN. Electrophysiologic substrate for ventricular tachycardia: correlation of properties in vivo and in vitro. *Circulation.* 1984;69:369–381.
12. Kadish A, Shinnar M, Moore EN, Levine JH, Balke CW, Spear JF. Interaction

of fiber orientation and direction of impulse propagation with anatomic barriers in anisotropic canine myocardium. *Circulation.* 1988;78:1478–1494.

13. Lesh M, Spear J, Simson M. A computer model of the electrogram: what causes fractionation? *J Electrocardiol.* 1988;21:S69–S73.

14. Lesh M, Goel A, Gibb W. Reentry in non-uniformly anisotropic ventricular myocardium: simulation and visualization in a computer model. *IEEE Trans Biomed Eng.* 1992;14:628–630.

15. Joyner R, Veenstra R, Rawling D, Chorro A. Propagation through electrically coupled cells: effects of a resistive barrier. *Biophys J.* 1984;45:1017–1025.

16. Moe G, Rheinboldt W, Abildskov J. A computer model of atrial fibrillation. *Am Heart J.* 1964;67:200–220.

17. Roberge F, Vinet A, Victorri B. Reconstruction of propagated electrical activity with a two-dimensional model of anisotropic heart muscle. *Circ Res.* 1986;58:461–475.

18. Van Capelle F, Durrer D. Computer simulation of arrhythmias in a network of coupled excitable elements. *Circ Res.* 1980;47:454–466.

19. Rudy Y, Quan W. A model study of the effects of the discrete cellular structure on electrical propagation in cardiac tissue. *Circ Res.* 1987;61: 815–823.

20. Wit A, Josephson M. Fractionated electrograms and continuous electrical activity: Fact or artifact. In: Zipes D, Jalife J, eds. *Cardiac Electrophysiology and Arrhythmias.* New York, NY: Grune & Stratton; 1985:343–351.

21. Lesh MD, Van Hare GF. Status of ablation in patients with atrial tachycardia and flutter. *Pacing Clin Electrophysiol.* 1994;17:1026–33.

22. Lesh MD, Van Hare GF, Epstein LM, et al. Radiofrequency catheter ablation of atrial arrhythmias: results and mechanisms. *Circulation.* 1994;89: 1074–1089.

23. Saoudi N, Atallah G, Kirkorian G, Touboul P. Catheter ablation of the atrial myocardium in human type I atrial flutter. *Circulation.* 1990;81:762–771.

24. Walsh EP, Saul JP, Hulse JE, et al. Transcatheter ablation of ectopic atrial tachycardia in young using radiofrequency current. *Circulation.* 1992;86: 1138–1146.

25. Haissaguerre M, Gencel L, Fischer B, et al. Successful catheter ablation of atrial fibrillation. *J Cardiovasc Electrophysiol.* 1994;5:1045–1052.

26. Chu E, Kalman JM, Kwasman MA, et al. Intracardiac echocardiography during radiofrequency catheter ablation of cardiac arrhythmias in humans. *J Am Coll Cardiol.* 1994;24:1351–1357.

27. Chu E, Fitzpatrick AP, Chin MC, Sudhir K, Yock PG, Lesh MD. Radiofrequency catheter ablation guided by intracardiac echocardiography. *Circulation.* 1994;89:1301–1305.

28. Olgin JE, Kalman JM, Fitzpatrick AP, Lesh MD. Role of right atrial endocardial structures as barriers to conduction during human type I atrial flutter: activation and entrainment mapping guided by intracardiac echocardiography. *Circulation.* 1995;92:1839–1848.

29. Spach MS, Josephson ME. Initiating reentry: the role of nonuniform anisotropy in small circuits. *J Cardiovasc Electrophysiol.* 1994;5:182–209.

30. Irisawa H, Giles W, Sinus and atrioventricular node cells: cellular electrophysiology. In: Zipes D, Jalife J, eds. *Cardiac Electrophysiology: From Cell to Bedside.* Philadelphia, Pa. WB Saunders Co; 1990:95–102.

31. Randall WC, Rinkema LE, Jones SB, Moran JF, Brynjolfsson G. Functional characterization of atrial pacemaker activity. *Am J Physiol.* 1982;242: H98–H106.

32. Joyner RW, van Capelle FJ. Propagation through electrically coupled cells: how a small SA node drives a large atrium. *Biophys J.* 1986;50(6):1157–64.

33. Lewis T, Drury A, Iliescu C. A demonstration of circus movement in clinical flutter of the auricles. *Heart.* 1921;8:341.

34. Rosenblueth A, Ramos G. Studies on flutter and fibrillation, II: the influence of artificial obstacles on experimental auricular flutter. *Am Heart J.* 1947;3: 677.

35. Frame LH, Page RL, Hoffman BF. Atrial reentry around an anatomic barrier with a partially refractory excitable gap: a canine model of atrial flutter. *Circ Res.* 1986;58:495–511.

36. Frame LH, Page RL, Boyden PA, Fenoglio JJJ, Hoffman BF. Circus movement in the canine atrium around the tricuspid ring during experimental atrial flutter and during reentry in vitro. *Circulation.* 1987;76:1155–1175.

37. Boyden PA. Models of atrial reentry. *J Cardiovasc Electrophysiol.* 1995;6: 313–324.

38. Puech P, Latour H, Grolleau R. Le flutter et ses limites. *Arch Mal Coeur.* 1970;63:116–144.

39. Klein G, Guiraudon G, Sharma A, Milstein S. Demonstration of macroreentry and feasibility of operative therapy in the common type of atrial flutter. *Am J Cardiol.* 1986;57:587–591.

40. Cosio FG, Lopez GM, Goicolea A, Arribas F. Electrophysiologic studies in atrial flutter. *Clin Cardiol.* 1992;15:667–673.

41. Olshansky B, Okumura K, Hess PG, Waldo AL. Demonstration of an area of slow conduction in human atrial flutter. *J Am Coll Cardiol.* 1990;16: 1639–1648.

42. Feld GK, Fleck RP, Chen PS, et al. Radiofrequency catheter ablation for the treatment of human type 1 atrial flutter: identification of a critical zone in the reentrant circuit by endocardial mapping techniques. *Circulation.* 1992; 86:1233–1240.

43. Kalman JM, Olgin J, Lee R, Saxon LA, Lesh MD. The anterior barrier in human atrial flutter: role of the tricuspid annulus. *Circulation.* 1995;92(suppl I):I-406. Abstract.

44. Kalman JM, Olgin J, Saxon LA, Lee R, Barnard D, Lesh MD. Electrophysiologic characteristics of atypical atrial flutter. *Circulation.* 1995;92(suppl I):I-406. Abstract.

45. Chen SA, Chiang CE, Yang CJ, et al. Sustained atrial tachycardia in adult patients: electrophysiological characteristics, pharmacological response, possible mechanisms, and effects of radiofrequency ablation. *Circulation.* 1994;90:1262–1278.

46. Kalman JM, Olgin J, Fitzpatrick AP, Lee R, Epstein LM, Lesh MD. "Cristal tachycardia": relationship of right atrial tachycardias to the crista terminalis identified using intracardiac echocardiography. *Pacing Clin Electrophysiol.* 1995;18:861.

47. Moe G. On the multiple wavelet hypothesis of atrial fibrillation. *Arch Int Pharmacodyn.* 1962;140:183–188.

48. Allessie M, Lammers WJEP, Bonke FI, Hollen J, Experimental evaluation of Moe's multiple wavelet hypothesis of atrial fibrillation. In: Zipes D, Jalife J, eds. *Cardiac Electrophysiology and Arrhythmias.* New York, NY: Grune and Stratton; 1985:265–275.

49. Konings KT, Kirchhof CJ, Smeets JR, Wellens HJ, Penn OC, Allessie MA. High-density mapping of electrically induced atrial fibrillation in humans. *Circulation.* 1994;89:1665–1680.

50. Spach MS, Dolber PC, Heidlage JF. Influence of the passive anisotropic properties on directional differences in propagation following modification of the sodium conductance in human atrial muscle: a model of reentry based on anisotropic discontinuous propagation. *Circ Res.* 1988;62:811–832.
51. Spach MS, Dolber PC. Relating extracellular potentials and their derivatives to anisotropic propagation at a microscopic level in human cardiac muscle: evidence for electrical uncoupling of side-to-side fiber connections with increasing age. *Circ Res.* 1986;58:356–371.

Chapter 6

Role of Discontinuous Conduction/Nonuniform Anisotropy in Clinical Arrhythmias

Charles J.H.J. Kirchhof, MD, PhD, and Mark E. Josephson, MD

Propagation of the cardiac impulse is based primarily on the successive generation of membrane action potentials in a syncytium of electrically coupled myocytes. Areas of local conduction delay or block may facilitate the initiation and perpetuation of reentrant excitation. These electrophysiological features have long been attributed to intrinsic or induced heterogeneities in sarcolemmal membrane kinetics or resting membrane potential leading to a decreased action potential upstroke, a prolonged action potential duration (APD), or diminished cellular excitability.

More recently, the structural anatomy and spatial arrangement of myocardial cells and fibers were shown to play an important role in normal and abnormal impulse conduction. Local conduction delay or block could occur as a direct consequence of tissue anisotropy and set the conditions for initiation and perpetuation of reentrant excitation in the absence of changes in cellular membrane kinetics or excitability.

Tissue Anisotropy

Tissue anisotropy can be subdivided into uniform and nonuniform types. Uniform anisotropy is a normal property of young myocardial

Dr. Kirchhof is supported by the Dutch Academic Cardiology Institute (ICIN) and the Cardiology Division of the Academic Hospital, University of Limburg, Maastricht, The Netherlands.

From: Spooner PM, Joyner RW, Jalife J (eds). *Discontinuous Conduction in the Heart.* Armonk, NY: Futura Publishing Company, Inc.; © 1997.

tissue and is based on the normal arrangement and quantity of intercellular gap junctions. This leads to a smooth and continuous propagation of the impulse in all directions but with a conduction velocity that is more rapid parallel to the fiber orientation. Nonuniform anisotropy occurs when the spatial distribution or function of the intercellular gap junctions is altered to such an extent that transverse conduction becomes so much slower than longitudinal conduction that adjacent muscle fibers are activated asynchronously. Anatomic factors such as hypertrophy, age-related fibrosis, and myocardial infarction and metabolic derangements such as ischemia and states of calcium overload all may result in nonuniform anisotropy by markedly influencing the quality and quantity of gap junctions and their positional relationship to the myocardial fiber axis.[1-4]

Since the development of nonuniform anisotropy is multifactorial, discontinuous conduction can have many causes, any one or all of which may be associated with clinical arrhythmias. The greater the degree of nonuniformities of electrical load imposed by nonuniform distribution or function of intercellular connections (gap junctions), the greater the window for inducing and maintaining reentrant arrhythmias. To understand what role discontinuous conduction plays in clinical arrhythmias, one needs to know the characteristic features of discontinuous conduction caused by nonuniform anisotrophy.

Electrophysiological Characteristics of Discontinuous Conduction in Nonuniform Anisotropic Tissue

Slow Conduction and Fragmented Electrograms

Nonuniform tissue anisotropy is histologically characterized by a sparsity of side-to-side gap junctions between cells or small group of cells due to the presence of a variable degree of collagenous septa or edema. As a result, impulse conduction transverse to the fiber orientation can be extremely slow (<5 cm/s) and is characterized by fractionated extracellular electrograms of low amplitude and long duration in the presence of normal transmembrane potentials. Experimental studies using isolated nonuniform anisotropic tissue specimens with fragmented extracellular electrograms revealed that the individual electrogram deflections represent the sequential activation of closely adjacent sites or fiber strands. This asynchronous activation of poorly coupled myocardial fibers is best described as saltatory or discontinuous conduction and is quite different from that in uniform anisotropic tissue, in which normal extracellular waveforms are recorded in all directions.[3,5,6]

Direction-Dependent Conduction and Refractoriness

Spach et al demonstrated in nonuniform anisotropic tissue that the conduction curve (A_1-A_2) of early premature beats often shows a distinct discontinuity caused by preferential conduction block in the longitudinal direction, whereas slow conduction in the transverse direction persists at shorter coupling intervals (shorter effective refractory period).[1-4] These conduction properties are illustrated in Figure 1 and imply that impulse conduction perpendicular to the fiber orientation is characterized by a higher safety factor for conduction than the more rapid conduction parallel to the fiber orientation. Nonuniform anisotropic tissue exhibits direction-dependent conduction block, which may easily provide the electrophysiological substrate for reentrant excitation (anisotropic reentry) and explain site-dependent initiation and termination of reentrant arrhythmias.

Capability of Small Reentrant Circuits

A consequence of the very slow discontinuous conduction in nonuniform anisotropic tissue is that the local wavelength of the electrical impulse in otherwise normal cardiac tissue can become very short (<5 mm). In human nonuniform anisotropic tissue, Spach et al showed that anisotropic microreentry may occur in an area of less than a few square millimeters of tissue. In these reentry circuits, average conduction velocities of <3 cm/s were found.[4]

Excitable Gap

Anisotropic reentrant ventricular tachycardia (VT) in canine infarct models revealed heterogeneous conduction properties within the reentry circuit. This was because some parts of the circuit demonstrated slow, discontinuous conduction, whereas other parts demonstrated rapid conduction parallel to the fiber orientation. In these anisotropic reentrant circuits, the presence of a fully excitable gap was demonstrated.[7] This forms an important difference from the "leading circle" type of reentry, which is based primarily on inhomogeneities in tissue repolarization and in which no fully excitable gap can be demonstrated.[8]

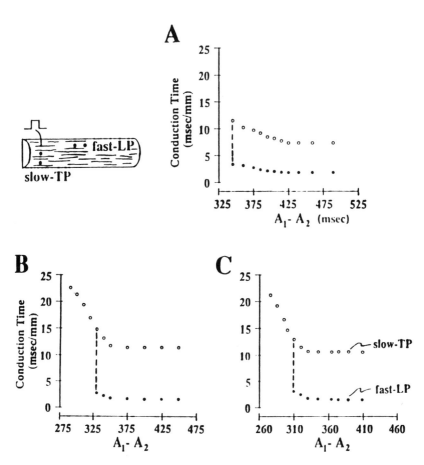

Figure 1. Anisotropic conduction time curves from (A) uniform anisotropic pectinate muscle of a 12-year-old child, (B) nonuniform anisotropic pectinate muscle of a 62-year-old men, and (C) atrial nonuniform anisotropic muscle of an adult dog. Drawing at upper left illustrates how longitudinal (LP) and transverse (TP) propagation of progressively premature extrastimuli were determined. Conduction times in ms/mm were measured from stimulus to steepest negative deflection in electrograms recorded by two pairs of extracellular electrodes. In preparation A, no discontinuity occurred in conduction curves, indicating that effective refractory periods of LP (solid circles) and TP (open circles) were equal. In nonuniform anisotropic bundles (B and C), a discontinuity occurred due to failure of fast LP at a longer refractory period than that of slow TP. Reprinted with permission from Reference 6.

Table 1
Characteristics of Nonuniform Anisotropy

1. Fast (FP) and slow (SP) pathways with different refractory periods are a general property of nonuniform anisotropic tissue.
2. Differences of FP and SP are due to nonuniformities of electrical load created by a heterogeneous distribution of cell-to-cell electrical coupling.
3. Slow, discontinuous conduction due to nonuniform anisotropy can be 10 times slower than the conduction velocity imposed through active membrane properties.
4. Extracellular electrograms in areas of slow conduction due to nonuniform anisotropy are characterized by long duration, low amplitude, and multiple components.
5. Manifestation of these characteristics depends on the direction of the wave front relative to the fiber orientation.

The characteristics of discontinuous conduction in nonuniform anisotropic tissue are summarized in Table 1.

Role of Discontinuous Conduction in Reentrant VT After Myocardial Infarction

Fractionated Electrograms

The hallmark of discontinuous conduction is fractionated extracellular electrograms of long duration and low amplitude, caused by asynchronous activation of adjacent tissue areas. In patients with VT and prior myocardial infarction, endocardial mapping of the left ventricle using 5- to 10-mm bipolar electrodes (40 to 500 Hz) has demonstrated fractionated low-amplitude electrograms in infarcted areas during sinus rhythm, ventricular pacing, and in diastole during sustained VT.[9–11] An example of such electrograms is given in Figure 2. During pacing, the width and degree of electrogram fractionation is closely related to both the site and the rate of stimulation.[10] Although the refractory period and degree of excitability of myocardial fibers may change during the acute and the healing phases of a myocardial infarction, the fragmented electrograms recorded from these chronically infarcted areas demonstrate the presence of discontinuous conduction in nonuniform anisotropic scar tissue. Even changes in local excitability have been related to the presence of these fractionated electrograms.[12]

It was thus important to demonstrate that these fragmented electrograms were directly related to the occurrence of VT in ischemic heart disease. Cassidy et al showed that the extent and duration of frag-

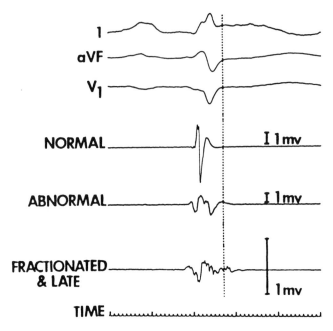

Figure 2. Various endocardial electrograms (normal, abnormal, and fractionated and late) can be recorded from different left ventricular regions in patients with a history of coronary disease. Dashed vertical line indicates end of surface ECG, of which three recordings are shown. Recording gain of electrograms is illustrated by mV bars. Note that terminal portion of low-amplitude fractionated electrogram extends beyond surface ECG. Reprinted with permission from Reference 9.

mented electrograms correlate best with the inducibility of the VT.[13] Moreover, they demonstrated that a higher incidence of abnormal endocardial electrograms was found in patients with a clinical history of sustained VT compared with patients without sustained VT. In endocardial resection preparations obtained during VT surgery, fractionated electrograms were recorded from the site of origin of the tachycardia as determined during endocardial mapping, whereas the action potentials from the muscle fibers in these sites showed a completely normal configuration.[14,15] Successful endocardial resection of the VT eliminates split and late potentials and decreases the number and extent of fractionated electrograms.[16] Morphological analysis of the resection preparations showed that in tissue from sites at which fragmented electrograms were recorded, the surviving myocardial fibers were separated by strands of fibrous tissue causing dissociated activation in areas less than a few square millimeters.[15,17,18]

The presence of slow conduction can be identified as late potentials in the signal-averaged ECG. Studies in patients after myocardial infarction with a history of VT have demonstrated that the late potentials are related to the extent and duration of fragmented electrograms extending beyond the QRS complex.[19] The incidence of positive signal-averaged ECGs in patients with sustained monomorphic VT is ≈85%, compared with ≈50% in patients with a history of cardiac arrest or nonsustained VT.[10]

Finally, critical areas of a VT circuit can be identified by the presence of diastolic fractionated electrograms that demonstrate a particular response to resetting or entrainment of the tachycardia, ie, a postpacing return cycle identical to the VT cycle length. By this criterion, areas of discontinuous conduction that are part of the reentrant circuit can be identified as a target for radiofrequency ablation so as to interrupt the VT circuit.[10,11]

Initiation of VT and Continuous Electrical Activity

During the initiation of sustained monomorphic VT by premature stimulation, the fragmented endocardial electrograms recorded at the site of VT origin often show a marked increase in duration and degree of fractionation compared with sinus rhythm. This suggests a further decrease in local conduction velocity of the premature impulse and an increase in local asynchronous activation due to nonuniform anisotropic tissue characteristics. A critical degree of slowing must be achieved to initiate sustained monomorphic tachycardia.[10]

The ultimate expression of delayed activation is the development of continuous electrical activity, which is necessary for initiation and maintainance of the VT. This can be demonstrated in ≈10% of the patients. An example is given in Figure 3. Continuous electrical activity is believed to be consistent with local reentrant excitation of a relatively "small" circuit.[10]

Sustained monomorphic VTs that are easily inducible with extrastimuli from one pacing site might not be inducible at all from another pacing site despite the ability to achieve comparable coupling intervals. This site-specific inducibility not only supports an underlying reentrant mechanism but also suggests that the occurrence of the functional barrier necessary for the initiation of reentry depends on the direction of the stimulated wave front in relation to the area providing the substrate for the functional barrier.[10]

Resetting of Clinical VT

Programmed electrical stimulation during hemodynamically tolerated sustained VT in patients with ischemic heart disease showed that

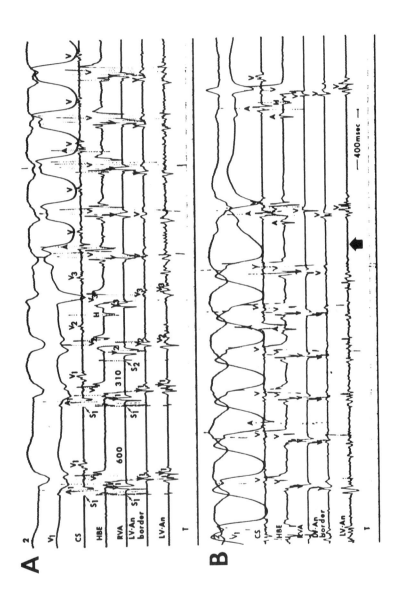

these tachycardias can be reset (often with fusion) by premature ventricular stimuli from different pacing sites.[10] This indicates the presence of an excitable gap and suggests that these VTs are based on an anatomic or anisotropic type of reentry (or a combination of both) but not of the "leading circle" type.

Resetting a VT by single or double extrastimuli may result in a flat, increasing, or combined (flat followed by increasing) reset curve. The flat portion of the curve represents orthodromic conduction of the resetting impulse without conduction delay. The increasing portion represents rate-dependent conduction delay of the resetting impulse due to encroachment on the refractory period defined by the APD, to poor cellular coupling in the setting of nonuniform anisotropy, or to stimulation-induced elongation of a functional conduction barrier and thus the entire path length. The total excitable gap, defined as the difference between the longest coupling interval that resets the VT and the coupling interval that results in termination of the VT, represents 30% to 35% of the VT cycle length.[10] In ≈50% of the VT cases, the reset response pattern is different in duration (excitable gap) and shape when stimulation from the right ventricular apex and outflow tract are compared.[20] This is illustrated in Figure 4 and may be explained by heterogeneous conduction properties of the reentry circuit whereby decremental conduction of the resetting impulse occurs in only a portion of the entire pathway. If a reentrant circuit includes different areas of discontinuous conduction, the site of entrance of the resetting impulse determines which area is first encountered and is mainly responsible for decremental conduction. The site dependency of resetting response patterns might also be explained by alteration of the size and location of the functional barrier and thus the length of the reentrant circuit due to penetration of the circuit from different sites. These findings practically exclude a purely anatomic reentry circuit as the mechanism underlying clinical VT in the setting of coronary artery disease (CAD).

Effects of Drugs

The action of drugs on VT cycle length, termination, and prevention and on the substrate of VT provides supporting evidence for the

---

Figure 3. Continuous electrical activity during initiation and maintenance of VT. Surface ECG leads II and V_1 are shown together with intracardiac electrograms from the CS, His bundle area (HBE), right ventricular apex (RVA), and at border of (LV-An border) and just inside (LV-An) a left ventricular aneurysm. Top, After delivery of an extrastimulus S_2 with a coupling interval of 310 ms (S_1-S_1, 600 ms), continuous electrical activity appears in electrogram recorded from LV-An, and VT is initiated. Bottom, When continuous activity stops (arrow), tachycardia terminates. Reprint with permission from Reference 10.

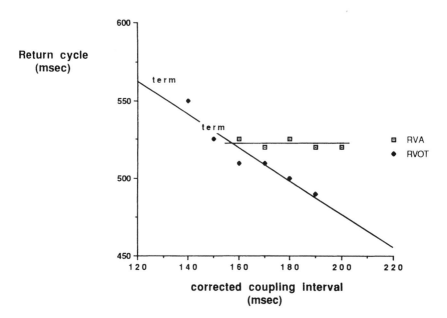

Figure 4. Different VT resetting response patterns during stimulation from right ventricular apex (RVA) and outflow tract (RVOT). Abscissa represents corrected coupling interval; ordinate, the corresponding return cycle. In this case, resetting from RVA resulted in a flat plus increasing curve, with duration of flat curve extending 80 ms. Resetting from RVOT showed a purely increasing curve lacking a flat portion. Slopes of increasing portions of both curves were not significantly different. Reprint with permission from Reference 20.

role of discontinuous conduction in reentrant VT due to CAD. Procainamide and lidocaine both have no effect on slow-response fibers but slow conduction in depressed fast fibers. They differ in that lidocaine has minimal effects on normally polarized fibers, which are dependent on normal sodium ion conductance. Procainamide alone affects conduction in normal tissue. In a study of lidocaine and procainamide on normal and abnormal (fractionated) left ventricular electrograms in patients with prior myocardial infarction and VT, Schmitt et al demonstrated that procainamide prolonged the duration of both types of electrograms, whereas lidocaine had no effect at all.[21] Furthermore, the fractionated electrograms showed a greater rate-dependent prolongation than the normal electrograms. This difference between lidocaine and procainamide confirms that slow conduction associated with fractionated electrograms is based on poorly coupled, normally polarized myocytes producing discontinuous conduction.

Procainamide causes marked prolongation (≈30%) of tachycardia cycle length, which correlates well with its effects on QRS width during

Table 2
Role of Nonuniform Anisotropy in Ventricular Tachycardia

1. Arrhythmogenic areas are characterized by fragmented electrograms, suggesting extremely slow conduction over a small area.
2. Inducibility of VT is closely related to the extent of these conduction abnormalities.
3. Histologically, nonuniform anisotropy is characterized by broad bands of fibrous tissue separating viable muscle fibers that show normal electrophysiological properties.
4. The presence of a fully excitable gap.
5. Stimulation-site–dependent resetting curves.

pacing at cycle lengths comparable to that of VT. The mechanism of slowing of VT by procainamide appears to be either a primary prolongation of conduction time or an extension of the proximal barriers around which the impulse circulates (increased tachycardia circuit size), because the QRS morphology remains the same. This is suggested by the persistence of a fully excitable gap, evidenced by a flat portion of the resetting curve during VT following procainamide, and indicates that the lengthening of VT cycle length is not mediated by prolongation of the refractory period.[22] Moreover, the relationship of QRS prolongation before VT cycle length prolongation favors primary conduction slowing as the mechanism of this response. Since the effects of procainamide are greatest in fractionated electrograms, prolongation of the tachycardia cycle length is most likely due to further depression of transverse conduction in areas of nonuniform anisotropy. Other drugs, such as quinidine, propafenone, flecainide, and amiodarone, also decrease the tachycardia rate, with persistence of a flat resetting curve. Thus, they all appear to act similarly. Therefore, termination of the tachycardia with procainamide or one of these other drugs is most likely caused by conduction block in an area of discontinuous impulse propagation.

In summary, overwhelming evidence exists that reentrant VT associated with CAD requires discontinuous conduction for its initiation and maintenance. This is provided by the structural tissue changes related to healed myocardial infarctions (Table 2).

AV Nodal Reentrant Tachycardia

The anatomic substrate of the AV junction and the response to programmed stimulation suggest that nonuniform anisotropic conduction may underlie AV nodal reentrant tachycardia (AVNRT).

'Dual AV Nodal Physiology' as a Manifestation of AV Nodal Anisotropy

In 10% to 15% of "normal" patients, AV nodal conduction (A-H interval) of premature atrial beats (APD) suddenly prolongs by ≥50 ms in response to a 10-ms increase in APD prematurity. It has been postulated that this discontinuity in AV nodal conduction curves, which is referred to as "dual AV nodal physiology," occurs because at a critical degree of prematurity, APDs block in a "fast (β) pathway" (FP) but propagate over a "slow (α) pathway" (SP) to the His bundle.[23,24] The refractory period of the SP is thus shorter than that of the FP. When anterograde conduction over the SP exceeds the refractory period of the FP, retrograde invasion of the latter may result in an AV nodal echo. If at that moment the SP is reexcitable, (sustained) AV nodal reentry can occur. These findings are comparable to those shown by Spach et al in nonuniform atrial tissue.[1-4]

Until recently, these AV nodal conduction phenomena were attributed to very slow conduction (<10 cm/s) in the AV node, where the action potential upstroke is based solely on slow calcium inward currents. Spach and Josephson recently suggested that dual AV nodal physiology could also be a manifestation of nonuniform anisotropic conduction in the AV node.[6] This hypothesis is supported by several lines of experimental evidence obtained from rabbit hearts. Morphological studies showed that the superficial transitional fibers of the posterior node are oriented parallel to the tricuspid annulus and arranged in small, irregular groups of cells separated by connective tissue.[25] Intracellular mapping of AV nodal reentry in rabbit hearts revealed dual intranodal pathways that were functionally rather than anatomically determined.[26] Furthermore, measurement of passive electrical properties in the rabbit AV node revealed a different electrotonic space constant in different directions.[27] Recent studies by Spach using high-resolution extracellular electrode arrays in the transitional zone of the AV node strongly supported the above hypothesis: uniphasic extracellular waveforms were recorded during relatively fast (39-cm/s) conduction parallel to the tricuspid annulus, whereas multiphasic waveforms of longer duration were seen during slow (6-cm/s) conduction perpendicular to the tricuspid annulus.[28,29]

Also in the clinical electrophysiology laboratory, several phenomena related to the induction and maintenance of AV nodal reentry have been observed that are difficult to understand without implicating mechanisms based on nonuniform anisotropy.

Direction-Dependent Initiation of Clinical AVNRT

Although never identified morphologically, the concept of "dual AV nodal physiology" may suggest the presence of distinct structures that are related to the AV nodal reentrant circuit. However, many clinical observations indicate that this is not the case. The site of stimulation can affect the ability to initiate dual AV nodal pathways and/or induce AVNRT (Figure 5). The conduction time (A-H) and refractory period in both the SP and FP often change with different sites of atrial stimulation.[30,31] Josephson observed that AVNRT is usually easier to induce by APDs from the high right atrium (HRA) than from the coronary sinus (CS).[31] Furthermore, the critical AV nodal delay (A-H) required to initiate reentry as well as the cycle length of the AVNRT are often different and depend on the site of stimulation. This site dependency

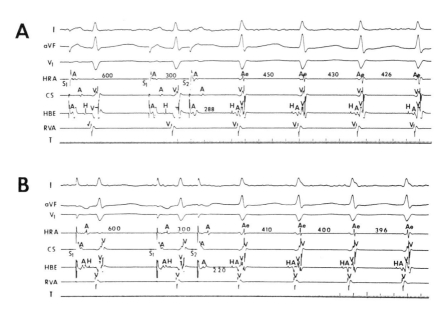

Figure 5. Initiation of AVNRT from different stimulation sites in same patient. Surface leads (I, aVF, and V_1) are shown together with intracardiac electrograms from HRA, CS, His bundle area (HBE), and right ventricular apex (RVA). Basic cycle length is 600 ms. Top, An extrastimulus (S_2) with a coupling interval of 300 ms during pacing from HRA results a marked increase in A-H interval (288 ms) followed by induction of AVNRT with a cycle length of ≈425 ms. Bottom, During stimulation from CS, an extrastimulus with a coupling interval of 300 ms causes a lesser degree of A-H prolongation (220 ms) followed by the induction of AVNRT with a cycle length of ≈395 ms. Reprint and adapted with permission from Reference 31.

could not be attributed to intra-atrial conduction delay. Monahan et al found that both the critical A-H interval for initiation of AVNRT and the initial H-A differed unpredictably between pacing from the SP and FP.[32] These observations suggest that the so-called "slow" and "fast" pathways are not anatomically fixed but rather are functional structures and that these direction-dependent effects of AVNRT-initiating APDs are due to nonuniform anisotropic properties of the AV node.[6]

Resetting of AVNRT

In patients, AVNRT can be reset or terminated by APDs from different pacing sites as well as by single or double ventricular premature depolarizations. This implies the presence of an excitable gap, which makes a leading-circle mechanism for AVNRT very unlikely. During resetting from the HRA, a progressive delay in the SP (prolongation of A-H) typically occurs with increased prematurity of the APDs. Comparison of the reset response curves from the SP and FP showed a greater antegrade conduction delay (A-H) during stimulation from the FP. In addition, Monahan et al found that the excitable gap was almost twice as long during pacing from the SP and the ventricle compared with stimulation at the FP (43 versus 26 ms).[33] Resetting from the ventricle showed no retrograde delay in the FP. These observations are compatible with a significant degree of slowing in response to resetting between the tendon of Todaro and the tricuspid ring. This direction of propagation is perpendicular to the fiber orientation of the transitional zone.

Atrial Activation During AVNRT

The role of the atrium in AVNRT remains controversial. Recent data obtained from our laboratory by simultaneous atrial mapping in the triangle of Koch and CS showed that there is either a broad band of simultaneous atrial activation (4 to 8 mm) and/or multiple sites of early breakthrough during AVNRT.[34] This pattern of activation differs from that during ventricular pacing. Similar findings were obtained by McGuire et al, who used high-resolution intraoperative mapping during AVNRT and demonstrated a relatively large elliptical epicardial breakthrough in the anterior triangle of Koch.[35] These different activation patterns are most likely to occur if atrial activation depends on rapid conduction parallel to the tricuspid ring with nearly simultaneous activation of the overlying atrial fibers. If the atrium were an essential part of the AVNRT circuit, the impulse would conduct more slowly and in a sequential manner around the tendon of Todaro, the CS ostium, and then parallel to the tricuspid annulus. This pattern has never been shown. Finally, the demonstration of atrial activation in the triangle of Koch by stimulated APDs without affecting the AVNRT cycle length further supports a subatrial level of AVNRT circuits.[31,36–38]

Effects of Aging

Since nonuniform anisotropy is a normal effect of aging,[39,40] AV nodal conduction may be altered in the elderly. Anselme et al retrospectively studied 45 patients of different ages and found that retrograde atrial activation in all regions of the low atrial septum except the SP was delayed during typical AVNRT.[41] Also, the tachycardia cycle length was significantly longer in the older patient group (>45 years of age), but only the A-H intervals were not significantly different. Furthermore, retrograde atrial activation along the tendon of Todaro showed, in all patients, either a single or multiple endocardial breakthrough sites unrelated to age. However, in the younger group (<45 years of age), an activation pattern more broad than sequential was present compared with the older group. This is compatible with a faster retrograde conduction in the younger group whereby the impulse almost simultaneously activates the superficial atrial tissue layer, as discussed above. These observations suggested an age-related slowing of retrograde conduction in the FP and overlying atrial transitional cells that is most likely due to age-related microfibrosis leading to enhanced nonuniform anisotropy.

Current experimental and clinical evidence strongly suggests that the AVNRT circuit is functionally rather than anatomically determined, the substrate for which is provided by nonuniform anisotropic properties of the AV node (Table 3).

Table 3

Evidence Supporting the Role of Local Anisotropy in AVNRT

---

1. Resetting from FP causes more AV nodal delay than from the SP.
2. Atrial activation during AVNRT shows more rapid conduction parallel to tricuspid annulus (longitudinal to local fiber orientation).
3. Stimulation-site–dependent "critical" A-H for initiation and AVNRT cycle length.
4. Stimulation-site–dependent duration of excitable gap.

Discontinuous Conduction in the Genesis of Atrial Flutter and AF

Specific atrial structures, such as the crista terminalis and pectinate muscle bundles, show uniform anisotropy. Also, along the mitral and tricuspid ring, the atrial fibers are oriented parallel to the annulus. Age-related nonuniform anisotropy may occur in all parts of the atrium.[6,39,40]

Fractionated Electrograms and Site-Dependent Initiation of Atrial Flutter

In the vast majority of patients, atrial flutter is based on reentrant excitation.[42,43] The occurrence of fractionated electrograms and site-dependent initiation of atrial flutter was first emphasized by Watson and Josephson.[44] Buxton et al[45] observed that APDs in patients with a history of atrial flutter or AF showed a higher degree of intra-atrial conduction delay, over a wider range of coupling intervals, than in normal subjects. In a large series of patients (n = 79) with a history of atrial flutter, Josephson recently showed that in 71%, the flutter was inducible by APDs from the HRA, but only in 44% by APDs from the CS. Induction of atrial flutter was often preceded by a wide range of coupling intervals of APDs showing fractionation of electrograms at the AV junction or CS ostium, and in most cases this fractionation was also required for initiation of atrial flutter (Figure 6). The absence of such fragmented electrograms during HRA or CS stimulation that failed to induce flutter suggests an important role of discontinuous conduction in the initiation of atrial flutter.[31]

Is the Inferoposterior Septum a Critical Area for Initiation and Maintainance of Atrial Flutter?

The most consistent finding in endocardial mapping of typical flutter is that fractionated electrograms can be recorded in the inferoposterior septum just before or at the onset of the negative component of the surface flutter wave.[31] Resetting from the CS required shorter coupling intervals than from the HRA. In most cases, reset response curves revealed the presence of a fully excitable gap. Taken in sum, these findings strongly suggest that the critical area for atrial flutter is located in the posterior triangle of Koch and that discontinuous conduction due to nonuniform anisotropy in this region provides an important electrophysiological substrate for the occurrence of atrial flutter.[31,46]

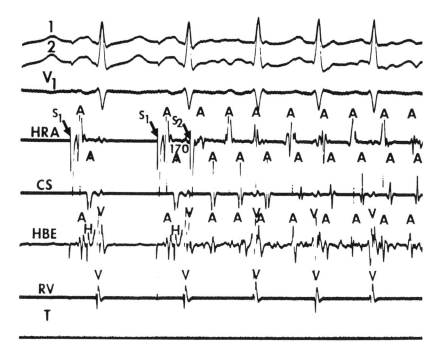

Figure 6. Induction of atrial flutter with a single extrastimulus. ECG leads I, II, and V₁ are shown together with intracardiac electrograms from HRA, CS, HBE, and RV. During a basic pacing cycle length of 600 ms, an extrastimulus (S₂) from HRA with a coupling interval of 170 ms induces a rapid atrial arrhythmia that became sustained atrial flutter after stabilization. Note initial irregularity in flutter intervals and fragmentation of His bundle electrogram. Similar recordings were found during initiation of AF. Reprinted with permission from Reference 31.

Nonuniform Anisotropy in AF

AF can be induced in otherwise healthy atria by premature or rapid stimulation (lone AF) and may occur secondary to other cardiac or systemic diseases. The overall incidence of AF shows a significant age-related increase that can be only partially attributed to an increased incidence of structural heart disease.

Patients with a history of AF often show increased intra-atrial conduction times in response to APDs, which favors the induction of AF.[45,47] It has also been recognized that AF inducibility is higher with APDs from the HRA than from the CS.[31,44] In patients without a documented history of AF, Papageorgiou et al[48] found that this site-specific induction from the HRA was related to a marked prolongation in conduction time to the posterior triangle of Koch and a significant fraction-

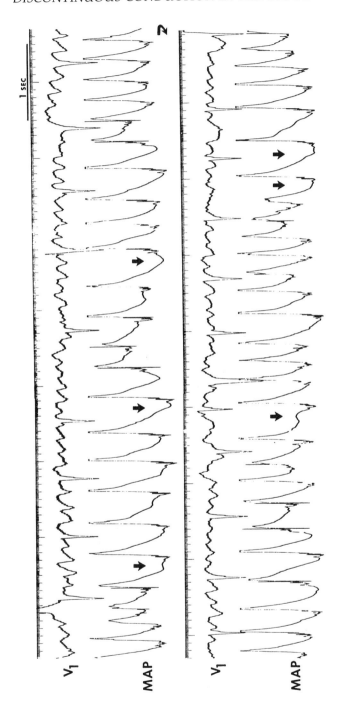

Table 4

Evidence Supporting a Role of Anisotropy in Atrial Flutter and AF

1. Initiation of atrial flutter or AF is easier from HRA than CS.
2. Presence of local conduction delay and electrogram fragmentation in low atrial septum during initiation of atrial flutter or AF; greater with HRA than CS stimulation.
3. Presence of an excitable gap.

ation of the local electrograms in that area compared with APDs from the CS. Analogous to atrial flutter, these observations suggest that nonuniform anisotropy in the posterior triangle of Koch plays an important role in the induction of AF (Table 4).

Intraoperative mapping in animals and humans confirmed Moe's multiple wavelet hypothesis for AF and demonstrated the occurrence of functionally determined arcs of conduction block and reentry.[49,50] It was recently demonstrated in canine hearts that during AF, a small but variable excitable gap exists.[51,52] Monophasic action potentials recorded during clinical AF also suggested the presence of a local excitable gap (Figure 7). On the one hand, this can be explained statistically by the limited number of simultaneously present fibrillation waves preventing atrial fibers from being reexcited immediately after they regained excitability.[52] Conversely, the presence of nonuniform anisotropy causing areas of discontinuous conduction and anisotropic reentry provides another explanation for the occurrence of a local excitable gap during AF. The presence of very short and very long intervals at a single site suggests functional block. Since the monophasic action potential configuration was normal, block would be more likely on the basis of discontinuous conduction. Further studies are necessary to elucidate the role of nonuniform anisotropy in the induction and perpetuation of AF.

Anisotropic Reentry in Nonischemic Substrates

As discussed above, discontinuous conduction plays an important role in the occurrence of sustained VT in patients with CAD. The ques-

◄————————————————————

Figure 7. Continuous recording during chronic AF in a patient. A precordial ECG lead (V$_1$) is shown together with a simultaneously recorded monophasic action potential (MAP) registration from right lateral atrial wall. Note continuous variation in local cycle length, duration, and shape of successive action potentials. Frequently, local fibrillation interval exceeded APD, leading to presence of an excitable gap during AF. Arrows indicate examples of a local excitable gap.

tion remains whether nonuniform anisotropy also provides an arrhythmogenic substrate for VT in patients with non–CAD-related cardiomyopathies. In a study by Watson et al in patients with hypertrophic cardiomyopathy and a history of VT/VF, local electrograms from both the right and left ventricles during pacing showed an abnormal degree of fractionation with a long duration and a normal amplitude (in contrast to fractionated electrograms from infarcted tissue).[53] These electrograms can be explained by an overall nonuniform anisotropy due to myocardial disarray and fibrosis as found in these patients and may provide the substrate for areas of slow, discontinuous conduction leading to lethal ventricular arrhythmias. Saumarez et al[54] believe that the relationship between degree of electrogram fractionation and coupling interval of ventricular premature depolarizations may be a useful indicator of the tendency toward malignant ventricular arrhythmias. Further investigations are necessary to better characterize the role of discontinuous conduction in hypertrophic and other cardiomyopathies.

References

1. Spach MS, Miller WT III, Geselowitz DB, et al. The discontinuous nature of propagation in normal canine cardiac muscle: evidence for recurrent discontinuities of intracellular resistance that affect the membrane currents. *Circ Res.* 1981;48:39–45.
2. Spach MS, Miller WT, Dolber PC, et al. The functional role of structural complexities in the propagation of depolarization in the atrium of the dog: cardiac conduction disturbances due to discontinuities of effective axial resistivity. *Circ Res.* 1982;50:175–191.
3. Spach MS, Dolber PC. The relation between discontinuous propagation in anisotropic cardiac muscle and the "vulnerable" period of reentry. In: Zipes DP, Jalife J, eds. *Cardiac Electrophysiology and Arrhythmias.* New York, NY: Grune & Stratton, Inc; 1985:241–252.
4. Spach MS, Dolber PC, Heidlage JF. Influence of the passive anisotropic properties on directional differences in propagation following modification of the sodium conductance in human atrial muscle: a model of reentry based on anisotropic discontinuous propagation. *Circ Res.* 1988;62:811–832.
5. Clerc L. Directional differences of impulse spread in trabecular muscle from mammalian heart. *J Physiol (Lond).* 1976;255:335–346.
6. Spach MS, Josephson ME. Initiating reentry: the role of nonuniform anisotropy in small circuits. *J Cardiovasc Electrophysiol.* 1994;5:182–209.
7. Wit AL, Dillon SM. Anisotropic reentry. In: Zipes DP, Jalife J, eds. *Cardiac Electrophysiology and Arrhythmias: From Cell to Bedside.* Philadelphia, Pa: WB Saunders Co; 1985:353–363.
8. Allessie MA, Bonke FIM, Schopman FJG. Circus movement in rabbit atrial muscle as a mechanism of tachycardia; III: the "leading circle" concept: a new model of circus movement in cardiac tissue without the involvement of an anatomical obstacle. *Circ Res.* 1977;41:9–18.
9. Cassidy DM, Vassallo JA, Buxton AE, et al. The value of catheter mapping

during sinus rhythm to localize the site of ventricular tachycardia. *Circulation.* 1984;69:1103–1110.

10. Josephson ME. *Clinical Cardiac Electrophysiology: Techniques and Interpretations.* 2nd ed. Philadelphia, Pa: Lea & Febiger; 1993:417–615.

11. Stevenson WG, Khan H, Sager P, et al. Identification of reentry circuit sites during catheter mapping and radiofrequency ablation of ventricular tachycardia late after myocardial infarction. *Circulation.* 1993;88:1647–1670.

12. Kienzle MG, Doherty JU, Cassidy D, et al. Electrophysiologic sequelae of chronic myocardial infarction: local refractoriness and electrographic characteristics of the left ventricle. *Am J Cardiol.* 1986;58:63–69.

13. Cassidy DM, Vassallo JA, Miller JM, et al. Endocardial catheter mapping in patients in sinus rhythm: relationship to underlying heart disease and ventricular arrhythmias. *Circulation.* 1986;73:645–652.

14. De Bakker JMT, van Capelle FJL, Janse MJ, et al. Reentry as a cause of ventricular tachycardia in patients with chronic ischemic heart disease: electrophysiologic and anatomic correlation. *Circulation.* 1988;77:589–606.

15. De Bakker JMT, Coronel R, Tasseron S, et al. Ventricular tachycardia in the infarcted, Langendorff-perfused human heart: role of the arrangement of surviving cardiac fibers. *J Am Coll Cardiol.* 1990;15:1594–1607.

16. Miller JM, Tyson GS, Hargrove WC III, et al. Effect of subendocardial resection on sinus rhythm endocardial electrogram abnormalities. *Circulation.* 1995;91:2385–2391.

17. Fenoglio JJ, Tuan Duc Pham, Harken AH, et al. Recurrent sustained ventricular tachycardia: structure and ultrastructure of subendocardial regions in which tachycardia originates. *Circulation.* 1983;68:518–533.

18. Wit AL, Fenoglio JJ, Tuan Duc Pham, et al. Fractionated electrograms in patients with sustained ventricular tachycardia: an indicator of arrhythmogenic microanatomy. *Circulation.* 1984;70(supp II):II-125. Abstract.

19. Vassallo JA, Cassidy D, Simson MB, et al. Relation of late potentials to site of origin of ventricular tachycardia associated with coronary artery disease. *Am J Cardiol.* 1985;55:985–989.

20. Callans DJ, Zardini M, Gottlieb CD, Josephson ME. The variable contribution of functional and anatomic barriers in human ventricular tachycardia: an analysis with resetting from two sites. *J Am Coll Cardiol.* 1996;27:1106–1111.

21. Schmitt CG, Kadish AH, Marchlinski FE, et al. Effects of lidocaine and procainamide on normal and abnormal intraventricular electrograms during sinus rhythm. *Circulation.* 1988;55:1030–1037.

22. Stamato NJ, Frame LH, Rosenthal ME, et al. Procainamide-induced slowing of ventricular tachycardia with insights from analysis of resetting response patterns. *Am J Cardiol.* 1989;63:1455–1461.

23. Kistin AD. Multiple pathways of conduction and reciprocal rhythm with interpolated ventricular premature systoles. *Am Heart J.* 1963;65:162–169.

24. Schuilenburg RM, Durrer D. Ventricular echo beats in the human heart elicited by induced ventricular premature beats. *Circulation.* 1969;40:337–347.

25. Anderson RH, Janse MJ, van Capelle FJL, et al. A combined morphological and electrophysiological study of the atrioventricular node of the rabbit heart. *Circ Res.* 1974;35:909–922.

26. Janse MJ, van Capelle FJL, Freud GE, et al. Circus movement within the AV node as a basis for supraventricular tachycardia as shown by multiple microelectrode recordings in the isolated rabbit heart. *Circ Res.* 1971;28:403–414.

27. Bukauskas FF, Veteikis RP. Passive electrical properties of the atrioventricular region of the rabbit heart. *Biofizika.* 1977;35:909–922.
28. Spach MS, Dolber PC. Relating extracellular potentials and their derivatives to anisotropic propagation at a microscopic level in human cardiac muscle: evidence for electrical uncoupling of side-to-side fiber connections with increasing age. *Circ Res.* 1986;58:356–371.
29. Spach MS, Heidlage JF, Darken ER, et al. Cellular Vmax reflects both membrane properties and the load presented by adjoining cells. *Am J Physiol.* 1992;263:H1855–H1863.
30. Ross DL, Brugada P, Bar FWHM, et al. Comparison of right and left atrial stimulation in demonstration of dual atrioventricular nodal pathways and induction of intranodal reentry. *Circulation.* 1981;64:1051–1058.
31. Josephson ME. *Clinical Cardiac Electrophysiology: Techniques and Interpretations.* 2nd ed. Philadelphia, Pa: Lea & Febiger; 1993:181–310.
32. Monahan KM, Zardini M, Boyle NG, et al. Site specific differences in conduction characteristics during initiation of reentry in AVNRT. *Pacing Clin Electrophysiol.* 1995;18:823.
33. Monahan KM, Boyle NG, Zardini M, et al. Resetting responses during atrioventricular nodal reentrant tachycardia suggest an anisotrophic mechanism. *J Am Coll Cardiol.* 1995;25:129-A. Abstract.
34. Hook BG, Callans DJ, Mitra RL, et al. Limitations to the concept of discrete AV nodal pathways. *J Am Coll Cardiol.* 1993;21:281.
35. McGuire MA, Bourke JP, Robotin MC, et al. High resolution mapping of Koch's triangle using sixty electrodes in humans with atrioventricular junctional (AV nodal) tachycardia. *Circulation.* 1993;88:2315–2328.
36. Josephson ME, Miller JM. AV nodal reentry: evidence supporting an intranodal location. *Pacing Clin Electrophysiol.* 1993;16:599–614.
37. Wellens HJJ, Wesdorp JC, Duren DR, et al. Second degree block during reciprocal atrioventricular nodal reentry. *Circulation.* 1976;53:595–599.
38. Ko PT, Naccarelli GV, Gulamhusein S, et al. Atrioventricular dissociation during paroxysmal junctional tachycardia. *Pacing Clin Electrophysiol.* 1981; 4:670–678.
39. Anderson RH, Becker AE, Brechenmacher C, et al. The human atrioventricular junctional area: a morphological study of the AV node and bundle. *Eur J Cardiol.* 1975;3:11–25.
40. Furberg CD, Manolio TA, Psaty BM, et al. Major electrocardiographic abnormalities in persons aged 65 years and older (the cardiovascular health study). *Am J Cardiol.* 1992;69:1329–1335.
41. Anselme F, Frederiks J, Papageorgiou P, et al. Nonuniform anisotropy is responsible for age-related slowing of atrioventricular reentrant tachycardia. *J Cardiovasc Electrophysiol.* 7(12):1145–1153.
42. Waldo AL, MacLean WAH, Karp RB, et al. Entrainment and interruption of atrial flutter with atrial pacing: studies in man following open heart surgery. *Circulation.* 1977;56:737–745.
43. Inoue H, Matsuo H, Takayanagi K, et al. Clinical and experimental studies of the effects of atrial extrastimuli and rapid pacing on atrial flutter cycle: evidence of macro-reentry with an excitable gap. *Am J Cardiol.* 1981;48: 623–631.
44. Watson RM, Josephson ME. Atrial flutter, I: electrophysiologic substrates and modes of initiation and termination. *Am J Cardiol.* 1980;45:732–741.
45. Buxton AE, Waxman HL, Marchlinski FE, et al. Atrial conduction: effects of extrastimuli with and without atrial dysrhythmias. *Am J Cardiol.* 1984; 54:755–761.

46. Almendral JM, Arenal A, Abeytus M, et al. Incidence and patterns of resetting during atrial flutter: role in identifying chamber of origin. *J Am Coll Cardiol*. 1987;9:153A. Abstract.
47. Cosio FG, Palacios J, Vidal JM, et al. Electrophysiologic studies in atrial fibrillation: slow conduction of premature impulses: a possible manifestation of the background for reentry. *Am J Cardiol*. 1983;51:122–130.
48. Papageorgiou P, Monahan K, Boyle N, et al. Site-dependent intra-atrial conduction delay: relationship to initiation of atrial fibrillation. *Circulation*. 1996;94:384–389.
49. Allessie MA, Lammers WJEP, Bonke FIM, et al. Experimental evaluation of Moe's multiple wavelet hypothesis of atrial fibrillation. In: Zipes DP, Jalife J, eds. *Cardiac Electrophysiology and Arrhythmias*. New York, NY: Grune & Stratton, Inc; 1985:265–276.
50. Konings KTS, Kirchhof CJHJ, Smeets JRLM, et al. High-density mapping of electrically induced atrial fibrillation in humans. *Circulation*. 1994;89: 1665–1680.
51. Allessie MA, Kirchhof CJHJ, Scheffer GJ, et al. Regional control of atrial fibrillation by rapid pacing in conscious dogs. *Circulation*. 1991;84: 1689–1697.
52. Kirchhof CJHJ, Chorro FJ, Scheffer GJ, et al. Regional entrainment of atrial fibrillation studied by high-resolution mapping in open-chest dogs. *Circulation*. 1993;88:736–749.
53. Watson RM, Schwartz JL, Maron BJ, et al. Inducible polymorphic ventricular tachycardia and ventricular fibrillation in a subgroup of patients with hypertrophic cardiomyopathy at high risk for sudden death. *J Am Coll Cardiol*. 1987;10:761–774.
54. Saumarez RC, Camm AJ, Panagos A, et al. Ventricular fibrillation in hypertrophic cardiomyopathy is associated with increased fractionation of paced right ventricular electrograms. *Circulation*. 1992;86:467–474.

Gating and Modulation
of Gap Junctions
Introduction

Eric C. Beyer MD, PhD

Gap junctions are sarcolemmal specializations that provide a major component of cardiac intercellular resistance, and the gating of these channels or the modulation of their number or distribution significantly affects the patterns and rates of cardiac conduction. Studies of the role of gap junctions in conduction have been facilitated by recent progress using molecular strategies following the cloning of subunit gap junction proteins and the development of powerful experimental models for the physiological evaluation of cardiac conduction.

This section includes five chapters devoted to the structure, function, and regulation of cardiac gap junctions. These chapters present a range of studies, from a detailed examination of individual channels through evaluation of conduction in cardiac muscle.

In chapter 7, Dr. Yeager considers the structure of the connexin protein and of the gap junctional channel. Data derived from x-ray scattering and electron microscopic analysis of isolated liver gap junctions have led to the development of a model of the structure of gap junctions. Dr. Yeager has extended the analyses to isolated cardiac gap junctions. He also presents new, higher-resolution data derived from electron cryocrystallography of an exogenously expressed truncated form of recombinant connexin43 (Cx43). These studies give our best views yet of structure and function derived directly from gap junction molecular architecture.

Gap junction channels are regulated by a number of cytoplasmic factors. Dr. Delmar and colleagues have focused on the regulation of Cx43 channels by intracellular pH. Using the paired *Xenopus* oocyte expression system and the expression of Cx43, these authors have identified two regions of the molecule involved in pH gating and they propose a ball-and-chain model for this process.

Passage of ions and small molecules through gap junctions can lead not only to current conduction but also to other important cellular consequences. Drs. ter Keurs and Zhang have studied isolated rat ventricular and human atrial trabeculae and present exciting data implicating gap junction-mediated transport of Ca^{2+} in the contractions and arrhythmias caused by acute damage to cardiac muscle. Their data suggest that local release of Ca^{2+} in a damaged region causes a Ca^{2+} transient that is conducted into intact muscle by the combination of Ca^{2+} diffusion through gap junctions and Ca^{2+}-induced Ca^{2+} release.

Although there is consensus that gap junction channels are important for intercellular passage of current-carrying ions, the magnitude of the importance of gap junction derangements in the development of reentrant arrhythmias has not been demonstrated. Dr. Kléber and colleagues have developed a tissue culture model in which neonatal cardiac myocytes can be grown in patterned arrays. Using high-resolution optical mapping, these authors assess microscopic conduction in such cultures. Their analyses emphasize the complexities of impulse propagation in the myocardium and the interactions of determining variables.

Dr. Spray and colleagues have performed extensive analyses of the physiological properties of cardiac gap junction channels. Their analyses include examination of the endogenous channels in cardiac myocytes as well as channels derived from the exogenous expression of cloned cardiac connexins. The physiological and biophysical properties of cardiac connexins are summarized. The authors also present a wide-ranging discussion of other issues related to these gap junctions, including potential explanations for the diversity of connexins and the potential for pharmacological manipulation of gap junction channels.

Chapter 7

Structure of Cardiac Gap Junction Membrane Channels:
Progress Toward a Higher Resolution Model

Mark Yeager, M.D., Ph.D.

Gap junctions are specialized regions of contact between cells that enable them to exchange nutrient and signal molecules and thereby coordinate their metabolic and electrical activities.[1] Gap junction protein subunits (connexins) assemble into a hemi-channel (called a connexon) that spans the lipid bilayer. The end-to-end interaction between the two connexons within the plasma membranes of adjacent cells occurs in the narrow extracellular gap, from which the name "gap junction" is derived (Figure 1). Hundreds of such intercellular channels are aggregated within a gap junction plaque.

Cardiac gap junctions reside in the intercalated disk[2] and maintain a functional syncytium in the heart by electrically coupling myocardial cells, thereby mediating intercellular propagation of the action potential.[3] The electrical coupling via cardiac gap junctions organizes the pattern of current flow, resulting in coordinated contraction of the muscle. In addition, altered gap junction current flow has been implicated in the genesis of potentially lethal arrhythmias.[4,5]

This study was supported by grants from the National Heart, Lung, and Blood Institute, a Grant-in-Aid from the American Heart Association, National Center, the Gustavus and Louise Pfeiffer Research Foundation, and the Donald E. and Delia B. Baxter Research Foundation. Dr. Yeager is an Established Investigator of the American Heart Association and Bristol-Myers Squibb.

The multigene family of gap junction proteins has been divided into two connexin types, α and β (Reference 21), on the basis of features in the amino acid sequences. An alternative nomenclature uses the molecular weight to specify individual connexins (Reference 19). In this article, we will include the CxMW designation in parentheses after the α and β designation.

From: Spooner PM, Joyner RW, Jalife J (eds). *Discontinuous Conduction in the Heart.* Armonk, NY: Futura Publishing Company, Inc.; © 1997.

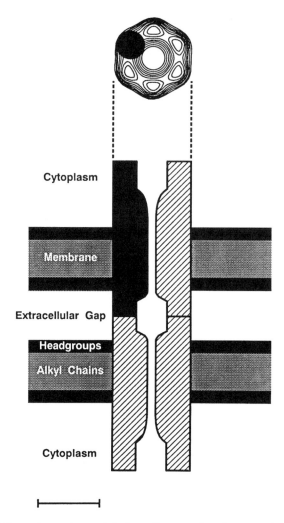

Figure 1. Schematic scale model of cardiac gap junction membrane channel (scale bar = 50 Å) based on planar density maps (shown above model) and edge-on density maps perpendicular to membrane plane provided by electron microscopy and image analysis of 2D crystals. In region of gap junction, plasma membranes of adjacent cells come into close contact via a narrow extracellular gap, from which name is derived. Gap junction is formed by aggregation of protein oligomers, called connexons, that are in register between cells, thereby forming a central channel that allows intercellular communication. Characteristic features of gap junction are closely apposed lipid bilayers, and connexons of adjacent membranes are in register to form central channel. Each connexon has a diameter of ≈65 Å and is formed by a hexameric cluster of connexin subunits. Detailed shape and transmembrane structure of channel have not been determined and are depicted here in a stylized fashion. Reprinted with permission from Reference 12.

Single-cell electrophysiology coupled with site-directed mutagenesis has provided a wealth of knowledge about the function of ion channels. However, there is a comparative paucity of experimental data about the structure of ion channels. As noted by Christopher Miller[6] in his appraisal of Bertil Hille's book, *Ionic Channels of Excitable Membranes,*[7] "The new edition makes it clear that future progress in the field will in addition depend upon a subject only recently relevant to ion channels—protein chemistry and macromolecular structure." With this in mind, we have been examining the structure of cardiac gap junction membrane channels for several years, using an integrated approach that employs complementary biophysical, biochemical, and spectroscopic techniques. Our ultimate goal is to delineate the molecular structure at a level of detail that will enable us to propose a chemically reasonable mechanism for channel gating. An atomic model for the channel will be fundamental for understanding the molecular basis of current flow in the heart and mechanisms of cardiac arrhythmias and will be essential for structure-based drug design. A complete understanding of arrhythmogenesis will also be contingent on knowledge about the expression and regulation of different connexin genes,[8] the biosynthesis and turnover of gap junctions,[9] the electrophysiological behavior of connexins,[10] and pathophysiological effects on the size, number, and location of gap junctions in the heart.[11]

In this chapter we summarize our results from negative stain and cryoelectron microscopy, indirect immunocytochemistry, and circular dichroism (CD) spectroscopy, which will be placed in the context of structural studies on other connexins. In addition, we will also present an integrated strategy that combines spectroscopic, x-ray, and electron crystallographic techniques to examine the structure and dynamics of integral membrane proteins. This chapter is based on our recent general summaries of gap junction structure.[12,13] Additional recent reviews on the structure and function of gap junctions include Reference 10 and References 14 through 18. Reviews on the multigene family of gap junction proteins have also been presented.[19–21]

Closely Apposed Lipid Bilayers are the 'Morphological Signature' of Gap Junctions

Conventional thin-section electron microscopy has served as a keystone for defining the "morphological signature" of gap junctions. Although the nuances of stain distribution may vary with the preparative technique,[22] the characteristic appearance is septalaminar, with stain exclusion in the hydrophobic domains of the lipid bilayers and stain accumulation in the extracellular gap and on the cytoplasmic faces. In contrast, tight junctions appear pentalaminar by thin-section electron microscopy.[22-25] The morphology of gap junctions has been further delineated by freeze-fracture microscopy, which has revealed that gap junctions appear to lack any connections with the cytoskeleton.[26]

Membrane Topology of Connexins Has Been Delineated by Immunocytochemistry and Protease Cleavage

Over the past decade, more than a dozen connexin gene products have been cloned and sequenced.[19-21] Hydropathy analyses of the amino acid sequences have shown considerable homology in the four hydrophobic domains (M1, M2, M3, and M4) as well as the two loops (E1 and E2) predicted to reside in the extracellular space (Figure 2). The carboxy-terminal domain and the hydrophilic loop connecting M2 and M3 are the most variable in size and sequence. The multigene family of connexins has been divided into two types, α and β.[21] Compared with the β-type connexins, the α-type connexins such as α_1 (Cx43), have a larger loop between M2 and M3 and a substantially larger carboxy-tail (Figure 2).

Detailed topological studies of three members of the connexin family—the principal gap junction protein in the heart, α_1 (Cx43); in rat liver, β_1 (Cx32); and in mouse liver, β_2 (Cx26)—have used a combination of labeling by site-specific, anti-peptide antibodies and treatments with highly specific proteases (Figure 2). The narrow extracellular gap is a feature that has been particularly useful for delineating the polypeptide topology, because macromolecular probes such as proteases and antibodies are excluded, unless specific treatments are used to separate the membranes.[27-29] In contrast, treatment of intact junctions with proteases has revealed that the carboxy-tail distal to M4 and the loop between M2 and M3 are accessible on the cytoplasmic membrane face.[30-33] In addition, sequences predicted by hydropathy analysis to reside on the cytoplasmic surface are readily accessible for labeling by site-specific peptide antibodies as demonstrated by indirect immunogold electron microscopy.[33-35]

The 2D Density Map Derived by Electron Microscopic Image Analysis Reveals That the Hexameric Quaternary Structure Is a Conserved Structural Motif of Connexons

Biochemically isolated liver gap junctions display hexagonal paracrystalline packing of the connexons. This critical feature has allowed

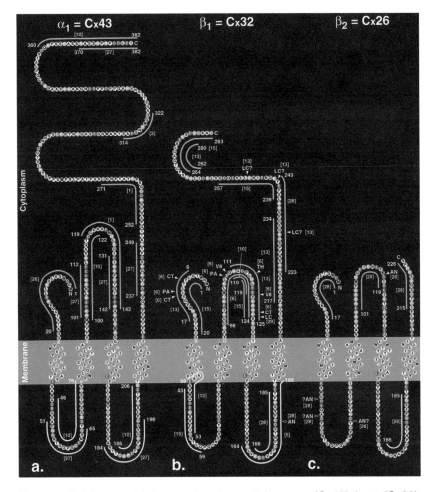

Figure 2. Folding models for gap junction proteins. a, α_1 (Cx43); b, β_1 (Cx32); and c, β_2 (Cx26). Amino-acid sequences of α_1 (Cx43),[102] β_1 (Cx32),[103,104] and β_2 (Cx26)[105] were deduced from cDNA analysis, and residues are coded as follows: hydrophobic in yellow, acidic in red, basic in blue, and cysteine in green. Hydropathy analysis predicts four membrane-spanning domains, referred to as M1, M2, M3, and M4, proceeding from N- to C-terminus. Predicted locations of extracellular and cytoplasmic regions were confirmed with site-directed antibodies (blue and yellow bars indicate cytoplasmic and extracellular epitopes, respectively) and proteases (solid arrowheads indicate sites accessible from cytoplasmic face; open arrowheads, sites accessible only after separation of membranes). CT indicates chymotrypsin; PA, proteinase A; V8, staphylococcal V8 protease; TH, thrombin; LC, Lys-C protease; and AN, Asp-N protease. Note three conserved cysteine residues (shown in green) located in each extracellular loop (designated E1 and E2) of three connexins.

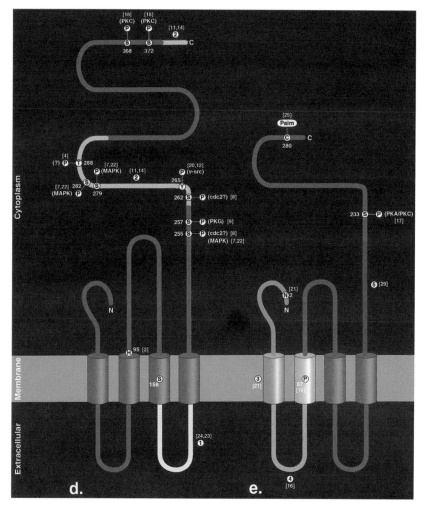

Figure 2. *(continued)* d, α_1 (Cx43) and e, β_1 (Cx32), indicating locations of various functionally important residues [Ser[158] and His[95] in α_1 (Cx43) and Asn[2] and Pro[87] in β_1 (Cx32)] and domains 1 (yellow) and 2 (blue) in α_1 (Cx43) and 3 (orange), 4 (green), and 5 (violet) in β_1 (Cx32) as determined by mutagenesis and chimera studies. Indicated sites of covalent modification are based on consensus sequences, modification of synthetic peptides in vitro, and mutagenesis studies. Significance of functional domains (circled numbers) and specifically mutated residues are as follows: Domain 1 (yellow) is the predominant determinant for specificity of heterotypic interactions between α_1 (Cx43), α_8 (Cx50), and α_3 (Cx46). [This result was based on chimeras of α_8 (Cx50) and α_3 (Cx46).] Domains 2 (blue) impart high sensitivity to pH gating of α_1 (Cx43). Gating by pH is also influenced by charge on His[95]. Domain 3 (orange) determines polarity of voltage sensor where an Asn[2] to Asp[2] change from β_1 (Cx32) to β_2 (Cx26) changes gating polarity. Domains 3 (orange) and 4 (green) deter-

the application of electron microscopy and digital image processing, first used by Caspar et al[36] to examine mouse liver gap junctions and subsequently by Zampighi and Unwin[37] to examine rat liver gap junctions. Gap junctions isolated from other tissues typically do not exhibit such a crystalline arrangement of the channels. Nevertheless, heart[33,38] and lens[39] gap junctions have been manipulated in order to grow 2D crystals amenable to electron microscopy and image analysis. As reviewed by Moody,[40] digital image processing of electron micrographs results in an enhanced reconstruction of a 2D crystalline specimen because (1) the diffraction pattern is generated by all molecules in the crystal, thereby improving the signal-to-noise ratio; (2) noise in the images is evident between the diffraction spots and can be removed by filtering; (3) symmetry relationships for the packing of molecules in the crystal may be used to further reduce noise; and (4) the phases for computing the density map by Fourier transformation are directly calculated from the images, unlike x-ray diffraction, in which the phase information is lost. The 2D projection density map is computed by inverse Fourier transformation and provides an enhanced view of the distribution of mass compared with the original unprocessed images.[41]

Several caveats regarding the method of electron microscopy and image analysis should be noted. The method is an averaging technique, so that the expression of multiple connexins within the cells of the same tissue could result in different types of molecular heterogeneity that could account for the limited resolution and some of the disorder observed in native gap junctions.[42] For instance, mouse liver gap junctions

---

mine voltage gating parameters; first extracellular loop, E1, is important in determining transjunctional voltage required for closure; Pro[87] serves as a critical feature of M2 involved in transduction of voltage response. [This observation was based on studies in β_2(Cx26) but has not been confirmed for other connexins]. Domain 5 (violet) constitutes potential calmodulin binding sites. Size and hydrophobicity of Ser[158] in α_1 (Cx43) influence permeability of larger dyes through gap junction pore (A.P. Moreno and D.C. Spray, personal communication). Numbered references are as follows: [1] Beyer et al[106]; [2] Ek et al[61]; [3] el Aoumari et al[107]; [4] Goldberg and Lau[108]; [5] Goodenough et al[109]; [6] Hertzberg et al[110]; [7] Kanamitsu and Lau[111]; [8] Kennelly and Krebs[112]; [9] Kwak et al[113]; [10] Laird and Revel[35]; [11] Liu et al[60]; [12] Loo et al[59]; [13] Milks et al[29]; [14] Morley et al[62]; [15] Rahman and Evans[114]; [16] Rubin et al[115]; [17] Saez et al[116]; [18] Saez et al[117]; [19] Suchyna et al[118]; [20] Swenson et al[58]; [21] Verselis et al[119]; [22] Warn-Cramer et al[120]; [23] White et al[121]; [24] White et al[51]; [25] Willecke et al[122]; [26] Yancey et al[34]; [27] Yeager and Gilula[33]; [28] Zhang and Nicholson[123]; and [29] Zimmer et al.[28] Reprinted with permission from Reference 12.

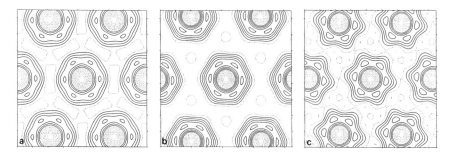

Figure 3. Comparison of 2D projection density maps for a, cardiac gap junction,[33,38] b, liver gap junctions,[54] and c, mouse gap junctions.[52] Although unit cell spacings varied (90, 84, and 81 Å, respectively), maps were all computed at 20-Å resolution. There is conservation in hexameric design of channels. However, there are notable differences in diameters of channels and shapes of hexameric connexons. Scale marks are 20 Å. Reprinted with permission from Reference 41.

not only contain β_1 (Cx32) but also β_2 (Cx26). At 15 to 20Å* resolution, subtle differences in the 2D projection density maps of homomeric channels formed by β_1 (Cx32) and β_2 (Cx26) would not be apparent in an averaged map derived from gap junctions containing a mixed population of channels.[43] Likewise, cardiac tissue contains multiple connexins.[44–47] In addition, an averaged map at 15Å resolution would also probably obscure heteromeric connexons in which oligomers are formed by different connexins. Evidence has been presented that lens gap junctions may indeed contain heteromeric connexons.[48] As another example, the acetylcholine receptor is formed by a heteropentamer containing β, δ, γ and two α subunits. Projection density maps at 17Å resolution do not reveal major differences between the homologous but different subunits.[49] Another type of heterogeneity would involve heterotypic channels[50,51] formed by homomeric connexons containing different connexins. Last, variability in the stoichiometry of the oligomer would also limit the resolution of the crystals. For instance, a small fraction of pentameric or heptameric connexons would be obscured in an averaged map at 15-Å resolution of a crystal containing predominantly hexamers. Even in a gap junction population containing just one connexin, there are additional sources of heterogeneity: conformational flexibility in the polypeptide, partial denaturation during isolation, the presence of nonconnexin proteins within the crystals, different degrees of posttranslational modification, fluid interactions at the protein-lipid interface that would allow rotational flexibility of the connexons in

---

* 10 Å = 1 nm.

the lattice, and lipid heterogeneity that may prevent precise chemical interactions at the protein-lipid interface that may be necessary for 2D crystallization of the connexons.

Despite these provisos, the projection density maps of different gap junction specimens at 20-Å resolution display intriguing differences that may relate to bona fide chemical differences in structure (Figure 3). For instance, the maps of mouse liver gap junctions[52] have shown density on the three-fold symmetry axis that has been interpreted as an arm of the connexin polypeptide.[53] Alternatively, this density may represent nonconnexin protein, but electrophoresis of isolated gap junctions does not suggest a substantial amount of nonconnexin protein. Maps of rat liver gap junctions[54] have not shown significant density on the threefold axis. In addition, a map has been derived for liver gap junctions from crude preparations of plasma membranes, thereby minimizing the effects of sarkosyl or alkali treatment and multiple centrifugation steps.[55] The projection density map displayed the characteristic hexameric connexons as well as an absence of density on the threefold axis. Interestingly, the density map of cardiac gap junctions[33,38] reveals a larger central channel compared with gap junctions containing β connexins. In addition, the reduced modulation of the subunits may be due to the larger carboxy-tail (compare Figure 4c with 4a). But such differences may also be related to differences in the isolation method or variability in negative staining. Cryoelectron microscopy of heart and liver gap junctions isolated by the same protocol should allow careful scrutiny of these differences.

Despite detailed differences in the projection density maps of different gap junction specimens, there are important conserved features. For instance, the oligomeric connexon with a central channel is a conserved motif in the design of gap junction membrane channels (Figure 3). Gap junction channels can also be simply viewed as having a modular design. Homology in the transmembrane sequences (Figure 2) suggests that there may be a common architecture for the transmembrane channel. Similarly, sequence homology in the extracellular domains suggests similar mechanisms for connexon-connexon interactions. However, it is clear that detailed differences in the extracellular loops place restrictions on the allowed pairing of different connexons. Last, the cytoplasmic loop between M2 and M3 and especially the carboxy-tail are the most divergent in sequence and size. Such divergence may confer unique functional properties. Indeed, the C-terminal domain of connexins plays an important role in regulating channel properties. For instance, differences in channel conductance were associated with C-terminal truncation[56] or phosphorylation.[57] Closure of α_1 (Cx43) channels was also effected by pp60v-src phosphorylation within the C-terminal domain[58,59] or by intracellular acidification.[60–62] Point mutations

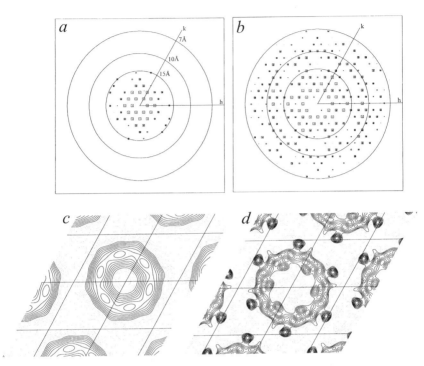

Figure 4. Computed diffraction patterns (a and b) and projection density maps (c and d) for gap junctions containing a recombinant form of rat heart α_1 (Cx43) in which majority of C-terminal domain has been deleted (truncation at Lys[263]).[87,88] a, Negatively stained crystals display diffraction to $\approx$15-Å resolution; b, When unstained crystals are examined by electron cryomicroscopy, diffraction patterns extend to $\approx$7-Å resolution. c, Projection density map at 15-Å resolution shows hexameric connexons, similar to maps at comparable resolution from rat heart gap junctions.[33,38] Diffraction patterns extend to a nominal resolution of $\approx$15 Å, and computed phases to this level of resolution are consistent with plane group symmetry p6, which has been enforced. d, Preliminary projection density map at 7-Å resolution displays three major features: a ring of circular densities centered at radius 17 Å interpreted as α-helices that line the channel, a ring of densities centered at 33-Å radius interpreted as α-helices that are most exposed to lipid, and a continuous band of density at 25-Å radius separating the two groups of helices. Hexagonal lattice had parameters $a = b = 79$ Å and $\gamma = 120°$. Spacing between grid bars is 40 Å. Reprinted with permission from Reference 12.

in the C-terminal domain of α_1 (Cx43) are also associated with developmental anomalies in the cardiovascular system.[63]

3D Electron Microscopy Reveals the Connexon Molecular Boundary

Despite the limiting resolution, electron microscopy and image analysis have been powerful methods for defining the 3D molecular envelope of the connexons in liver gap junctions. The approach relies on the ability to tilt the membrane crystals via the rotation stage of the electron microscope.[64] The projected views represent planar sections through the 3D density map. The 2D sections are combined in Fourier space, and the 3D Fourier transform is interpolated in the regions for which sections were not obtained. The 3D density map is then obtained by inverse Fourier transformation. This approach was pioneered by Henderson and Unwin[65] in their analysis of bacteriorhodopsin membrane crystals.

3D density maps have been derived for rat liver gap junctions either stained with uranyl acetate[66] or in the frozen-hydrated state.[67] Specimens imaged by negative stain microscopy are sensitive to beam-induced shrinkage,[68] and the thickness of the liver gap junction determined by 3D electron microscopy[66] was adjusted to match the membrane thickness measured from x-ray scattering of hydrated specimens.[69] Since the stain puddles around the perimeter of the specimen, the images are a representation of the molecular envelope. In the case of cryoelectron microscopy of unstained specimens, the derived maps reveal not only the surface contours of a structure but also the internal organization (eg, see Reference 70). Cryoelectron microscopy of unstained samples also minimizes the potential specimen shrinkage and distortion encountered with negative-stain microscopy. Nonetheless, the overall low-resolution maps obtained by negative-stain and cryoelectron microscopy are quite similar.

The rat liver gap junction connexon is formed by a cluster of six rodlike subunits oriented roughly perpendicular to the membrane plane. The subunits have a diameter of ≈ 25 Å and surround a central channel that has a diameter of ≈ 20 Å. At a resolution of 18 Å, the contours of the channel within the hydrophobic interior of the bilayer are not revealed. The connexon extends ≈ 20 Å into the extracellular space so that the gap is ≈ 40 Å thick. Interestingly, the 3D maps only resolve density extending ≈ 10 Å into the cytoplasmic space. This is substantially less than would be expected, knowing that the amino terminal loop, the carboxy-tail, and the loop between M2 and M3 should all reside on the cytoplasmic face and account for more than one third of the mass of β_1 (Cx32), the predominant connexin in rat liver gap junctions. One possible explanation is that the cytoplasmic domains exhibit conformational flexibility so that their density would be smeared out during crystallographic averaging. Another explanation is that the map is less well resolved in the z direction perpendicular to the membrane because the specimens can only be tilted up to ≈60°. The resulting "missing cone" of data tends to smear the map in the z direction. A comparison of the x-ray-scattering density profiles of native and trypsin-treated mouse liver gap junctions showed that protein extends 85 to 90 Å from the center of the gap.[53] The lipid headgroup region on the cytoplasmic leaflet of the bilayer is centered ≈64 Å from the center of the gap. Assuming a head-group region ≈10 Å thick, the cytoplasmic protein extends 15 to 20 Å beyond the membrane surface, which should certainly be sufficient to accommodate the connexin domains predicted to reside on the cytoplasmic face, particularly given the higher complement of β_2 (Cx26) in mouse liver gap junctions. Cardiac gap junctions have a thickness of ≈250 Å (Figure 1) so that the protein on the cytoplasmic face may extend 40 to 50 Å from the membrane surface, as was suggested by freeze-etched images[71] and which is consistent with the larger size of the α_1 (Cx43) carboxy-tail and the loop connecting M2 and M3 (Figure 2) compared with the β connexins.

Indirect Evidence Suggests That the Transmembrane Domains May Be α-Helical

The 3D density map of the liver gap junction connexon at 18-Å resolution defines the molecular boundary of the cylindrical connexin subunits and the hexameric quaternary structure.[67] However, the map is not of sufficient resolution to define the folding of the polypeptide chain. Analysis of membrane topology confirms the cytoplasmic location of the N- and C-termini and the presence of four conserved hydrophobic domains, consistent with transmembrane regions. Although the transmembrane domains can be modeled as α-helices, direct evidence for this secondary structure is lacking. Hypothetical working models for the secondary structure have been based on inferences from (1) the topological mapping of the primary sequence (see above) combined with the 3D density maps provided by electron image analysis,[29,67] (2) x-ray diffraction patterns,[53,72] and (3) CD spectroscopy.[73,74]

1. The topological studies described above support a folding model with four transmembrane domains of sufficient length that they could be folded as α-helices. By analogy with soluble proteins having four anti-parallel α-helices, a model was proposed by Milks et al[29] in which the four transmembrane domains of β_1 (Cx32) are folded as a

four-helix bundle that could be accommodated within the cross-sectional area of each connexin, estimated as 500Å^2 from 3D density maps of the liver gap junction connexon. Six M3 transmembrane domains from each of the six subunits were proposed to form the boundary of the aqueous channel, because M3 contains a series of polar amino acids spaced so that they could form an amphipathic α-helix.

2. The x-ray diffraction patterns recorded from oriented liver gap junction membranes display sharp fringes centered at ≈ 4.7 Å on the meridian and diffraction centered at ≈ 11 Å on the equator. These patterns were initially interpreted as β-sheets with the strands running more parallel than perpendicular to the surface.[75] To test this hypothesis, connexon models were built that contained a transmembrane core based on known soluble protein structures that were formed by α-helical bundle and β-sheet conformations.[72] In fact, the predicted diffraction patterns for purely α-helical conformations were in closer agreement with the x-ray diffraction data. For α-helices packed perpendicular to the membrane plane, a diffraction fringe at ≈ 5 Å would have been predicted. However, in four-helix-bundle proteins, the helices are tilted with respect to each other, resulting in a shift of the fringe to ≈ 4.7 Å.

3. From 190 to 240 nm, CD spectra of proteins are sensitive to molecular geometry and are therefore quite useful for determining protein secondary structure and monitoring conformational changes.[76–80] CD spectra recorded from suspensions of rat liver and heart gap junction membranes display considerable similarity to the spectra for a polypeptide with an α-helical conformation, and the estimated content of α-helix (40% to 50%) is sufficient so that the four transmembrane domains may be folded as α-helices.

Expression of Recombinant Connexins Combined with Cryoelectron Microscopy Is Yielding Higher-Resolution Structural Data

To obtain direct experimental evidence for the presence of α-helices, crystals have to be coherently ordered to better than 10-Å resolution. Three membrane proteins have been crystallized in lipid bilayers and examined in three dimensions at near-atomic resolution by electron diffraction (bacteriorhodopsin,[81] bacterial porin,[82] and the light harvesting complex II of photosynthetic membranes[83]). In each case, the protein was highly purified and homogeneous. On the basis of this experience, growth of high-resolution 2D crystals of connexons will require chemically pure protein. However, the source to date for 2D crystallization studies of gap junctions have been preparations isolated from heart, liver, and the lens of the eye. For example, isolated cardiac gap junctions possess very little inherent crystallinity compared with liver gap junctions. A strategy for in situ crystallization is to expose the isolated junctions to low concentrations of nonionic detergents to extract lipid and concentrate the protein in the membrane plane.[38]

Because of the possible molecular heterogeneity in gap junctions from native tissues, it is probable that growth of high-resolution 2D crystals will be quite difficult. An alternative approach is to overexpress a single recombinant connexin by use of SF9 insect cells and the baculovirus vector, with synthesis driven by the polyhedrin promotor.[84] Overexpressed membrane proteins often form insoluble inclusion bodies because of improper folding. The ability of overexpressed connexins to self-assemble as recognizable gap junction structures in infected cells is convincing evidence that the recombinant protein folds in a native conformation. Initial 3D crystallization trials were encouraging,[84] but high-resolution crystals for x-ray analysis have not been forthcoming. Compared with other polytopic membrane proteins, the pairing of connexon hemichannels in the double-membrane structure of the gap junction is unique and may result in that are relatively unstable in hemichannels detergent solution. Although paired connexons may be more stable, crystallization of such a large complex with two hydrophobic "belts" of detergent is likely to pose a difficult 3D crystallization task. Alternatively, detergent-solubilized and purified connexons may be amenable to in vitro reconstitution with lipids to grow high-resolution 2D crystals.[85]

More recently, recombinant connexins have been expressed in a stably transfected baby hamster kidney cell line under control of the inducible metallothionin promotor.[86] A recombinant rat α_1 (Cx43) that lacks most of the large C-terminal domain (truncation at Lys^{263}) assembles into gap junctions having the characteristic septalaminar morphology. Freeze-fracture images revealed that the gap junctions form small 2D crystals, and the crystallinity could be improved by extraction with nondenaturing detergents such as Tween20,[87,88] an approach similar to that taken for crystallization of native rat heart gap junctions.[38]

A projection density map derived from negatively stained recombinant α_1 Cx crystals (Figure 4c) closely resembles the maps for native cardiac gap junction membranes.[33,38] The recombinant connexon has a diameter of ≈ 65 Å and is formed by a hexameric cluster of connexin subunits. The preliminary density map at 7-Å resolution (Figure 4d) reveals distinct structural features related to each connexin subunit. In particular, at 17-Å radius, the channel is lined by circular densities that have the characteristic appearance of transmembrane α-helices oriented perpendicular to the membrane plane.[81] A similar appearance for densities at 33-Å radius suggests that α-helices are at the interface with the membrane lipids. The continuous band of density at 25-Å radius separates the two rings. Definitive interpretation of these densities will of course require further analysis of the 2D crystals as well as a 3D structure analysis by tilt reconstruction.

Constraints on Possible Molecular Models for Gap Junction Intercellular Channels

The pattern of the α-helices that are resolved in the projection map places constraints on possible structural models for the intercellular channel. For instance, the model shown in Figure 5 is in agreement with the projection density map in Figure 4d, which shows superposition of the resolved α-helices. The superposition of the helices and this rotation dictate that the α-helices within one connexin will be superimposed with helices within two connexin subunits in the apposed connexon. Note that this model predicts that each subunit in one connexon will make contact with two connexin subunits in the apposing connexon. Such an arrangement may confer stability in the docking of the connexons. As a consequence of the 30° displacement between the inner and outer rings of α-helices, the two connexons forming the channel are rotationally staggered with respect to each other (as shown by the arcs in Figure 5). Models that are inconsistent with the projection map in-

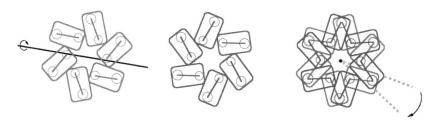

Figure 5. Schematic model for packing of α-helices, connexins, and connexons in gap junction intercellular channel.[88] Each connexin subunit is represented by a rectangle, and transmembrane α-helices are depicted as circles. Two-fold symmetry axes located in extracellular gap generate views of apposed connexons in cell 1 (red) and cell 2 (blue) that form intercellular channel. Superposition is in accordance with observed projection density map (Figure 4d) and predicts that connexons within channel will be rotationally staggered, as shown by dashed lines and arc. Superposition of helices and this rotation dictate that α-helices within one connexin will be superimposed with helices within two connexin subunits in apposed connexon (ie, one red subunit makes contact with two blue subunits and vice versa). Reprinted with permission from Reference 88.

clude those with $<30°$ of rotational stagger between the connexons, which would tend to generate 12 rather than 6 peaks in the outer ring of densities. In addition, the 30° displacement between the rings of helices is not consistent with models in which the α-helices are collinear through the center of the channel (eg, see Figure 6a in Milks et al[29]).

With the positions of two putative transmembrane α-helices within each subunit of a recombinant cardiac gap junction channel having been resolved, additional transmembrane domains may reside within the continuous band of density at a 25-Å radius. The three distinct domains within this continuous band of density cannot be interpreted unambiguously. However, it is likely that the three domains represent a superposition of projections of additional transmembrane α-helices and polypeptide density arising from the extracellular and intracellular loops within each connexin subunit. A definitive interpretation of these densities and further scrutiny of the model proposed in Figure 5 will only be possible by a 3D analysis based on images recorded from tilted crystals.

An Integrated Strategy for Structure Analysis of Membrane Proteins Combines Spectroscopy, X-Ray Crystallography, and Cryoelectron Microscopy

Useful spectroscopic techniques for examining membrane protein structure include (1) CD spectroscopy (described above), (2) Fourier transform infrared (FTIR) spectroscopy, (3) fluorescence spectroscopy, (4) electron paramagnetic resonance (EPR) spectroscopy, and (5) nuclear magnetic resonance (NMR) spectroscopy.

The advantage of FTIR spectroscopy is that spectra can be recorded from stacked membrane pellets that are fully hydrated so that information can be obtained about the angular orientation of α-helices with respect to the membrane surface.[89–92]

Time-resolved fluorescence spectroscopy is a powerful method for examining conformational dynamics.[93,94,95a] This approach may be particularly useful to detect conformational changes that occur during gating of membrane channel proteins. Given the advancing expertise in mutagenesis of connexins, it may be possible to replace all but one of the tryptophan residues with phenylalanine.[96] The remaining tryptophan residue could then serve as a reporter of local environment and dynamics during channel gating. In addition, energy transfer between donor and acceptor chromophores attached to macromolecules can be used to determine proximity relationships.[95a,97,98]

EPR spectroscopy is another powerful method to study protein structure and dynamics.[99-101] For instance, cysteine substitution mutagenesis can be used to introduce spin labels at particular sites in membrane proteins, and the EPR spectrum reveals amino acid side-chain dynamics, solvent accessibility, polarity and electrostatic potential.

Although proteins of fairly sizable molecular weight can now be examined by NMR spectroscopy, it is still not feasible to attempt to carry out NMR studies of membrane proteins in detergent micelles. The tumbling rate of the protein-detergent complex would be so slow that the spectral lines would exhibit substantial line broadening, precluding interpretation. Nevertheless, small soluble regions of membrane proteins may be amenable to NMR spectroscopy. For instance, NMR spectroscopy has been used to examine the structure of the third cytoplasmic loop and the carboxy-terminal domain of bovine rhodopsin.[92a,93a] The synthesized peptides were biologically active, suggesting that the conformation of the peptides is relevant to the native protein structure. For connexins, candidate domains are the extracellular loops, the cytoplasmic loop between M2 and M3, the amino tail, and the carboxy-tail.

Needless to say, such soluble domains, which could be readily expressed in bacterial or insect systems, may also be more amenable to conventional 3D crystallization and examination by x-ray crystallography than the full-length protein. This has certainly been a fruitful strategy in several other systems in which the hydrophilic, water-soluble domains of bitopic membrane proteins were expressed, purified, and examined at atomic resolution.[94a,95,96a] However, this approach does not allow examination of transmembrane domains. An integrated strategy that combines NMR or crystallographic analyses of expressed water-soluble domains with 2D crystallization and electron cryocrystallography of membrane domains should be of general utility in the higher-resolution structure analysis of polytopic membrane proteins.

Summary

Cardiac gap junctions play an essential functional role in the heart by electrically coupling adjacent cells to synchronize the contraction of the muscle. Gap junctions in the heart are intimately involved not only in the normal coordinated depolarization of muscle but also with cardiac arrhythmias responsible for sudden death. The structure of 2D crystals of cardiac gap junction channels in their native membrane environment has been examined by electron microscopy and image analysis. Projection density maps reveal that the connexon in cardiac gap junctions is formed by a hexameric cluster of highly asymmetric subunits, called α_1 connexin (Cx43). Membrane topology of the α_1(Cx43) subunits has been mapped by use of seven site-specific peptide antibodies and selective protease cleavage. The results support a model in which α_1(Cx43) spans the lipid bilayer four times with an $\approx$5.1 kD loop and $\approx$13 kD carboxy-tail accessible on the cytoplasmic membrane face. CD spectra suggest that protease-cleaved α_1(Cx43) contains sufficient α-helix so that the transmembrane hydrophobic domains can be folded as α-helices. A working model is that the cardiac gap junction channel is formed by paired hexamers $\approx$65 Å in diameter with subunits ($\approx$25 Å in diameter and $\approx$125 Å long) having transmembrane domains folded as a four-α-helical bundle. This model is being further examined by cryoelectron microscopy and image analysis of truncated α_1(Cx43) that has been expressed and crystallized in the membranes of BHK cells. A preliminary projection density map at 7-Å resolution reveals a ring of transmembrane α-helices that lines the aqueous pore and a second ring of α-helices in close contact with the membrane lipids. This is the first example in which an approach that uses the overexpression of a recombinant membrane protein combined with electron cryocrystallography has been successfully used to explore the secondary structure of the transmembrane domains of a polytopic integral membrane protein. An integrated strategy that combines spectroscopic techniques for examining conformational dynamics, high resolution NMR and/or x-ray crystallographic analyses of expressed water-soluble domains, and 2D crystallization and electron cryomicroscopy of membrane domains should be of general utility in the exploration of membrane protein structure and dynamics.

References

1. Loewenstein WR. Junctional intercellular communication: the cell-to-cell membrane channel. *Physiol Rev.* 1981;61:829–913.
2. McNutt NS, Weinstein RS. The ultrastructure of the nexus: a correlated thin-section and freeze-cleave study. *J Cell Biol.* 1970;47:666–688.
3. Barr L, Dewey MM, Berger W. Propagation of action potentials and the structure of the nexus in cardiac muscle. *J Gen Physiol.* 1965;48:797–823.
4. Spach MS. The role of cell-to-cell coupling in cardiac conduction disturbances. *Adv Exp Med Biol.* 1983;161:61–77.
5. Spach MS. Changes in the topology of gap junctions as an adaptive structural response of the myocardium. *Circulation.* 1994;90:1103–1106.
6. Miller C. Ion channels, all in one place. *Cell.* 1992;69:579.
7. Hille B. *Ionic Channels of Excitable Membranes*, 2nd ed. Sunderland, Mass: Sinauer Assoc; 1992.
8. Fishman GI, Vink MJ, Spray DC. Can we learn about conduction using genetic approaches? This volume.
9. Beyer EC, Saffitz JE, Davis LM, et al. Molecular and biochemical regulation of connexins: potential targets for modulation of cardiac intercellular communication. This volume.
10. Beyer EC, Veenstra RD. Molecular biology and electrophysiology of car-

diac gap junctions. In: *Handbook of Membrane Channels.* New York, NY: Academic Press, Inc; 1994:379–401.

11. Saffitz JE, Beyer EC, Darrow BJ, et al. Gap junction structure, conduction, and arrhythmogenesis: directions for future research. This volume.

12. Yeager M, Nicholson BJ. Structure of gap junction intercellular channels. *Curr Opin Struct Biol.* 1996;6:183–192.

13. Yeager M, Nicholson BJ. Structure and biochemistry of gap junctions. In: Hertzberg E, ed. *Advances in Molecular and Cell Biology.* JAI Press. In press.

14. Spray DC, Burt JM. Structure-activity relations of the cardiac gap junction channel. *Am J Physiol.* 1990;258:C195–C205.

15. Bennett MVL, Barrio LC, Bargiello TA, Spray DC, Hertzberg E, Saez JC. Gap junctions: new tools, new answers, new questions. *Neuron.* 1991;6: 305–320.

16. Paul DL. New functions for gap junctions. *Curr Opin Cell Biol.* 1995;7: 665–672.

17. Kumar NM, Gilula NB. The gap junction communication channel. *Cell.* 1996;84:381–388.

18. Goodenough DA, Goliger JA, Paul DL. Connexins, connexons, and intercellular communication. *Ann Rev Biochem.* 1996;65:475–502.

19. Beyer EC, Paul DL, Goodenough DA. Connexin family of gap junction proteins. *J Membr Biol.* 1990;116:187–194.

20. Willecke K, Hennermann H, Dahl E, et al. The diversity of connexin genes encoding gap junctional proteins. *Eur J Cell Biol.* 1991;56:1–7.

21. Kumar NM, Gilula NB. Molecular biology and genetics of gap junction channels. *Semin Cell Biol.* 1992;3:3–16.

22. Brightman MW, Reese TS. Junctions between intimately apposed cell membranes in the vertebrate brain. *J Cell Biol.* 1969;40:648–667.

23. Trelstad R, Revel J-P, Hay E. Tight junctions between cells in the early chick embryo as visualized by electron microscopy. *J Cell Biol.* 1966;31: C6–C10.

24. Revel J-P, Karnovsky MJ. Hexagonal array of subunits in intercellular junctions in the mouse heart and liver. *J Cell Biol.* 1967;33:C7–C12.

25. Friend DS, Gilula NB. Variations in tight and gap junctions in mammalian tissues. *J Cell Biol.* 1972;53:758–776.

26. Hirokawa N, Heuser J. The inside and outside of gap-junction membranes visualized by deep etching. *Cell.* 1982;30:395–406.

27. Manjunath CK, Goings GE, Page E. Detergent sensitivity and splitting of isolated liver gap junctions. *J Membr Biol.* 1984;78:147–155.

28. Zimmer DB, Green CR, Evans WH, Gilula NB. Topological analysis of the major protein in isolated intact rat liver gap junctions and gap junction-derived single membrane structures. *J Biol Chem.* 1987;262:7751–7763.

29. Milks LC, Kumar NM, Houghton R, et al. Topology of the 32-kD liver gap junction protein determined by site-directed antibody localizations. *EMBO J.* 1988;7:2967–2975.

30. Gros DB, Nicholson BJ, Revel J-P. Comparative analysis of the gap junction protein from rat heart and liver: is there a tissue specificity of gap junctions? *Cell.* 1983;35:539–549.

31. Manjunath CK, Goings GE, Page E. Proteolysis of cardiac gap junctions during their isolation from rat hearts. *J Membr Biol.* 1985;85:159–168.

32. Manjunath CK, Nicholson BJ, Teplow D, et al. The cardiac gap junction protein (M_r 47,000) has a tissue-specific cytoplasmic domain of M_r 17,000 at its carboxy-terminus. *Biochem Biophys Res Commun.* 1987;142:228–234.

33. Yeager M, Gilula NB. Membrane topology and quaternary structure of cardiac gap junction ion channels. *J Mol Biol.* 1992;223:929–948.
34. Yancey SB (I), John SA (II), Lal R (III), Austin BJ, Revel J-P. The 43-kD polypeptide of heart gap junctions: immunolocalization (I), topology (II), and functional domains (III). *J Cell Biol.* 1989;108:2241–2254.
35. Laird DW, Revel J-P. Biochemical and immunochemical analysis of the arrangement of connexin43 in rat heart gap junction membranes. *J Cell Sci.* 1990;97:109–117.
36. Caspar DLD, Goodenough DA, Makowski L, Phillips WC. Gap junction structures, I: correlated electron microscopy and x-ray diffraction. *J Cell Biol.* 1977;74:605–628.
37. Zampighi G, Unwin PNT. Two forms of isolated gap junctions. *J Mol Biol.* 1979;135:451–464.
38. Yeager M. *In situ* two-dimensional crystallization of a polytopic membrane protein: the cardiac gap junction channel. *Acta Crystallogr.* 1994;D50: 632–638.
39. Lampe PD, Kistler J, Hefti A, et al. *In vitro* assembly of gap junctions. *J Struct Biol.* 1991;107:281–290.
40. Moody M. Image analysis of electron micrographs. In: Hawkes PW, Valdræ U. eds. *Biophysical Electron Microscop: Basic Concepts and Modern Techniques.* London, UK: Academic Press; 1990:145–287.
41. Yeager M. Electron microscopic image analysis of cardiac gap junction membrane crystals. *Microsc Res Tech.* 1995;31:452–466.
42. Sosinsky GE, Baker TS, Caspar DLD, Goodenough DA. Correlation analysis of gap junction lattice images. *Biophys J.* 1990;58:1213–1226.
43. Sosinsky G. Mixing of connexins in gap junction membrane channels. *Proc Natl Acad Sci USA.* 1995;92:9210–9214.
44. Kanter HL, Saffitz JE, Beyer EC. Cardiac myocytes express multiple gap junction proteins. *Circ Res.* 1992;70:438–444.
45. Kanter HL, Laing JG, Beau SL, Beyer EC, Saffitz JE. Distinct patterns of connexin expression in canine Purkinje fibers and ventricular muscle. *Circ Res.* 1993;72:1124–1131.
46. Kanter HL, Laing JG, Beyer EC, Green KG, Saffitz JE. Multiple connexins colocalize in canine ventricular myocyte gap junctions. *Circ Res.* 1993;73: 344–350.
47. Gros D, Jarry-Guichard T, Ten Velde I, et al. Restricted distribution of connexin40, a gap junctional protein, in mammalian heart. *Circ Res.* 1994; 74:839–851.
48. Jiang JX, Goodenough DA. Heteromeric connexons in lens gap junction channels. *Proc Natl Acad Sci USA.* 1996;93:1287–1291.
49. Toyoshima C, Unwin N. Ion channel of acetylcholine receptor reconstructed from images of postsynaptic membranes. *Nature.* 1988;336: 247–250.
50. Barrio LC, Suchyna T, Bargiello T, et al. Gap junctions formed by connexins 26 and 32 alone and in combination are differently affected by applied voltage. *Proc Natl Acad Sci USA.* 1991;88:8410–8414. Published erratum appears in *Proc Natl Acad Sci USA.* 1992;89:4220.
51. White TW, Paul DL, Goodenough DA, Bruzzone R. Functional analysis of selective interactions among rodent connexins. *Mol Biol Cell* 1995;6: 459–470.
52. Baker TS, Sosinsky GE, Casper DLD, Gall C, Goodenough DA. Gap junction structures VII. Analysis of connexon images obtained with cationic and anionic negative stains. *J Mol Biol.* 1985;184:81–98.

53. Makowski L, Caspar DLD, Phillips WC, Goodenough DA. Gap junction structures V: structural chemistry inferred from x-ray diffraction measurements on sucrose accessibility and trypsin susceptibility. *J Mol Biol.* 1984; 174:449–481.
54. Gogol E, Unwin N. Organization of connexons in isolated rat liver gap junctions. *Biophys J.* 1988;54:105–112.
55. Sikerwar SS, Unwin N. Three-dimensional structure of gap junctions in fragmented plasma membranes from rat liver. *Biophys J.* 1988;54:113–119.
56. Fishman GI, Moreno AP, Spray DC, Leinwand LA. Functional analysis of human cardiac gap junction channel mutants. *Proc Natl Acad Sci USA.* 1991;88:3525–3529.
57. Moreno AP, Saez JC, Fishman GI, Spray DC. Human connexin43 gap junction channels: regulation of unitary conductances by phosphorylation. *Circ Res.* 1994;74:1050–1057.
58. Swenson KI, Piwnica-Worms H, McNamee H, Paul DL. Tyrosine phosphorylation of the gap junction protein connexin43 is required for the pp60v-src-induced inhibition of communication. *Cell Regul.* 1990;1: 989–1002.
59. Loo LWM, Berestecky JM, Kanemitsu MY, Lau AF. pp60[src]-mediated phosphorylation of connexin 43, a gap junction protein. *J Biol Chem.* 1995; 270:12751–12761.
60. Liu SG, Taffet S, Stoner L, et al. A structural basis for the unequal sensitivity of the major cardiac and liver gap junctions to intracellular acidification-the carboxyl tail length. *Biophys J.* 1993;64:1422–1433.
61. Ek JF, Delmar M, Perzova R, Taffet SM. Role of His95 in pH gating of cardiac gap junction protein, connexin 43. *Circ Res.* 1994;74:1058–1064.
62. Morley GE, Taffet SM, Delmar M. Intramolecular interactions mediate pH regulation of connexin 43 channels. *Biophys J.* 1996;70:1294–1302.
63. Britz-Cunningham SH, Shah MM, Zuppan CW, Fletcher WH. Mutations of the connexin43 gap-junction gene in patients with heart malformations and defects of laterality. *N Engl J Med.* 1995;332:1323–1329.
64. Amos LA, Henderson R, Unwin PNT. Three-dimensional structure determination by electron microscopy of two-dimensional crystals. *Prog Biophys Mol Biol.* 1982;39:183–231.
65. Henderson R, Unwin PNT. Three-dimensional model of purple membrane obtained by electron microscopy. *Nature.* 1975;257:28–32.
66. Unwin PNT. Zampighi G. Structure of the junction between communicating cells. *Nature.* 1980;283:545–549.
67. Unwin PN, Ennis PD. Two configurations of a channel-forming membrane protein. *Nature.* 1984;307:609–613.
68. Sosinsky GE, Jesior JC, Caspar DLD, Goodenough DA. Gap junction structures. VIII. Membrane cross-section. *Biophys J.* 1988;53:709–722.
69. Makowski L, Caspar DLD, Phillips WC, Goodenough DA. Gap junction structures, II: analysis of the x-ray diffraction data. *J Cell Biol.* 1977;74: 629–645.
70. Yeager M, Berriman JA, Baker TS, Bellamy AR. Three-dimensional structure of the rotavirus haemagglutinin VP4 by cryo-electron microscopy and difference map analysis. *EMBO J.* 1994;13:1011–1018.
71. Shibata Y, Manjunath CK, Page E. Differences between cytoplasmic surfaces of deep-etched heart and liver gap junctions. *Am J Physiol.* 1985;249: H690–H693.
72. Tibbits TT, Caspar DLD, Phillips WC, Goodenough DA. Diffraction diag-

nosis of protein folding in gap junction connexons. *Biophys J.* 1990;57: 1025–1036.

73. Cascio M, Gogol E, Wallace BA. The secondary structure of gap junctions: influence of isolation methods and proteolysis. *J Biol Chem.* 1990;265: 2358–2364.

74. Yeager M. Structure and design of cardiac gap-junction membrane channels. In: Hall JE, Zampighi GA, Davis RM. eds. *Progress in Cell Research, vol 3: Gap Junctions.* Amsterdam, Netherlands: Elsevier; 1993:47–55.

75. Makowski L. X-ray diffraction studies of gap junction structure. *Adv Cell Biol.* 1988;2:119–158.

76. Johnson WC. Secondary structure of proteins through circular dichroism spectroscopy. *Annu Rev Biophys Biophys Chem.* 1988;17:145–166.

77. Johnson WC. Protein secondary structure and circular dichroism. *Proteins.* 1990;7:205–214.

78. Fasman GD. Distinguishing transmembrane helices from peripheral helices by circular dichroism. *Biotechnol Appl Biochem.* 1993;18:111–138.

79. Bloemendal M, Johnson WC. Structural information on proteins from circular dichroism spectroscopy-possibilities and limitations. *Pharm Biotechnol.* 1995;7:65–100.

80. Woody RW. Circular dichroism. *Methods Enzymol.* 1995;246:34–71.

81. Henderson R, Baldwin JM, Ceska TA, Zemlin F, Beckmann E, Downing KH. Model for the structure of bacteriorhodopsin based on high-resolution electron cryo-microscopy. *J Mol Biol.* 1990;213:899–929.

82. Jap BK, Walian PJ, Gehring K. Structural architecture of an outer membrane channel as determined by electron crystallography. *Nature.* 1991; 350:167–170.

83. Kühlbrandt W, Wang DN, Fujiyoshi Y. Atomic model of plant light-harvesting complex by electron crystallography. *Nature.* 1994;367:614–621.

84. Stauffer KA, Kumar NM, Gilula NB, Unwin N. Isolation and purification of gap junction channels. *J Cell Biol.* 1991;115:141–150.

85. Kühlbrandt W. Two-dimensional crystallization of membrane proteins. *Quart Rev Biophys.* 1992;25:1–49.

86. Kumar NM, Friend DS, Gilula NB. Synthesis and assembly of human β_1 gap junctions in BHK cells by DNA transfection with the human β_1 cDNA. *J Cell Sci.* 1995;108:3725–3734.

87. Unger VM, Kumar NM, Klier G, et al. 2-D crystallization and projection map of a recombinant truncated form of the α_1 cardiac gap junction channel. *Biophys J.* 1996;70:A207. Abstract.

88. Unger VM, Kumar NM, Gilula NB, Yeager M. Projection map of a recombinant gap junction channel at 7Å resolution. *Nat Struct Biol.* 1997;4:39–43.

89. Braiman MS, Rothschild KJ. Fourier transform infrared techniques for probing membrane protein structure. *Annu Rev Biophys Biophys Chem.* 1988;17:541–570.

90. Cooper EA, Knutson K. Fourier transform infrared spectroscopy investigations of protein structure. *Pharm Biotechnol.* 1995;7:101–143.

91. Haris PI, Chapman D. The conformational analysis of peptides using Fourier transform IR spectroscopy. *Biopolymers.* 1995;37:251–263.

92. Jackson M, Mantsch HH. The use and misuse of FTIR spectroscopy in the determination of protein structure. *Crit Rev Biochem Mol Biol.* 1995;30: 95–120.

92a. Yeagle PL, Alderfer JL, Albert AD. Structure of the carboxy-terminal domain of bovine rhodopsin. *Nat Struct Biol.* 1995;2:832–834.

93. Stryer L. Fluorescence spectroscopy of proteins. *Science.* 1968;162:526–533.
93a. Yeagle PL, Alderfer JL, Albert AD. Structure of the third cytoplasmic loop of bovine rhodopsin. *Biochemistry.* 1995;34:14621–14625.
94. Somogyi B, Lakos Z. Protein dynamics and fluorescence quenching. *J Photochem Photobiol.* 1993;18:3–16.
94a. Wang J, Yan Y, Garrett TPJ, et al. Atomic structure of a fragment of human CD4 containing two immunoglobulin-like domains. *Nature.* 1990; 348:411–418.
95. De Vos AM, Ultsch M, Kossiakoff AA. Human growth hormone and extra-cellular domain of its receptor: crystal structure of the complex. *Science.* 1992;255:306–312.
95a. Jiskoot W, Hlady V, Naleway JJ, Herron JN. Application of fluorescence spectroscopy for determining the structure and function of proteins. *Pharm Biotechnol.* 1995;7:1–63.
96. Menezes ME, Roepe PD, Kaback HR. Design of a membrane transport protein for fluorescence spectroscopy. *Proc Natl Acad Sci USA.* 1990;87: 1638–1642.
96a. Shapiro L, Fannon AM, Kwong PD, et al. Structural basis of cell-cell adhesion by cadherins. *Nature.* 1995;374:327–337.
97. Wu CW, Stryer L. Proximity relationships in rhodopsin. *Proc Natl Acad Sci USA.* 1972;69:1104–1108.
98. Clegg RM. Fluorescence resonance energy transfer. *Curr Opin Biotechnol.* 1995;6:103–110.
99. Todd AP, Cong J, Levinthal F, et al. Site-directed mutagenesis of colicin E1 provides specific attachment sites for spin labels whose spectra are sensitive to local conformation. *Proteins.* 1989;6:294–305.
100. Hubbell WL, Altenbach C. Investigation of structure and dynamics in membrane proteins using site-directed spin labeling. *Curr Opin Struct Biol.* 1994;4:566–573.
101. Voss J, Hubbell WL, Kaback HR. Distance determination in proteins using designed metal ion binding sites and site-directed spin labeling: application to the lactose permease of *Escherichia coli. Proc Natl Acad Sci USA.* 1995;92:12300–12303.
102. Beyer EC, Paul DL, Goodenough DA. Connexin 43: a protein from rat heart homologous to a gap junction protein from liver. *J Cell Biol.* 1987; 105:2621–2629.
103. Paul DL. Molecular cloning of cDNA for rat liver gap junction protein. *J Cell Biol.* 1986;103:123–134.
104. Kumar NM, Gilula NB. Cloning and characterization of human and rat liver cDNAs coding for a gap junction protein. *J Cell Biol.* 1986;103: 767–776.
105. Zhang J-T, Nicholson BJ. Sequence and tissue distribution of a second protein of hepatic gap junctions, Cx26, as deduced from its cDNA. *J Cell Biol.* 1989;109:3391–3401.
106. Beyer EC, Kistler J, Paul DL, Goodenough DA. Antisera directed against connexin43 peptides react with a 43-kD protein localized to gap junctions in myocardium and other tissues. *J Cell Biol.* 1989;108:595–605.
107. el Aoumari AE, Fromaget C, Dupont E, et al. Conservation of a cyto-plasmic carboxy-terminal domain of connexin 43, a gap junctional protein, in mammal heart and brain. *J Membr Biol.* 1990;115:229–240.
108. Goldberg GS, Lau AF. Dynamics of connexin43 phosphorylation in pp60v-src-transformed cells. *Biochem J.* 1993;295:735–742.

109. Goodenough DA, Paul DL, Jesaitis L. Topological distribution of two connexin32 antigenic sites in intact and split rodent hepatocyte gap junctions. *J Cell Biol.* 1988;107:1817–1824.
110. Hertzberg EL, Disher RM, Tiller AA, Zhou Y, Cook RG. Topology of the Mr 27,000 liver gap junction protein: cytoplasmic localization of amino- and carboxyl termini and a hydrophilic domain which is protease-hypersensitive. *J Biol Chem.* 1988;263:19105–19111.
111. Kanemitsu MY, Lau AF. Epidermal growth factor stimulates the disruption of gap junctional communication and connexin43 phosphorylation independent of 12-O-tetradecanoylphorbol 13-acetate-sensitive protein kinase C: the possible involvement of mitogen-activated protein kinase. *Mol Biol Cell* 1993;4:837–848.
112. Kennelly PJ, Krebs EG. Consensus sequences as substrate specificity determinants for protein kinases and protein phosphatases. *J Biol Chem.* 1991; 266:15555–15558.
113. Kwak BR, Saez JC, Wilders R, et al. cGMP-dependent phosphorylation of connexin 43: influence on gap junction channel conductance and kinetics. *Pflugers Arch.* 1996; in press.
114. Rahman S, Evans WH. Topography of connexin32 in rat liver gap junctions: evidence for an intramolecular disulphide linkage connecting the two extracellular peptide loops. *J Cell Sci.* 1991;100:567–578.
115. Rubin JB, Verselis VK, Bennett MVL, Bargiello TA. A domain substitution procedure and its use to analyze voltage dependence of homotypic gap junctions formed by connexins 26 and 32. *Proc Natl Acad Sci USA.* 1992; 89:3820–3824.
116. Saez JC, Nairn AC, Czernik AJ, et al. Phosphorylation of connexin 32, a hepatocyte gap-junction protein, by cAMP-dependent protein kinase, protein kinase C and Ca^{2+}/calmodulin-dependent protein kinase II. *Eur J Biochem.* 1990;192:263–273.
117. Saez JC, Nairn AC, Czernik AJ, Spray DC, Hertzberg EL. Rat connexin 43: regulation by phosphorylation in heart. In: Hall JE, Zampighi GA, Davis RM, eds. *Progress in Cell Research, vol 3: Gap Junctions.* Amsterdam, Netherlands: Elsevier; 1993:275–282.
118. Suchyna TM, Xu LX, Gao F, et al. Identification of a proline residue as a transduction element involved in voltage gating of gap junctions. *Nature.* 1993;365:847–849.
119. Verselis VK, Ginter CS, Bargiello TA. Opposite voltage gating polarities of two closely related connexins. *Nature.* 1994;368:348–351.
120. Warn-Cramer BJ, Lampe PD, Kurata WE, et al. Characterization of the mitogen activated protein kinase phosphorylation sites on the connexin 43 gap junction protein. *J Biol Chem.* 1996;271:3779–3786.
121. White TW, Bruzzone R, Wolfram S, et al. Selective interactions among the multiple connexin proteins expressed in the vertebrate lens: the second extracellular domain is a determinant of compatibility between connexins. *J Cell Biol.* 1994;125:879–892.
122. Willecke K, Traub O, Look J, Stutenkemper R, Dermietzel R. Different protein components contribute to the structure and function of hepatic gap junctions. In: Hertzberg EL, Johnson RG, eds. *Modern Cell Biology, vol 7: Gap Junctions.* New York, NY: Alan R. Liss; 1988:41–52.
123. Zhang J-T, Nicholson BJ. The topological structure of connexin-26 and its distribution compared to connexin 32 in hepatic gap junctions. *J Membr Biol.* 1994;139:15–29.

Chapter 8

Major Cell Biological Issues and Strategies in Discontinuous Conduction

David C. Spray, PhD, Monique J. Vink, MD, and Glenn I. Fishman, MD

Impulse conduction in the heart is microscopically discontinuous, in that action potentials are regenerated in each cell, passing from one cell to the next with measurable delay. This discontinuity is due to the connection of each cardiac myocyte to neighboring cells through gap junction channels, and it results in anisotropic conduction due to nonuniform cellular geometry as well as nonuniform gap junction distribution between myocytes. Because gap junctions are the organelles largely responsible for this expression of discontinuous conduction, regulation of gap junctions is fundamental to understanding conduction in both normal and pathologically diseased hearts. The purpose of this chapter is to outline what is now known regarding the physiology of cardiac gap junction channels and to highlight what needs to be known at the basic cell biological level to begin to consider whether therapeutic approaches for rhythm disturbances could be developed based on principles of altering gap junction function.

Overview of Gap Junction Structure

Gap junctions are aggregates of intercellular channels; at sites of gap junctional contact between cells, membranes of contiguous cells tend to be planar, so that gap junctions viewed in thin section or as freeze-fracture replicas generally appear as plaques between cells.[1] Gap

From: Spooner PM, Joyner RW, Jalife J (eds). *Discontinuous Conduction in the Heart.* Armonk, NY: Futura Publishing Company, Inc.; © 1997.

junction plaques can be quite large (up to several micrometers across in ventricular myocytes) or quite small. Each gap junction channel is made of two mirror-symmetrical components contributed by each cell, called connexons or hemichannels.[2] Each connexon, or hemichannel, in turn is made up of six homologous subunits, each one consisting of a single connexin protein molecule. More than a dozen different connexins have been cloned and sequenced from rodents and humans.[3] Most are encoded by a single gene family with common structure consisting of a single intron separating a small upstream exon from an exon containing the entire connexin coding sequence. In the human and mouse, single copies of different connexin genes map to at least four chromosomes, including Chromosome X (see chapter 16, by Fishman et al). Connexin family members are quite similar in structure, with ≈50% of their amino acid sequences showing identity despite a diverse pattern of tissue distribution. Three main connexins are expressed by mammalian cardiac myocytes: Cx40, Cx43, and Cx45.[4]

Each connexin molecule crosses the membrane four times (segments M1, M2, M3, and M4) and has both its amino-terminal (NT domain) and carboxyl-terminal (CT domain) on the cytoplasmic face of the membrane. Extracellular loops (C1, C2) are structurally conserved, with three cysteine residues in each loop positioned identically in all 12 connexins. Presumably, this feature accounts for the high-affinity interactions between many, but not all, different connexin molecules when connexons are paired end to end. The part of the connexin molecule between M2 and M3 forms a loop or hinge region in the cytoplasm whose length is used to separate different connexins into group I (β) and group II (α) subfamilies.[2,5] The cardiac gap junction proteins Cx40, Cx43, and Cx45 are all members of group II (α). The third transmembrane domain (M3) is the most amphipathic, with charged amino acid residues occurring at every third or fourth position in an otherwise predominantly hydrophobic sequence. Six M3 regions are believed to provide the hydrophilic face lining the lumen of the channel[2,6] (but see Reference 7 for evidence that other sequences also participate).

The regions of greatest divergence between different connexins are the cytoplasmic loop region between M2 and M3 and the carboxyl-terminal tail beyond M4. The latter contain unique peptide sequences that have proved quite useful in generating connexin-specific antibodies.

What Gap Junctions Do and How They Do It

Cardiac Gap Junction Channels as K⁺ Channels

In excitable tissues, the preeminent role of gap junctions is to permit electrotonic spread of current facilitating rapid signal relay from one cell to the next. In some regions of the heart, such as the Purkinje fibers, it is the actual rapidity that is most important, whereas in others, such as nodal structures, a paucity of channels results in a delay that provides the timing necessary for rhythmic muscular contracture. Current spread from one cardiac myocyte to the next is mediated by the flow of ions. Because K^+ is the most abundant and most mobile intracellular ion, it is responsible for carrying most current between cells. Thus, in their role as electrotonic synapses, gap junctions functionally operate as K^+ channels.

Cardiac Gap Junction Channels as Ca^{2+} and Second Messenger Channels

Gap junction channels are also permeable to larger ions and molecules, admitting the dye molecule lucifer yellow (M_r 457.2), which is generally used to detect gap junction function, as well as molecules such as cAMP, cGMP, IP_3, ATP, and ADP. Despite an abundant literature implicating Ca^{2+} ions in causing uncoupling between cardiac cells, it is now recognized that Ca^{2+} can diffuse between cells through gap junction channels. Ca^{2+} waves, traveling at a velocity of 20 to 50 $\mu m/s$, distinct from the thousandfold faster waves of contracture that are propagated by regenerative electrical events, have been demonstrated in cells from many tissues.[8,9] Recent work from our laboratory has shown that a similar phenomenon can be demonstrated under Ca^{2+}-overload conditions in cardiac myocytes from rodent heart.[10] This phenomenon may be mediated by diffusion of Ca^{2+} between myocytes, which would then be regenerative through Ca^{2+}-induced Ca^{2+} release, or it might involve IP_3 generation, its diffusion through the gap junctions, and secondary Ca^{2+} release at IP_3 receptors. Although localization of IP_3 receptors in intercalated disk regions of adult ventricular myocytes[11] provides an anatomic organization that might be ideal for such intercellular signaling, actual mechanisms remain poorly explored.

Which Gap Junction Proteins Are Expressed in Cardiovascular Tissues?

Identification of connexins in the cardiovascular system began with the cloning of DNA encoding Cx43, the major gap junction protein of rat and human cardiac tissue and of bovine smooth muscle.[12–14] These studies conclusively demonstrated that the junctional protein in heart was distinct from but closely related to the gap junction proteins of liver, which are primarily Cx32 and Cx26.[2] Additional work showed that chick heart expresses two additional gap junction proteins,[15] and it has now become clear that their mammalian homologues, Cx40 and Cx45, are also expressed in bovine, canine, human, and rodent cardiovascular systems.[4,16–27] Moreover, Cx37, initially characterized in lung,[28] has also been localized to the vessel wall.[29] Thus, although Cx43 is the most abundant gap junction protein in adult mammalian heart, especially in ventricular tissue,[25] Cx40 contributes to the junctional complement in the cardiac conduction system, adult atrium, and vascular smooth muscle and endothelium[4,16,18–23]; Cx45 is abundant throughout the heart early during development and persists in adulthood,[30] and Cx37 contributes to junctions between endothelial cells.[28,29]

Why Are There Multiple Cardiovascular Connexins?

Three reasons for the diversity of gap junction proteins have been proposed.

1. Different connexins have different affinities for one another: This would allow communication between diverse cell populations or their segregation into isolated communication compartments. Although coupling is readily established between cells of different types in coculture,[31,32] this might be due to similar connexins being expressed by different cells. Functional coupling between cells expressing different connexin has also been confirmed by exogenous expression studies using *Xenopus* oocytes injected with connexin cRNAs[33] and with communication-deficient cells stably transfected with connexin cDNAs.[34] These studies have shown that Cx43 can pair with Cx37 and Cx45, but not with Cx40, to form functional channel.[18,35] From the standpoint of the cardiovascular system, cell interfaces that would permit Cx40-Cx43 heterologous pairings could occur between endothelial and smooth muscle cells in the vessel wall. As Bruzzone et al[18] pointed out, nonfunctional myoendothelial Cx40-Cx43 pairings could serve to separate endothelial and smooth muscle compartments in the vasculature. Perhaps more significantly, predominant expression of Cx40 by cells of the conduction system and of Cx43 by the ventricular mass would be expected to restrict dispersion of excitation,[36] while favoring pathways of contact between Purkinje cells and ventricular muscle, the P-V$_j$ junctions.[37] Cx45 has higher affinity for Cx43 than either connexin has

for itself,[35] and heterologous Cx43-Cx45 pairings might cause unidirectional block, because this combination shows strong asymmetrical voltage sensitivity.[35,38]

2. Channels formed by different connexins have different functional and gating properties. Gap junction channels open and close in response to various stimuli, including transjunctional voltage difference, intracellular pH, connexin phosphorylation, and exposure to any of a wide variety of lipophilic molecules.[39] From the standpoint of cardiac pathophysiology, each of these factors may play a significant roles. For example, during ischemia, appreciable transjunctional voltage gradients may develop, intracellular pH is radically lowered, phosphorylation substrates are reduced, and phosphatases may be activated.[40] Moreover, lipophilic fatty acids with uncoupling action are produced through lipid peroxidation and activation of phospholipases.[41] It is now quite clear that gap junction channels formed of different connexins are differentially sensitive to transjunctional voltage, to intracellular pH, and to phosphorylating agents. Furthermore, it has been suggested recently that the sensitivity to certain lipophiles of gap junction channels formed of Cx40 may differ from that of Cx43.[42] In addition, the size of gap junction channels formed by different connexins differs, evaluated on the basis of either unitary conductance of individual channels or size limit and charge selectivity. Because conductance determines current-carrying capacity, attenuation of conductance could have significant effects on synchronicity and speed of conduction. Recordings from cardiovascular tissue have detected unitary junctional currents corresponding to different channel sizes.[43] Although some of this diversity results from subconductance or alternate conductance states of the junctional channels,[39] diversity may also arise from the expression of multiple gap junction proteins. Finally, although it has been assumed that all gap junction channels were similarly permeable to molecules below a size limit of $\approx$1 kD, it is now clear that the gap junction channels formed of the cardiac connexins have markedly different permeabilities for anions than for cations. Thus, whereas Cx43 channels are freely permeable to lucifer yellow and other anions, Cx37 and Cx40 channels show more restricted diffusion, and Cx45 channels are virtually anion-impermeable.[44–46]

3. Different connexins are differentially affected by transcrip-

tional and posttranscriptional control mechanisms. Numerous drugs, growth factors, and hormones affect connexin mRNA and protein levels and perhaps coupling over a time course of hours to days.[47–53] Both transcriptional and mRNA stabilizing signals differ among the few connexin proteins in which gene regulatory sequences have been mapped or mRNA stability has been measured.[54–61] These mechanisms could allow differential regulation of the same connexin in different cells and different connexins in the same cellular environment.

Physiological and Biophysical Properties of Cardiac Connexins

The strategy that permitted stable expression of individual gap junction proteins in communication-deficient cell lines that we introduced in 1990[14,62] allowed the characterization of the connexins present in cardiac cells at the single-channel level and their comparison with properties of intact mammalian cardiac myocytes determined almost 10 years ago.[63,64] Moreover, exogenous expression of mutant connexins in *Xenopus* oocytes and in mammalian cell lines is beginning to permit localization of gating domains within individual connexin molecules. Biophysical properties of channels formed by each of the cardiovascular connexins are summarized below.

Unitary Conductances

Connexin43

Human and rat Cx43 channels have been examined in a number of mammalian cells and cell lines in which Cx43 is the predominant or sole gap junction protein expressed. These include stably transfected SKHep1 hepatoma and pc12 adrenal medullary tumor cells.[14,65,66] In each of these cell types, Cx43 displays two conduct states at low driving forces (60 to 70 pS and 90 to 110 pS in CsCl internal solution[67]), whereas at high transjunctional voltages, a lower-conductance state is induced (30 pS[68]). These unitary conductances are comparable to values obtained in cardiac myocytes and other cells in which Cx43 is expressed.[65,69] The higher-conductance states are interconvertible on phosphorylation and dephosphorylation, and for the rat sequence, the conductance substate may also be favored after activation of specific protein kinases (see below).

Connexin37

Cx37 channels have been studied in N2A neuroblastoma cells transfected with rat[44,70] and human[46] sequences, and both exhibit a maximally open state of 250 to 300 pS at low transjunctional voltages and a conductance state of ~75 pS at high driving forces. At intermediate-voltage driving forces, intermediate conductances are also observed. For the rat but not the human sequence, channels show saturation at moderate transjunctional voltages and at cation concentrations within the physiological range.

Connexin40

Cx40 channels have been recorded in stably transfected HeLa cells,[71] in N2A cells,[72] and in certain tumor cells in which rat or human Cx40 appears to be expressed exclusively.[73] In all cases, the main state of the channel appears to have a unitary conductance of ≈200 pS, with at least one additional state (≈50 pS) at higher voltages.

Connexin45

We have characterized the properties of the human isoform of Cx45 using a subclone of SKHep1 cells with uniform expression. Cx45 was identified on the basis of Northern blots, Western blots of immunoprecipitated material, and immunostaining.[74] Cx45 forms the lowest-conductance channels of all the cardiovascular connexins; the fully open state has a unitary conductance of ≈30 pS[45,74] and a substate of 15 to 20 pS at higher transjunctional voltages.

Selective Permeability of Cardiovascular Gap Junction Channels

Through ion substitution experiments, it has been estimated that relative anion/cation permeabilities are between 0.1 for Cx45 and 0.4 for Cx37.[45,46] Although our hCx45 channel measurements are consistent with this, we have recently found through symmetrical replacement of CsCl or KCl with chloride salts of quaternary ammonium ions that the anion permeability of rat Cx37 is vanishingly low.[44] Preliminary experiments on Cx40 indicate that the anion/cation permeability ratio is at least 0.3: measurable anion permeability of Cx40 is also suggested by diffusion of lucifer yellow in well-coupled Cx40-expressing cell lines.[26,73] Thus, the studies performed to date strongly suggest that anion permeabilities of Cx37 and Cx45 are markedly lower than for Cx43 and Cx40. This could suggest that flow of anionic second messenger molecules (eg, cAMP, cGMP, IP$_3$) could be impeded even though current, which is carried predominantly by K$^+$ ions in situ, may be similar in anion-permeant and impermeant channels.

A question that inevitably arises is whether ionic permeabilities differ in different electrical conductance states. For Cx37 and Cx43, our studies indicate that conductances of all states are similarly affected by ionic substitutions; furthermore, the ratio g_{min}/g_{max} in different solutions appears to be constant, implying that main and substate permeabilities are not radically different.[44,68]

Voltage Sensitivity of Gap Junction Channels Differs According to Connexin Type

Voltage sensitivity of Cx43 measured in mammalian cells is substantially different from results obtained in *Xenopus* oocyte expression studies, in which Cx43 voltage sensitivity had not been observed at all until recently (cf References 75 and 76). In transfectants and in rat cardiac myocytes,[68] conductance (g_j) was maximal at zero transjunctional voltage (V_j) and declined exponentially with pulses of either polarity. Equilibrium g_j values decreased symmetrically about the 0-mV axis, with V_0 (V_j at which the voltage-sensitive component is reduced by half) about ± 60 mV, g_{min} (the minimal g_j value obtained at high V_j) about 40% g_{max}, and n (the equivalent number of gating charges) ≈ 2. Cx40 is slightly more voltage sensitive, with $V_0 < 50$ mV and g_{min}/g_{max} ≈ 0.2.[73] Human Cx45 and both rodent and human Cx37 are much more voltage sensitive, with V_j as low as ± 10 mV substantially affecting g_j.[77] Chick Cx45 is markedly less voltage sensitive than its mammalian homologue (cf References 45 and 74). The residual voltage-insensitive conductance, g_{min}, has recently been shown to be due to a channel subconductance state at high V_j. Higher g_{min} values for some connexins than others is ascribable to relative unitary conductance and relative open time of the substates at high voltages compared with the state at low voltages.[78]

Such varied voltage sensitivity may be functionally important in regions of the cardiovascular system in which different connexins are expressed at interfaces between compartments, suggesting that heterotypic pairings might be expected at such junctions. Most heterotypic combinations have been examined in oocytes, in which results are largely as expected for additive interaction of separate voltage-sensitive gates.[76] Few such pairings have been attempted in transfected mammalian cells, although our recent studies on Cx45-Cx43 are illustrative of functional consequences.[35] Phenomena predicted by these studies have now been observed in developing chick heart.[38] These heterotypic junctions displayed marked rectification, such that depolarization of the Cx43 side resulted in rapid channel closure. Unidirectional block from Cx45 to Cx43 at heteromeric Cx43-Cx45 channels would be expected under conditions of even weak sustained depolarization of the Cx43 side and might favor retrograde ventricular-Purkinje conduction during arrhythmogenesis.

Differential Sensitivity of Cardiac Connexins to Phosphorylating Treatments

Connexin43

Junctional conductance can be increased, decreased, or unchanged when cells are exposed to phosphorylating or dephosphorylating conditions. However, at the single-channel level, all Cx43-containing cells respond similarly. We have shown that the unitary conductance of rat and human Cx43 channels is predominantly 60 to 70 pS under phosphorylating conditions (exposure of cells to okadaic acid, cAMP, or tumor-promoting phorbol esters) and is predominantly 90 to 100 pS when cells are exposed to dephosphorylating treatments (staurosporine, phosphatase in pipettes). We have further shown that, under conditions mimicking those used for most electrophysiological studies, phosphate incorporation into Cx43 is increased.[67,79]

Connexin45

We found no strong effects on Cx45 when we added phosphorylating agents as a control for studies on Cx43.[67] Although dephosphorylating agents were not explicitly tested, no shifts in the background currents were detected in experiments in which phosphatase was added to the pipette.

Connexin40

Surprisingly, our recent experiments using intracellular solutions containing phosphatase on Cx40 transfectants indicate that dephosphorylated Cx40 may exhibit a very low unitary conductance (M.J. Vink, L.K. Moore, and D.C. Spray, unpublished observations). This is opposite to the effect on Cx43 and leads us to hypothesize that cardiac cells isolated from wild-type and Cx43 knockout animals will respond differently to phosphorylating and dephosphorylating conditions. Moreover, such differential action would predict that acute dephosphorylation, as might occur during ischemia, would lower g_j in regions of the heart in which Cx40 expression predominates, whereas Cx43-rich areas would be spared initially.

Can There Be a Useful Pharmacology of Cardiac Gap Junction Channels?

There are several avenues of drug discovery that might be pursued to develop pharmacological strategies that increase or decrease coupling in cardiac tissue. Gating mechanisms that are already partially understood might be targeted, with the goal of affecting conductance of individual connexins and thereby selectively altering conduction in certain cardiac regions. For example, gating by transjunctional voltage induces occupancy of a partially conducting substate of gap junction channels that does not occur in response to other gating stimuli (except possibly by cGMP activation in rodent Cx43[80]). Because the substate conductance is a different fraction of main-state conductance for each cardiac connexin (40% of main-state conductance in Cx43, 20% in Cx40, and 5% in Cx45), pharmacological agents that would induce this substate would reduce conductance more in the conduction system than in contractile tissue. Alternatively, certain lipophiles may be more potent in reducing open times of some gap junction channels than others, as suggested by studies with oleic acid.[42] Although general depression of other ion channel activities is currently a severe drawback of this and other lipophilic compounds, pharmacokinetic studies should be pursued. In addition, the ball-and-chain domain docking model proposed by Delmar and colleagues to explain pH gating (see chapter 9) implies that unique polypeptides should interact with each connexin, further suggesting that targetable binding sites should exist that may be accessible to action by membrane-permeant drugs. Finally, the differential effects of phosphorylation of each cardiovascular connexin by specific protein kinases may offer the possibility of selectively affecting conduction velocity or contraction synchrony through pharmacological activation of α or β-adrenergic receptors with pharmacological agents.

A different strategy for drug discovery might combine the serendipitous reports of actions of novel compounds in heart or in other systems with analytic approaches to refine specificity and potency. For example, clinically useful antiarrhythmic agents might be screened for effects on junctional conductance with the goal of either establishing novel modes of action or identifying more potent agents. Although minimal effects were detected in a preliminary screening of these compounds,[81] two recent abstracts by Miyachi et al[82] and Uchiyama et al[83] indicate increased coupling by the class III agents sotalol and tedesimil that they attribute to β-adrenergic agonistic properties of these agents. Another approach is currently being pursued by Dhein and colleagues, who are studying the mode of action and structure-activity relationships of antiarrhythmic peptides (AAPs). Synchronization of beating of chick heart cell cultures by hexapeptides isolated from bovine atria was reported in 1980 by Kohana and colleagues.[84] These peptides have subsequently been reported by the Kohana and Dhein groups[85,86] to be antiarrhythmic in aconitine-induced arrhythmias in mice, ventricular fibrillation in dogs and rats, and reperfusion arrhythmias. Although the mechanism of action of AAPs has not been unambiguously identified, recent voltage-clamp studies of pairs of guinea pig ventricular myocytes using 10-nmol/L concentrations of the synthetic AAP10 has revealed a junctional conductance increase by as much as 25% to 30%. It was proposed that this increase in coupling may be responsible for decreased susceptibility to arrhythmias.[87] Because of the problems inherent in clinical use of polypeptides, one strategy to extend this work would be to determine whether these agents exhibit high-affinity binding to a receptor and then explore the pharmacology of the receptor.

Finally, there are both environmental toxins such as dieldrin[88] and active ingredients in herbal remedies, such as the glycyrrhetinic acid derivatives found in licorice,[89] that are potent inhibitors of gap junction channels in other systems but for which the mechanism of action is presently unknown. The latter compounds are effective at micromolar concentrations and have been experimentally useful in studies of gap junction channels in noncardiac tissues.[90]

Overall, the prospects for specifically targeting cardiac gap junctions within individual cardiac tissues with pharmacological compounds that increase or decrease electrical coupling are not as bleak as they once were. However, it seems clear that further rational development of effective strategies must rely on additional mechanistic understanding of gap junction gating and, in particular, of differences in gating mechanisms of channels formed by distinct gap junction proteins. For such studies, exogenous expression systems, in which individual connexins can be singly expressed, will be useful experimentally, but ultimately such studies must necessarily be extended to mammalian cardiac cells to verify efficacy and therapeutic potential.

References

1. Page E, Manjunath CK. Communicating junctions between cardiac cells. In: Fozzard H, Haber E, Jennings RB, Katz A, Morgan H, eds. *The Heart*

and *Cardiovascular System: Scientific Foundations.* New York, NY: Raven Press; 1986;1:573–600.

2. Bennett MVL, Barrio LC, Bargiello TA, Spray DC, Hertzberg E, Saez JC. Gap junctions: new tools, new answers, new questions. *Neuron.* 1991;6: 305–320.

3. Bennett MVL, Zheng X, Sogin ML. The connexins and their family tree. In: Fambrough D, ed. *Molecular Evolution of Physiological Processes.* 47th Annual Symposium of the Society of General Physiologists. New York, NY: Rockefeller Press; 1994;49:223–233.

4. Kanter HL, Laing JG, Beau SL, Beyer EC, Saffitz JE. Distinct patterns of connexin expression in canine Purkinje fibers and ventricular muscle. *Circ Res.* 1993;72:1124–1131.

5. Kumar NM, Gilula NB. The gap junction communication channel. *Cell.* 1996;84:381–388.

6. Yaeger, M, Gilula NB. Membrane topology and quaternary structure of cardiac gap junction ion channels. *J Mol Biol* 1992;223:929–948.

7. Pfahnl A, Zhou X-W, Tian J, Werner R, Dahl G. Mapping of the pore of gap junction channels by cysteine scanning mutagenesis. *Biophys J.* 1996; 70:A31. Abstract.

8. Saez JC, Connor JA, Spray DC, Bennett MVL. Hepatocyte gap junctions are permeable to the second messenger, inositol 1,4,5-trisphosphate, and to calcium ions. *Proc Natl Acad Sci U S A.* 1989;86:2708–2712.

9. Sneyd J, Charles AC, Sanderson MJ. A model for the propagation of intercellular calcium waves. *Am J Physiol.* 1994;266:C293–C302.

10. Spray DC, Vink MJ. Cardiac gap junctions as K^+ (and Ca^{2+}) channels. In: Vereecke J, Verdonck F, van Bogaert R-P, eds. *Potassium Channels in Normal and Pathological Conditions.* Leuven, Belgium: University Press; 1996. In press.

11. Kijima Y, Saito A, Jetton TL, Magnuson MA, Fleischer S. Different intracellular localization of inositol 1,4,5-triphosphate and ryanodine receptors in cardiomyocytes. *J Biol Chem.* 1993;268:3499–3506.

12. Beyer EC, Paul DL, Goodenough DA. Connexin43: a protein from rat heart homologous to the gap junction protein from liver. *J Cell Biol.* 1987;105: 2621–2629.

13. Lash JA, Critser ES, Pressler ML. Cloning of a gap junctional protein from vascular smooth muscle and expression in two-cell mouse embryos. *J Biol Chem.* 1990;265:13113–13117.

14. Fishman G, Spray DC, Leinwand LA. Molecular characterization and functional expression of the human cardiac gap junction channel. *J Cell Biol.* 1990;111:589–598.

15. Beyer EC. Molecular cloning and developmental expression of two chick embryo gap junction proteins. *J Biol Chem.* 1990;265:14439–14443.

16. Beyer EC, Reed KE, Westphale EM, Kanter HL, Larson DM. Molecular cloning and expression of rat connexin40, a gap junction protein expressed in vascular smooth muscle. *J Membr Biol.* 1992;127:69–76.

17. Haefliger JA, Bruzzone R, Jenkins NA, et al. Four novel members of the connexin family of gap junction proteins. *J Biol Chem.* 1992;25:2057–2064.

18. Bruzzone R, Haefliger J-A, Gimlich RL, Paul DL. Connexin40, a component of gap junctions in vascular endothelium, is restricted in its ability to interact with other connexins. *Mol Cell Biol.* 1993;4:7–20.

19. Kanter HL, Laing JG, Beyer EC, Green KG, Saffitz JE. Multiple connexins

colocalize in canine ventricular myocyte gap junctions. *Circ Res.* 1993;73: 344–350.

20. DeMaziere A, Analbers L, Jongsma HJ, Gros D. Immunoelectron microscopic visualization of the gap junction protein connexin40 in the mammalian heart. *Eur J Morphol.* 1992;30:305–308.

21. Haefliger JA, Bruzzone R, Jenkins NA, Gilbert DJ, Copeland NG, Paul DL. Four novel members of the connexin family of gap junction proteins. *J Biol Chem.* 1992;267:2057–2064.

22. Gourdie R, Green C, Severs N, Thompson R. Immunolabelling patterns of gap junction connexins in the developing and mature rat heart. *Anat Embryol.* 1992;185:363–378.

23. Kanter HL, Saffitz JE, Beyer EC. Cardiac myocytes express multiple gap junction proteins. *Circ Res.* 1992;70:438–444.

24. Laing JG, Westphale EM, Engelmann GL, Beyer EC. Characterization of the gap junction protein, connexin45. *J Membr Biol.* 1994;139:1–40.

25. Haefliger JA, Bruzzone R, Jenkins NA, Gilbert DJ, Copeland NG, Paul DL. Four novel members of the connexin family of gap junction proteins: molecular cloning, expression, and chromosome mapping. *J Biol Chem.* 1992;267:2057–2064.

26. Hennemann H, Suchyna T, Lichtenberg-Frate H, et al. Molecular cloning and functional expression of mouse connexin40, a second gap junction gene preferentially expressed in lung. *J Cell Biol.* 1992;117:1299–1310.

27. Hennemann H, Schwarz H-J, Willecke K. Characterization of gap junction genes expressed in F9 embryonic carcinoma cells: molecular cloning of mouse connexin31 and − 45 cDNAs. *Eur J Cell Biol.* 1992;57:51–58.

28. Willecke K, Heynkes R, Dahl E, Stutenkemper R, Hennemann H, Jungbluth S, Suchyna T, Nicholson BJ. Mouse connexin 37: cloning and functional expression of a gap junction gene highly expressed in lung. *J Cell Biol.* 1991; 114:1049–1057.

29. Reed KE, Westphale EM, Larson DM, Wang HZ, Veenstra RD, Beyer EC. Molecular cloning and functional expression of human connexin37, an endothelial gap junction protein. *J Clin Invest.* 1993;91:997–1004.

30. Saffitz JE, Kanter HL, Green KG, Tolley TK, Beyer EC. Tissue-specific determinants of anisotropic conduction velocity in canine atrial and ventricular myocardium. *Circ Res.* 1994;74:1065–1070.

31. Michalke W, Loewenstein WR. Communication between cells of different type. *Nature.* 1971;232:121–123.

32. Epstein ML, Gilula NB. A study of communication specificity between cells in culture. *J Cell Biol.* 1977;75:769–787.

33. Nicholson BJ, Suchyna T, Xu LX, et al. Divergent properties of different connexins expressed in Xenopus oocytes. *Prog Cell Res.* 1993;3:3–14.

34. Elfgang C, Eckert R, Lichtembderg-Fiate H, et al. Specific permeability and selective formation of gap junction channels in connexin-transfected HeLa cells. *J Cell Biol.* 1995;129:805–817.

35. Moreno AP, Fishman GI, Beyer EC, Spray DC. Voltage dependent gating and single channel analysis of heterotypic gap junction channels formed of Cx45 and Cx43. In: Kanno Y, ed. *Gap Junctions. Prog Cell Biol.* 1995; 405–408.

36. Bastide B, Neyses L, Ganten D, Paul M, Willecke K, Traub O. Gap junction protein connexin40 is preferentially expressed in vascular endothelium and

conductive bundles of rat myocardium and is increased under hypertensive conditions. *Circ Res.* 1993;73:1138–1149.

37. Rawling DA, Joyner RW. Characteristics of the junctional regions between Purkinje and ventricular muscle cells of the canine ventricular subendocardium. *Circ Res.* 1987;60:580–585.

38. Chen Y-H, DeHaan RL. Asymmetric voltage dependence of embryonic cardiac gap junction channels. *Am J Physiol.* 1996;270:C276–C285.

39. Spray DC. Physiological and pharmacological regulation of gap junction channels. In: Citi S, ed. *Molecular Mechanisms of Epithelial Cell Junctions: From Development to Disease.* Austin, Tex: RG Landes Co; 1994:195–215.

40. McHowat J, Yamada KA, Wu J, Yan GX, Corr PB. Recent insights pertaining to sarcolemmal phospholipid alterations underlying arrhythmogenesis in the ischemic heart. *J Cardiovasc Electrophysiol.* 1993;4:288–310.

41. Wu J, McHowat J, Saffitz JE, Yamada KA, Corr PB. Inhibition of gap junctional conductance by long-chain acylcarnitines and their preferential accumulation in junctional sarcolemma during hypoxia. *Circ Res.* 1993;: 879–889.

42. Hirschi KK, Minnich BN, Moore LK, Burt JM. Oleic acid differentially affects gap junction-mediated communication in heart and vascular smooth muscle cells. *Am J Physiol.* 1993 5(6 pt 1):C1517–1526.

43. Spray DC, Rook M, Moreno AP, et al. Cardiovascular gap junctions: gating properties, function and dysfunction. In: Spooner PM, Brown AM eds. *Ion Channels in the Cardiovascular System: Function and Dysfunction.* Mt Kisco, NY: Futura Publishing Co; 1994:185–217.

44. Waltzman M, Spray DC. Anionic permeability of Cx37 channels is vanishingly low. *Biophys J.* 1995;68:A227. Abstract.

45. Veenstra RD, Wang H-Z, Beyer E, Brink PR. Selective dye and ionic permeability of gap junction channels formed by connexin45. *Circ Res.* 1994;75: 483–490.

46. Veenstra RD, Wang HZ, Beyer EC, Ramanan SV, Brink PR. Connexin37 forms high conductance gap junction channels with subconductance state activity and selective dye and ionic permeabilities. *Biophys J.* 1994;66: 1915–1928.

47. Saez JC, Berthoud VC, Moreno AP, Spray DC. Gap junctions: multiplicity of controls in differentiated and undifferentiated cells and possible implications. In: Shenolikar S, Nairn AC, eds. *Advances in Second Messenger and Phosphoprotein Research.* Vol. 27 1993;27:163–198.

48. Weiner EC, Loewenstein WR. Correction of cell-cell communication defect by introduction of a protein kinase into mutant cells. *Nature.* 1983;305: 433–435.

49. Kessler JA, Spray DC, Sáez JC, Bennett MVL. Determination of synaptic phenotype: insulin and cAMP independently initiate development of electrotonic coupling between cultured sympathetic neurons. *Proc Natl Acad Sci U S A.* 1984;81:6235–6239.

50. DeMaziere AMGL, Scheuermann DW. Morphological analysis of gap-junctional area in parenchymal cells of the rat liver after administration of dibutyryl cAMP and aminophylline. *Cell Tissue Res.* 1988;252:611–618.

51. Cole WC, Garfield RE. Evidence for physiological regulation of myometrial gap junction permeability. *Am J Physiol.* 1986;251:C411–C420.

52. Mehta PP, Rose B. Expression of connexin43 and of functional cell-to-cell

channels in a Morris hepatoma cell line is regulated by cAMP. *J Cell Biol.* 1990;111:154a. Abstract.

53. Stagg RB, Martinez AM, Green LM, Fletcher WH. cAMP regulation of connexin43 (Cx43) transcription in a variety of cell types: evidence for de novo transcription in a communication deficient mouse fibroblast cell line (CL-1D). *J Cell Biol.* 1990;111:155a. Abstract.

54. Yancey SB, John SA, Ratneshwar L, et al. The 43-kD polypeptide of heart gap junctions: immunolocalization, topology, and functional domains. *J Cell Biol.* 1989;108:2241–2254.

55. Miller T, Dahl G, Werner R. Structure of a gap junction gene: connexin32. *Biosci Rep* 1988;8:455–464.

56. Bai S, Spray DC, Burk R. Characterization of rat connexin32 gene regulatory elements. In: Hall J, Zampighi G, Davis RE, eds. *Gap Junctions.* New York, NY: Elsevier; 1993;291–297.

57. Sáez JC, Gregory WA, Watanabe T, et al. cAMP delays disappearance of gap junctions between pairs of rat hepatocytes in primary culture. *Am J Physiol.* 1989;257:C1–C11.

58. Yu W, Dahl G, Werner R. The connexin43 gene is responsive to oestrogen. *Proc R Soc Lond B Biol Sci.* 1994;255:125–132.

59. Kren BT, Kumar NM, Wang SQ, Gilula NB, Steer CJ. Differential regulation of multiple gap junction transcripts and proteins during rat liver regeneration. *J Cell Biol.* 1993;123:707–718.

60. Mehta PP, Yamamoto M, Rose B. Transcription of the gene for the gap junctional protein connexin43 and expression of functional cell-to-cell channels are regulated by cAMP. *Mol Biol Cell.* 1992;3:839–850.

61. Lee SW, Tomasetto C, Paul D, Keyomarsi K, Sager R. Transcriptional down-regulation of gap-junction proteins blocks junctional communication in human mammary tumor cells. *J Cell Biol.* 1992;118:1213–1221.

62. Eghbali B, Kessler JA, Spray DC. Expression of gap junction channels in a communication incompetent cell line after transfection with connexin32 cDNA. *Proc Natl Acad Sci U S A.* 1990;87:1328–1331.

63. Burt JM, Spray DC. Single channel events and gating behavior of the cardiac gap junction channel. *Proc Natl Acad Sci U S A.* 1988;85:3431–3434.

64. Rook MB, Jongsma HJ, van Ginneken ACG. Properties of single gap junctional channels between isolated neonatal rat heart cells. *Am J Physiol.* 1988; 255:H770–H782.

65. Moreno AP, Fishman GI, Spray DC. Phosphorylation shifts unitary conductance and modifies voltage dependent kinetics of human connexin43 gap junction channels. *Biophys J.* 1992;62:51–53.

66. Spray DC, Moreno AP, Eghbali B, Fishman GI, Chanson M. Gating of gap junction channels as revealed in cells stably transfected with wild type and mutant connexin cDNAs. *Biophys J.* 1992;62:48–50.

67. Moreno AP, Saez JC, Fishman GI, Spray DC. Human connexin43 gap junction channels: regulation of unitary conductances by phosphorylation of the channel protein. *Circ Res.* 1994;74:1050–1057.

68. Moreno AP, Rook MB, Fishman GI, Spray DC. Gap junction channels: distinct voltage-sensitive and insensitive conductance states. *Biophys J.* 1994; 67:113–119.

69. Campos de Carvalho AC, Roy C, Moreno AP, et al. Gap junctions formed of connexin43 are found between smooth muscle cells of human *corpus cavernosum. J Urol.* 1993;149:1568–1575.

70. Waltzman M, Bai S, Spray DC. Stable transfection and functional expression of a gap junction protein, rat connexin 37 (rCx37) in a communication-deficient cell line. *Biophys J.* 1994;66:1260.

71. Bukauskas FF, Elfgang C, Willecke K, Weingart R. Biophysical properties of gap junction channels formed by mouse connexin40 in induced pairs of transfected human HeLa cells. *Biophys J.* 1995;68:2289–2298.

72. Beblo DA, Wang H-Z, Beyer EC, Westphale E, Veenstra RD. Unique conductance, gating and selective permeability properties of gap junction channels formed by connexin40. *Circ Res.* 1995;77:813–822.

73. Hellmann P, Winterhager E, Spray DC. Properties of connexin40 gap junction channels endogenously expressed and exogenously overexpressed in human choriocarcinoma cell lines. *Pflugers Arch* 1996;432:501–509.

74. Moreno AP, Laing JG, Beyer EC, Spray DC. Properties of gap junction channels formed of connexin45 endogenously expressed in human hepatoma (SKHep1) cells. *Am J Physiol.* 1995;268:C356–C365.

75. Swenson KI, Jordan JR, Beyer EC, et al. Formation of gap junctions by expression of connexins in *Xenopus* oocyte pairs. *Cell.* 1989;57:145–155.

76. White TW, Bruzzone R, Wolfram S, Paul DL, Goodenough DA. Selective interactions among the multiple connexin proteins expressed in the vertebrate lens: the second extracellular domain is a determinant of compatibility between connexins. *J Cell Biol.* 1994;125:879–892.

77. Waltzman MN, Spray DC. Exogenous expression of connexins for physiological characterization of channel properties: comparison of methods and results. In: Kanno Y, ed. *Gap Junctions. Prog Cell Res.* 1995;4:9–17.

78. Spray DC. Gap junction channels: yes, there are substates, but what does that mean? *Biophys J.* 1994;67:491–492.

79. Saez JC, Nairn A, Spray DC, Hertzberg EL. Rat connexin43: regulation by phosphorylation in heart. In: Hall J, G. Zampighi G, Davis RM, eds. *Gap Junctions.* New York, NY: Elsevier; 1993:275–281.

80. Kwak BR, Sáez JC, Wilders R, et al. Effects of cGMP-dependent phosphorylation on rat and human connexin43 gap junction channels. *Eur J Physiol.* 1995;430:770–778.

81. Moore LK, Burt JM. Antiarrythmic drugs have a minor effect on gap junction conductance. *Biophys J.* 1990;57:246a. Abstract.

82. Miyachi E, Manoach M, Uchiyama H, Watanabe Y, Thormaehlen D. Tedisamil enhances intercellular coupling: a new explanation of its ventricular defibrillating action. *2nd Workshop on Antiarrhythmic Drugs and Self Ventricular Defibrillation.* September, 1995:28. Abstract.

83. Uchiyama H, Manoach M, Miyachi E, Watanabe Y. Sotalol facilitates spontaneous ventricular defibrillation by enhancing intercellular coupling: an entirely new mechanism for its antiarrythmic action. *2nd Workshop on Antiarrhythmic Drugs and Self Ventricular Defibrillation.* September, 1995:49. Abstract.

84. Aonuma S, Kohama Y, Akai K, et al. Studies on heart, 19: isolation of an atrial peptide that improves the rhythmicity of cultured myocardial cell clusters. *Chem Pharm Bull.* 1980;28:3340–3346.

85. Aonuma S, Kohana, Y, Makino T, et al. Studies on heart 22: inhibitory effect of an atrial peptide on several drug induced arrhythmias in vivo. *Yakugaku Zasshi.* 1983;103:662–666.

86. Dhein S, Tudyka T. Therapeutic potential of antiarrhythmic peptides: cellular coupling as a new antiarrhythmic target. *Drugs.* 1995;49:851–855.

87. Dhein S, Tudyka T, Schott M, et al. Enhancement of cellular coupling as a possible new antiarrhythmic mechanism. *Naunyn Schmiedebergs Arch Pharmacol.* 1995;351(suppl):R106. Abstract.
88. Matesic DF, Rupp HL, Bonney WJ, Ruch RJ, Trosko JE. Changes in gap-junction permeability, phosphorylation, and number mediated by phorbol ester and non-phorbol-ester tumor promoters in rat liver epithelial cells. *Mol Carcinog.* 1994;10:226–236.
89. Davidson JS, Baumgarten IM. Glycyrrhetinic acid derivatives: a novel class of inhibitors of gap-junctional intercellular communication: structure-activity relationships. *J Pharmacol Exp Ther.* 1988;246:1104–1107.
90. Munari-Silem Y, Lebrethon MC, Morand I, Rousset B, Saez JM. Gap junction-mediated cell-to-cell communication in bovine and human adrenal cells: a process whereby cells increase their responsiveness to physiological corticotropin concentrations. *J Clin Invest.* 1995;95:1429–1439.

Molecular Analysis of the pH Regulation of the Cardiac Gap Junction Protein Connexin43

Mario Delmar, MD, PhD,
Gregory E. Morley, PhD,
and Steven M. Taffet, PhD

A mature heart is composed of millions of highly specialized cells. In isolation, each one of those cells is capable of contracting upon stimulation. Individual pacemaker cells are also capable of beating spontaneously when separated from the rest of the tissue. Yet the heart as a functional unit is an amazing example of synchrony: A normal beat travels rapidly in a defined sequence to all cells. As a result, the microscopic mechanical effort of individual myocytes is translated into a powerful stroke capable of pumping blood for the entire body. This "team effort" requires a highly efficient cell-to-cell information system to coordinate contraction. This is provided by the passage of electrical charge across low-resistance intercellular pathways called gap junctions.

Gap Junction Regulation in the Heart

For the most part, cardiac gap junctions are perceived as passive elements, yet the evidence shows that gap junction conductance is not always the case. Indeed, gap junction conductance can be regulated by

This work was supported by grants PO1-HL39707 and RO1-HL52812 from the National Institutes of Health, Heart Lung and Blood Institute. Mario Delmar is an Established Investigator of the American Heart Association.

From: Spooner PM, Joyner RW, Jalife J (eds). *Discontinuous Conduction in the Heart*. Armonk, NY: Futura Publishing Company, Inc.; © 1997.

a variety of factors in the intracellular environment, including intracellular proton concentration (pH$_i$),[1-3] ATP,[4] accumulation of long-chain acylcarnitines,[5] and activation of kinases.[6] The physiological significance of gap junction regulation in the normal adult mammalian heart has not been well established. However, it has been suggested that changes in gap junction conductance may occur during ischemia, thus setting the stage for life-threatening arrhythmias.[7-10] Indeed, myocardial ischemia is known to trigger some of the very changes associated with gap junction channel closure. The specific contribution of electrical uncoupling to the development of ischemia-induced malignant ventricular arrhythmias has been difficult to assess, partly because ischemia causes global changes in the physiology of cardiac myocytes.[8-10] Nevertheless, the evidence available shows a good correlation between the onset of some of the cardiac arrhythmias observed in whole-animal models of ischemia and the time course of electrical uncoupling as demonstrated in isolated preparations.[9,10]

Gap junction channels also seem to play an important role in cardiac development. Indeed, recent studies have shown that transgenic mice lacking the gene that codes for the major cardiac gap junction protein, connexin43 (Cx43), complete their development in utero but die shortly after birth, victims of a failure in pulmonary gas exchange.[11] Anatomic inspection shows an enlargement of the conus region overlying the right ventricular outflow tract. Many questions that stem from these results remain unanswered. However, the data strongly suggest that molecular signals travel across the junctions to synchronize proper cardiac formation during development. In addition, one might speculate that gap junction permeability can in itself be finely regulated, so that only selected molecules reach the neighboring cells at the appropriate stages of embryogenesis. This seems to be supported by the recent studies of Britz-Cunningham et al,[12] who linked some (though not all)[13,14] cases of human visceroatrial heterotaxia (a congenital cardiac malformation involving problems of lateralization) with mutations in the carboxyl-terminal end of Cx43. Noticeably, most of these mutations alter the phosphorylation state of the protein in vitro. Phosphorylation is a well-known regulator of gap junction channel conductance.[15-17] Thus, it is possible that during embryogenesis, gap junctions act as regulators of intercellular signaling.

If cardiac gap junctions are involved in normal development, it is conceivable that they are also involved in the transmission of chemical messages in the adult heart. Recent studies by Rourke et al[18] show that the heart is subject to metabolic oscillations that synchronize with the cardiac cycle. It is possible that those oscillations occur in the heart in situ. In that case, gap junctions would allow for the synchronization of metabolic oscillations between cells as in other systems (eg, secretory cells).[19]

Finally, one may speculate that if gap junctions are necessary for the harmonic development of the embryonic heart, they may also be involved in morphological changes that occur to the adult heart. A case in point is the development of cardiac hypertrophy. In particular, one may ask whether the molecular signals that command the hypertrophic response of the heart travel across junctions to achieve a homogeneous response across the ventricles. Further studies on the pathological involvement of gap junctions in this and other conditions are clearly warranted.

At this time, the evidence suggests that gap junction channels are not just passive conduits of electrical charge but rather dynamic entities that regulate the communication of essential molecular messages between neighboring cells. Modulation of gap junction channel conductance could therefore be an essential component of normal function and, if altered, a potential mechanism of disease. The importance of understanding the molecular bases for gap junction channel regulation can be readily appreciated. A mounting number of connexins have already been cloned,[20] and at least three of these are present in the adult mammalian heart.[21] The level of expression of each connexin apparently may vary during development.[22]

Our approach to this problem has been to focus our attention on the regulation of one specific connexin (Cx43) by one specific factor (pH_i). Our goal is to formulate a molecular model for the pH gating of Cx43, which could be used as a reference point to study regulation of other connexins by multiple factors. In this chapter, we review our hypothesis that pH gating of Cx43 can be modeled as an intramolecular particle-receptor interaction similar to the ball-and-chain mechanism of voltage-dependent gating.[23,24] In addition, we provide new evidence to further validate certain methodological aspects of our experimental preparation; and finally, we pose some of the unanswered questions that stem from the data collected so far.

Recent Studies on pH Gating of Cx43: Methodological Considerations

Our approach involves the use of the oocyte expression system to examine pH sensitivity of Cx43 and its mutants. Pairs of connexin-expressing oocytes are progressively acidified by superfusion with increasing concentrations of CO_2. Junctional conductance is measured electrophysiologically while at the same time, pH_i is recorded by optical methods.

Measurement of pH_i: Optical Methods versus pH-Sensitive Microelectrodes

In our earlier studies,[25] intracellular pH was measured by means of a proton-sensitive microelectrode. This technique, although reliable, is more cumbersome than the optical approach. A critical issue in the use of pH-sensitive microelectrodes is that the calibration at the end of the experiment should be identical to that measured at the beginning. In our experience, however, electrode properties tend to be altered at or during the impalement, thus causing a shift in electrode calibration. As a result, the success rate of experiments involving pH-sensitive electrodes is rather low. Moreover, pH-sensitive electrodes cannot be used when intracellular acidification is achieved by CO_2 because of artifactual changes in pH calibration.[25,26] In addition, the pH_i measurement recorded by the microelectrode is even more limited in space than the one obtained by the use of fluorophores. Finally, optical methods do not require the disruption of the membrane by impalement with an additional electrode, which reduces the chances of cell damage. In general, we have found that optical methods provide a more flexible and far more efficient system for intracellular pH recording than the pH-sensitive electrode.

Selection of the Appropriate Fluorophore

A number of proton-sensitive fluorophores are currently available. We have chosen a single-excitation, dual-emission dye called seminaphthorhodafluor (SNARF). This dye is available in a dextran form that can be easily injected into oocytes. The emission spectra shown in Figure 1 were recorded from an oocyte previously injected with 50 nL of a 357-μmol/L solution of SNARF. The cell was excited with monochromatic light at a wavelength of 534 nm. The spectrum depicted by a continuous line was obtained while the oocyte was maintained in a bicarbonate-buffered solution at a pH of 7.2. The broken line shows the spectrum following acidification to a pH_o of 6.1. Both spectra are normalized to the intensity recorded at the isosbestic point for SNARF (611 nm). Clearly, acidification caused an increase in the emission intensity at 580 to 590 nm and a decrease in the intensity at $\approx$640 nm. A qualitatively similar shift in the emission spectra is obtained when the dye is simply dissolved in a saline solution.

An acetoxymethyl derivative of SNARF (SNARF-AM) is also available. In principle, these molecules can enter the cytoplasm if the cells are simply incubated in a dye-containing solution.[27] Once inside, the lipophilic groups are cleaved by cytoplasmic esterases, yielding a

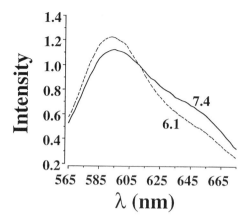

Figure 1. Emission spectra obtained from a single *Xenopus laevis* oocyte injected with dextran form of proton-sensitive dye SNARF. Spectrum depicted by solid line was obtained while oocyte was maintained in a saline solution buffered with 18 mmol/L NaHCO$_3$ and gassed with 95% O$_2$/5% CO$_2$ at pH 7.4. Trace denoted by dashed line was obtained while solution was gassed with 100% CO$_2$ (pH 6.1). Abscissa shows emission wavelength (λ); ordinate, emission intensity plotted relative to the isosbestic point for SNARF. Details of protocol are given in Morley et al.[30]

charged free acid that cannot cross the cell membrane. Such a form of the dye has been used successfully in cardiac myocytes.[27] Accordingly, one may predict that this method would be simpler to use than the microinjection of the dextran form; the possibilities of cell damage caused by the injection would also be avoided. In our experience, however, the spectral properties of SNARF-AM in oocytes did not conform to what has been described for this same dye in other cells or in vitro or with the properties of dextran-SNARF in oocytes. Indeed, as shown in Figure 2, the maximum intensity of emission was recorded at around 605 nm, and a peculiar "hump" in the emission spectra at lower wavelengths is seen both at normal and at a lower pH. The reasons why SNARF-AM did not show the same emission spectra as dextran-SNARF (or as SNARF in solution) in our system are unknown. Our data, however, warn against the use of AM forms of ion-sensitive dyes in oocytes unless appropriate controls are used. The data also stress the importance of recording full emission spectra as a part of the initial characterization process.

BCECF is a pH-sensitive dye that has been previously used in oocytes.[28] This is a dual-excitation, single-emission dye. The dynamic range of this dye is also well suited for pH$_i$ measurements at near-physiological range. But the advantage of dual-emission dyes is that they allow for measurements of emission in real time, whereas dual

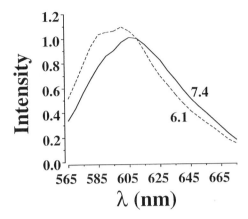

Figure 2. Emission spectra recorded from a single oocyte incubated in a saline solution containing 1 μmol/L SNARF-AM. Same experimental protocol as for Figure 1. Although emission properties of dye are still pH dependent, shape of spectra is different from that obtained from dextran-SNARF in oocytes as well as from SNARF in vitro[27] or in other cells.[27] Traces as in Figure 1.

excitation requires the use of alternating excitation signals. This is important when the rate of acquisition becomes the limiting factor for the study of time-dependent phenomena.

Calibration of the Proton-Sensitive Fluorophore in Oocytes

Calibration of SNARF emission signals requires an independent measurement of proton concentration while emission intensities are recorded simultaneously. For this purpose, some investigators[28] have used a combination of nigericin (a potassium/proton antiporter) and valinomycin, either alone or together with the protonophore FCCP.[27,28] The basic assumption with this method is that the concentration of protons inside the cell is the same as that outside. We failed in our attempt to use this calibration system with oocytes. As shown in Figure 3, shifting the pH of the superfusate from 7.4 (solid line) to 8.0 (dashed line) in the presence of the protonophore caused an increase in the 590-nm peak with reduction in the 640-nm peak. Such a change in SNARF emission is expected as a result of acidification and is therefore exactly opposite to what would be predicted after alkalinization of the intracellular space. Although the mechanism responsible for this shift was not studied further, it is very possible that the proton concentration inside

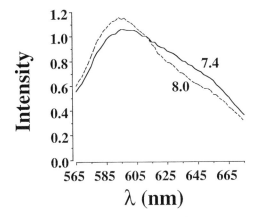

Figure 3. Emission spectra recorded from an oocyte maintained in a solution containing (in mmol/L): KCl 100, MgSO₄ 0.82, CaCl₂ 0.74, and HEPES 10. pH of solution was adjusted to 7.4 (solid line) or 8.0 (dashed line). Solution also contained nigericin (50 μmol/L), valinomycin (50 μmol/L), and FCCP (50 μmol/L) in an attempt to equilibrate intracellular and extracellular concentrations of protons.[27,28] Contrary to what would be expected, emission spectrum changed toward acidic direction, despite alkalinization of extracellular environment. These results indicate that this calibration procedure is not applicable to our experimental conditions.

the cell was not the same as that outside. Inconsistent results were also obtained when the "null point" procedure[29] was used to calibrate the dye.

Our laboratory has previous experience with pH-sensitive microelectrodes. We therefore decided to calibrate the optical system by simultaneously recording emission spectra of dextran-SNARF and intracellular pH with the microelectrode. The calibration curve, shown in Figure 4 is similar to that obtained in cardiac myocytes.[27] As with the myocytes, the curve was different from that obtained when SNARF was calibrated in solution, illustrating the importance of obtaining a calibration curve in the cell system under study.

These results show that optical measurement of light emission by use of dextran-SNARF is a reliable method for estimating intracellular pH in oocytes. One limitation of SNARF is reduced resolution at pH$_i$ values <6.35. We have measured lower pH$_i$ values in oocytes by means of a different dye, rhodol green. This dye, also available in dextran form, yields intense and very stable signals when injected into oocytes. As shown in Figure 5, the dynamic range of rhodol green is more acidic than that of SNARF, allowing measurement of pH$_i$ in the range at which SNARF is no longer sensitive.

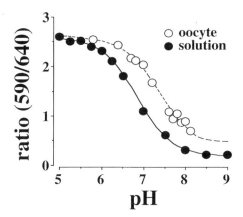

Figure 4. Calibration curves for dextran-SNARF in oocytes and in solution. pH_i was measured with an intracellular pH-sensitive microelectrode.[25] Measurements are ratios of emission intensity at 590 nm to that at 640 nm. Reprinted with permission from Reference 30.

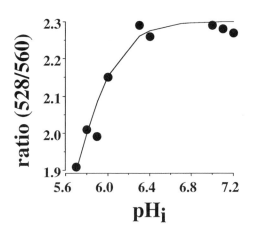

Figure 5. Calibration curve of proton-sensitive dye rhodol green (dextran form) in oocytes. pH_i was measured with a proton-sensitive microelectrode.[25] pH sensitivity was determine as ratio of intensity of emission at 528 nm to that at 560 nm. Measurements <5.7 could not be obtained because of cell damage. Dye shows good resolution up to a pH_i of ≈6.4.

Rate of Acidification Can Alter the Apparent pH Sensitivity of Cx43

These data validated our choice of techniques to measure pH_i in oocytes. Next, we developed a procedure that would allow us to change pH_i in oocytes in a slow, reproducible manner. The latter is important because the apparent dependence of gap junction channels on pH_i could be affected by the rate at which intracellular acidification is achieved (see also below). To address this problem, we developed an experimental paradigm that allows us to change pH_i in a ramp-like fashion at a slow rate that is reproducible between experiments. A diagram of the experimental set-up is presented in Figure 6. An O_2/CO_2 gas mixture saturates a bicarbonate-buffered solution used to superfuse the oocyte pair. The pH of the superfusate is changed precisely in a manner predicted by the Henderson-Hasselbach equation. Although the proportion of CO_2 in the gas mixture is increased stepwise, changes in pH_i take longer to develop and are controlled by the number of steps used, their duration, and the proportion of CO_2 in the mix.

Figure 7 shows effects on an oocyte pair acidified by the proce-dures described.[30] In this case, five steps of 10 minutes each were used to change intracellular pH from 7.2 to 6.4. Junctional conductance (G_j) was recorded simultaneously. As intracellular acidification progressed, G_j progressively decreased until uncoupling ensued. The point-by-point correlation depicted in Figure 7B shows a smooth, sigmoidal func-tion, with a pKa (ie, the pH_i at which G_j reaches 50% of maximum) of ≈6.7. Acidification ramps like this one were highly reproducible, thus allowing for comparison of results obtained from oocytes expressing different connexin constructs.

It is important that acidification be done carefully to minimize distortions caused by delay in the time course of uncoupling. A case in point is illustrated in Figure 8A. Under control conditions, the cells were constantly superfused with a bicarbonate-buffered solution gassed with 5% CO_2. The proportion of CO_2 in the gas mixture was then abruptly increased to 100%. Rapid acidification of the intracellular space ensued, followed by a reduction in G_j. However, G_j adapted more slowly, reaching 50% of maximum at the rather acidic pH_i of 6.6. Moreover, the "pH-sensitivity" curve fell almost vertically at a pH_i of 6.5 while G_j continued changing, despite a constant pH_i. A similar case is shown in Figure 8B, where five steps of 5 minutes each were used to acidify the cells. Although the point-by-point correlation showed a smoother function, a vertical fall at a pH_i of 6.5 was still apparent. Again, this vertical drop was consequent to the fact that G_j was trailing after the changes in pH_i. This type of G_j-versus-pH_i correlation clearly

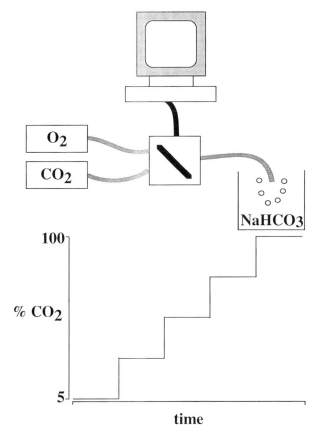

Figure 6. Diagram of experimental setup for slow acidification of connexin-expressing cells. Central box with solid diagonal line represents a solenoid valve, which is controlled by a computer (top). Valve regulates proportions of O_2 and CO_2 that are used to bubble bicarbonate-containing superfusate. Bottom diagram indicates that proportion of CO_2 is increased with time in a stepwise manner. Computer controls amplitude and duration of each step.

indicates that G_j was not at steady state at the time pH_i reached a new value. Therefore, the correlation between the two variables is not an indication of the changes in G_j that result as a function of pH_i only. Indeed, the results indicate participation of a time-dependent component of unknown magnitude.

The mechanism responsible for the delay in uncoupling presented in Figure 8 is unknown. There are at least three possibilities. The first is that pH gating (ie, the change in junctional conductance in response to changes in pH_i) may in itself be a slow process; this would be analogous to what could occur if we were to study voltage dependence of

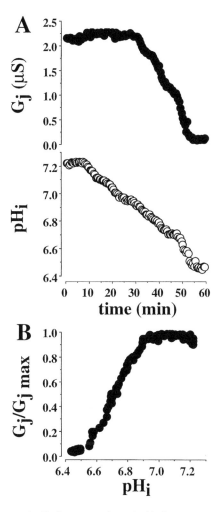

Figure 7. A, Changes in G_j (top trace) and pH_i (bottom trace) recorded from an oocyte pair expressing Cx43. B, Plot obtained by correlating pH_i and G_j at each point in time. With slow acidification, correlation can be used as a representation of pH sensitivity of connexin under study. Reprinted with permission from Reference 30.

Cx43 using voltage ramps. Since voltage gating is time dependent,[31] the currents elicited by a fast voltage ramp would yield an inaccurate representation of the steady-state current-voltage dependence of Cx43. A second possibility is that triggering of pH gating requires slow intermediary steps. It has previously been proposed that pH gating of gap junctions actually results from calmodulin-mediated, calcium-initiated

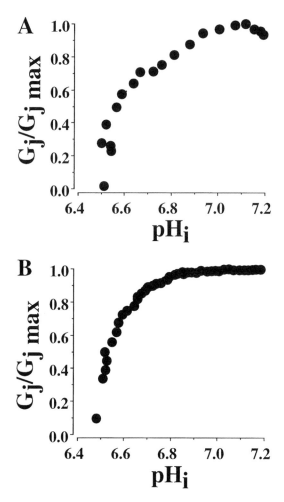

Figure 8. G_j vs pH_i curves obtained from two different oocyte pairs that were rapidly acidified. Vertical drop observed at $pH_i \approx 6.5$ is indicative that changes in G_j lagged behind changes in pH_i; consequently, G_j continued to change after pH_i reached a stable value. The latter suggests that for these pairs, acidification protocols were too fast to determine pH sensitivity of the connexin studied.

changes in G_j.[26,32] From this perspective, intracellular acidification would act only as a trigger for the increase in intracellular calcium, although this hypothesis has not been tested with Cx43. However, the recent results of Terstal-Kortekaas et al[33] indicate that Cx43-transfected cells develop acidification-induced uncoupling even in the presence of calcium chelators in the recording pipettes. Those observations are consistent with ours showing that susceptibility to acidification-induced uncoupling of Cx43 is not affected by the injection of dextran-

BAPTA into the oocytes. Further experiments would be necessary to study the interaction between protons and other ions in the pH-gating process. Although the two possibilities described above cannot be discarded, it is important to note that the pH_i that we measure may differ from the pH_i at the mouth of the gap junction channel. Thus, a third possibility we should consider is that the uncoupling delay may result from the time it takes for the protons to diffuse from the area under the cell membrane where our recordings are obtained to the actual site of cell-cell apposition. In that regard, slower acidification ramps allow more time for equilibration of ion concentrations within the intracellular space. Whether ramps such as the one presented in Figure 7 are slow enough to avoid pH_i gradients remains to be determined, but by applying the same protocol in all experiments, we minimize the possibility that differences between groups are affected by differences in the time course and extent of acidification. With this protocol, we consistently obtain smooth, sigmoidal functions and do not observe abrupt changes in the slope of the pH-sensitivity curve. Although slower ramps would be technically possible, an increase in the acidification time would enhance the chances of oocyte damage. Moreover, with the acidification protocol used for Figure 7, the possibility of G_j lagging behind pH_i is unlikely.

In experiments in which the acidification ramp has been stopped before complete uncoupling, no changes in G_j have been observed for as long as pH_i remains at a constant value. An example is shown in Figure 9. These recordings were obtained from an oocyte pair coexpressing a mutant form of Cx43 named M257 and, as a separate protein, the carboxyl-terminal domain of Cx43.[30] In this case, acidification was induced with a faster protocol. In ≈25 minutes, pH_i dropped from 7.2 to 6.4. G_j showed a small initial increase, followed by a drop to a value near 50% below maximum. Interestingly, the rate of uncoupling followed the rate of acidification, and as pH_i reached an asymptotic value, G_j also stabilized. As a result, a cluster of points at a pH_i near 6.4 was recorded in the G_j-versus-pH_i plot (Figure 9B). These results show that in this experiment, G_j was not trailing after changes in pH_i. Similar results have been obtained in other experiments in which the acidification protocol was interrupted before complete uncoupling was achieved. These results suggest that when a slow acidification ramp is used, changes in G_j occur synchronously with changes in pH_i and support our recent findings[30] on the pH sensitivity of different connexins.

A Particle-Receptor Hypothesis for the pH Gating of Cx43

We have previously shown that truncation of the carboxyl-terminal domain of Cx43 significantly impairs acidification-induced uncoup-

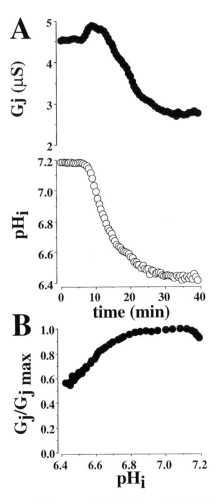

Figure 9. Time course of changes in G_j (top) and pH_i (bottom) recorded from an oocyte pair expressing a mutated form of Cx43 (M257) and its carboxyl-terminal domain (see Figure 10 and Reference 30 for more details). Despite relatively fast drop in pH_i, changes in G_j closely follow pH_i changes. In contrast to G_j-vs-pH_i curves shown in Figure 8, here the pH-sensitivity curve shows a cluster of values at asymptotic pH_i.

ling.[25] In other studies, we found that mutations of histidine 95 (located near the interface between the second membrane-spanning domain and the beginning of the cytoplasmic loop) also alter pH sensitivity.[34] We therefore proposed that pH gating results from the interaction between the carboxyl-terminal, acting as a gating particle, and a separate domain, acting as a receptor for the particle. Upon acidification, the parti-

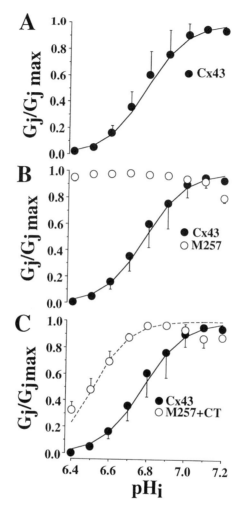

Figure 10. A, Average pH-sensitivity curve obtained from Cx43-expressing oocytes. B, Truncation of carboxyl-terminal end of Cx43 at amino acid 257 (M257) prevented acidification-induced uncoupling in the pH range tested. C, Coexpressing M257 with mRNA coding for the missing carboxyl-terminal (CT) region partly restored pH sensitivity of gap junction channels (M257 + CT). These results demonstrate that pH gating results from interaction of carboxyl-terminal, acting as an independent domain, with another region of protein affiliated with pore-forming structure. See Morley et al[30] for further details. Reprinted with permission from Reference 30.

cle would noncovalently bind to its receptor, causing the channel to close. A similar mechanism has been proposed for the voltage-dependent inactivation of sodium and potassium channels.[23,24,35]

The results in Figure 10 support this hypothesis. Cx43 or its mutants were expressed in antisense-injected *Xenopus* oocyte pairs, and G_j and pH_i recorded. Figure 10A shows the pH sensitivity of the wild-type protein. The open circles in 10B depict a lack of pH sensitivity with a Cx43 mutant truncated at amino acid 257. The open circles in C are data obtained when the truncation mutant was coexpressed with mRNA coding exclusively for the carboxyl-terminal domain. Clearly, the carboxyl-terminal domain recognized the rest of the connexin molecule and interacted with it, so that the pH sensitivity of the gap junction channels was partly restored. The data do not establish whether the particle-receptor interaction is direct or mediated through an intermediary molecule.

Future Directions

Determination of the role of gap junctions in physiological and pathophysiological processes has been limited by, among other things, the lack of a specific agent that could either prevent pH gating or induce channel closure at normal pH. Although various "uncouplers" have been described,[36] none have demonstrated enough selectivity to isolate effects unique to just gap junctions, and not other channels. By showing which parts of the molecule participate, our studies may help in the development of just such an agent. Indeed, characterization of functionally important primary structures has been instrumental for drug design in other systems. More importantly, the demonstration that pH gating involves the interaction of the carboxyl-terminal with a separate domain allows us to approach pH gating as a ligand-receptor interaction. Accordingly, we postulate that channel closure could be prevented by molecules that, although analogous to the particle, may bind to the receptor but not induce the gating response. Conversely, mutations in the particle may increase its affinity for the receptor, so that channel closure could occur at a normal pH_i. Further studies will be necessary to address these possibilities.

Recently, using site-directed mutagenesis, we identified two specific regions in the carboxyl-terminal domain that, when absent, prevent acidification-induced uncoupling.[37] One of these regions is between residues 261 and 300, and the other includes the last nine amino acids. Interestingly, substitution of one amino acid (aspartate 379) for its corresponding amide also prevents acidification-induced uncoupling. Other mutations having similar effects are currently under study. Why these mutated channels loose pH gating remains to be determined. One possibility is that some mutated form still recognize the receptor but cannot trigger gating. If that were the case, they may act as competitive antagonists of the normal particle-receptor binding reaction.

Our results also provide new insight into molecular mechanisms of pH regulation of rat cardiac Cx43 but raise other questions as well. For example, What is the stoichiometry of the particle-receptor interaction? Is pH gating mediated by an intermediary molecule or does it involve only the connexin channel and its carboxyl-terminal CT domain? Is acidification just the trigger, or is binding of the particle and the receptor dependent on increased proton concentration? Is this particle-receptor mechanism of pH gating common to other connexins and to the chemical regulation of other channels? Finally, could regulation of gap junction conductance by other mechanisms (eg, phosphorylation) be mediated by similar mechanisms?

Modern optical, electrophysiological, and molecular biological methods provide new approaches to add such issues. Yet we are still a long way from integrating these kinds of data with the actual gap junction channel function and its regulation in the heart. Perhaps newer genetic approaches using transgenic animals[11] or the transfer of genes into adult tissues[38,39] hold the key to understanding the reductionist connexin molecules in isolation and their importance in the physiology of highly complex integrated organisms.

Acknowledgments   We thank Dr. José Jalife for his advice and support throughout this project. The assistance of Dr. Harvey Penefsky in the implementation of the optical recording technique is greatly appreciated. We are also grateful to Wanda Coombs, Christine Burrer, and Christine Kapuscinski for their excellent technical support and to LaVerne Gilbert for her excellent secretarial support.

References

1. White RL, Doeller JE, Verselis VK, Wittenberg BA. Gap junctional conductance between pairs of ventricular myocytes is modulated synergistically by H^+ and Ca^{++}. *J Gen Physiol.* 1990;95:1061–1075.
2. Burt JM. Block of intercellular communication: interaction of intracellular H^+ and Ca^{2+}. *Am J Physiol.* 1987;253:C607–C612.
3. Firek L, Weingart R. Modification of gap junction conductance by divalent cations and protons in neonatal rat heart cells. *J Mol Cell Cardiol.* 1995;27:1633–1643.
4. Sugiura H, Toyama J, Tsuboi N, Kamiya K, Kodama I. ATP directly affects junctional conductance between paired ventricular myocytes isolated from guinea pig heart. *Circ Res.* 1990;66:1095–1102.
5. Wu J, McHowat J, Saffitz JE, Yamada KA, Corr PB. Inhibition of gap junctional conductance by long-chain acylcarnitines and their preferential accumulation in junctional sarcolemma during hypoxia. *Circ Res.* 1993;72:879–889.

6. Strasser RH, Braun-Dullaeus R, Walendzik H, Marquetant R. α_1-Receptor-independent activation of protein kinase C in acute myocardial ischemia. *Circ Res*. 1992;70:1304–1312.
7. Gettes LS, Buchanan JW, Saito T, Kagiyama Y, Oshita S, Fujino T. Studies concerned with slow conduction. In: Zipes DP, Jalife J, eds. *Cardiac Electrophysiology and Arrhythmias*. Orlando, Fla: Grune & Stratton Inc; 1985:81–87.
8. Gettes LS, Cascio WE. Effect of acute ischemia on cardiac electrophysiology. In: Fozard H, et al, eds. *The Heart and Cardiovascular System*. New York, NY: Raven Press; 1992:2021–2054.
9. Kleber AG, Riegger CB, Janse MJ. Electrical uncoupling and increase of extracellular resistance after induction of ischemia in isolated, arterially perfused rabitt papillary muscle. *Circ Res*. 1987;61:271–279.
10. Janse MJ, Wit AL. Electrophysiological mechanisms of ventricular arrhythmias resulting from myocardial ischemia and infarction. *Physiol Rev*. 1989; 69:1049–1169.
11. Reaume AG, de Sousa PA, Kulkarni S, et al. Cardiac malformation in neonatal mice lacking connexin43. *Science*. 1995;267:1831–1834.
12. Britz-Cunningham SH, Shah MM, Zuppan CW, Fletcher WH. Mutations of the connexin43 gap-juntion gene in patients with heart malformations and defects of laterality. *N Engl J Med*. 1995;332:1323–1329.
13. Casey B, Ballabio A. Connexin43 mutations in sporadic and familial defects of laterality. *N Engl J Med*. 1995;333:941. Letter.
14. Splitt MP, Burn J, Goodship J. Connexin43 mutations in sporadic and familial defects of laterality. *N Engl J Med*. 1995;333:941. Letter.
15. Moreno AP, Saez JC, Fishman GI, Spray DC. Human connexin43 gap junction channels: regulation of unitary conductances by phosphorylation. *Circ Res*. 1994;74:1050–1057.
16. Kwak BR, Van Veen TAB, Analbers LJS, Jongsma HJ. TPA increases conductance but decreases permeability in neonatal rat cardiomyocyte gap junction channels. *Exp Cell Res*. 1995;220:456–463.
17. Kwak BR, Saez JC, Wilders R, et al. Effects of cGMP-dependent phosphorylation on rat and human connexin43 gap junction channels. *Pflugers Arch*. 1995;430:770–778.
18. Rourke B, Ramza BM, Marban E. Oscillations of membrane current and excitability driven by metabolic oscillations in heart cells. *Science*. 1994;265: 962–966.
19. Meda P, Vozzi C, Ullrich S, et al. Gland cell connexins. In: Kanno Y, et al, eds. *Intercellular Communication Through Gap Junctions*. Amsterdam, Netherlands: Elsevier; 1995:281–287.
20. Bennett MVL, Zheng X, Sogin ML. The connexin family tree. In: Kanno Y, et al, eds. *Intercellular Communication Through Gap Junctions*. Amsterdam, Netherlands: Elsevier; 1995:3–8.
21. Kanter HL, Saffitz JE, Beyer EC. Cardiac myocytes express multiple gap junction proteins. *Circ Res*. 1992;70:438–444.
22. van Kempen MJA, Fromaget C, Gros D, Moorman AFM, Lamers WH. Spatial distribution of connexin43, the major cardiac gap junction protein, in the developing and adult rat heart. *Circ Res*. 1991;68:1638–1651.
23. Hoshi T, Zagotta WN, Aldrich RW. Biophysical and molecular mechanisms of Shaker potassium channel inactivation. *Science*. 1990;250:533–538.
24. Zagotta WN, Hoshi T, Aldrich RW. Restoration of inactivation in mutants of Shaker potassium channels by a peptide derived from ShB. *Science*. 1990; 250:568–571.

25. Liu S, Taffet S, Stoner L, Delmar M, Vallano ML, Jalife J. A structural basis for the unequal sensitivity of the major cardiac and liver gap junctions to intracellular acidification: the carboxyl tail length. *Biophys J.* 1993;64: 1422–1433.
26. Peracchia C. Increase in gap junction resistance with acidification in crayfish septate axons is closely related to changes in intracellular calcium but not hydrogen ion concentration. *J Membr Biol.* 1990;113:75–92.
27. Blank PS, Silverman HS, Chung OY, et al. Cytosolic pH measurements in single cardiac myocytes using carboxy-seminaphtorhodafluor-1. *Am J Physiol.* 1992;263:H267–H284.
28. Sasaki S, Ishibashi K, Nagai T, Marumo F. Regulation mechanisms of intracellular pH of Xenopus laevis oocyte. *Biochim Biophys Acta.* 1992;1137:45–51.
29. Eisner DA, Kenning NA, O'Neill SC, Pocok G, Richards CD, Valdeomillos M. A novel method for absolute calibration of intracellular pH indicators. *Pflugers Arch.* 1989;413:553–558.
30. Morley GE, Taffet SM, Delmar M. Intramolecular interactions mediate pH regulation of connexin43 channels. *Biophys J.* 1996;70:1294–1302.
31. Rook MB, Jongsma HJ, van Ginneken ACG. Properties of single gap junctional channels between isolated neonatal rat heart cells. *Am J Physiol.* 1988; 255:H770–H782.
32. Arellano RO, Ramon F, Rivera A, Zampighi G. Calmodulin acts as an intermediary for the effects of calcium on gap junctions from crayfish lateral axons. *J Membr Biol.* 1988;101:119–131.
33. Terstal-Kortekaas P, Hermans MMP, Rook MB, Jongsma HJ. The role of histidines 126 and 142 on pH sensitivity of connexin43. *Pflugers Arch.* 1995; 430:R174. Abstract.
34. Ek JF, Delmar M, Perzova R, Taffet SM. Role of histidine 95 on the pH gating of the cardiac gap junction protein connexin43. *Circ Res.* 1994;74: 1058–1064.
35. Armstrong CM, Bezanilla F. Inactivation of the sodium channel, II: gating current experiments. *J Gen Physiol.* 1977;70:567–590.
36. Spray DC, Burt JM. Structure-activity relations of the cardiac gap junction channel. *Am J Physiol.* 1990;258:C195–C205.
37. Ek-Vitorin JF, Calero G, Morley GE, Coombs W, Taffet SM, Delmar M. pH regulation of connexin43: molecular analysis of the gating particle. *Biophys J.* 1996;71:1273–1284.
38. Johns DC, Nuss B, Chiamvimonvat N, Ramza BM, Marban E, Lawrence JH. Adenovirus-mediated expression of a voltage-gated potassium channel in vitro (rat cardiac myocytes) and in vivo (rat liver). *J Clin Invest.* 1995;95: 1152–1158.
39. Guzman RJ, Lemarchand P, Crystal RG, Epstein SE, Finkel T. Efficient gene transfer into myocardium by direct injection of adenovirus vectors. *Circ Res.* 1993;73:1202–1207.

Chapter 10

Triggered Propagated Contractions and Arrhythmias Caused by Acute Damage to Cardiac Muscle

Henk E.D.J. ter Keurs, MD, PhD,
and Ying Ming Zhang, MSc

Extrasystoles and Arrhythmias

Arrhythmias commonly arise as the oscillatory response to an extrasystole by a reentry pathway in nonuniform working myocardium or conduction tissue. In the human heart, the nonuniformity of conduction is often a result of myocardial ischemia or infarction due to coronary artery disease. Nonuniformity caused by ischemic damage may be aggravated by cardiac remodeling during development of congestive heart failure, which may explain why fatal arrhythmias are often found in patients with congestive heart failure. Most concepts of arrhythmias emphasize the importance of electrical nonuniformity, but it is evident that myocardium that has been rendered nonuniform may also suffer from variations of stresses and strains from cell to cell and in addition may show differences in excitation-contraction coupling between cells.

Little is known about the role played by nonuniform myocardial stress and strain distributions and by nonuniform excitation-contraction coupling in mechanisms underlying extrasystoles that initiate an

This work was supported by grants from the Janssen Research Foundation and the Alberta Heart and Stroke Foundation. Dr. H.E.D.J. ter Keurs is a Medical Scientist of the Alberta Heritage Foundation for Medical Research (AHFMR). Ying Ming Zhang holds a studentship of the AHFMR.

From: Spooner PM, Joyner RW, Jalife J (eds). *Discontinuous Conduction in the Heart.* Armonk, NY: Futura Publishing Company, Inc.; © 1997.

arrhythmia. Still, this knowledge is essential to the choice of treatment aimed at prevention of an extrasystole versus treatment aimed at suppression of reentry. A typical scenario in which arrhythmias occur is acute damage of myocardium commonly due to ischemia. Such damage may lead to extrasystoles as a result of Ca^{2+} overload of the damaged cells and their neighbors. Hence, it is conceivable that damage-induced extrasystoles may set up the initiating event for reentry arrhythmias.

Aftercontractions and Afterdepolarizations

It has been known for half a century[1-5] that two types of oscillations in membrane potential may follow an action potential of cardiac muscle: (1) early afterdepolarizations and (2) delayed afterdepolarizations. Widespread interest in delayed afterdepolarizations resulted in the early 1970s from the observation that these afterdepolarizations could be induced by digitalis intoxication.[6,7] Triggered arrhythmias appeared to result from delayed afterdepolarizations.[8] A clue to their mechanism was provided by the observation that afterdepolarizations in Purkinje fibers and the accompanying aftercontractions occurred when the muscle was "loaded" with Ca^{2+}. Both the latency after the last twitch and the time course of these transients accelerated if either $[Ca^{2+}]_o$ or the stimulation rate was increased. Digitalis accelerated the afterdepolarizations even further than high $[Ca^{2+}]_o$ and a high stimulus rate.[6,7]

Like any arrhythmia, triggered arrhythmias are oscillations in which the action potentials of the arrhythmia both result from the previous impulse and lead to subsequent impulse generation. It has been shown that the delayed afterdepolarizations are based on a spontaneous increase in $[Ca^{2+}]_i$ leading to a transient inward current on the one hand and to activation of the contractile filaments on the other.[9,10] The $[Ca^{2+}]_i$ transient was assumed to be due to "spontaneous" Ca^{2+} release from the sarcoplasmic reticulum (SR). Fabiato's work[11] on the properties of the SR of cardiac muscle provided a potential explanation for such spontaneous Ca^{2+} release. He observed that in skinned cardiac muscle in which the SR was intact, excessive Ca^{2+} loading of the SR caused spontaneous Ca^{2+} release. Intact cells with a high Ca^{2+} load of the SR show a similar phenomenon.[12,13] Hence, in myocardium with a high cellular Ca^{2+} load, the oscillatory character of a triggered arrhythmia may be based on the effect of an action potential to carry more Ca^{2+} into the cells, causing even more Ca^{2+} loading of the SR. Consequently, as soon as the release process has recovered, the overloaded SR releases a fraction of its Ca^{2+}. The requirement that the Ca^{2+} release mechanism has to recover first would explain the delay between the preceding twitch and the aftercontractions and afterdepolarizations. A sufficiently high Ca^{2+} load of the SR would create an unstable state in which the Ca^{2+} release may become so large that the resulting transient inward current depolarizes the cells enough to trigger a new action potential, which perpetuates itself as a triggered arrhythmia.[8]

Triggered Propagated Contractions

In the following, we will discuss observations that suggest that aftercontractions in cardiac trabeculae occur as the combined result of local damage and elevated cellular Ca^{2+} levels and may give rise to triggered arrhythmias. The properties of the aftercontractions that can be elicited in this manner are similar to many of the properties of aftercontractions and depolarizations that have been described before. However, a unique aspect of the aftercontractions that arise in damaged regions is that they are initiated by stretch of the damaged region during the regular twitch and appear to propagate into neighboring myocardium. Most of the observations discussed in this chapter have been made on isolated rat ventricular and human atrial trabeculae. Our observations suggest that arrhythmias may be caused by Ca^{2+} release from the SR in the cells of the damaged region. Local release of Ca^{2+} in the damaged region causes a Ca^{2+} transient, which is conducted into intact muscle by the combination of Ca^{2+} diffusion and Ca^{2+}-induced Ca^{2+} release. The elevation of $[Ca^{2+}]_i$ that accompanies this process causes propagating contractions, which we have called triggered propagated contractions (TPCs).[14,15] The $[Ca^{2+}]_i$ transient also causes a depolarization of the cell membrane that may reach threshold and becomes responsible for action potential generation.[6] Damage-induced aftercontractions may therefore serve as the mechanism that couples regional damage with the initiation of extrasystoles and consequent arrhythmias in the adjacent myocardium.

TPCs appeared to arise in the ends of trabeculae,[14,15] which are often damaged by dissection and mounting of the muscle. This provided us with a means to induce and control the extent of the damage and study the consequences of acute injury on myocardium. Figure 1 shows a typical example of a TPC.

It is clear from Figure 1 that the local contraction of TPCs propagates along trabeculae with a constant velocity (V_{prop}). This wavelike character is thought to be consistent with a model of Ca^{2+}-induced Ca^{2+} release from the SR mediated by Ca^{2+} diffusion down its concentration gradient to adjacent sarcomeres and adjacent cells.[12,14–19] Theoretical simulation of the Ca^{2+} transport process has provided support for this

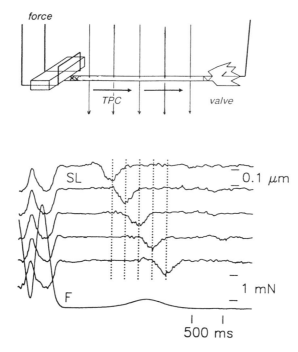

Figure 1. Sarcomere length (SL) recordings at five different sites (each 300 μm apart) along a 2.94-mm-long trabecula during a TPC with a propagation velocity of 1.4 mm/s. Interval between peak sarcomere shortening due to TPCs (vertical dashed lines) was constant from site to site, indicating that propagation velocity remained constant along preparation. F indicates force. $[Ca^{2+}]_o$ 1.0 mmol/L, temperature 21°C. Initial sarcomere length varied <0.05 μm between sites of measurement. Modified with permission from Reference 22.

hypothesis.[20] The observation that local contractions propagate in saponin-skinned trabeculae after rapid local exposure of the fiber to a Ca^{2+}-containing solution supports the notion that the SR is essential for the phenomenon.[16]

TPCs: Damage and the Initiating Event

TPCs arise invariably in damaged regions of cardiac muscle, as is shown in Figure 2. It is well known that damage causes loss of integrity of the cell membrane. Increased membrane permeability allows Ca^{2+} entry into damaged cells, which induces Ca^{2+} overload and asynchronous spontaneous activity.[15] Ca^{2+} will then diffuse into adjacent cells with intact sarcolemma in a border zone via gap junctions, which remain open for some time after the damage,[21] depending on the internal

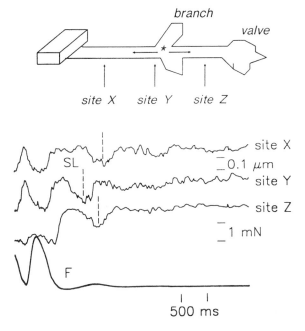

Figure 2. Schematic of muscle in which TPCs started from a centrally located damaged region (asterisk) near two cut side branches. Bottom, Sarcomere length (SL) recordings at three sites of preparation, illustrating that TPC propagated away from damaged region in both directions. Modified with permission from Reference 22.

environmental conditions of the cell, including temperature.[22] Spontaneous activity in the damaged zone is random; hence, the accompanying Ca^{2+} transients will be small and may not be propagated throughout the muscle but can cause Ca^{2+} overload and spontaneous activity in border zone. This process continues until the $[Ca^{2+}]$ gradient is too small between cells or gap junctions close.[15] The existence of spontaneous contractions increases resting tension and decreases twitch force.[13,23] Thus, the damaged cells and the border zone may be weaker during the twitch than the center region of the trabeculae. When the central part of the trabeculae contracts, the damaged region is stretched and subsequently rapidly released during the relaxation phase of the twitch. Thus, it is reasonable to assume that stretch or quick release of damaged ends of trabeculae during the preceding twitch triggers TPCs,[14] and this may provide an explanation for the triggering mechanism. We have recently described that elimination of the stretch of the damaged region and the border zone during the twitch and hence the quick release during the relaxation phase prevents the induction of

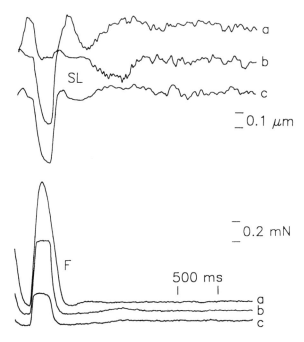

Figure 3. Sarcomere length (SL) and force (F) recordings of last of electrically stimulated twitches and a TPC at different afterloads in one muscle. $[Ca^{2+}]_o$ 2.50 mmol/L. Initial sarcomere length 2.15 μm. All sarcomere length recordings were made at one site of preparation. Both sarcomere length and force tracings were artificially shifted. A decrease in afterload delayed initiation of TPC significantly. Modified with permission from Reference 14.

TPCs. Figure 3 shows an example of such an experiment in which we have used a servomotor control to impose an afterload on the muscle. When the afterload is reduced, the stretch of the damaged areas decreases while the shortening of the sarcomeres in the center of the trabeculae increases. It appeared that reduction of the afterload to <20% of the isometric force eliminated the TPCs completely, an effect that was immediately reversed by forcing the muscle to contract again at a high afterload. Thus, apparently the probability of triggering a TPC depends on the degree of stretch of the damaged area during the twitch or on the subsequent shortening during the relaxation phase of the twitch. We have found that the initiation process of TPCs is unaffected by Gd^{3+} ions, suggesting that stretch-activated channels play little or no role in the initiation of damage-induced TPCs.[24] Also, the observation that the TPCs always start shortly after the rapid shortening of the damaged areas suggests that it is actually the shortening that initiates a TPC. Housmans et al[25] and others[26–29] indeed have described that a rapid shortening of a contracting muscle causes rapid release of Ca^{2+} ions from the myofilaments. It follows that TPCs may be initiated by Ca^{2+} ions that dissociate from the contractile filaments due to the quick release of these areas during relaxation. At that time, the SR has already recovered sufficiently[30] to allow Ca^{2+}-induced Ca^{2+} release to amplify the initial Ca^{2+} transient in the damaged region and/or the border zone.

Propagation of TPCs

Figure 1 shows a characteristic TPC in a rat cardiac trabecula. The displacement of the TPC occurs at a linear rate (see Figure 1). V_{prop} found in these preparations at room temperature varied from 0.1 to 15 mm/s[15] and correlated tightly with the amplitude of the twitch preceding the TPC, suggesting that the Ca^{2+} load of the SR dictates V_{prop}.[22] Studies of the effects of interventions such as varied $[Ca^{2+}]_o$ and Ca^{2+} channel agonists and antagonists support the idea that the Ca^{2+} load of the SR is the main determinant of V_{prop}.[31] On the other hand, interventions that cause a leak of Ca^{2+} from the SR (caffeine and ryanodine) suggest that V_{prop} also depends on the diastolic cytosolic Ca^{2+} level.[31] The rate of initiation of TPCs and their V_{prop} in all these studies was tightly correlated, suggesting that the triggering process and the propagation process are determined by similar mechanisms.

The observation that TPCs travel at constant velocity through undamaged muscle led us to postulate that they are caused by Ca^{2+}-induced Ca^{2+} release from the SR mediated by diffusion of Ca^{2+} to adjacent SR.[15] Model simulation (see below) of propagation of TPCs on the basis of Ca^{2+}-induced Ca^{2+} release mediated by diffusion of Ca^{2+} to adjacent SR within the cell and to SR in adjacent cells[15,20] predicted a range of V_{prop} that was in agreement with the observed data. Propagation, usually at 0.05 to 0.2 mm/s, of spontaneous localized contractions as well as Ca^{2+} waves in single cells[18,19,32–38] has also been explained on the basis of Ca^{2+}-induced Ca^{2+} release from SR mediated by diffusion of Ca^{2+} to adjacent SR.[39,40] It is interesting to note here that Ca^{2+} waves have been observed to travel at V_{prop} as high as 3 mm/s (M. Miura, personal communication). This range of V_{prop} is similar to that in isolated trabeculae, suggesting that the mechanism of propagation in isolated cells and in multicellular preparations is the same. The observed spatial and temporal patterns of propagation of $[Ca^{2+}]_i$ waves by Takamatsu and Wier[35] are consistent with this hypothesis.

Ca^{2+}-Induced Ca^{2+} Release by the SR as a Mechanism Underlying TPCs

The observation that the TPCs travel at a constant velocity and with a constant amplitude through the myocardium is an important clue to the mechanism of propagation. Diffusion of Ca^{2+} alone would clearly be too slow by at least two to three orders of magnitude and would be accompanied by a decline of the observed TPC amplitude. On the other hand, the propagation of electrical activity is much faster, 1 m/s for the action potential in ventricular myocardium, and electrotonic conduction is also too fast to be compatible with the observed values for V_{prop}. We therefore propose that a combination of Ca^{2+} diffusion and Ca^{2+}-induced Ca^{2+} release could be responsible. We have modeled the behavior of a myofibril accompanied by its SR during a sudden focal Ca^{2+} release in Figure 4.[20] The method of solution involved writing the diffusion equation as a difference equation in the spatial coordinates. The resultant coupled ordinary differential equations in time with banded coefficients were solved with Gear's sixth-order predictor-corrector algorithm for stiff equations with reflective boundaries. It appeared that Ca^{2+} fluctuations propagate through the cytosol at a rate modified by binding to troponin and calmodulin and sequestration by the SR as well as by the rate of Ca^{2+} release from adjacent release sites of the SR (Figure 5). V_{prop} appeared to increase in the model from 0.1 to 15 mm/s owing to the combined effects of a rise of (1) the diastolic $[Ca^{2+}]_i$, (2) the rate of rise of the Ca^{2+} release, and (3) the amount of Ca^{2+} released by the SR.[20] This combination of changes in Ca^{2+} levels in the cytosol and in the SR would be expected to result from loading of cardiac cells with Ca^{2+} during repetitive stimulation or from exposure to high $[Ca^{2+}]_o$ or Ca^{2+} agonists.[15]

Important to the viability of the proposed model of TPCs was a high conductance of the Ca^{2+} channel in the SR, while the expected open time for the Ca^{2+} channel in the SR would have to be on the order of 0.5 ms to allow for the highest V_{prop}. At the time of formulation of the model, these properties of the SR Ca^{2+} channels seemed extremely rapid. Nowadays, reports on extremely fast Ca^{2+} transients such as sparks recorded by use of confocal microscopy and fast and sensitive fluorescent Ca^{2+} dyes such as Fluo 3^{41} suggest that our assumption may not have been excessive. Nevertheless, it is clear that our understanding of TPCs requires further study of Ca^{2+} transient at a high spatial and temporal resolution.

The model of a myofibril together with SR over a length of 50 sarcomeres accurately predicted the propagation velocities observed in muscles. This accuracy is somewhat surprising because in the real muscle, the Ca^{2+} transient has to travel not only from sarcomere to sarcomere but also from cell to cell. The high propagation velocity suggests that the barrier for Ca^{2+} diffusion imposed by gap junctions between cells is minor compared with the other parameters in the model, such as Ca^{2+} binding to ligands in the cell and Ca^{2+} extrusion and sequestration processes. We tested the importance of gap junctions

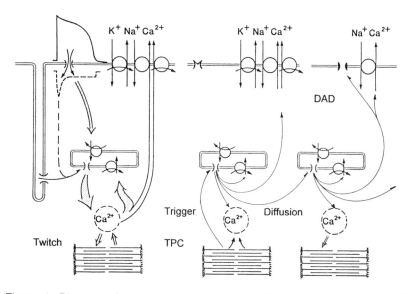

Figure 4. Diagram of excitation-contraction coupling system in cardiac cell and its role during TPCs. Left, Events during twitch. During action potential, a large transient Ca^{2+} influx enters cells followed by a maintained component of slow inward current (dashed line). Ca^{2+} entry does not lead directly to force development, because Ca^{2+} that enters is rapidly bound to binding sites on SR. Rapid influx of Ca^{2+} via T tubuli is thought to induce release of Ca^{2+} from a release compartment in SR by triggering opening of Ca^{2+} channels in terminal cisternae, thus activating contractile filaments to contract. Rapid relaxation follows because cytosolic Ca^{2+} is sequestered rapidly in an uptake compartment of SR and partly extruded through cell membrane by Na^{+}/Ca^{2+} exchanger and by low-capacity, high-affinity Ca^{2+} pump. This process loads SR. It is important to note that process of Na^{+}/Ca^{2+} exchange is electrogenic, so that Ca^{2+} extrusion through exchanger leads to a depolarizing current. Middle, Events near a damaged region during triggering of TPC. Rapid shortening of this region occurs during relaxation of twitch following stretch by normal and therefore stronger myocardium during contraction. This rapid release of sarcomeres leads to dissociation of Ca^{2+} from contractile filaments during relaxation phase. SR is recovered enough to respond to increase in $[Ca^{2+}]_i$ by Ca^{2+}-induced Ca^{2+} release, leading to an aftercontraction. Resultant elevation of $[Ca^{2+}]_i$ also causes diffusion of Ca^{2+} to adjacent sarcomeres. Right, Arrival of diffusing Ca^{2+} after release in damaged region leads to Ca^{2+}-induced Ca^{2+} release by SR in adjacent sarcomeres. Ca^{2+} diffuses next sarcomere while causing a local contraction as well as a delayed afterdepolarization (DAD) due to electrogenic Na^{+}/Ca^{2+} exchange and activation of Ca^{2+}-sensitive nonselective channels in sarcolemma. Diffusion of Ca^{2+} along its gradient maintains propagation of TPC.

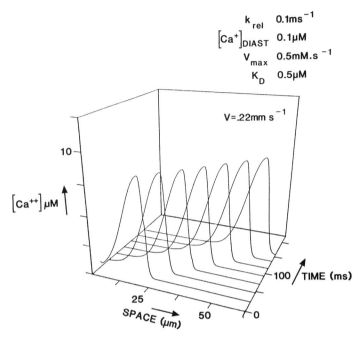

Figure 5. Ca^{2+} transients as a function of distance along preparation at different times. Propagating nature of Ca^{2+} wave is evident from figures. Modified with permission from Reference 20.

to the properties of the TPCs by exposing the trabeculae to the gap junction blockers heptanol and octanol. Although these compounds, like many drugs, probably have numerous side effects, their main effect is assumed to be reduction of the open frequency of gap junctions. Exposure of the muscles to these alcohols showed a unique effect on TPCs that we have not encountered with other drugs; ie, the rate of initiation and V_{prop} decreased without a noticeable decrease in twitch force. This suggests that closure of gap junctions reduces the rate of initiation and V_{prop} by reducing the effective rate of diffusion from cell to cell.

Our model suggests that the rate of propagation of TPCs should be reduced by active extrusion of Ca^{2+} from the cytosol. Therefore, we tested whether the rate of propagation of contractions that can be induced in skinned fibers would be faster than or at least as fast as those in intact trabeculae. Trabeculae were investigated in a way similar to the procedure depicted in Figure 1; the trabeculae were skinned in this study to eliminate the contribution of the sarcolemma. Then the skinned muscle was exposed to a skinned fiber solution, which allowed loading of the SR, and subsequently Ca^{2+}-induced Ca^{2+} release was induced by use of a microelectrode to squirt a small amount of Ca^{2+}-containing solution onto the fiber. The rapid local exposure to a high $[Ca^{2+}]$ led to a local contraction followed by a propagated contraction. This propagated contraction traveled at a velocity ranging from $\approx$50 to 300 μm/s. We did not succeed in creating conditions under which the contraction traveled faster than 300 μm/s either by enhancing or reducing the SR load with Ca^{2+} or restricting Ca^{2+} diffusion to the bathing medium by placing the fibers in silicon oil. It is possible that a crucial condition for rapid propagation is a high $[Ca^{2+}]$ around the myofibrils so that most of the cytosolic Ca^{2+}-binding sites are occupied; this possibility remains to be tested.

Propagated Ca^{2+} Release Induces Extrasystoles

Whenever a TPC arises, it is accompanied by a depolarization. These depolarizations are remarkably similar to delayed afterdepolarizations. It appeared that the duration of the depolarizations correlated exactly with the time during which the TPCs travel through the trabeculae. Also, the amplitude of the afterdepolarizations correlated exactly with the amplitude of the TPCs.[16] This is shown in Figure 6. The tight correspondence between the time course of TPCs and those of the depolarizations suggests that the depolarization is elicited by a Ca^{2+}-dependent current that exists as long as the $[Ca^{2+}]_i$ persists. In the small trabeculae that we used for these studies, this depolarization can be recorded over a distance of a few millimeters without much decrement because of the cable properties of these fibers.[16] This assumption could be verified experimentally by interrupting the propagation process of the TPC by locally heating the muscle over a length of a few hundred micrometers by a few degrees, as is shown in Figure 7. Local heating of the muscle caused the TPC to stop at the site of heating, whereas the concomitant depolarization could still be measured at a distance of $\approx$1 mm distal to the heating site.[16] This observation clearly indicates that the depolarization cannot be the source of the TPC but must be induced by the TPC. The effect of local heating also makes it unlikely that TPCs are induced as a result of spontaneous Ca^{2+} release along the muscle, which exhibit pseudopropagation because of a linear gradient of Ca^{2+} overload along the muscle, which is maximal at the damaged region and minimal at the other end of the muscle.

Triggered Arrhythmias Resulting From TPCs

TPCs always can be noticed directly after damage to the muscle. This is usually evident shortly after a muscle is mounted in an experi-

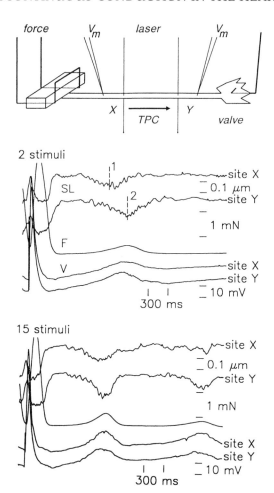

Figure 6. Parallel changes in characteristics of TPCs and delayed afterdepolarizations (DADs) after two (middle) and 15 (bottom) conditioning stimuli. Top, Trabecula with ventricular end positioned in a cradle attached to a force transducer and valvular side attached to a hook. Sarcomere length and membrane potential were monitored at two sites along preparation (X and Y). Records in middle and bottom panels show force (F), sarcomere length (SL), and membrane potential (V) of last stimulated twitch and a subsequent TPC and DAD in a representative muscle. Preparation hyperpolarized slightly during stimulation, accounting for depolarizing drift upon which DADs occurred. At two measuring sites, membrane potential tracings were virtually identical. With an increase in number of conditioning stimuli from 2 to 15, TPC propagation velocity increased from 2.4 to 9.5 mm/s. Furthermore, TPC force and DAD amplitude increased, while TPC latency, DAD latency, and duration of both TPC force and DAD decreased. After 15 stimuli, a second TPC and DAD were induced. $[Ca^{2+}]_o$ 1.0 mmol/L, temperature 20.8°C, resting membrane potential −68 and −64 mV at sites X and Y, respectively. Muscle length, 2.23 mm; initial sarcomere length, 2.10 μm. Reprinted with permission from Reference 16.

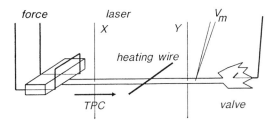

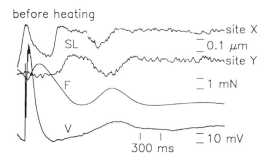

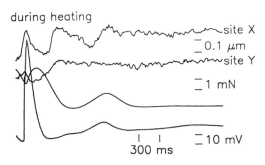

Figure 7. Effect of local heating of muscle on a TPC and delayed afterdepolarization (DAD). Top, Schematic muscle with free right ventricular wall attachment positioned in cradle of a force transducer (left) and valvular side (right). TPCs propagated in direction opposite to superfusing flow. Measurements of sarcomere length were made both proximal (X) and distal (Y) to heating wire; membrane potential was monitored only at Y. Middle, During control phase, recordings of sarcomere length (SL) at both X and Y, force (F), and membrane potential (V) of last stimulated twitch and a TPC and DAD, with local contraction in X preceding that in Y, indicative of propagating character of TPC. Resting membrane potential −64 mV, [Ca^{2+}]$_o$ 1.25 mmol/L, temperature 19.8°C, TPC propagation velocity 3.0 mm/s. During local heating (bottom), a local contraction due to a TPC still occurred at site X, but propagation of TPC was interrupted at heating wire and no unstimulated contraction was visible at Y, despite a local depolarization. Note accelerated relaxation of last stimulated twitch and decreased latency of both TPC and DAD. Decrease in distance of TPC propagation is responsible for decrease in TPC duration and amplitude. Reprinted with permission from Reference 16.

A

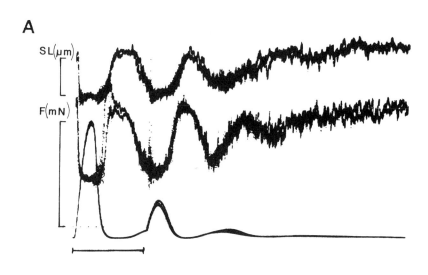

B

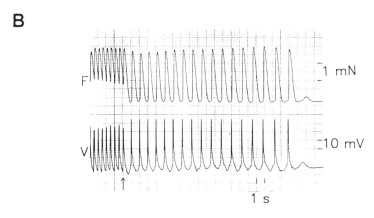

Figure 8. Spontaneous contractions cause development of twitches and arrhythmias. A, Example of development of spontaneous twitch that is triggered by a propagating aftercontraction. Note acute increase of rate of rise of force during development of first aftercontraction (arrow) and similarity of time course of subsequent twitch and that of electrically elicited twitch. Modified with permission from Reference 15. B, Force (F) and membrane potential (V) recordings during a train of conditioning stimuli (ending at arrow) and a subsequent triggered arrhythmia. Note initial slow upstroke in both force and membrane potential of triggered twitches, suggestive of an underlying TPC and DAD. Triggered arrhythmia terminated spontaneously with an increase in interval between triggered beats, followed by a TPC and DAD. Temperature 20.4°C, $[Ca^{2+}]_o$ 2.25 mmol/L. Resting membrane potential -71 mV. Modified with permission from Reference 22.

mental setup. The acute Ca^{2+} load to the damaged cells and their neighbors is then apparently so large that virtually every electrically paced beat is followed by TPCs. We usually observe that the TPCs are accompanied by delayed afterdepolarizations sufficiently large to elicit action potentials and synchronized contractions, shown in Figure 8A. As discussed above, the addition of Ca^{2+} by the action potential that follows the TPC may be so large that a triggered arrhythmia arises, as is shown in Figure 8B. Triggered arrhythmias occur in the damaged muscle when the Ca^{2+} load of the SR is large. We have observed these triggered arrhythmias at room temperature during the first hour after damage to the muscle has occurred. In such a case, the full-blown arrhythmia is usually preceded by the repeated occurrence of single extrasystoles. At 37°C, the time span over which these damage-related events occur is much shorter, and the cause of the extrasystoles (ie, the TPCs) disappears in <10 minutes.[42] Under those conditions, it is likely that their occurrence is limited by rapid closure of gap junctions as a result of persistently elevated Ca^{2+} levels in the damaged cells and/or a lowered pH in these cells, which must sustain an enormous metabolic load as a result of intense ion movement across their membranes or across membranes in the vicinity.

These observations make it likely that extrasystoles that initiate an arrhythmia in acutely damaged myocardium may result from an intracellular Ca^{2+} oscillation in the damaged region. The resulting $[Ca^{2+}]_i$ transient propagates into adjacent myocardium and induces delayed afterdepolarizations and TPCs. If the $[Ca^{2+}]_i$ transient is large enough, it will lead to action potential formation. Clearly, damage initiates a chain of subcellular events leading to oscillations of $[Ca^{2+}]_i$ that may cause macroscopic arrhythmias in the damaged heart. Few studies have addressed possible pharmacological interventions aimed at this source of extrasystoles. Thus far, we have succeeded only in reducing the chance of development of TPCs, without simultaneously causing a negative inotropic effect, by using R56865, a Na^+ and Ca^{2+} overload inhibitor.[43]

References

1. January CT, Fozzard HA. Delayed afterdepolarizations in heart muscle: mechanisms and relevance. *Pharmacol Rev.* 1988;40:219–227.
2. January CT, Riddle JM, Salata JJ. A model for early afterdepolarizations: induction with the calcium channel agonist Bay K 8644. *Circ Res.* 1988;62: 563–571.
3. January CT, Riddle JM. Early afterdepolarizations: mechanism of induction and block: a role for L-type Ca^{2+} current. *Circ Res.* 1989;64:977–990.
4. Wit AL, Rosen MR. Afterdepolarizations and triggered activity. In: Fozzard

HA, Haber E, Jennings RB, Katz AM, Morgan HE, eds. *The Heart and Cardiovascular System.* New York, NY: Raven Press; 1986:1449–1490.

5. Rosen MR, Danilo PJ. Digitalis-induced delayed afterdepolarizations. In: Zipes DP, Bailey JC, Elharrar V, eds. *The Slow Inward Current and Cardiac Arrhythmias.* The Hague/Boston/London: Martinus Nijhoff; 1980:417–435.

6. Ferrier GR, Saunders JH, Mendez C. A cellular mechanism for the generation of ventricular arrhythmias by acetylstrophanthidin. *Circ Res.* 1973;32: 600–609.

7. Ferrier GR. Digitalis arrhythmias: role of oscillatory afterpotentials. *Prog Cardiovasc Res.* 1977;19:459–474.

8. Cranefield PF. Action potentials, afterpotentials, and arrhythmias. *Circ Res.* 1977;41:415–423.

9. Ferrier GR. The effects of tension on acetylstrophanthidin-induced transient depolarizations and aftercontractions in canine myocardial and Purkinje tissues. *Circ Res.* 1976;38:156–162.

10. Kass RS, Lederer WJ, Tsien RW et al. Role of calcium ions in transient inward currents and aftercontractions induced by strophanthidin in cardiac Purkinje fibres. *J Physiol.* 1978;281:187–208.

11. Fabiato A. Spontaneous versus triggered contractions of "calcium-tolerant" cardiac cells from the adult rat ventricle. *Basic Res Cardiol.* 1985;80(suppl 2):83–88.

12. Capogrossi MC, Lakatta EG. Frequency modulation and synchronization of spontaneous oscillations in cardiac cells. *Am J Physiol.* 1985;248:H412–H418.

13. Kort AA, Lakatta EG. Calcium-dependent mechanical oscillations occur spontaneously in unstimulated mammalian cardiac tissues. *Circ Res.* 1984; 54:396–404.

14. Daniels MCG, ter Keurs HEDJ. Spontaneous contractions in rat cardiac trabeculae: trigger mechanism and propagation velocity. *J Gen Physiol.* 1990; 95:1123–1137.

15. Mulder BJM, de Tombe PP, ter Keurs HEDJ. Spontaneous and propagated contractions in rat cardiac trabeculae. *J Gen Physiol.* 1989;93:943–961.

16. Daniels MCG, Fedida D, Lamont C, et al. Role of the sarcolemma in triggered propagated contractions in rat cardiac trabeculae. *Circ Res.* 1991;68: 1408–1421.

17. ter Keurs HEDJ, Backx PH, de Tombe PP et al. Aftercontractions and excitation-contraction coupling in rat cardiac muscle. *Can J Physiol Pharmacol.* 1988;66:1239–1245.

18. Kort AA, Capogrossi MC, Lakatta EG. Frequency, amplitude, and propagation velocity of spontaneous calcium-dependent contractile waves in intact adult rat cardiac muscle and isolated myocytes. *Circ Res.* 1985;57:844–855.

19. Rieser G, Sabbadini R, Paolini P, et al. Sarcomere motion in isolated cardiac cells. *Am J Physiol.* 1979;236:C70–C77.

20. Backx PH, de Tombe PP, van Deen JHK, et al. A model of propagating calcium-induced calcium release mediated by calcium diffusion. *J Gen Physiol.* 1989;93:963–977.

21. Sedovy JD, White RL. Modulation of gap junctional permeability in whole perfused rat heart. *Biophys J.* 1994;66:A259. Abstract.

22. Daniels MCG. *Mechanism of Triggered Arrhythmias in Damaged Myocardium.* Utrecht, The Netherlands: the University of Utrecht; 1991. PhD Thesis.

23. Stern MD, Kort AA, Bhatnagar GM, et al. Scattered-light intensity fluctuations in diastolic rat cardiac muscle caused by spontaneous calcium-dependent cellular mechanical oscillations. *J Gen Physiol.* 1983;82:119–153.

24. Zhang Y, ter Keurs HEDJ. Effects of gadolinium on twitch force and triggered propagated contractions in rat cardiac trabeculae. *Cardiovasc Res.* 1996;32:180–188.

25. Housmans PR, Lee NKM, Blinks JR. Active shortening retards the decline of the intracellular calcium transient in mammalian heart muscle. *Science.* 1983;221:159–161.

26. Allen DG, Kentish JC. The cellular basis of the length-tension relation in cardiac muscle. *J Mol Cell Cardiol.* 1985;17:821–840.

27. Allen DG, Kurihara S. The effects of muscle length on intracellular calcium transients in mammalian cardiac muscle. *J Physiol.* 1982;327:79–94.

28. Allen DG, Kentish JC. Calcium concentration in the myoplasm of skinned ferret ventricular muscle following changes in muscle length. *J Physiol.* 1988;407:489–503.

29. Backx PH, Gao WD, Azan-Backx MD, et al. The relationship between contractile force and intracellular [Ca^{++}] in intact rat cardiac trabeculae. *J Gen Physiol.* 1995;105:1–19.

30. Banijamali HS, Gao WD, MacIntosh BR, ter Keurs HEDJ. Force-interval relations of twitches and cold contractures in rat cardiac trabeculae: influence of ryanodine. *Circ Res.* 1991;69:937–948.

31. Daniels MCG, ter Keurs HEDJ. Propagated contractions in rat cardiac trabeculae: effects of caffeine, ryanodine, Bay K 8644, and D-600. *Biophys J.* 1990;57:170a. Abstract.

32. Golovina VA, Rozenshtraukh LV, Solov'ev BS, et al. Wavelike spontaneous contractions of isolated cardiomyocytes. *Biophysics.* 1986;31:311–318.

33. Wier WG, Cannell MB, Berlin JR, et al. Cellular and subcellular heterogeneity of intracellular calcium concentration in single heart cells revealed by fura-2. *Science.* 1987;235:325–328.

34. Stern MD, Capogrossi MC, Lakatta EG. Spontaneous calcium release from the sarcoplasmic reticulum in myocardial cells: mechanisms and consequences. *Cell Calcium.* 1988;9:247–256.

35. Takamatsu T, Wier WG. Calcium waves in mammalian heart: quantification of origin, magnitude, waveform and velocity. *FASEB J.* 1990;4:1519–1525.

36. Wier WG, Blatter LA. Ca-oscillations and Ca-waves in mammalian cardiac and vascular smooth muscle cells. *Cell Calcium.* 1991;12:241–254.

37. Ishide N, Urayama T, Inoue K, et al. Propagation and collision characteristics of calcium waves in rat myocytes. *Am J Physiol.* 1990;259:H940–H950.

38. Wier WG, Beuckelmann DJ, Barcenas-Ruiz L. [Ca^{++}]i in single isolated cardiac cells: a review of recent results obtained with digital imaging microscopy and fura-2. *Can J Physiol Pharmacol.* 1988;66:1224–1231.

39. Stern MD, Capogrossi MC, Lakatta EG. Propagated contractile waves in single cardiac myocytes modeled as regenerative calcium induced calcium release from the sarcoplasmic reticulum. *Biophys J.* 1984;45:94a. Abstract.

40. Regirer SA, Tsaturyan AK, Chernaya GG. Mathematical model of propagation of activation waves in an isolated cardiomyocyte. *Biophysics.* 1986;31:725–730.

41. Harrison SM, Bers DM. Influence of temperature on the calcium sensitivity of the myofilaments of skinned ventricular muscle from the rabbit. *J Gen Physiol.* 1989;93:411–428.

42. Daniels MCG, Kieser T, ter Keurs HEDJ. Triggered propagated contractions in human atrial trabeculae. *Cardiovasc Res.* 1993;27:1831–1835.

43. Daniels MCG, ter Keurs HEDJ. The suppressive effects of the novel drug R 56865 on triggered propagated contractions in rat cardiac trabeculae. *J Cardiovasc Pharmacol.* 1992;20:187–196. Abstract.

Chapter 11

Microscopic Conduction in Cell Cultures Assessed by High-Resolution Optical Mapping and Computer Simulation

André G. Kléber, MD, Vladimir G. Fast, PhD, and Stephan Rohr, MD

Mechanisms of cardiac arrhythmias are usually divided into disturbances of impulse formation and impulse conduction. Whereas the mechanisms and excitation patterns in some arrhythmias have been well characterized, delineation of mechanisms of arrhythmias originating from small foci is more difficult because of the small size of the reentrant circuits. It is generally agreed that some of the clinically relevant arrhythmias are due to oscillations at the level of the cardiac membrane (delayed and early afterdepolarizations), with mismatch between repolarizing and depolarizing currents at different levels of membrane potentials.[1,2] However, some of the focal arrhythmias may also arise from circus movement or reflection reentry confined to microscopic structures.[3,4]

The specific architecture of cardiac muscle includes the anisotropic cellular shape, the discrete distribution of connexons, and the arrangement of individual cells as cell bundles and of cell bundles as larger fibers separated by blood vessels and by connective tissue sheets.[5] This architecture, which is known to be modified by growth, the aging process, and disease (hypertrophy, infarction, myopathy), may form the substrate for unidirectional conduction block and reentry. In the past, it has been difficult to assess experimentally the specific importance of the individual structural elements for propagation in vivo because of

From: Spooner PM, Joyner RW, Jalife J (eds). *Discontinuous Conduction in the Heart.* Armonk, NY: Futura Publishing Company, Inc.; © 1997.

the spatial and temporal limitations of available mapping techniques. Computer modeling using sophisticated models with multiple excitable elements representing a single cell and taking into account the stochastic variability in cell shape and gap junction distribution has provided a tentative insight into conduction at the cellular level.[6-8] In particular, such models suggest a discontinuous spatial distribution of the transmembrane voltage during the upstroke of the action potential. Whether and to what extent the discontinuities at the various levels of tissue organization may form the substrate for microreentrant circuits has not yet been established.

Over the past years, our laboratory has made an effort to develop methods allowing the experimental assessment of cardiac conduction at a microscopic level, which involves patterned or anisotropic growth of neonatal cardiac myocytes and the fluorimetric measurement of transmembrane voltage at high temporal and spatial resolution. Moreover, a computer model of propagation has been developed to assess the changes in transmembrane ionic and electrotonic currents underlying the experimentally observed changes in voltage. This work, insofar as it concerns the mechanisms involved in anisotropic conduction and conduction block, is summarized in this chapter.

Methods Used to Produce Patterned or Anisotropic Growth of Cultured Neonatal Rat Heart Cells and to Perform High-Resolution Optical Mapping of Transmembrane Potential

Methods to fabricate growth patterns of cultured cell monolayers were first described in neurobiology.[9] In heart tissue, Liebermann and colleagues[10-13] produced cablelike cardiac structures (so-called "synthetic strands") by culturing cells using either a nylon thread as growth backbone or grooves etched into the agar coating of a coverslip (for review see Reference 14). The technique developed in our laboratory to pattern the growth of cells is shown in Figure 1 and is described in detail elsewhere.[15] In brief, dissociated cells from neonatal rat ventricles are seeded on specially processed coverslips at a density of $\approx 1.3 \times 10^{-3}$ cells/mm^2. The coverslips are processed in such a way that a layer of Photoresist (Kodak KTRF) is applied to one surface and spun to a thickness of a few micrometers. Subsequently, a microfilm depicting the growth pattern at a 1:1 scale is tightly applied to the Photoresist-coated coverslip and exposed to light, as shown in Figure 1. The nonexposed parts are dissolved with xylol, thereby producing a pattern consisting of either glass surface (cell adherence) or Photoresist surface (no cell

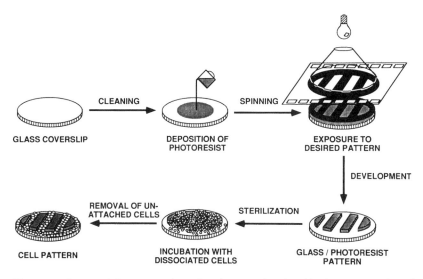

Figure 1. Sequential presentation of main steps involved in the preparation of cell cultures exhibiting directed growth. Glass coverslips are cleaned (top left), covered with Photoresist (top middle), and spun and contact-exposed to desired pattern with UV light (top right). After development, patterned coverslips (bottom right) are sterilized and incubated with freshly dissociated neonatal ventricular rat heart cells (bottom middle). Final pattern (bottom left) is obtained by removal of nonadhering cells. Reprinted with permission from Reference 14.

adherence). An advantage of this technique is that virtually any growth pattern can be easily obtained with a conventional graphics program on a PC. A technique for producing 2D anisotropic cell monolayers is illustrated in Figure 2 and described in detail elsewhere.[16] Collagen type IV (20 to 50 μg/mL) is applied to coverslips, which subsequently are dried. Afterward, a parallel alignment of the collagen fibers is obtained by gentle rubbing of the surface with a fine brush. The cell cultures obtained in such a way exhibit a typical anisotropic appearance, the mean cell length being 66 ± 13 μm and the transverse diameter 12 ± 3 μm.[16]

For optical measurements, coverslips are transferred to an experimental chamber mounted on a vibration-isolation table. Voltage-sensitive dyes (RH-237 or di-8-ANEPPS, Molecular Probes) are used to measure transmembrane potential changes.[17,18] The optical system used to measure transmembrane potential has been described in detail previously.[16,17] It consists of an inverted microscope (Axiovert 35M, Zeiss) equipped for epifluorescence with a 100-W arc mercury lamp as a light source. Fluorescence measurements with RH-237 are performed with

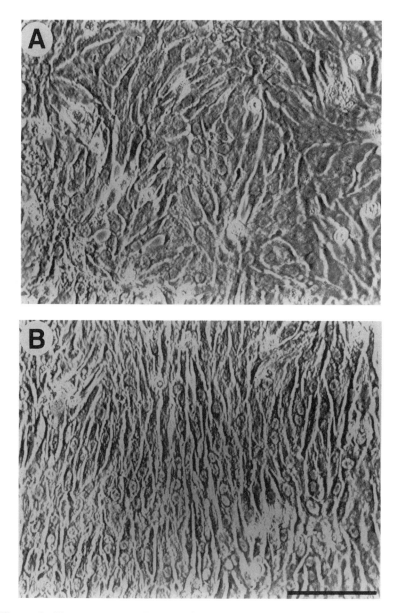

Figure 2. Phase-contrast pictures of isotropic (A) and anisotropic (B) cell monolayers. Calibration bar = 50 μm. Anisotropic pattern was obtained by gently rubbing collagen-coated surface with a fine brush. Reprinted with permission from Reference 16.

a filter set with a band-pass excitation filter (530 to 585 nm), a dichroic mirror (600 nm), and a low-pass emission filter (>615 nm). The spatial resolution is determined by the magnification of the objectives ($\times 40$, $\times 63$, $\times 86$, and $\times 100$). The fluorescence emitted by the dye is measured by photodiodes, with a either a row of three diodes or a 10×10 diode array (Centronic) located in the image plane of the microscope. In the "row detector," the diodes are separated by 30 μm, with each diode monitoring the signal from a membrane area of 6.5 μm at $\times 100$ magnification. On the 10×10 diode array, each diode monitors an area of 14×14 μm^2 at $\times 40$ magnification. The photocurrents from the diodes are converted to voltage by I/V convertors built with operational amplifiers (OPA 121, BurrBrown) and 100-MΩ feedback resistors (Eltec Instruments Inc). These voltages are directed into second-stage amplifiers with a sample-and-hold circuit for subtraction of DC signals. Subsequently, signals are converted by data acquisition cards (NB-A2000, National Instruments). The sampling rate is 25 to 100 kHz per channel. A personal computer (MacIntosh IIfx Apple Computer) is used for data storage and analysis. To eliminate high-frequency noise, signals are digitally filtered with a gaussian low-pass filter with a cutoff frequency of 1.5 to 2 kHz. During the measurements, cells are superfused at a rate of 2 mL/min with a solution containing (in mmol/L) NaCl 150, KCl 5, 1.2 CaCl$_2$ 1.2, MgCl$_2$ 1, NaHCO$_3$ 5.8, HEPES 5, and glucose 5. pH was 7.4, and temperature was 34°C to 35°C.

Effect of Cell Boundaries on Impulse Conduction and dV/dt$_{max}$ in Patterned Cell Cultures

To investigate the possibility that cell-to-cell connections introduce discontinuities in conduction, myocytes were grown in single cell strands, as shown in Figure 3.[17,18] Since cells in such strands exhibit only end-to-end but no side-to-side connections, the conduction times along the cell strands are determined solely by action potential propagation within the cells and through the connexons located in the end-to-end connections. The optical upstrokes and conduction times obtained in these strands are shown in Figure 3B for a single experiment.[17] The cytoplasmic conduction time along 30 μm is relatively short (30 μs), whereas the conduction time along the same distance is significantly longer (110 μs) if an end-to-end cell connection is interposed. The differences between the two conduction times correspond to the transfer time at the junction between the two cells. The histograms of the collected data in Figure 3C yield an average cytoplasmic conduction time (along a distance of 30 μm) of 38 μs, and the average conduction time from one cell to the following cell amounts to 118 μs. The differ-

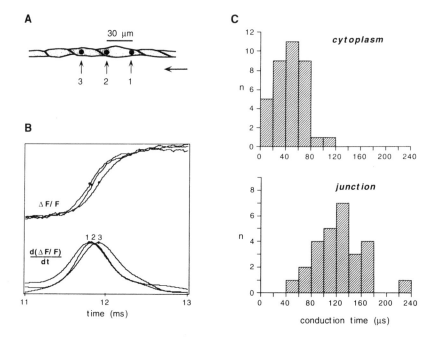

Figure 3. Impulse propagation in 1D cell chains. A, Picture of a portion of a cell chain, reproduced from bright-field illumination photograph. Positions and sizes of membrane areas sensed by three diodes are indicated by solid circles. Dark arrow indicates direction of propagation. B, Potential-dependent fluorescence change ∆F/F recorded by diodes shown in A and their superimposed derivatives d(∆F/F)/dt. Dots indicate activation times. Cytoplasmic conduction time = 30 μs, junctional conduction time = 110 μs. C, Histograms of conduction times from all experiments. Average cytoplasmic conduction time (t = 38 ± 25 μs, n = 37) was markedly shorter than average junctional conduction time (t = 118 ± 40 μs, n = 27, P<.0001). Mean difference, attributed to conduction delay induced by gap junctions, amounted to 80 μs, which is 51% of overall conduction time. Reprinted with permission from Reference 17.

ence of 80 μs corresponds to the conduction time through an end-to-end cell connection. An experiment analogous to the one shown in Figure 3 but carried out in a cell strand consisting, on average, of 5 or 6 cells in parallel is illustrated in Figures 4A and 4B; the collected data are shown in Figure 4C. In the wider strands, the average cytoplasmic conduction time is longer than in the single cell chains and the average cell-to-cell conduction time is shorter, the mean transfer time across an end-to-end cell connection amounting to 88 μs (versus 118 μs in the single cell chain). It is important to note that the macroscopic conduction velocities in single cell chains are not significantly different from the wider cell strands in such types of experiments (34 versus 36 cm/s).

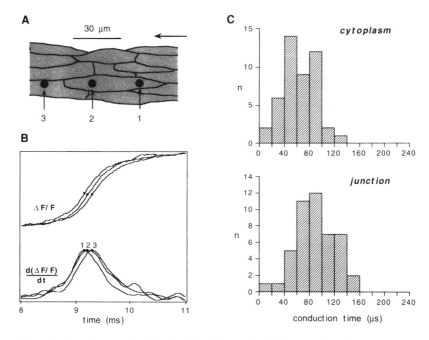

Figure 4. Impulse conduction in 2D cell strands. A, Picture of a wide cell strand (four to six cells wide) reproduced from a bright-field illumination photograph. Positions and sizes of membrane areas sensed by three diodes are indicated by solid circles. Dark arrow indicates direction of propagation. B, Fluorescence changes ΔF/F and their superimposed derivatives d(ΔF/F)/dt recorded by diodes shown in A. Cytoplasmic conduction time = 60 μs, junctional conduction time = 80 μs. C, Histograms of conduction times from all experiments. Average cytoplasmic conduction time was 57 ± 26 μs (n = 46); junctional conduction time was 89 ± 39 μs (n = 48, *P*<.001). Gap junctional conduction delay amounted to 32 μs, which is 22% of overall conduction time. Reprinted with permission from Reference 17.

Comparison between the data obtained in the two types of structures therefore indicates that the lateral apposition of cell chains to a cell strand has an averaging effect, ie, it partially cancels the discontinuities in conduction caused by the connexons located at the cell ends. So far, the investigation of impulse propagation at the microscopic scale is confined to the measurement of membrane potential, while analysis of electrotonic and ionic current flow in this situation requires computer simulation. Therefore, this so-called "lateral averaging" effect has been further investigated in a computer model representing (1) a chain of single cells and (2) a wide strand consisting of five rows of cells, each cell being interconnected by two resistors to the neighboring row.[17] In this model, the single cell is represented by eight excitable elements

(Beeler and Reuter type with Ebihara-Johnson modification of fast Na^+ current kinetics), and the individual cells are connected by a single gap junctional resistor.[19] The parameters of the model are chosen such that the simulation closely fits the experimentally obtained values for propagation in the single cell chains. The effect of the lateral apposition of cell rows is followed by varying the value of the lateral coupling resistors. Conduction times obtained with this model confirmed the experimental results and are shown in Figure 5. Starting at the right from a very low degree of lateral coupling and a large difference in cytoplasmic versus cell-to-cell conduction times, the two values approach each other when the lateral coupling resistance (Ry) is decreased, supporting the experimental finding that lateral coupling decreases the average degree of discontinuity during longitudinal conduction. The model also predicts that tissue with a very high degree of anisotropy

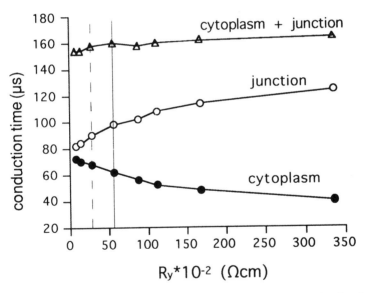

Figure 5. Simulation of junctional, cytoplasmic, and overall conduction times in a computer model in which electrical parameters were adapted to behavior of neonatal rat heart cells, with cytoplasmic and cell-to-cell conduction times as in Figure 3. Five cell chains were connected by lateral resistivity, R_y. The interrupted line denotes an anisotropic ratio, R_y/R_i, of 10, taken for simulation of results shown in Figure 8B. Solid line corresponds to an R_y/R_i of 20. At this ratio, experimental and simulated degrees of inhomogeneity introduced by end-to-end cell connections (22% of overall conduction times) are equal. Above an R_y/R_i of ≈60, averaging affect of lateral connections is absent. Note that variation of lateral coupling resistance has almost no effect on overall propagation time or velocity. Reprinted with permission from Reference 17.

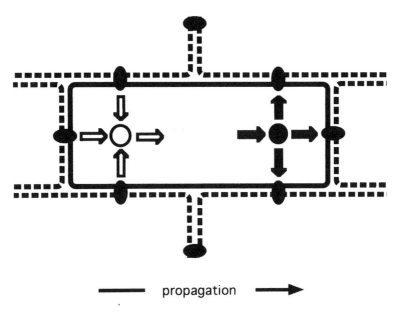

propagation →

Figure 6. Schematic showing local current flow in a cell of a 2D strand coupled to six neighboring cells. Solid ovals indicate gap junctions. Electrotonic currents flowing in wavefront of propagation (horizontal arrows) and between laterally apposed cells (vertical arrows) are depicted at instants of local activation for a point distal to end-to-end cell connection (open symbols) and at a point proximal to end-to-end connection (solid symbols). Direction of these currents is given by computed potential distribution at two instances of activation. At distal point, lateral convergence of local current accelerates activation; at proximal point, lateral divergence delays activation. Both divergence and convergence of local currents through lateral connections are responsible for reduced inhomogeneity of propagation in 2D strands. Reprinted with permission from Reference 17.

(eg, crista terminalis) will show relatively large discontinuities due to cell borders.

The effect of "lateral averaging" can best be explained by looking at the magnitude and direction of electrotonic current flow at the time when a given membrane site reaches threshold for rapid Na^+ inward current, as explained in Figure 6. If the wave front of propagation reaches a point immediately beyond an end-to-end connection, the wave front will lag slightly behind the front in the two neighboring cells, because these two cells do not encounter a resistive barrier at that site. Consequently, this point will receive local electrotonic current from both neighboring rows in addition to the normal electrotonic current flowing in the direction of the wave front (current sink). Sites immediately beyond an end-to-end connection will therefore depolarize earlier if the lateral coupling is low, and consequently, the transition time across the longitudinal cell-to-cell connection will become shorter and the cytoplasmic conduction time will become longer. The opposite process takes place at the cell end, where local current from this site is fed to the two neighboring cells (current source). As a result, shortening of the transition time across the longitudinal cell-to-cell connection and prolongation of the cytoplasmic conduction time occurs.

Several precautions have to be taken into account when extrapolating these data to the situation in vivo. (1) Comparison of mean conduction times provides knowledge about the average behavior of the cellular network. Diversity in conduction times, as suggested from the histograms in Figures 3 and 4, is expected from the variability in cell shape, the variability in lateral apposition of individual cells, and the variability in connexin distribution. This diversity was simulated recently in a computer model that took the stochastic architecture of adult myocytes into account.[8] (2) The relative shortness of neonatal rat myocytes ($\approx$60% of the length of adult canine myocytes) will influence the degree of discontinuity imposed by the connexons. For the case of a single row, it is anticipated that cytoplasmic acceleration is faster in the longer adult myocytes (and the degree of discontinuity larger) for the same degree of longitudinal and lateral connectivity. (3) In most cardiac tissues, propagation occurs as a 3D event. Consequently, lateral averaging will concern all myocytes surrounding a given myocyte during propagation. In canine ventricular myocardium, 11.3 myocytes on average are connected to an individual myocyte, with both abundant end-to-end and side-to-side connections (Figure 4 of Saffitz et al[20]). Therefore, the "lateral averaging" will be significantly higher in 3D tissue than in 2D slices or cultures, thereby cancelling the effects of discrete distribution of gap junctions.

Most experiments performed in isolated ventricular and atrial tissue have shown that the maximal upstroke velocity of the transmembrane action potential, dV/dt_{max}, is higher during transverse than during longitudinal propagation.[21–24] This difference was taken to indicate a different mechanism for propagation in the longitudinal versus transverse direction and related to the intrinsic arrhythmogenic substrate of anisotropic tissue. Whether or not this difference is explained by the specific arrangement of the gap junctions in the part of the tissue that consists of densely coupled cells or by the presence of connective-tissue sheets and blood vessels separating fiber bundles cannot be answered from experiments in isolated tissue because of methodological limitations. An experiment showing anisotropic conduction in a dense network of cultured cells (devoid of large extracellular clefts) is illustrated in Figure 7.[16] Such types of experiments have shown that, in contrast to the in vivo experiments, average dV/dt_{max} in the transverse and

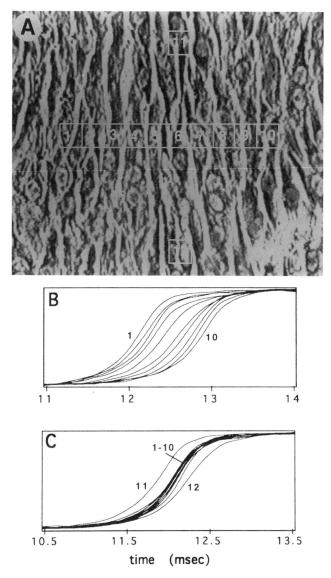

Figure 7. Activation sequences of transverse and longitudinal conduction in an anisotropic cell culture. A, Phase-contrast image of cell culture and photodiodes. Numbers within rectangles indicate photodiode numbers. B, Normalized optical upstrokes recorded by photodiodes shown in A during transverse conduction. C, Normalized optical upstrokes recorded from same localization during longitudinal conduction. Action potential upstrokes during both longitudinal and transverse conduction show variability in maximal upstroke velocity indicating local variability in current flowing into membrane capacitance. However, no significant difference between mean values in transverse versus longitudinal direction can be detected.[16] Reprinted with permission from Reference 16.

longitudinal directions are not different, although there is a considerable variability in dV/dt_{max} during both longitudinal and transverse propagation spread. These results suggest that at a moderate degree of anisotropy (eg, ventricular tissue), with relatively well-preserved lateral coupling, the discrete arrangement of gap junctions at the cell borders is not directly responsible for the direction-dependent differences in dV/dt_{max}. Similar findings have recently been obtained by computer simulations.[25] They indirectly attribute a crucial importance to the resistive discontinuities at a higher structural level for explaining direction-dependent differences in dV/dt_{max} and arrhythmogenicity. Modification of gap junctional coupling will nevertheless modulate the effects of large resistive barriers, as discussed below.

Effects of Large Resistive Discontinuities on Propagation in Cellular Networks

In heart tissue, structural discontinuities exist at several levels. In addition to discontinuities imposed by cell borders (as described in the paragraph above), connective tissue sheets and microvessels may act as resistive barriers. A propagating impulse is expected to (1) collide with such a barrier and (2) travel around resistive barriers wherever it encounters excitable tissue. The sites at which these microscopic deviations of the wave fronts from linearity occur are known to be susceptible to conduction block because of current-to-load mismatch. Several geometries leading to current-to-load mismatch have been described, such as single-ended obstacles or pivoting points forcing the wave front to curve around the end,[26] a narrow "isthmus" of excitable tissue where the propagation has to emerge into a large tissue area,[27] or a narrow "street" of excitable tissue emerging into a larger area.[25,28,29] Current-to-load mismatch has been implicated in the mechanisms of transition of the impulse from Purkinje fibers to the ventricular muscle, from the sinoatrial node to the atrium, and between fibers surviving in scars after chronic infarction.[30-33]

A simple model used to investigate the effect of current-to-load mismatch and obtained by the technique of patterned growth of cultured cells (described above) is shown in Figure 8[25] (see also Reference 28). In this model, the impulse traveling along the narrow strand has to excite the large tissue mass beyond the expansion and therefore has to furnish local excitatory current to a large surface of excitable membranes downstream. As a consequence, local slowing of conduction is to be expected, and eventually, conduction block occurs if the width of the strand reaches a critical diameter, h_c. Typically, the action potentials exhibit a biphasic upstroke resulting from the impedance

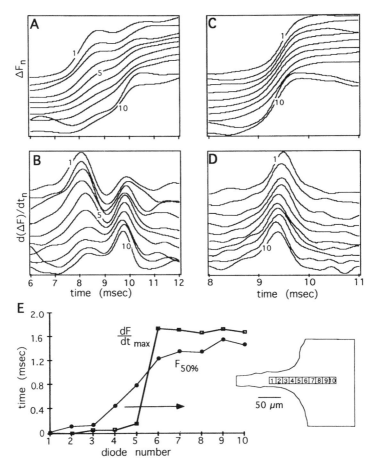

Figure 8. Anterograde and retrograde impulse conduction across an abrupt expansion in a cell culture. Bottom right, Schematic of an abrupt tissue expansion. Width of small cell strand merging with large area (corresponding to geometry shown in Figure 7A) is 22 μm. Grid shows localization of photodiodes with numbers. An individual diode covers a cell membrane area of 14×14 μm². Interdiode spacing is 1 μm. A and C, Normalized optical upstrokes (ΔF_n) of transmembrane action potentials recorded during anterograde conduction (A) from strand into large area and during retrograde conduction (C). Numbers on traces indicate corresponding photodiode numbers. Time was measured from beginning of recording interval. Stimulation pulse was delivered at t = 5 ms. B and D, Normalized first time derivatives of corresponding optical signals, dF/dt_n. Two rising phases can be seen on optical upstrokes ΔF_n corresponding to the two maxima on derivative traces dF/dt_n. E, Time sequences of dF/dt_{max} (squares) and $F_{50\%}$ (circles) calculated from recordings in A and B. Data are plotted relative to moment of dF/dt_{max} at site number 10, which was considered to be zero. Note that geometric expansion induces a conduction delay during anterograde spread (A), whereas propagation is fast during spread from large area into strand (C). Reprinted with permission from Reference 25.

mismatch at the geometric transition. Conduction velocity at such expansions becomes smaller with decreasing "street" width until it occasionally blocks if the streets are only one to two cells wide. Because of the asymmetry of the tissue, conduction in the inverse direction accelerates locally with decreasing street width.[25] Although this type of tissue geometry is the most simple representation of a current-to-load mismatch, it shares common characteristics with the so-called "isthmus" geometry or with a "pivoting," ie, an end of a resistive barrier, as described above.

The questions relevant to discussing anisotropic conduction are whether such resistive obstacles take part in impulse deviation and discontinuous conduction in vivo and whether they contribute to anisotropy, ie, whether their effects depend on the direction of spread of the wave front. An important role for connective tissue sheets separating bundles of excitable myocytes, which are longitudinally aligned and thus show anisotropy, was given by Spach and Josephson,[34] who observed discontinuities in action potential upstrokes and extracellular electrograms during transverse but not during longitudinal direction in such tissue. In particular, it was emphasized that such structural remodeling appears in human hearts with age.[35] Comparing discontinuities at a relatively large scale (obstacles introduced by connective tissue separating whole cell bundles or carrying blood vessels) with discontinuities introduced by the discrete gap junction distribution, one might argue that the larger the discontinuity, the larger the susceptibility to occurrence of conduction block in a stage of depressed excitability. As discussed in the previous paragraph, the situation is likely to be far more complex because of interaction between the macroscopic tissue geometry, gap junctional coupling, and activation of ionic membrane currents.

Interaction Between Structural Discontinuities, Active Membrane Properties, and Changes in Gap Junctional Conductance

Experimental data and computer simulations suggest mutual and complex interactions between the discontinuities at smaller (cellular) and larger (connective tissue, vasculature) scales. An example of the effect of an abrupt tissue expansion on the activation of membrane currents is shown in Figure 9, which depicts the simulated time course of the fast Na^+ inward current, I_{Na^+}, at consecutive sites along the tissue expansion.[29] As can be seen, there is a significant increase of I_{Na^+}, at the sites at which the conduction delay is maximal. The increase in

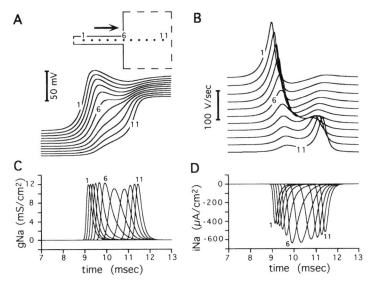

Figure 9. Computer simulation of impulse conduction in a structure with an abrupt expansion. Transmembrane action potentials, V (A); first time derivative of action potential, dV/dt (B); sodium conductance, gNa (C); and sodium current, iNa (D) calculated during impulse propagation from a narrow strand into a large area are shown. Time was measured from onset of stimulus. Geometric structure is depicted in inset of A (analogue geometry to Figures 7A and 8). The 11 recording points were 30 μm apart. Arrow indicates direction of propagation. Strand width was 120 μm. Strand length was 3 mm (only a short strand portion is shown). Length and width of large area were 3 and 2 mm, respectively. Note that there is an increase in maximum sodium current at tissue expansion, demonstrating a feedback effect of tissue geometry on activation of local ionic currents. Reprinted with permission from Reference 25.

depolarizing current contributes to maintenance of conduction at the expansion and to prevention of conduction block. It is explained by the slower rate of depolarization at the expansion with respect to steady-state conduction, which allows the Na^+ channels enough time to fully activate. Also, it has recently been shown that, in contrast to normal steady-state propagation, the slow inward Ca^{2+} current may be of critical importance for conduction if the macroscopic structure imposes a conduction delay.[36] Thus, it appears not only that primary changes in ionic current flow at the level of the cell membranes will determine conduction or block at a site of a change in macroscopic tissue architecture but also that the macroscopic tissue architecture will itself exert a feedback interaction on the activation of ionic membrane channels. An example of the interaction between changes in average cell-to-cell coupling and macroscopic tissue architecture is shown in

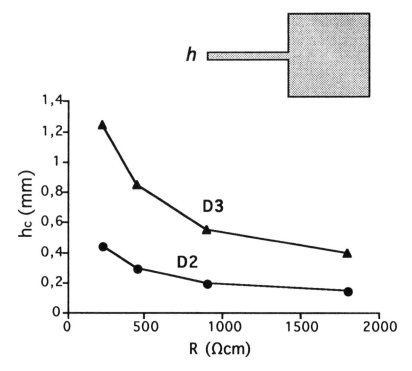

Figure 10. Dependence of critical strand width, h_c, on intracellular resistivity, R. Inset, Schematic of an abrupt tissue expansion. A small strand of width h merges with a large cell area. If h decreases, unidirectional conduction block occurs at critical width h_c. Graph, Critical width, h_c, is plotted as a function of intracellular resistivity R given in Ω·cm for a 2D expansion (D2) and a 3D expansion (D3). This simulation demonstrates that an event at the molecular level (cellular uncoupling) can modulate effect of macroscopic tissue geometry to produce conduction block at critical width, h_c. Reprinted with permission from Reference 29.

Figure 10.[29] In this figure, a simulated geometric expansion contains a network of excitable elements in which both the resistive interconnections and the membrane ionic currents can be modified. These modifications do affect the minimal width of the "street," h_c, at which conduction block occurs. If the resistors between the excitable elements (simulating cell-to-cell coupling) are increased within a certain range, h_c decreases, ie, propagation across the site of impedance-to-load mismatch becomes safer and the probability for occurrence of conduction block lower. The resistors responsible for this phenomenon are those located in the large area and oriented in the y direction. The safer propagation is explained by the higher resistances decreasing the amount of electrotonic current loss downstream of the abrupt geometric tissue transition. The occurrence of conduction block in Figure 10 at larger strand diameters than observed in vivo is most likely due to the slight taper, which is inevitably present in all cultures. There is a close match of the simulated minimal strand width with the one observed experimentally if the taper is included in the simulations.[29]

The above examples illustrate that impulse propagation in heart is a complex process, in which many variables show mutual interaction: (1) the ionic currents responsible for discharging membrane capacity (causing the upstroke of the action potential) and for the excitatory current in the head of the propagating wave front; (2) the type, biophysical properties, density, and geometric arrangement of connexons between closely apposed cells; and (3) the arrangement of the cellular network into a more complex structure, consisting of cells, connective tissue sheets, and the vascular tree. All of these elements are known to undergo changes in a diversity of pathophysiological settings.

References

1. Luo CH, Rudy Y. A dynamic model of the cardiac ventricular action potential, II: afterdepolarizations, triggered activity, and potentiation. *Circ Res.* 1994;74:1097–1113.
2. January CT, Riddle JM. Early afterdepolarizations: mechanism of induction and block: a role for L-type Ca^{2+} current. *Circ Res.* 1989;64:977–990.
3. Jalife J, Moe GK. Excitation, conduction, and reflection of impulses in isolated bovine and canine cardiac Purkinje fibers. *Circ Res.* 1981;49:233–247.
4. Wit AL, Cranefield PF, Hoffman BF. Slow conduction and reentry in the ventricular conducting system, II: single and sustained circus movement in networks of canine and bovine Purkinje fibers. *Circ Res.* 1972;30:11–22.
5. Sommer JR, Scherer B. Geometry of cell and bundle appositions in cardiac muscle: light microscopy. *Am J Physiol.* 1985;248:H792–H803.
6. Leon LJ, Roberge FA. Directional characteristics of action potential propagation in cardiac muscle: a model study. *Circ Res.* 1991;69:378–395.
7. Muller-Borer BJ, Erdman DJ, Buchanan JW. Electrical coupling and impulse propagation in anatomically modeled ventricular tissue. *IEEE Trans Biomed Eng.* 1994;41:445–454.
8. Spach MS, Heidlage JF. The stochastic nature of cardiac propagation at a microscopic level: electrical description of myocardial architecture and its application to conduction. *Circ Res.* 1995;76:366–380.
9. Kleinfeld D, Kahler KH, Hockberger PE. Controlled outgrowth of dissociated neurons on patterned substrates. *J Neurosci.* 1988;8:4098–4120.
10. Purdy J, Liebermann M, Roggeveen AE, Kirk R. Synthetic strands of cardiac muscle: growth and physiological implications. *J Cell Biol.* 1972;65:563–578.
11. Lieberman M, Sawanabori T, Kootsey JM, Johnson EA. A synthetic strand of cardiac muscle: its passive electrical properties. *J Gen Physiol.* 1975;65:527–550.
12. Lieberman M, Roggeveen AE, Purdy JE, Johnson EA. Synthetic strands of cardiac muscle: growth and physiological implications. *Science.* 1972;175:909–911.

13. Horres C, Lieberman M, Purdy J. Growth orientation of heart cells on nylon monofilament. *J Membr Biol.* 1977;34:313–329.
14. Rohr S. Determination of impulse conduction characteristics at a microscopic scale in patterned growth heart cell cultures using multisite optical mapping of transmembrane voltage. *J Cardiovasc Electrophysiol.* 1995;6: 551–568.
15. Rohr S, Schölly DM, Kléber AG. Patterned growth of neonatal rat heart cells in culture: morphological and electrophysiological characterization. *Circ Res.* 1991;68:114–130.
16. Fast VG, Kléber AG. Anisotropic conduction in monolayers of neonatal rat heart cells cultured on collagen substrate. *Circ Res.* 1994;75:591–595.
17. Fast VG, Kléber AG. Microscopic conduction in cultured strands of neonatal rat heart cells measured with voltage-sensitive dyes. *Circ Res.* 1993; 73:914–925.
18. Rohr S, Salzberg BM. Discontinuities in action potential propagation along chains of single ventricular myocytes in culture: multiple site optical recording of transmembrane voltage (MSORTV) suggests propagation delays at the junctional sites between cells. *Biol Bull.* 1992;183:342–343.
19. Rudy Y, Quan W. A model study of the effects of the discrete cellular structure on electrical propagation in cardiac tissue. *Circ Res.* 1987;61: 815–823.
20. Saffitz JE, Kanter HL, Green KG, Tolley TK, Beyer EC. Tissue-specific determinants of anisotropic conduction velocity in canine atrial and ventricular myocardium. *Circ Res.* 1994;74:1065–1070.
21. Delmar M, Michaels DC, Johnson T, Jalife J. Effects of increasing intercellular resistance on transverse and longitudinal propagation in sheep epicardial muscle. *Circ Res.* 1987;60:780–785.
22. Kadish AH, Spear JF, Levine JH, Moore EN. The effects of procainamide on conduction in anisotropic canine ventricular myocardium. *Circulation.* 1986;74:616–625.
23. Tsuboi N, Kodama I, Tayama J, Yamada K. Anisotropic conduction properties of canine ventricular muscles. *Jpn Circ J.* 1985;49:487–498.
24. Spach MS, Miller WTI, Gezelowitz DB, Barr RC, Kootsey JM, Johnson EA. The discontinuous nature of propagation in normal canine cardiac muscle: evidence for recurrent discontinuities of intracellular resistance that affect the membrane currents. *Circ Res.* 1981;48:39–54.
25. Fast VG, Kléber AG. Cardiac tissue geometry as a determinant of unidirectional conduction block: assessment of microscopic excitation spread by optical mapping in patterned cell cultures and in a computer model. *Cardiovasc Res.* 1995;29:697–707.
26. Schalij MJ, Lammers WJEP, Rensma PL, Allessie MA. Anisotropic conduction and reentry in perfused epicardium of rabbit left ventricle. *Am J Physiol.* 1992;263:H1466–H1478.
27. Cabo C, Pertsov AM, Baxter WT, Davidenko JM, Gray RA, Jalife J. Wavefront curvature as a cause of slow conduction and block in isolated cardiac muscle. *Circ Res.* 1994;75:1014–1028.
28. Rohr S, Salzberg BM. Characterization of impulse propagation at the microscopic level across geometrically defined expansions of excitable tissue: multiple site optical recording of transmembrane voltage (MSORTV) in patterned growth heart cell cultures. *J Gen Physiol.* 1994;104:287–309.
29. Fast VG, Kléber AG. Block of impulse propagation at an abrupt tissue expansion: evaluation of the critical strand diameter in 2- and 3-dimensional computer models. *Cardiovasc Res.* 1995;30:449–459.

30. Joyner RW, Veenstra R, Rawling D, Chorro A. Propagation through electrically coupled cells: effects of a resistive barrier. *Biophys J.* 1984;45:1017–1025.
31. Joyner RW, Overholt ED, Ramza B, Veenstra R. Propagation through electrically coupled cells: two inhomogeneously coupled cardiac tissue layers. *Am J Physiol.* 1984;247:H596–H609.
32. Joyner RW, Overholt ED. Effects of octanol on canine subendocardial Purkinje-to-ventricular transmission. *Am J Physiol.* 1985;249:H1228–H1231.
33. Joyner RW, van Capelle FJL. Propagation through electrically coupled cells: how a small SA node drives a large atrium. *Biophys J.* 1986;50:1157–1164.
34. Spach MS, Josephson ME. Initiating reentry: the role of nonuniform anisotropy in small circuits. *J Cardiovasc Electrophysiol.* 1994;5:182–209.
35. Spach MS, Dolber PC. Relating extracellular potentials and their derivatives to anisotropic propagation at a microscopic level in human cardiac muscle: evidence for electrical uncoupling of side-to-side fiber connections with increasing age. *Circ Res.* 1986;58:356--371.
36. Rohr S, Kucera J. The calcium inward current can play a critical role for the success of impulse propagation across abrupt expansions of cardiac tissue in presence of the sodium inward current. *Circulation.* 1995;92(suppl I):I-432. Abstract.

Waves and Arrhythmias
Introduction

José Jalife, MD

This section deals with aspects of discontinuous wave propagation in cardiac muscle that may be explained by generic models of excitable media. The basic postulates may be summarized as follows: (1) The curvature of the wave front is an important factor leading to slow conduction and block. (2) The interaction of a cardiac electrical wave with macroscopic anatomic or functional obstacles in its path may lead to the initiation of the reentrant process as the result of fragmentation of the propagating wave front. The dynamics of such fragmented wave fronts ("wavebreaks") are dependent on the conditions of excitability and refractoriness of the tissue, which will establish the final outcome after a wavebreak has formed. (3) The rapidly rotating activity that seems to be responsible for functional reentry in the heart may be explained on the basis of the formation of wavebreaks that give rise to self-organized rotors, manifested as vortices of electrical waves. (4) The size scale of the structural discontinuities that lead to wavebreaks is usually >1 mm and depends on the width of the wave front. In the following, I will briefly introduce some of the concepts that are relevant to such postulates.

Wave Front Curvature and Propagation

Curvature is a relatively new concept in cardiac electrophysiology. It has been brought to light only recently by studies[1-4] on the applica-

Supported by Grant PO1-HL39707 from the National Institutes of Health, National Heart, Lung, and Blood Institute

From: Spooner PM, Joyner RW, Jalife J (eds). *Discontinuous Conduction in the Heart.* Armonk, NY: Futura Publishing Company, Inc.; © 1997.

tion of spiral wave theory to cardiac excitation dynamics and by the development of optical mapping techniques, particularly video imaging of voltage-sensitive dye fluorescence.[5-8] Such techniques have greatly increased our ability to record cardiac excitation waves from the surface of the heart with very high spatial resolution. As a result, electrophysiologists can now think in terms of 2D or 3D waves rather than just impulses. Studies of cardiac arrhythmias using such techniques in very thin pieces of cardiac tissue[5,6] have demonstrated that reentrant excitation waves are nonlinear waves that self-organize as elongated spirals and whose curvature varies with the distance to the spiral core. Curvature is largest near the core and decreases toward the periphery. Because the larger the curvature is, the slower the conduction velocity, it follows that the velocity of propagation of a reentrant wave is slowest near the center of rotation. These simple concepts may have important implications for the understanding of the mechanisms of reentry, particularly with regard to the use of such parameters as conduction velocity, wavelength, and excitable gap when we are trying to determine sustainability of reentry.

Wavebreaks and Lateral Instabilities

The concept of "wavebreak" is an important contribution of the theory of wave propagation in excitable media.[9,10] During the propagation of a wave initiated by a point source (ie, a circular wave) or by a linear source (ie, a planar wave), the wave front is always followed by a recovery tail of finite dimensions. The distance between the front and the tail corresponds to the wavelength of excitation. In other words, the edge of the wave front and the edge of the wave tail never meet each other. In contrast, rotating waves show a unique phenomenon whereby the wave front and wave tail actually touch each other at a specific point, or wavebreak.[9] Under these conditions, wave-front velocity decreases toward the wavebreak, at which velocity is supposed to be zero. A pronounced curvature is established in close proximity to the wavebreak so that the wave fails to activate the tissue ahead and instead rotates around a small region (ie, the core), which, although excitable, remains unexcited. Under these conditions, the wavebreak becomes analogous to a hinge that pivots around the core and forces the wave to rotate. Hence, a self-sustained rotating wave may be initiated simply by inducing a wavebreak.[10,11]

The concept of wavebreak is important not only for the understanding of reentry initiation but also for the understanding of the interactions of wave fronts with anatomic as well as functional obstacles in their paths. Indeed, it has been shown in experiments with the cesium-catalyzed Belousov-Zhabotinsky (BZ) reaction[9] that under certain conditions, the broken ends of wave fronts do not curve to form spiral waves but rather keep their elongated shape and contract. Even though the broken ends of those wave fronts do not progress laterally but shrink, forward propagation is similar to planar. Eventually, as a result of the progressive shrinking of the broken ends, the excitation wave collapses after exhibiting a robust decremental propagation. Using a generic model of an excitable medium, Pertsov et al[12,13] studied the conditions in which a propagating wave breaks after colliding with an obstacle. They concluded that a wavebreak leads to lateral instabilities and that the onset of such instabilities was associated with the existence of a critical curvature for propagation in the medium. When the curvature of the wave front in the area of the break was higher than critical, the wave would shrink, resulting in 2D decremental conduction.[10] If the curvature of the front was lower than critical, the wave would expand. If the expansion was slow and the size of the obstacle was large enough, the broken end might curve and give rise to vortexlike activity.[9,10] Inhomogeneities in cardiac muscle may cause a break in a propagating wave, leading to lateral instabilities. In addition, changes in excitability may be used to fine-tune such instabilities[14] in such a way that when excitability is low, a broken wave should contract and disappear (ie, conduction block). However, at an intermediate level of excitability, a broken wave may either remain unchanged and propagate or curve and expand, resulting in initiation of vortexlike activity.[10] As predicted by experiments in the BZ reaction and by simulations,[8,12–14] the dynamics of lateral instabilities should be determined not only by the critical curvature of the wave front (ie, the curvature at which propagation ceases[15]) but also by the excitability of the medium and the frequency of wave succession, which if high would have the effect of decreasing the excitability.

As discussed in the chapter by Pertsov, the characteristics of the obstacle with which the wave front interacts also play a role in determining the formation of wavebreaks and vortexlike activity, including its shape and size. Indeed, it has been shown in the BZ reaction that for rotating waves to be initiated in the vicinity of an inexcitable barrier, the barrier must have sharp corners, because a wavebreak will not detach from a slowly curving barrier. In numerical simulations using the FitzHugh-Nagumo equations, Pertsov et al[13] demonstrated that a wave propagates much more readily through the distal end of a long channel than through a narrow slit in an inexcitable screen. In the former case, the distal end of the channel is equivalent to a slowly curving obstacle (90°), whereas in the latter, the slit corresponds to an obstacle with sharp curvature (180°). Hence, the necessary conditions for initiation of vortices by the interaction of a wave with an obstacle interposed in its path are a sufficiently short period of stimulation (ie, sufficiently low excitability) and an obstacle of sufficient size and sufficiently sharp corners. As shown by Agladze et al,[15] if the size of the obstacle is too small or the stimulation period is too long, a planar wave initiated proximal to the obstacle will split at the obstacle into two waves with free ends, each of which will circumnavigate the obstacle. Subsequently, the two wave ends will meet again to form a single wave. However, when the size of the obstacle is large enough or the excitation period becomes shorter than some critical value, the wave splits and the ends remain separated from the obstacle and from each other. As discussed above, depending on the conditions of excitability, a pair of counterrotating waves may be formed beyond the obstacle.

Are Wavebreaks Important in Discontinuous Propagation and Reentry?

Exploration of the significance of wavebreaks in the context of propagation of electrical waves in cardiac muscle has just begun. From studies in other excitable media,[12–15] Starmer and Starobin hypothesize that under normal conditions of excitability and cycle length, collision of an excitation wave with an obstacle in the atrium or ventricle should not cause a wavebreak. As shown recently[14] and also discussed in the chapter by Davidenko et al, it is only when the excitability of the tissue is relatively low that the broken wave front may become laterally unstable (ie, its broken ends do not progress laterally) after its interaction with an appropriate anatomic or functional obstacle.

But what constitutes an appropriate obstacle? The complicated anatomic structure of the subendocardium of the normal atria and ventricles is probably an important substrate for the establishment of reentrant arrhythmias. Indeed, the natural orifices of the caval and pulmonary veins, the atrioventricular rings, and the highly heterogeneous tissue type distributions and geometric arrangements of cardiac cells have all been implicated in the mechanisms of the arrhythmias. However, sustained arrhythmias do not occur under normal circumstances and can only be induced by high-frequency or premature stimulation and facilitated by the presence of certain neurotransmitters (eg, acetylcholine in the atrium) or drugs. On the other hand, in the diseased heart, there has been ample speculation about the histopathological substrate for reentrant arrhythmias in patients with congestive heart failure or myocardial infarction.[16] Sclerotic patches, diffuse fibrotic displacement of cardiac muscle, or both are commonly found, particularly in elderly patients who are most vulnerable to these arrhythmias. In addition, in some of these patients the onset of arrhythmias has been ascribed to increased dispersion of refractoriness secondary to uneven chamber enlargement.[17,18] Such increased dispersion would set the stage for functionally determined obstacles that would interfere with the propagation of wave fronts. Wavebreaks and lateral instabilities may result from such interference and may be one of the initiating causes of reentrant activation. Indeed, it is well known that in heart muscle and other excitable media, wavebreaks leading to rotating wave initiation may be a consequence of the interaction of two waves.[19] During stable vortexlike reentry, the broken wave front rotates around the functional core without shortcutting the circuit. However, broken ends of the wave front do not always lead to reentrant activity (see above), and it is possible that the unstable and fragmented activation fronts that are frequently observed during the apparently turbulent activity that characterizes fibrillation are, in fact, waves that have been broken by interaction with other wave fronts or with obstacles. As a result of their lateral instability, some such waves may shrink and undergo decremental conduction; other broken waves may propagate unchanged until they are annihilated by collision with another wave or boundary; and still other waves will undergo curling at their broken end to create new rotors and spiral waves. The final result would be, as originally postulated by Moe and Abildskov,[20] the fragmentation of the wave fronts into multiple independent daughter wavelets giving rise to new wavelets that sometimes may lead to new rotors and new wavebreaks, and so on in a self-perpetuating motion that characterizes atrial fibrillation. In these three chapters, the postulate is made that wavebreaks and lateral instabilities are an essential ingredient in the initiation of functional reentrant activity. The studies presented here represent the initial attempts to test such a conjecture and provide analyses that bring together underlying mechanistic approaches and the powerful nonlinear dynamics tools used to predict or describe complex nonlinear behavior in excitable media.

2D Vortexlike Reentry: Rotors and Spirals

Recent advances in the understanding of vortexlike rhythms have come from studies that apparently have nothing to do with the heart. Indeed, it has recently become clear that vortexlike reentry is not unique to abnormal cardiac rhythms. Phenomena that have very much in common with vortexlike reentry have been observed in other biological systems such as the brain and retina,[21] the social amoeba *Dyctiostelium*,[22] and calcium waves in *Xenopus laevis* oocytes[23] and single ventricular myocytes,[24] as well as in autocatalytic chemical reactions.[25] The common feature of all these systems is excitability, because, just as in myocardial tissue, in any of these systems a local excitation above a certain threshold results in the initiation of a propagating wave akin to the cardiac action potential. These systems are called excitable media[26] and are governed by a mathematical description that is very similar to the well-known models of cardiac propagation.[27,28] We should point out, however, that there are enormous differences in time and space scales in the various excitable media; for example, the conduction velocity of calcium waves in the oocyte is ≈30 μm/s, whereas in heart muscle, the normal velocity of action potential propagation is ≈0.3 to 0.5 m/s. Yet in all types of excitable media studied thus far, it has been demonstrated that a particular perturbation of the excitation wave may result in vortexlike activity. During such activity, the excitation wave acquires the shape of an archimedean spiral[2] and is called a spiral wave or vortex, organized by its center of rotation, or rotor. As in the case of functional reentry, spiral waves do not require a discontinuity, and their rotation period is close to the refractory period of the medium. The hypothesis that functional reentry is the result of a rotor giving rise to vortices of electrical wave was formulated many years ago.[2] Only recently, however, has this hypothesis been supported by direct evidence.[5-7,28,29] Such evidence was obtained by use of a newly developed high-resolution optical mapping technique that allows direct visualization of the excitation wave in cardiac muscle.

Drifting Spirals Give Rise to Complex Excitation Patterns

The traditional electrophysiological concepts see functional reentry as a strictly stationary phenomenon: an "arc of block" in the center of a reentrant loop acts as a functional obstacle and does not provide any mechanism for reentry drift, which is not the case for rotors. Like other vortices, such as hurricanes and tornados, rotating waves in the heart would rather drift than stay in the same place. Drifting may either be intrinsic[30] or appear as a result of heterogeneity of the medium,[31-33] an external electrical field,[34] or boundary effects.[35] Often, drifting rotors hit the border of the medium and disappear[31]; sometimes they become attached to heterogeneities (obstacles), giving rise to stable rhythms[5] whose periodicity depends on the size of the obstacle around which they rotate.

The concept of drifting rotors provides new insight into the mechanisms of variability and termination of reentry.[5,6,28,29,36,37] Drifting of a reentrant circuit consistent with the theory of wave propagation in excitable media has been demonstrated in isolated rabbit heart in relation to ventricular tachycardia and fibrillation.[38] Similar effects were observed in isolated rabbit ventricle[6,36,37] and in thin layers of sheep ventricular epicardial muscle by optical mapping techniques.[5,6,28,29] In the latter case, however, the observation of drifting was not the result of drug effects or any other external influence but rather was caused by intrinsic heterogeneities in the epicardial muscle itself. Moreover, by use of a simulated electrocardiogram in such preparations, it was demonstrated that drifting spirals can yield an undulating QRS pattern very similar to that of torsade de pointes.[6,36] Finally, sustained rotating activity has been amply demonstrated in the atrium, and in their study using the sterile pericarditis model of the dog atrium, Ortiz et al[39] considered the possibility that the dynamics of drifting and anchoring rotors may be involved in the conversion of atrial flutter to atrial fibrillation and vice versa.

Spiral Breakup and Fibrillation

A number of mathematicians and theoretical biologists have interpreted the degeneration of ordered reentrant tachycardia into disordered fibrillation in the context of the theory of wave propagation in excitable media as the breakup of a spiral into multiple rotors, giving rise to waves propagating in complex pathways.[40–44] These investigators used various 2D and 3D models of propagation in the heart to investigate and make predictions about the conditions leading to spiral breakup and fibrillation.

The chapters that follow deal explicitly with all of the above issues and provide interesting new ideas regarding discontinuous propagation and mechanisms of arrhythmia initiation and perpetuation. The chapter by Starmer and Starobin provides us with an introduction to the use of nonlinear reaction-diffusion models of homogeneous excitable media for the study of action potential propagation in the heart. They begins with a historical review of the most relevant literature dealing with models of excitable membranes and the mechanisms of sodium channel blockade. They then illustrate how very simple generic models of wave propagation in 2D excitable media can help to provide insight into the mechanisms of initiation of reentry in the heart. They explore the dynamics involved in the formation of wavebreaks when a propagating wave collides with an anatomic obstacle. They then demonstrate how changes in the characteristics of the obstacle or in a relevant parameter such as excitability can lead to separation of the wavebreak from the obstacle, with the consequent initiation of spiral wave activity. They conclude with several novel ideas relating spiral wave dynamics with reentrant arrhythmias and their manifestation in the electrocardiogram.

The chapter by Davidenko et al reviews some very recent results demonstrating that, in two dimensions, the curvature of the wave front can be used as a parameter to quantify the safety factor for propagation: a convexly curved wave front has a lower safety factor for propagation than a planar wave front.[4,8] Specifically, if the curvature of the wave front is larger than a certain critical value, propagation will stop.[4,8,14] Accordingly, since one of the necessary requirements for initiation of reentrant activity is unidirectional block, in nonhomogeneous cardiac muscle conduction block can be caused by local differences in electrophysiological properties, particularly refractory period[45-48] and excitability.[48,49] In more homogeneous tissue (minimal spatial differences in electrophysiological properties), geometric factors such as branching sites[50-52] or isthmuses[8,53] might create the conditions for a lowering of the safety factor for propagation and cause block. Thus, Davidenko et al go on to explore five different conditions under which wave fronts with large curvature are expected: (1) initiation of propagation by a point source on the surface of the heart, (2) propagation through a narrow isthmus, (3) collision of waves with obstacles with sharp borders, (4) propagation near the core of a spiral wave, and (5) interactions of two counterrotating waves (figure-eight reentry). The data presented by Davidenko et al provide compelling evidence for the role of wavefront curvature in discontinuous propagation.

Finally, the chapter by Pertsov provides us with a theorist's perspective on the problem of discontinuous propagation. This chapter is concerned with the appropriate scale at which the collision of wave fronts with anatomic obstacles leads to the formation of wavebreaks. Pertsov's ultimate goal is to analyze how structural discontinuities in the heart may affect the dynamic properties of functional reentrant circuits in two and three dimensions. He uses numerical simulations to test the hypothesis that "macroscopic" discontinuities (ie, at a scale >1 mm) are more important than microscopic discontinuities in the formation of wavebreaks leading to unidirectional block and reentry.

References

1. Gul'ko FB, Petrov AA. Mechanism of the formation of closed pathways of conduction in excitable media [in Russian]. *Biofizika.* 1972;17:271–282.
2. Krinsky VI. Mathematical models of cardiac arrhythmias (spiral waves). *Pharmacol Ther.* 1978;3:539–555.
3. Winfree AT. *When Time Breaks Down.* Princeton, NJ: Princeton University Press; 1987.
4. Zykov VS. *Simulation of Wave Processes in Excitable Media.* Manchester, England: Manchester University Press; 1987.
5. Davidenko MJ, Pertsov AM, Salomonsz R, et al. Stationary and drifting spiral waves of excitation in isolated cardiac muscle. *Nature.* 1991;355: 349–351.

6. Pertsov AM, Davidenko JM, Salomonsz R, et al. Spiral waves of excitation underlie reentrant activity in isolated cardiac muscle. *Circ Res.* 1993;72: 631–650.

7. Gray RA, Jalife J, Panfilov AV, et al. Mechanisms of cardiac fibrillation. *Science.* 1995;270:1222–1223.

8. Cabo C, Pertsov AM, Baxter WT, et al. Wave-front curvature as a cause of slow conduction and block in isolated cardiac muscle. *Circ Res.* 1994;75: 1014–1028.

9. Nagy-Ungvarai Z, Pertsov AM, Hess B, et al. Lateral instabilities of a wave front in the Ce-catalyzed Belousov-Zhabotinsky reaction. *Physica D.* 1992; 61:205–212.

10. Panfilov AV, Pertsov AM. Mechanism of spiral wave initiation in active media connected with critical curvature phenomenon. *Biofizica.* 1982;27: 886–888.

11. Tyson JJ, Keener JP. Singular perturbation theory for travelling waves in excitable media (a review). *Physica D.* 1988;32:327–361.

12. Pertsov AM, Panfilov AV, Medvedeva FU. Instability of autowaves in excitable media associated with the phenomenon of critical curvature. *Biofizica.* 1983;28:100–102.

13. Pertsov AM, Ermakova EA, Shnol EE. On the diffraction of autowaves. *Physica D.* 1990;44:178–190.

14. Cabo C, Pertsov AM, Davidenko JM, et al. Vortex shedding as a precursor of turbulent electrical activity in cardiac muscle. *Biophys J.* 1996;70:1105–1111.

15. Agladze K, Keener JP, Müller SC. Rotating spiral waves created by geometry. *Science.* 1994;264:1746–1748.

16. Rossi L. Histopathologic correlates of atrial arrhythmias. In: Touboul P, Waldo AL, eds. *Atrial Arrhythmias: Current Concepts and Management.* St Louis, Mo: Mosby Year Book; 1990:27–41.

17. Kaseda S, Zipes DP. Contraction-excitation feedback in the atria: a cause of changes in refractoriness. *J Am Coll Cardiol.* 1988;11:1327–1336.

18. Klein LS. Effect of atrioventricular interval during pacing or reciprocating tachycardia on atrial size, pressure and refractory period: contraction-excitation feedback in human atrium. *Circulation.* 1990;82:60–68.

19. Winfree AT. Electrical instability in cardiac muscle: phase singularities and rotors. *J Theor Biol.* 1989;138:353–405.

20. Moe GK, Abildskov JA. Atrial fibrillation as a self-sustaining arrhythmia independent of focal discharge. *Am Heart J.* 1959;58:59–70.

21. Gorelova NA, Bures J. Spiral waves of spreading depression in the isolated chicken retina. *Neurobiology.* 1983;14:353–363.

22. Gerisch G. Stadienspezifische Aggregationsmuster bei *Distyostelium discoideum. Wilhelm Roux Archiv Entwick Org.* 1965;156:127–144.

23. Lechleiter J, Girard S, Peralta E, et al. Spiral calcium wave propagation and annihilation in *Xenopus laevis oocytes. Science.* 1991;252:123–126.

24. Lipp P, Niggli E. Microscopic spiral waves reveal positive feedback in subcellular calcium signaling. *Biophys J.* 1993;65:2272–2276.

25. Winfree AT. Spiral waves of chemical activity. *Science.* 1972;175:634–636.

26. Krinsky VI, ed. *Self-Organization: Autowaves and Structures Far From Equilibrium.* Berlin, Germany: Springer Verlag; 1984.

27. Luo C, Rudy Y. A model of the ventricular cardiac action potential: depolarization, repolarization and their interaction. *Circ Res.* 1991;68:1501–1526.

28. Davidenko JM, Kent P, Chialvo DR, et al. Sustained vortex-like waves in normal isolated ventricular muscle. *Proc Natl Acad Sci U S A.* 1990;87:8785.

29. Davidenko JM, Kent P, Jalife J. Spiral waves in normal isolated ventricular muscle. *Physica D.* 1991;49:182–197.
30. Skinner GS, Swinney HL. Periodic to quasiperiodic transition of chemical spiral rotation. *Physica.* 1991;48:1–16.
31. Pertsov AM, Ermakova EA. Mechanism of the drift of spiral wave in an inhomogeneous medium. *Biophysics.* 1988;33:338–341.
32. Zou X, Levine H, Kessler DA. Interaction between a drifting spiral and defects. *SO Phys Rev E Stat Phys Plasma Fluids Relat Interdiscip Top (USA).* 1993;47:R800–R803.
33. Rudenko AN, Panfilov AV. Drift and interaction of vortices in two-dimensional heterogeneous active medium. *Stud Biophys.* 1983;98:183–188.
34. Steinbock O, Schütze J, Müller SC. Electric field-induced drift and deformation of spiral waves in an excitable medium. *Phys Rev Lett.* 1992;68:248–251.
35. Yermakova YA, Pertsov AM. Interaction of rotating spiral waves with a boundary. *Biophysics.* 1986;31:932–940.
36. Gray RA, Jalife J, Panfilov A, et al. Nonstationary vortexlike reentrant activity as a mechanism of polymorphic ventricular tachycardia in the isolated rabbit heart. *Circulation.* 1995;91:2454–2469.
37. Fast VG, Pertsov AM. Drift of a vortex in the myocardium. *Biophysics.* 1990; 35:489–494.
38. Gray RA, Jalife J, Panfilov AV, et al. Mechanisms of cardiac fibrillation: drifting rotors as a mechanism of cardiac fibrillation. *Science.* 1995;270: 1222–1223.
39. Ortiz J, Niwano S, Abe H, et al. Mapping the conversion of atrial flutter to atrial fibrillation and atrial fibrillation to atrial flutter: insights into mechanisms. *Circ Res.* 1994;74:882–894.
40. Panfilov AV, Holden AV. Spatiotemporal irregularity in a two-dimensional model of cardiac tissue. *Int J Bifurc Chaos.* 1991;1:219–225.
41. Ito H, Glass L. Spiral breakup in a new model of discrete excitable media. *Phys Rev Lett.* 1991;66:671–674.
42. Panfilov A, Hogeweg P. Spiral breakup in a modified Fitzhugh-Nagumo model. *Phys Lett.* 1993;176:295–299.
43. Courtemanche M. *Reentrant Waves in Excitable Media.* Tucson, Az: University of Arizona; 1993. PhD dissertation.
44. Winfree AT. Theory of spirals. In: Zipes DP, Jalife J, eds. *Cardiac Electrophysiology: From Cell to Bedside.* 2nd ed. Philadelphia, Pa: WB Saunders; 1995; 379–389.
45. Allessie MA, Bonke FIM, Schopman FJG. Circus movement in rabbit atrial muscle as a mechanism of tachycardia, II: the role of nonuniform recovery of excitability in the occurrence of unidirectional block, as studied with multiple electrodes. *Circ Res.* 1976;39:168–177.
46. Han J, Moe GK. Nonuniform recovery of excitability in ventricular muscle. *Circ Res.* 1964;14:44–60.
47. Allessie MA, Bonke FIM, Schopman FJC. Circus movement in rabbit atrial muscle as a mechanism of tachycardia, III: the "leading circle" concept: a new model of circus movement in cardiac tissue without the involvement of an anatomical obstacle. *Circ Res.* 1977;41:9–18.
48. Gough WB, Mehra R, Restivo M, et al. Reentrant ventricular arrhythmias in the late myocardial infarction in the dog, 13: correlation of activation and refractory maps. *Circ Res.* 1985;57:432–442.
49. Cranefield PF, Klein HO, Hoffman BF. Conduction of the cardiac impulse, I: delay, block, and one-way block in depressed Purkinje fibers. *Circ Res.* 1971;28:199–219.

50. Cranefield PF, Hoffman BF. Conduction of the cardiac impulse, II: summation and inhibition. *Circ Res.* 1971;28:220–233.
51. Spach MS, Miller WT III, Dolber PC, et al. The functional role of structural complexities in the propagation of depolarization in the atrium of the dog: cardiac conduction disturbances due to discontinuities of effective axial resistivity. *Circ Res.* 1982;50:175–191.
52. Spach MS, Miller WT III, Geselowitz DB, et al. The discontinuous nature of propagation in normal canine cardiac muscle: evidence of recurrent discontinuities of intracellular resistance that affect the membrane currents. *Circ Res.* 1981;48:9–54.
53. de la Fuente D, Sasyniuk B, Moe GK. Conduction through a narrow isthmus in isolated canine atrial tissue: a model of the W-P-W syndrome. *Circulation.* 1971;44:803–809.

Chapter 12

Scale of Geometric Structures Responsible for Discontinuous Propagation in Myocardial Tissue

Arkady Pertsov, PhD

It has been demonstrated that severe propagation disturbances leading to dangerous cardiac arrhythmias, including fibrillation, often occur in patients with a history of myocardial infarction.[1-3] A border zone of healed myocardial infarction is known to be the most likely source of these arrhythmias. Intracellular recordings of electrical activity from the border zone are usually not significantly different from those in normal tissue.[4] In contrast, the propagation pattern changes dramatically as a result of structural changes that occur during the healing process.[5-10] This explains increasing interest in studying the role of geometric factors in propagation, particularly in relation to specific mechanisms leading to propagation disturbances and arrhythmias. Another factor that fuels interest in structural effects is the possible application in therapy of cardiac arrhythmias by radiofrequency ablation. Better understanding of arrhythmogenic sources may lead to significant advances in identifying targets for ablation and minimizing damage to myocardial tissue.

Experimental studies of structural effects on propagation are extremely difficult. The major reason is that tissue morphology cannot be easily modified as, for example, ionic channels, which can be blocked or activated by pharmacological agents. Accordingly, separation of geometric effects from other factors is very difficult in experimental

This work was partially supported by National Heart and Blood Institute grant HL39707 and American Heart Association Grant-in-Aid 94016950.

From: Spooner PM, Joyner RW, Jalife J (eds). *Discontinuous Conduction in the Heart.* Armonk, NY: Futura Publishing Company, Inc.; © 1997.

conditions. There have been significant advances recently in experimental control of tissue organization by so-called patterned growth in tissue culture[11-14] and methods of molecular biology.[15-17] Thus far, however, these studies are the exception rather than the rule. The experimental difficulties mentioned above make mathematical modeling an important tool in studying geometric problems of propagation.

This chapter presents data from mathematical modeling studies designed to determine the relevant scale of structures responsible for discontinuous propagation. This question is not as abstract as it may seem. Indeed, structural organization of myocardial tissue is so complex that it is not immediately clear what particular feature of this structure is the most important. The data presented here indicate that the relevant scale is the width of the depolarization front, W. This scale is relatively large, ≈1 mm. This means that only structures of this size or larger should be able to significantly perturb propagation and lead to arrhythmia. All examples of computer modeling results presented in this chapter were generated with the FitzHugh-Nagumo model, which is often used in studies of excitable media and simulations of excitation propagation in cardiac muscle.[18]

Width of the Front as a Spatial Scale

The width of the wave front, W, characterizes the size of the area in which transition from the resting to the fully depolarized state occurs. The simplest way of estimating W is by multiplying the duration of the action potential upstroke by propagation velocity. For normal myocardial tissue, this estimate gives a value of W of ≈1 mm for longitudinal propagation. Indeed, for upstroke duration of 2 ms and propagation velocity measured along fibers of 0.5 m/s, we obtain $W = 2$ ms $\times 0.5$ mm/ms $= 1$ mm. W can be measured directly from a single snapshot of a propagating wave obtained by the optical mapping technique with sufficient spatial and temporal resolution. Figure 1A shows a snapshot of a wave front in the FitzHugh-Nagumo model[18] (see also chapter 14), scaled to fit the cardiac action potential amplitude and propagation velocity.

It is reasonable to hypothesize that W is the scale at which the perturbations to the propagation occur. To illustrate this, let us consider two computational examples in which obstacles of sizes L≫W and L≈W are introduced in the path of the propagating wave (see Figures 1B and 1C). As can be clearly seen, the small obstacle in Figure 1B does not noticeably disturb the propagation, whereas for the larger obstacle in Figure 1C (L≈W), the perturbation is significant. Subsequently, the ends of the break reconnect, restoring normal propagation within 1 ms (middle and right panels).

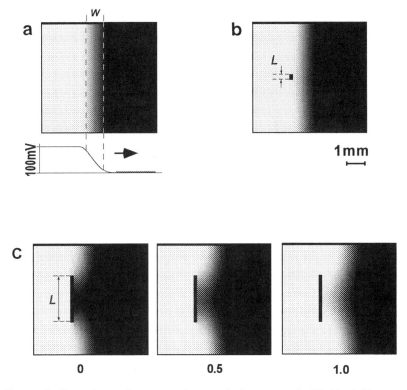

Figure 1. Snapshots of propagating excitation wave in FitzHugh-Nagumo model.[18] Model is scaled to fit characteristics of cardiac action potential. Gray levels correspond to different levels of membrane potential. White and black correspond to fully depolarized and fully repolarized states, respectively. Profile of wave is shown at bottom. Dashed lines indicate width of wavefront (left and right lines are at levels 10 and 90 mV. A, Continuous propagation; B, propagation in presence of small obstacle (black bar in center); C, perturbation of wave front by an obstacle comparable to width of wave-front L>W. Three sequential snapshots are shown at intervals of 0.5 ms (numbers at bottom).

How can this example be related to real myocardium? Let us see what myocardial structures can be observed at a scale L≈W≈1 mm. This scale significantly exceeds the size of single cardiac myocytes. Structures that fall into this range are bundles of cardiac myocytes, layers of connective tissue, and coronary vessels. Figure 2 shows a myocardial slice from normal sheep right ventricle at low magnification. For comparison, in this figure we also show schematically a depolarization front at approximately the correct scale. As one can see, the largest and most abundant objects are clefts (shown as black lines) between adjacent bundles (shown in gray). The length, L, of the clefts

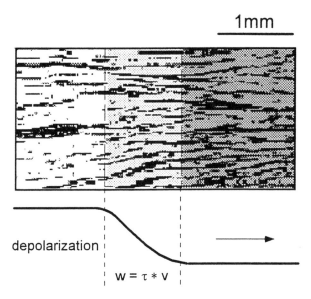

Figure 2. Binarized inverted image of a histological slice from normal sheep right ventricle at low magnification with a superimposed wave profile propagating from left to right (schematic). Black areas correspond to gaps between fibers. Gray levels in background correspond to different levels of depolarization. White, fully depolarized; dark gray, fully recovered. Dashed lines indicate width of depolarization front. Width of front, W, is equal to duration of upstroke, τ, multiplied by propagation velocity, v.

characterizes the distance between lateral connections from one bundle to another. L can be quite long and often exceeds 1 mm. According to histological data, in certain areas of ventricular myocardium L may reach 3 to 5 mm.[19] Much larger values have been reported for infarcted tissue.[7] It will be demonstrated below that in terms of propagation, these clefts can be considered to be obstacles. The spatial pattern of these obstacles (called "texture" below) may determine the anisotropic properties of the tissue. Perturbation of the excitation wave caused by this macroscopic texture (L≥W) is the likely mechanism of discontinuous propagation.

Discontinuous Propagation

Experimental evidence accumulated during the past two decades indicates that the traditional uniform-cable (core-conductor) models are not sufficient to explain many aspects of excitation propagation in myocardial tissue.[20–23] These multiple experimental observations that do not agree with the uniform-cable theory are usually unified under the single term "discontinuous propagation." The most studied effect of discontinuous propagation is anisotropy in the rate of depolarization, $(dV/dt)_{max}$. This effect was first reported by Spach et al[20-22] and then confirmed in other laboratories.[23] Spach and colleagues showed that the rate of rise of action potentials recorded at the same site depends on the direction of propagation. It is faster if the wave propagates perpendicular to fiber orientation and slower when propagation is along the fibers. Another well-established example of discontinuous propagation is fractionation of the electrogram: in certain conditions, instead of the characteristic biphasic shape, extracellular electrodes record a very complex fractionated signal. Fractionated electrograms are usually observed in the border of chronic myocardial infarction and correlate with severe rhythm disturbances.[24]

It is generally agreed that the discrepancies between the model and experimental observations are due to the discrete (discontinuous) nature of myocardial tissue, which is neglected in the core-conductor model. Major efforts have been undertaken to refine the core-conductor model by introducing specific features of myocardial structure, such as the shape of cardiac myocytes, geometry of intercellular junctions,[25] variation in fiber orientation, etc.[26-30] Thus far, the studies of discontinuous propagation have focused primarily on intercellular communication at a microscopic scale.[31-33] The analysis presented below indicates that discontinuous propagation is most likely caused by macroscopic textures (see Figure 2) and cannot be observed when L/W becomes <1.

Simplest Model of Discontinuous Propagation

Before considering a realistic geometry of myocardial tissue, let us first illustrate the role of scaling in a much simpler example. Let us consider again a uniform, continuous 2D excitable medium in which a thin cut of length L>W has been made. We will show that, in this geometry, phenomena that are very similar to experimental manifestation of discontinuous propagation[20-23] can be reproduced. Specifically, (1) the rate of depolarization, $(dV/dt)_{max}$, recorded near the cut is greater when the wave propagates perpendicular to the cut than when it propagates along the cut, and (2) the extracellular potential is fractionated when the wave propagates perpendicular to the cut and is smooth for longitudinal propagation. Varying L from L/W≪1 to L/W≫1 shows that the effects listed above are very sensitive to the relative length of the cut and completely disappear when L/W becomes <1.

Figure 3 depicts traces of the transmembrane potential (V_m), its derivative dV_m/dt, and the extracellular potential V_{ex} for longitudinal (dashed line) and transverse (solid line) propagation in this simplified

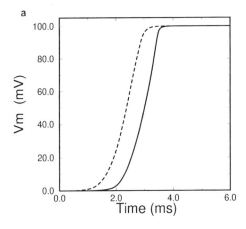

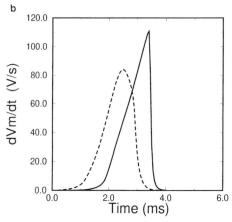

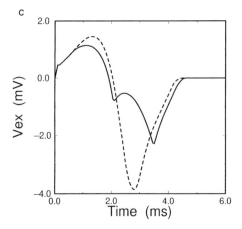

Figure 3. Differences in rate of depolarization and shape of electrogram observed near a cut with L/W>1 during longitudinal and transverse propagation. Dashed and solid lines correspond to longitudinal and transverse propagation, respectively. a, Transmembrane potentials (V_m); b, depolarization rate, dV_m/dt; c, extracellular potentials (V_{ex}) recorded at same location.

model (see Figure 1c). The maximum rate of depolarization $(dV_m/dt)_{max}$ is much greater for transverse than for longitudinal propagation (Figure 3b). Increased depolarization rates for transverse propagation are due to the collision of the wave-front ends behind the obstacle. In the case of longitudinal propagation, $(dV_m/dt)_{max}$ is not different from the control value (see Figure 1a), which is not surprising because, in this case, the cut does not cause any apparent perturbation of the wave front.

The effects of orientation on extracellular potential are depicted in Figure 3c. As with (dV_m/dt), the shape of the extracellular potential recorded near the obstacle is also sensitive to the orientation of propagation. For transverse propagation, the electrogram splits, forming two distinct peaks. The first peak corresponds to the moment of the first collision of the wave front with the obstacle. The second peak coincides with the moment when the ends of the wavebreak reconnect. For longitudinal propagation, the extracellular potential is indistinguishable from the potential recorded in a uniform medium.

Varying the obstacle size shows that intracellular and extracellular manifestations of discontinuous propagation can be observed only for obstacles comparable to the width of the wavefront, W. Figure 4a shows the rate of rise of transmembrane potential for obstacles with relative sizes $L/W = 0.25, 0.5, 0.75,$ and 1.0. No increase in $(dV_m/dt)_{max}$ can be observed for obstacles $<W/2$ $(L/W<0.5)$. As the relative size of the obstacle increases, $(dV_m/dt)_{max}$ increases, reaching saturation at $L/W \approx 3$ (see Figure 4). Similarly, the fragmentation of the electrogram in this example is also determined by the L/W ratio and disappears when L becomes small (see Figure 4c).

Discontinuous Propagation in a More Realistic Model: Textures

To further verify our hypothesis, we now consider a more realistic model that mimics the macroscopic structure of interconnected multicellular strands in myocardial tissue (texture).[34] Texture can be simulated by use of an approach similar to the one described in the previous section. A texture model can be designed with a continuous 2D sheet (or 3D excitable cube) in which multiple insulating cuts following a given pattern are made. Similar models were used earlier by Leon and Roberge[35] and later by Maglaveras et al.[36] Examples of 2D and 3D textures are depicted in Figure 5. The texture in Figure 5a is reminiscent of a parallel slice of myocardial tissue (see Figure 2). To simulate a 3D structure of the myocardium, cuts similar to the one shown in Figure 5a are applied along both vertical and horizontal axes (see Figure 5b).

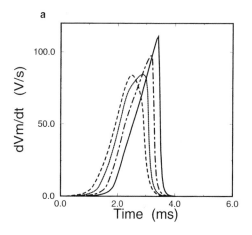

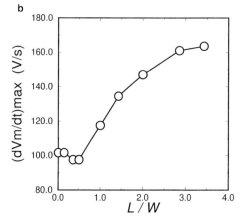

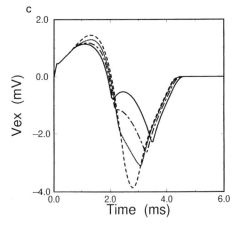

Figure 4. dV_m/dt and extracellular potentials near obstacle as a function of L/W during transverse propagation. A, dV_m/dt traces for L/W = 0, 0.15, 0.5, and 1.0 are shown by broken, dotted, dashed, and solid lines, respectively. B, $(dV_m/dt)_{max}$ as a function of L/W. C, Extracellular potential as a function of L/W.

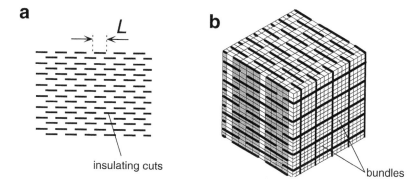

Figure 5. Textures used to simulate discontinuous anisotropic propagation in myocardial syncytium. Black bars show location of insulating cuts mimicking separation between separate multicellular strands. a, 2D texture; b, 3D texture. Black bars show geometry of insulating cuts within cube. As one may see, cuts result in formation of a 3D structure of interconnecting isolated bundles reminiscent of structure of myocardial tissue (compare left, right, and top faces of cube).

As a result of this procedure, a pattern of isolated bundles typical of transverse slices of myocardial tissue is formed in a cross section.

Discontinuous Propagation in Texture Models

One of the interesting results that immediately follows from the analysis of the texture model is that anisotropy is not determined only by the shape of myocardial cells and spatial distribution of intercellular junctions: the important factor that determines anisotropy in myocardial tissue is the macroscopic texture. Figure 6 show examples of excitation propagation in a 3D textured model with different periodic textures. A propagating wave was initiated by point stimulation in the center of the cube. Each snapshot shows a horizontal slice through the point of stimulation.

Figure 6a is a control with no texture applied. Excitation (shown in white) is isotropic, forming a spherical wave. Figure 6b and 6c show the propagation patterns after application of two different textures. The right texture was obtained by scaling the middle one by a factor of 3. One may see that application of the texture results in anisotropic propagation. The wave front is now elliptical, with the main axis parallel to the "bundle orientation." The anisotropy occurs because the discontinuities introduced by the texture do not allow rectilinear propagation in the transverse direction, thus reducing transverse conduction

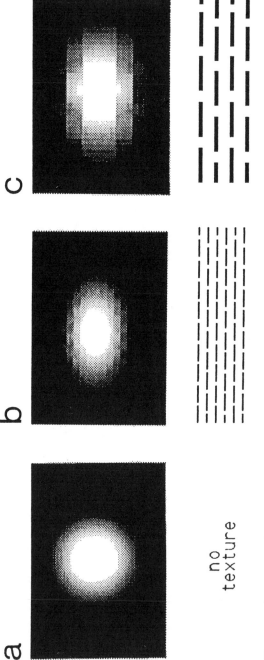

Figure 6. Snapshots of excitation wave initiated in center of array in uniform and textured models. Gray levels correspond to different levels of depolarization (10 mV<V_m<100 mV) from fully depolarized (white) to fully recovered (black). a, Isotropic propagation in absence of texture. b, Introduction of texture results in slowing of propagation in direction perpendicular to fiber orientation. Excitation wave acquires an elliptical shape, and spatial distribution of potential becomes discontinuous. c, Proportional increase in texture size by a factor of 3 does not affect anisotropy.

velocity. In both cases presented in Figure 3, the anisotropic ratio of conduction velocities is ≈ 2. Anisotropy can be controlled by varying the length, L, of the individual cut. The anisotropy increases when L becomes larger.

By scaling the size of the texture up and down, one can explore the effects of discontinuous propagation. The results of such analysis appear to be very similar to those obtained in the model with a single cut. Indeed, the depolarization front propagating perpendicular to fiber orientation has a greater rate of rise $[(dV_m/dt)_{max}]$ than the front propagating along the fibers if the length of each texture element is comparable to the width of the propagating front. Similarly, fractionation of the electrogram in a textured model occurs only when the wave propagates perpendicular to the fiber orientation and when the scale of the texture is large.

The texture model provides an explanation for the correlation between high anisotropy and discontinuous propagation that is usually observed in areas of healed myocardial infarction.[7,37] Such a correlation is most likely a result of the reduced number of lateral connections between bundles (increase in L) that is usually observed in infarcted tissue. Indeed, according to the texture model, an increase in L increases anisotropy and amplifies the effects of discontinuous propagation. It should be noted, however, that there is no direct relation between discontinuous propagation and anisotropy. Indeed, discontinuous propagation completely disappears when the texture size is scaled down sufficiently, whereas anisotropy in conduction velocities is not affected by scaling the texture size. Anisotropy is preserved even at very small L/W, when the model becomes indistinguishable from a continuous anisotropic cable model.

Rentry in Textured Model

It has been demonstrated that the surviving epicardial rim of healed myocardial infarction is highly anisotropic and susceptible to reentrant arrhythmias.[7,37] Analysis of 2D continuous anisotropic models shows, however, that except for significant deformation of the excitation wave and the reentry circuit, the anisotropy itself does not affect either the rotation cycle or the excitable gap between the front and tail of the circulating wave.[18] In the presence of discontinuous anisotropy, this is not necessarily the case. Indeed, the analysis of the textured model shows that the rotation cycle of reentry at L$\approx$W can be 20% to 30% shorter than one in a continuous system (L$\ll$W). The ability of an impermeable barrier to accelerate rotation of vortexlike reentry has been demonstrated earlier[38] and is related to reduced electrotonic load near the center of rotation.

In a 3D medium, this effect may lead to different frequencies of rotation depending on the orientation of the reentry circuit with respect to the fiber direction. Figure 7 shows a 3D vortexlike reentry, a so-called scroll wave,[39] in a textured model with scaling L/W>1. Figures 7a and 7b depict scroll waves with longitudinal and transverse orientations of the rotation axes, respectively. It should be noted that the size of the reentry circuit is shorter for the longitudinal (7a) than for the transverse (7b) orientation of the rotation axis. That means that a reentry circuit is most likely to occur in this orientation. On the myocardial surface, this type of reentry should manifest itself as an elongated breakthrough (see Figure 7b)

In addition to their effect on the rotation cycle, the large-scale macroscopic discontinuities may play an important role in the initiation of reentry due to the so-called "vortex-shedding" effect.[40–43] Near the edge of the cut, the wave front may detach (shed) from the obstacle, forming a vortex-like reentry. This effect has been demonstrated recently in myocardial tissue[44] and is discussed in detail in chapters 13 and 14.

"Fibrillation" in Textured Model: Role of Scaling Factor

Textured models are not limited to the simplified periodic textures described above. Precise structural information can be incorporated in the model by using genuine textures derived from different experimental techniques such as serial histological slices, 3D magnetic resonance imaging, or confocal microscopy. Analysis of these models shows that at very large texture sizes, discontinuities may significantly perturb propagation and lead to very complex irregular activation patterns and self-sustained activity: "fibrillation." To illustrate this statement, we use a realistic texture derived from a real histological slice (see Figure 8). To simulate pathological conditions, L/W is significantly increased compared with normal scale. Perturbations of the wave front that occur at normal scale are sufficient to cause anisotropy in $(dV_m/dt)_{max}$; however, they are too small to be "arrhythmogenic."

Figure 8 shows examples of excitation propagation in the presence of such magnified texture. The difference between Figures 8a and 8b is that the scaling factor L/W in 8a is ≈4 times smaller than in 8b. In both cases, a single excitation wave was initiated near the bottom. As shown by the four consecutive frames in Figure 8a, the excitation front is significantly perturbed, but the wave reaches the upper boundary without initiating self-sustained activity. Calculated extracellular potentials manifest fragmentation (not shown). In Figure 8b, in which the

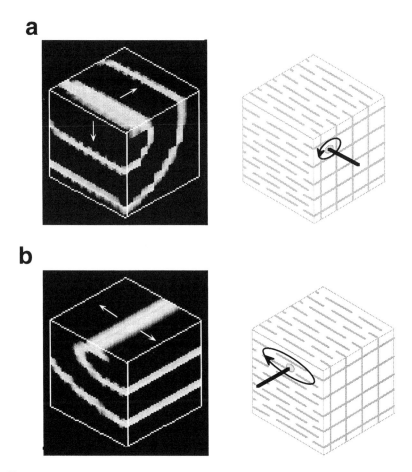

Figure 7. 3D vortexlike reentry (scroll wave) in textured model. a and b show two different orientations of rotation axis. In all cases, top surface represents epicardium and bottom surface endocardium. Left, snapshots of excitation wave. Right, Relative orientation of rotation axis (solid line) with respect to texture. Black arrows indicate direction of rotation; white arrows, direction of propagation. a, Intramural scroll wave with rotation axis oriented along fibers. A spiral shape characteristic of vortexlike reentry can be seen on right lateral surface. No reentrant activity can be seen on epicardial surface (top). Multiple small distortions of wave front are introduced by texture. b, Scroll wave with rotation axis perpendicular to fiber orientation. Due to anisotropy in propagation velocity, spiral is elongated (compare with panel a, in which spiral is isotropic).

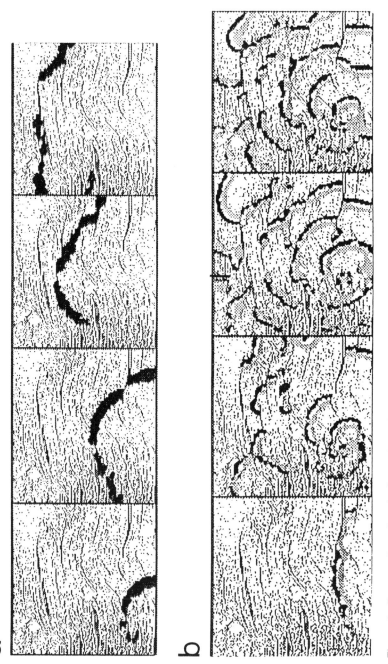

Figure 8. Propagation of excitation at large L/W. Texture derived from a longitudinal slice of rabbit right ventricle. Wave fronts are shown in dark gray. a, L/W increased 4 times compared with control. b, In addition to further increase in L/W, action potential duration was significantly reduced.

scaling factor is greater, perturbations of the excitation wave are more severe. Multiple wavebreaks and reentry loops are formed that lead to self-sustained activity reminiscent of fibrillation. These two examples clearly illustrate that the major factor determining the overall effect on propagation is the relative size of the discontinuity rather than the presence of the discontinuity itself.

We would like to emphasize, however, that in addition to large L/W, other conditions must be satisfied for a discontinuity to become a substrate for arrhythmia. For example, the initiation of reentry requires that L be comparable to the wavelength of excitation. This chapter does not discuss the specific mechanisms of initiation of arrhythmias due to structural effects. These mechanisms are discussed in part in chapters 13 and 14.

Elements that Affect Scaling Factor

One important factor that may affect the L/W ratio is the tissue resistance, R. Indeed, according to cable theory,[45,46] W is proportional to $1/\sqrt{R}$, where R is determined by the extracellular resistance, R_o, the resistance of the axoplasm, R_i, and the intercellular or junctional resistance, R_j. In pathological conditions, R usually increases, leading to amplification of L/W and to an increase in the propensity for arrhythmias. An increase in R is usually related to increases in R_j and R_o. An increase in R_j can be the result of a reduced number of intercellular junctions[47] as well as an increase in single channel resistance due to low pH or high intercellular calcium.[48,49] The mechanisms of regulation of junctional resistance via modification of channel proteins (connexins) and their expression have been extensively studied during the past decade, both in general and specifically in relation to myocardial ischemia, hypertrophy, and other pathological conditions leading to propagation abnormalities (for review, see chapter 9). Increase in tissue resistivity, R_o, can be a result of changes in the extracellular matrix occurring in the area of infarction scar during tissue remodeling.[50] Indeed, areas of chronic infarction are characterized by slow propagation velocity and sharp upstrokes,[7,37,50] which indicates significant increase in R and leads to reduction in W.

Another determinant of the L/W ratio is the characteristic length of discontinuity, L. The parameter L is fixed by tissue geometry, although it may be affected during tissue remodeling that usually occurs with age[22] or as a result of disease.[6–10] Histological studies of infarcted tissue show that muscle fibers in the border zone are sparse and have lower connectivity (longer distance between connections) than normal tissue.[7] An increase in L in addition to a reduction in W at the border zone of

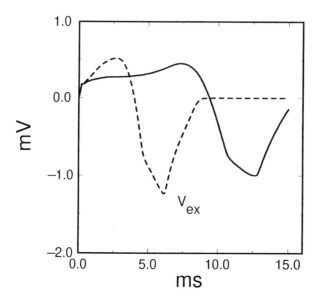

Figure 9. Extracellular potentials at two different levels of excitability. $(dV_m/dt)_{max}$ was changed from 100 V/s (dashed line) to 70 V/s (solid line).

chronic infarction further increases the ratio L/W, creating a substrate for discontinuity-related arrhythmias.

It should be noted that changes in excitability do not necessarily affect L/W. As we already mentioned, $W = \tau \cdot v$, where τ is the upstroke duration and v is the propagation velocity. Usually, τ and v vary in opposite directions. Reduction in excitability increases τ, while v becomes smaller. As a result, W may change very little because the increase in τ is compensated by the decrease in v. This suggests that depression of $(dV_m/dt)_{max}$ and resulting reduction in propagation velocity may not lead to discontinuous propagation. Figure 9 illustrates this statement using the simplest model with a single cut. To make the demonstration more distinct, the size of the cut (L/W = 0.75) was chosen slightly below critical so that even a small increase in L/W would result in a split of the electrogram. The solid line shows the extracellular potential after a twofold reduction in $(dV_m/dt)_{max}$ compared with normal conditions (dashed line). The conspicuous effect is the reduced amplitude and widening of the electrogram due to reduced propagation velocity; however, fractionation does not occur.

Microscopic Discontinuities

To give a full picture of the effects of discontinuous propagation, I would like to indicate the role of discontinuities at the cellular and subcellular levels. As was already mentioned in the previous section, microscopic factors may affect intracellular resistance, R, resulting in variation in L/W. Otherwise, microscopic discontinuities usually average out[25] and do not manifest themselves at the macroscopic scale.

However, this may not always be the case. Mathematical models predict that increasing the coupling resistance may not only reduce propagation velocity, as predicted by the core-conductor model, but may completely block propagation when intercellular resistance exceeds a certain critical value.[31–33] (According to continuous models, an increase in intercellular resistance can only slow down propagation without causing block.) The major difference between these models and a core-conductor model is that the former assume that intercellular resistance is localized at the intercellular junctions rather than uniformly distributed.

It has been hypothesized that propagation block due to increase in intercellular resistance may occur during acute ischemia; however, the relevance of this mechanism has not yet been validated. Experimental studies indicate that even during severe pathological conditions causing propagation impairment, such as anoxia and metabolic blockade, the critical value for block may not be reached.[51,52] Indeed, by simultaneously recording action potential propagation and R_j during anoxia, Riegger et al[51] demonstrated that in most instances, propagation failure occurs before any detectable changes in R_j. Similar results were reported in cell pairs during pharmacological inhibition of aerobic metabolism with the mitochondrial uncoupler 2,4-dinitrophenol,[52] increasing intracellular concentration of Ca^{2+}, or reduced ATP concentration.[52] Increases in R_j in these experiments were preceded by a drop in membrane resistance, R_m, caused by the dinitrophenol. The observed increase in R_j was not sufficient to cause a measurable delay in cell-to-cell propagation, whereas the drop in R_m consistently led to failure of cell excitation.

Macroscopic Versus Microscopic Discontinuities

Recent experimental observations indicate that indeed, macroscopic rather than microscopic discontinuities at a cellular level are responsible for discontinuous propagation. The strongest support for this concept comes from studies using monolayers of cardiac myocytes.[11–14] Such monolayers can manifest anisotropy in propagation velocity;[13] however, they do not show any significant directional differences in $(dV_m/dt)_{max}$. Indeed, monolayers of cultured cells do not have distinct macroscopic (L/W≈1) structures and thus should not manifest features of discontinuous propagation.

More evidence in favor of the macroscopic concept comes from studies of fractionation of the electrogram in healed myocardial infarction. Using high-density electrode arrays, de Bakker et al[7] electrophysiologically estimated the distance between lateral connections between parallel bundles in explanted human infarcted tissue (equivalent to L). According to their estimates, this distance may be as large as 9 mm, which agrees well with the predictions of the model.

Conclusions

In this short review, I propose a unifying concept that allows the determination of the role of particular geometric structures constituting myocardial tissue in propagation using a single dimensionless parameter, L/W. The nominator and denominator in this ratio are the characteristic length of the structure, L, and the width of the depolarization front, W, respectively. The analysis presented here indicates that only macroscopic structures with L/W>1 contribute directly to discontinuous propagation, whereas microscopic factors can only modulate it. This emphasizes the importance of studying the macroscopic organization of myocardial tissue, which may lead to better understanding of mechanisms of reentrant arrhythmias.

Acknowledgments   I am very grateful to my collaborators Drs Michael Vinson and Sergey Mironov for helping with generating computational examples for this chapter.

References

1. Poole JE, Bardy GH. Sudden cardiac death. In: Zipes DP, Jalife J, eds. *Cardiac Electrophysiology: From Cell to Bedside.* 2nd ed. Philadelphia, Pa: WB Saunders; 1995:812–832.
2. Epstein AE, Ideker RE. Ventricular fibrillation. In: Zipes DP, Jalife J, eds. *Cardiac Electrophysiology: From Cell to Bedside.* 2nd ed. Philadelphia, Pa: WB Saunders; 1995:927–933.
3. Stevenson WG. Catheter mapping of ventricular tachycardia. In: Zipes DP, Jalife J, eds. *Cardiac Electrophysiology: From Cell to Bedside.* 2nd ed. Philadelphia, Pa: WB Saunders; 1995:1093–1112.
4. Ursell PC, Gardner PI, Albala A, et al. Structural and electrophysiological changes in the epicardial border zone of canine myocardial infarcts during infarct healing. *Circ Res.* 1985;56:436–451.
5. Stevenson WG, James NW, Wiener I, et al. Slow conduction in the infarct scar: relevance to the occurrence, detection, and ablation of ventricular reentry circuits resulting from myocardial infarction. *Am Heart J.* 1989;117:452–467.
6. Gardner PI, Ursell PC, Duc Pham T, et al. Experimental chronic ventricular

tachycardia: anatomic and electrophysiologic substrates. In: Josephson ME, Wellens HJJ, eds. *Tachycardias: Mechanisms, Diagnosis, Treatment.* Philadelphia, Pa: Lea & Febiger; 1984:29–60.

7. De Bakker JMT, van Capelle FJL, Janse MJ, et al. Slow conduction in the infarcted human heart: "zigzag" course of activation. *Circulation.* 1993;88:915–926.

8. De Bakker JMT, van Capelle FJL, Janse MJ, et al. Reentry as a cause of ventricular tachycardia in patients with chronic ischemic heart disease: electrophysiologic and anatomic correlation. *Circulation.* 1988;77:589–606.

9. Fenoglio JJ, Pham TD, Harken AH, et al. Recurrent sustained ventricular tachycardia: structure and ultrastructure of subendocardial regions in which tachycardia originates. *Circulation.* 1983;68:518–533.

10. Gardner PI, Ursell PC, Pham TD, et al. Experimental chronic ventricular tachycardia: anatomic and electrophysiologic substrates. In: Josephson ME, Wellens HJJ, eds. *Tachycardias: Mechanisms, Diagnosis, Treatment.* Philadelphia, Pa: Lea & Febiger; 1984:29–60.

11. Rohr S. Schölly DM, Kléber AG. Patterned growth of neonatal rat heart cells in culture: morphological and electrophysiological characterization. *Circ Res.* 1991;68:114–130.

12. Fast VG, Kléber AG. Microscopic conduction in monolayers of neonatal rat heart cells measured with voltage-sensitive dyes. *Circ Res.* 1993;73:914–925.

13. Fast VG, Kléber AG. Anisotropic conduction in monolayers of neonatal rat heart cells cultured on collagen substrate. *Circ Res.* 1994;75:591–595.

14. Rohr S. Determination of impulse conduction characteristics at a microscopic scale in patterned growth heart cell cultures using multiple site optical recording of transmembrane voltage. *J Cardiovasc Electrophysiol.* 1995;6:551–568.

15. Rossant J. Mouse mutants and cardiac development: new molecular insights into cardiogenesis. *Circ Res.* 1996;78:349–353.

16. Chien KR. Cardiac muscle diseases in genetically engineered mice: evolution of molecular physiology. *Am J Physiol.* 1995;269:H755–H766.

17. Reaume AG, de Sousa PA, Kulkarni S, et al. Cardiac malformation in neonatal mice lacking connexin43. *Science.* 1995;267:1831–1834.

18. Pertsov AM, Davidenko JM, Salomonsz R, Baxter W, Jalife J. Spiral waves of excitation underlie reentrant activity in isolated cardiac muscle. *Circ Res.* 1993;72:631–650.

19. LeGrice IJ, Smaill BH, Chai LZ, et al. Laminar structure of the heart: ventricular myocyte arrangement and connective tissue architecture in the dog. *Am J Physiol.* 1995;269:H571–H582.

20. Spach MS, Miller WT III, Geselowitz DB, et al. The discontinuous nature of propagation in normal canine cardiac muscle: evidence for recurrent discontinuities of intracellular resistance that affect the membrane currents. *Circ Res.* 1981;48:39–54.

21. Spach MS, Miller WT III, Dolber PC, et al. The functional role of structural complexities in the propagation of depolarization in the atrium of the dog: cardiac conduction disturbances due to discontinuities of effective axial resistivity. *Circ Res.* 1982;50:175–191.

22. Spach MS, Dolber PC. Relating extracellular potentials and their derivatives to anisotropic propagation at a microscopic level in human cardiac muscle: evidence for electrical uncoupling of side-to-side fiber connections with increasing age. *Circ Res.* 1986;58:356–371.

23. Delgado C, Steinhaus B, Delmar M, et al. Directional differences in excitabil-

ity and margin of safety for propagation in sheep ventricular epicardial muscle. *Circ Res.* 1990;67:97–110.

24. Josephson ME, Wit AL. Fractionated electrical activity and continuous electrical activity: fact or artifact? *Circulation.* 1984;70:529–532.

25. Spach MS, Heidlage JF. The stochastic nature of cardiac propagation at a microscopic level: electrical description of myocardial architecture and its application to conduction. *Circ Res.* 1995;76:366–380.

26. Barr RC, Plonsey R. Propagation of excitation in idealized anisotropic two-dimensional tissue. *Biophys J.* 1984;45:1191–1202.

27. Pollard AE, Burgess MJ, Spitzer KW. Computer simulations of three-dimensional propagation in ventricular myocardium: effects of intramural fiber rotation and inhomogeneous conductivity on epicardial activation. *Circ Res.* 1993;72:744–756.

28. Henriquez C. Simulating the electric behavior of cardiac tissue using the bidomain model. *Crit Rev Bioeng.* 1993;21:1–77.

29. Panfilov AV, Keener JP. Generation of reentry in anisotropic myocardium. *J Cardiovasc Electrophysiol.* 1993;4:412–421.

30. Rogers JM, McCulloch AD. Nonuniform muscle fiber orientation causes spiral wave drift in a finite element model of cardiac action potential propagation. *J Cardiovasc Electrophysiol.* 1994;5:496–509.

31. Joyner RW. Effects of the discrete pattern of electrical coupling on propagation through an electrical syncytium. *Circ Res.* 1982;50:192–200.

32. Rudy Y, Quan W-L. A model study of the effects of the discrete cellular structure on electrical propagation on cardiac tissue. *Circ Res.* 1987;61:815–823.

33. Keener JP. Propagation and its failure in coupled systems of discrete excitable cells. *SIAM J Appl Math.* 1987;47:556–572.

34. Pertsov AM, Davidenko JM, Jalife J. Simulation of anisotropic propagation and reentry in a 3-dimensional network of multicellular branching strands. *Circulation* 1992;86(suppl I):I-751. Abstract.

35. Leon LJ, Roberge FA. Directional characteristics of action potential propagation in cardiac muscle: a model study. *Circ Res.* 1991;69:378–395.

36. Maglaveras N, Bakker JMT, Van Capelle FJL, et al. Activation delay in healed myocardial infarction: a comparison between model and experiment. *Am J Physiol.* 1995;269:H1441–H1449.

37. Dillon SM, Allessie MA, Ursell PC, et al. Influences of anisotropic tissue structure on reentrant circuits in the epicardial border zone of subacute canine infarcts. *Circ Res.* 1988;63:182–206.

38. Pertsov AM, Emarkova EA, Panfilov AV. Rotating spiral waves in modified FitzHugh-Nagumo model. *Physica D.* 1984;14:117–124.

39. Pertsov AM, Jalife J. Three-dimensional vortex-like reentry. In: Zipes DP, Jalife J, eds. *Cardiac Electrophysiology: From Cell to Bedside.* 2nd ed. Philadelphia, Pa: WB Saunders; 1995:403–410.

40. Panfilov A, Pertsov AM. Mechanism of spiral waves initiation in active media connected with critical curvature phenomenon. *Biophysics.* 1982;27:931–934.

41. Pertsov AM, Ermakova EA, Shnol EE. On the diffraction of autowaves. *Physica D.* 1990;44:178–190.

42. Panfilov A, Keener JP. Effects of high frequency stimulation on cardiac tissue with an inexcitable obstacle. *J Theor Biol.* 1993;163:439–448.

43. Starobin JM, Zilberter YI, Rusnak EM, Starmer CF. Wavelet formation in excitable cardiac tissue: the role of wavefront-obstacle interactions in initiating high-frequency fibrillatory-like arrhythmias. *Biophys J.* 1996;70:581–594.

44. Cabo C, Pertsov AM, Davidenko JM, Baxter WT, Gray RA, Jalife J. Vortex-shedding as a precursor of turbulent electrical activity in cardiac muscle. *Biophys J.* 1996;70:1105–1111.
45. Weidmann S. Electrical constants of trabecular muscle from mammalian heart. *J Physiol.* 1970;210:1041–1054.
46. Clerc L. Directional differences of impulse spread in trabecular muscle from mammalian heart. *J Physiol.* 1976;255:335–346.
47. Peters NS, Green CR, Poole-Wilson PA, Sivers NJ. Cardiac arrhythmogenesis and the gap junction. *J Mol Cell Cardiol.* 1995;27:37–44.
48. Kléber AG, Riegger CB, Janse MJ. Electrical uncoupling and increase of extracellular resistance after induction of ischemia in isolated, arterially perfused rabbit papillary muscle. *Circ Res.* 1987;61:271–279.
49. Firek L, Weingart R. Modification of gap junction conductance by divalent cations and protons in neonatal rat heart cells. *J Mol Cell Cardiol.* 1995;27:1633–1643.
50. Spear JF, Michelson EL, Moore EN. Reduced space constant in slowly conducting regions of chronically infarcted canine myocardium. *Circ Res.* 1983;53:176–185.
51. Riegger CB, Alperovich G, Kléber AG. Effect of oxygen withdrawal on active and passive electrical properties of arterially perfused rabbit ventricular muscle. *Circ Res.* 1989;64:532–541.
52. Morley GE, Anumonvo JMB, Delmar M. Effects of 2,4-dinitrophenol or low [ATP]$_i$ on cell excitability and action potential propagation in guinea pig ventricular myocytes. *Circ Res.* 1992;71:821–830.

Chapter 13

Wave-Front Curvature Leads to Slow Conduction and Block in Two-Dimensional Cardiac Muscle

Jorge M. Davidenko, MD,
Candido Cabo, PhD, and José Jalife, MD

In a linear cable composed of electrically interconnected excitable cells, impulse propagation is determined primarily by the ratio between the current available to excite cells downstream (the "source") and the current required by those cells to be excited (the "sink").[1–3] Among the factors that influence the source, we can include the maximum rate of rise of the action potential upstroke, the action potential amplitude, and under certain conditions, the action potential duration. Passive membrane properties such as axial resistivity may also modulate the amount of excitatory current delivered by the source. The factors that influence the sink include the membrane resistance, the voltage threshold, and the difference between voltage threshold and membrane potential. Thus, the "safety factor" for propagation in a 1D cable is proportional to the excess of source current over to the sink needs. Normal conduction, slow conduction, and block may result from a progressive decrease in the safety factor. Geometric factors may lead to an "impedance mismatch" between sink and source that will result in propagation disturbances. For instance, an action potential may effectively propagate through a cable but block at branching sites as a result of a sudden increase of the repolarizing load.[4–7] Similar rules apply for the initiation

Supported in part by grants P01-HL39707, R01-HL29439 and R01-HL46148 from the National Heart, Lung, and Blood Institute, National Institutes of Health.

From: Spooner PM, Joyner RW, Jalife J (eds). *Discontinuous Conduction in the Heart.* Armonk, NY: Futura Publishing Company, Inc.; © 1997.

of a propagated response. In this case, a "liminal length" of cable has to be excited simultaneously to overcome the repolarizing ("loading") effect of resting cells.[1-3]

When propagation of the impulse occurs in two dimensions, other factors come into play. Indeed, in a 2D medium, the shape (ie, curvature) of the wave front is thought to be a major determinant of the success or failure of propagation.[8-11] The more convexly curved a wave front is, the lower its velocity of propagation. In fact, beyond a certain critical curvature, propagation of the wave front cannot proceed. The relationship between curvature and propagation has been confirmed experimentally in a chemically excitable medium.[12,13] Its study has just begun in cardiac muscle.[14,15]

There are several conditions under which cardiac electrical wave fronts with pronounced curvature are expected to occur and thus influence the propagation of the impulse: (1) initiation of a propagating wave from a small source, (2) propagation through a narrow isthmus, (3) propagation of a wave front around an anatomic obstacle with sharp borders, (4) propagation near the tip of a rotating spiral wave, and (5) interaction between two or more waves. This chapter discusses recent numerical and experimental studies[14-16] in which these conditions have been recreated and studied.

Initiation of a Propagating Wave From a Small Source

Computer simulations have shown that the velocity of a wave front progressively increases toward its steady-state value as the wave propagates away from a point source.[17,18] A linear relation between the wave-front velocity and its curvature has been found in various theoretical[8-11] and experimental[19] models of excitable media. In a recent study from our laboratory,[15] we were able to reproduce such results using an ionic model of cardiac tissue. We used a continuous 2D anisotropic array of excitable elements in which the membrane impedance consisted of a single capacitance in parallel with the ionic currents described by the phase 1 Luo-Rudy model.[20] The liminal area for propagation was obtained from the minimum number of nodes that needed to be stimulated (stimulation was effected by bringing the membrane potential to 50 mV) before a propagating wave ensued. Critical curvature was defined as the reciprocal of the critical radius of the area occupied by those nodes. The critical radius for propagation was between 0.2 and 0.225 mm (ie, critical curvature of 44.4 cm^{-1}). When the number of nodes being activated was larger than critical, a propagating wave front with a circular shape ensued. Obviously, for a wave front with circular shape, the curvature is constant along the front and equal to the reciprocal of its radius. Therefore, by measuring the reciprocal of the distance between the head of the activation front and the stimulating node as well as the time required for the wave front to travel from one node to the next (activation time was determined at the moment in which the total ionic current became negative), one can obtain the relation between curvature and velocity of propagation for that medium. In Figure 1 velocity (in cm·s^{-1}) is plotted as a function of curvature (in cm^{-1}). The data points can be well fitted with a straight line, as predicted by other models of excitable media.[8-11] Three important parameters can be estimated from the linear fit to the data: (1) velocity at 0 curvature (ie, planar wave front), which in this case was 75 cm·s^{-1}; (2) the value of curvature at which velocity was expected to be 0 (ie, critical curvature), which was 40 cm^{-1}; and (3) the slope of the linear fit, 2.04 cm^2·s^{-1}, which was a good estimate of the diffusion coefficient of the medium (h/2R$_i$C$_m$). The relation between velocity of propagation and curvature was independent of the stimulus strength and duration used. Given that all cells in the model had the same characteristics, it is clear from Figure 1 that the increase in conduction velocity that was observed at progressively greater distances from the site of stimulation was the result of a gradual decrease in the wave-front curvature.

Propagation Through a Narrow Isthmus

Following the propagation of a wave across a narrow isthmus of cardiac tissue allows the study of wave-front curvature and its influence on conduction velocity.[14] De la Fuente et al[21] were first in studying propagation through a narrow isthmus in canine atrial tissue. Although they did not measure precisely the critical isthmus size, the anatomic width at which they demonstrated conduction block at slow frequency was 0.5 to 1 mm. More recently, Fast and Kléber[22] studied propagation through narrowing groups of cells in patterned rat myocyte cultures and found that an action potential emerging from a strand 5 to 8 cells wide always propagated to a large growth area, albeit at a reduced velocity. The latter would suggest that in that case, the critical isthmus was < 65 to 130 μm. A recent study from our laboratory[14] used both a 2D array of the Luo-Rudy model and thin slices of sheep epicardial muscle to investigate the characteristics of propagation through an isthmus as well as the influence of anisotropy, as discussed below.

Computer Simulations

An isthmus was simulated in the 2D array described above by placing an impermeable screen with a hole at the center of the medium

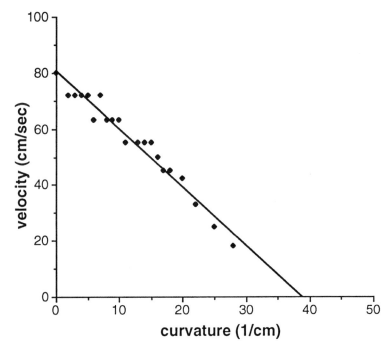

Figure 1. Relation between velocity and curvature for point stimulation. Curve was calculated from propagation of a single beat. Electrical activity was originated by stimulation from a point source. Spatial and time discretization steps were 0.05 mm and 0.002 ms, respectively. Equation of linear fit was: velocity $= 79.91 - 2.04 \times$ curvature. Extracellular resistance was set to 0. Membrane current, I_m, is expressed as $I_m = (1/S_V)[(1/R_{ix})(V_m)_{xx} + (1/R_{iy})(V_m)_{yy}] = I_{ion} + C_m(V_m)_t$, where I_m is transmembrane current at a certain patch of membrane (in $\mu A/cm^2$), S_v is surface/volume ratio of preparation (2000 cm^{-1}), R_{ix} is intracellular resistance in longitudinal direction ($0.5 k\Omega \cdot cm$), R_{iy} is intracellular resistance in transverse direction (8 $k\Omega \cdot cm$), V_m is transmembrane potential (in mV), I_{ion} is total ionic current (in $\mu A/cm^2$), and C_m is specific membrane capacitance (1 $\mu F/cm^2$). Boundary nodes in sheet are considered sealed (ie, no intracellular current flowing out of domain), so boundary conditions are $\partial V_m/\partial x = 0$ and $\partial V_m/\partial y = 0$. Differential equations were integrated by finite-element method, interpolating with fifth-degree polynomials and using a spatial discretization step of 133 μm and a time step of 100 μs. Reprinted with permission from Reference 15.

(Figure 2). The anisotropic ratio, measured as the difference between longitudinal and transverse conduction velocities, was 3:1 (for further details see Reference 14). Propagation was initiated by planar stimulation in the proximal side, with the resulting wave front being parallel to the screen. The velocity of propagation of the planar wave in the longitudinal direction was 41 cm/s. The size of the isthmus was reduced gradually until the wave failed to propagate from the proximal to the distal side. The critical width of the isthmus was shown to be a function of the direction of propagation. In the longitudinal and transverse directions, the critical widths were 200 and 600 μm, respectively. It is interesting that the width of the critical isthmus scales in the same way as the anisotropic ratio. The critical size of the isthmus for propagation was strongly dependent on the excitability of the medium. A decrease in the maximum value of the sodium conductance from 11.5 (considered normal) to 6.9 mS/cm^2 resulted in a decrease in the velocity of a

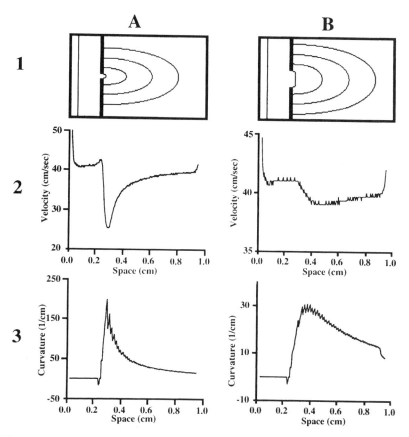

Figure 2. Numerical experiment showing longitudinal propagation through narrow (width, 250 μm, panel A 1–3) and wide (width, 950 μm, panel B, 1–3) isthmuses. A1 and B1 show isochronal maps for each condition; A2 and B2 are changes in velocity of propagation along a line in direction of propagation (left to right) through middle of isthmus; A3 and B3 are changes in curvature of wave front along same line. Simulations correspond to a case with normal excitability. Reprinted with permission from Reference 14.

planar wave (longitudinal conduction velocity = 31 cm/s) and an increase in the size of the critical isthmus to 500 μm. In Figure 2A, we summarize our numerical study of the relation between curvature and conduction velocity during longitudinal propagation across a 250-μm isthmus. Panel A1 shows an isochronal map with isochrones displayed every 5 ms. Panel A2 depicts the local conduction velocity along a line in the direction of propagation through the center of the isthmus. Proximal to the isthmus, the velocity of the wave front increased as it approached the isthmus. The velocity decreased to a minimum (25 cm/s) after the isthmus and then progressively increased again toward the value of the velocity of a planar wave. Panel A3 shows the changes in wave-front curvature as a function of space. Clearly, the changes in the curvature correlated very well with changes in the conduction velocity: Because of the high resistivity at the barrier, the increase in the conduction velocity just before the isthmus corresponded to that of a wave front of negative curvature (concave). Conversely, the decrease in the conduction velocity beyond the isthmus corresponded to wave fronts of positive curvature (convex). The minimum velocity occurred at a distance of 0.5 mm from the isthmus and coincided with the site of maximum curvature.

Propagation through a wider isthmus (950 μm) is presented in Figure 2B. Qualitatively, the results are similar to those shown in Figure 2A: Velocity and curvature were again related to each other. However, there were some quantitative differences: Minimum velocity and maximum curvature occurred farther away from the isthmus and over a wider range of distances. Data obtained during transverse propagation with an isthmus wider than critical (width, 950 μm) were similar to those shown here for longitudinal propagation.[14]

It is important to indicate at this point that the above results would be difficult to explain on the basis of the 1D concept of impedance mismatch.[4–7] It is in fact unlikely that the impedance mismatch at the isthmus had any influence on the velocity of propagation far from the isthmus. If an impedance mismatch had any effect at the isthmus, then it would be expected that changes in conduction velocity should have occurred right at the isthmus and not far away from it. Yet propagation velocity through the isthmus was normal because the wave front was flat; the minimum velocity of propagation occurred far away from the isthmus where the curvature of the wave front was maximal. Farther away from the isthmus, the velocity was still slower than that of a planar wave because the wave front was curved. Thus, according to the model results, the most important effect of the isthmus was to diffract the planar wave front into an elliptical curvature. The local changes in curvature themselves were responsible for the corresponding changes in velocity. It follows from these results that, since a large curvature of the wave front causes a reduction in the velocity of propagation (see Figures 2A and 2B), it is reasonable to propose that propagation will be possible only for wave fronts whose curvature is less than critical. This would mean that there should be a critical curvature for propagation in cardiac tissue as well.

Relation Between Velocity of Propagation, Curvature, and Isthmus Size

As shown above, the minimum velocity of propagation occurred when the curvature of the wave front was maximal. In Figure 3A, we have plotted the velocity of the wave front as a function of the local curvature for the case of propagation through a 250-μm isthmus (same as Figure 2A). The data were well fitted by a straight line whose slope of 0.102 cm²/s (95% confidence interval, 0.096 to 0.108 cm²/s) is equivalent to the so-called "diffusion coefficient." When we calculated the average velocity of propagation after the isthmus for isthmuses of different sizes, we obtained the plot presented in Figure 3B. The average velocity was calculated from the distance traveled by the wave in 5 ms from the isthmus. The maximum curvature of the wave front imposed by a certain isthmus is given by $(AR) \times (2/w)$, where AR is anisotropic ratio and w is the width of the isthmus. Therefore, given the linear relation between curvature and propagation velocity (Figure 3A), it is not surprising that the points in 3B could be well fitted by a straight line.

The value of the curvature at which the velocity is zero is an estimate of the critical curvature for propagation. From the line in Figure 3A, the critical curvature in the longitudinal direction is 414.5 cm⁻¹ (intercept/slope = 41.45/0.102). Considering the errors in the estimation of the intercept and the slope, the 95% confidence interval for the critical curvature was estimated to be between 381 and 435 cm⁻¹. The value expected from the parameters of the model is 372.7 cm⁻¹ (velocity of a planar wave/diffusion = 41/0.11). The value of the critical curvature for propagation can also be estimated from the value of the critical isthmus as $(AR) \times (2/w)$.[14] In that case, the critical curvature is estimated to be 300 cm⁻¹ ($3 \times 2/0.02$). Differences might be due to the spatial discretization step used in the model (50 μm).

Isolated Tissue Experiments

We tested the above model predictions in a series of optical mapping experiments. We used voltage-sensitive dyes and a CCD video

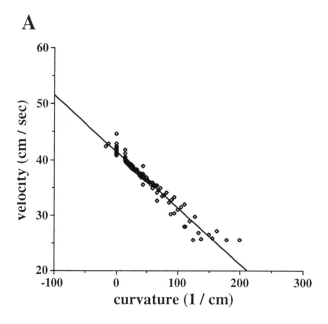

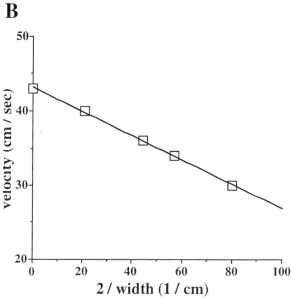

Figure 3. A, Relation between propagation velocity and wave front curvature in simulation of propagation through narrow isthmus. B, Relation between average velocity of propagation after isthmus and width of isthmus. Reprinted with permission from Reference 14.

camera to record the transmembrane electrical activity from the surface of thin (≈0.5 mm thick) slices of sheep epicardial muscle. Detailed description of the technique appears elsewhere.[14] Qualitatively, all model predictions were borne out by the experimental results. An example of longitudinal propagation through an isthmus is presented in Figure 4. The top left frame shows the image of the tissue to illustrate the two cuts produced horizontally across the fibers in the middle of the preparation. The other five frames show video images of the dye fluorescence taken once every 16 ms after subtraction of the background image during quiescence. Activation was initiated at the top border of the preparation (proximal side of the isthmus) at a basic cycle length of 500 ms. Depolarized cells appear in white and repolarized cells in black. The wave appeared as an elliptical wave front as it emerged from the isthmus, thus reflecting the fiber orientation: the velocity was much faster in the vertical direction (ie, longitudinal) than orthogonally.

Effect of the Isthmus on Conduction Velocity

As predicted by the computer simulations, isthmuses of different widths diffract planar waves to elliptical shapes having different curvatures (see Figure 2). We tested such a prediction in additional experiments in which we quantified the changes in the velocity of propagation produced by changes in the width of the isthmus. Figure 5 shows a case of propagation in the longitudinal direction; basic cycle length was 500 ms in all panels. Panel A shows an isochrone map obtained in the absence of an isthmus. The preparation was stimulated on the left border. As shown by the 16-ms isochrone lines, the wave front had a very small curvature and propagated rapidly toward the right border. Panels B and C show the isochrone maps for isthmuses of 2.26 and 0.88 mm, respectively. Clearly, the smaller the isthmus, the steeper the curvature of the elliptical wave front and the slower the velocity. Panel D shows the numerical values of the velocities plotted versus twice the reciprocal of the width of the isthmus (as in Figure 5B) in this experiment. The velocity was calculated as the spatial distance between the last isochrone before the isthmus and the first isochrone after the isthmus divided by the time between isochrones (16.67 ms) and averaged over three consecutive beats. It is clear that the velocity of propagation through the isthmus decreased with a decrease in the width of the isthmus (increasing 2/w), which corresponded to an increase in the curvature of the wave front after the isthmus. This strongly suggests that, as in the computer simulations, the slowing of conduction was caused by the pronounced curvature caused by propagation through the isthmus.

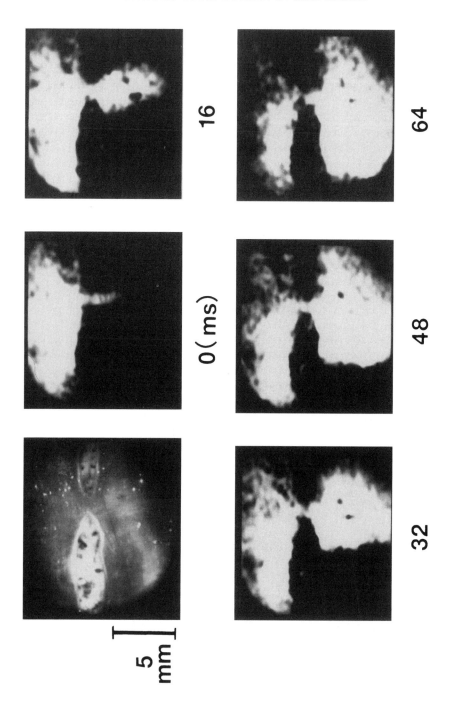

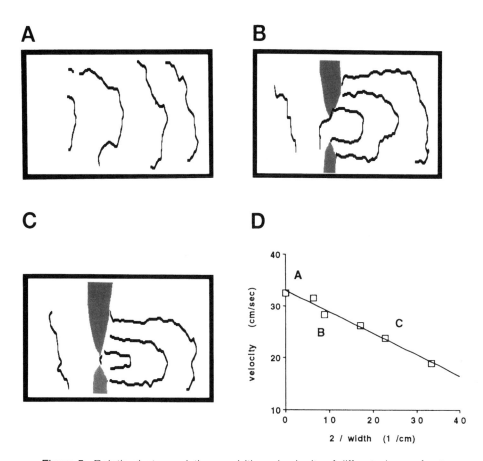

Figure 5. Relation between isthmus width and velocity of diffracted wave front in sheep epicardial muscle. A, Isochronal map before any isthmus was created. Stimulation from left at basic cycle length of 500 ms. Propagation is longitudinal; time between isochrones is 16.67 ms. B, Isochronal map when width of isthmus was 2.26 mm. C, Isochronal map after width of isthmus was reduced to 0.88 mm. D, Conduction velocity plotted versus twice reciprocal of width of isthmus. Velocity was calculated as spatial distance between last isochrone before isthmus and first after isthmus, divided by time between ischrones (16.67 ms) and averaged over three consecutive beats. Velocities measured from isochrones in A, B, and C were used to calculate velocities labeled A, B, and C in panel D. Reprinted with permission from Reference 14.

◄──────────────────────────────────────

Figure 4. Experiment in a sheep epicardial preparation showing longitudinal propagation through a 1.09-mm isthmus. Stimulation was applied to top (basic cycle length, 500 ms). See text for details. Reprinted with permission from Reference 14.

Propagation of a Wave Front Around an Anatomic Obstacle With Sharp Borders

A wave front may be forced to develop a pronounced curvature during the activation of the tissue surrounding an obstacle (ie, inexcitable barrier) with sharp borders. Figure 6A shows three snapshots and the complete isochronal map obtained during propagation around an obstacle in a 2D array of Luo-Rudy cells. In this case, an impermeable barrier was connected to one of the sides (left side) of the array. A stimulus was applied to the bottom half of the same side. The propagating wave activated the left lower quadrant at a normal velocity. Upon reaching the edge of the barrier, the wave front developed a pronounced curvature (see snapshots at 12 and 15 ms). The wave front proceeded to activate the bottom half of the array with no major delays (see distance between isochrones 10 to 40 ms in the isochronal map). Propagation of the upper half of the near edge of the barrier, however, was slightly delayed as a result of the curvature. Thus, in this example, a pronounced curvature of the wave front led to only a slight slowing of propagation (ie, there was no propagation block), which indicates that the curvature was less than critical for this particular medium. As previously discussed, the value of the critical curvature is a function of the excitability of the medium. Thus, if the excitability decreases, wave fronts with less curvature may fail to propagate. Figure 6B shows the effects of reducing the excitability of the medium. In this example, the conductance for sodium (g_{Na}) was reduced to 25% of the normal value. As a result, the velocity of the planar wave decreased, as reflected by the reduced distance separating isochrones 0 and 10 ms. At the end of the barrier, the curvature developed by the wave front was greater than critical, which resulted in regional block in the upper direction (see snapshots at 17 and 30 ms). In fact, a unique phenomenon took place whereby the wave front detached from the barrier and traveled as a discontinuous wave front or wavebreak. Note that the whole array was homogeneous and that there were no differences in refractoriness, because activation was started after complete quiescence. Therefore, local block was the result of critical curvature for propagation that developed at the edge of an obstacle. Upon reaching the right border (isochrones 60 to 70 ms), the wave front turned and activated the upper part of the array (isochrones 80 to 110 ms).

Very similar dynamics of propagation were observed in isolated slices of sheep epicardial muscle. Figures 6C and 6D show the isochronal map obtained from one of our experiments in which a barrier (black area) was created by cutting the tissue with fine scissors. Stimulation was initiated from the lower left quadrant, indicated by the aster-

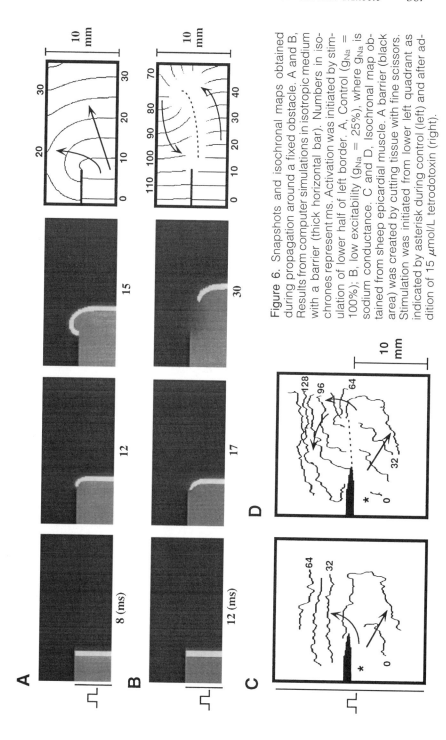

Figure 6. Snapshots and isochronal maps obtained during propagation around a fixed obstacle. A and B, Results from computer simulations in isotropic medium with a barrier (thick horizontal bar). Numbers in iso-chrones represent ms. Activation was initiated by stimulation of lower half of left border. A, Control (g_{Na} = 100%); B, low excitability (g_{Na} = 25%), where g_{Na} is sodium conductance. C and D, Isochronal map obtained from sheep epicardial muscle. A barrier (black area) was created by cutting tissue with fine scissors. Stimulation was initiated from lower left quadrant as indicated by asterisk during control (left) and after addition of 15 μmol/L tetrodotoxin (right).

isk. Under control conditions (panel C), the wave front turned around the edge of the cut and rapidly activated the complete preparation. During superfusion with tetrodotoxin (15 μmol/L), however, there was detachment of the wave front, which traveled rectilinearly toward the right, as predicted by the computer simulation, and then turned upward upon approaching the right border of the tissue.

In summary, the presence of fixed obstacles with sharp edges may destabilize the propagation of cardiac excitation waves. As discussed elsewhere,[23] depending on the excitability, such destabilization may lead to decremental propagation and functional blockade (see Figure 6) or to the formation of self-sustained vortices and turbulent electrical activity.

Wave Front of Rotating Spiral Waves

Recent theoretical and experimental studies suggest that functionally determined reentrant activity in the heart may be the result of self-sustaining spiral wave activity. Spiral waves are found in a wide variety of homogeneous physical,[24] chemical,[25,26] and biological[27-29] excitable media even in the absence of barriers or any other discontinuities. Such media include, among others, the so-called Belousov-Zhabotinski (B-Z) reaction, which also represents the cleanest and best-understood example yet of oscillatory chemical reaction occurring under conditions that are far from equilibrium. The B-Z reaction and the cardiac tissue seem to be analogous in various crucial aspects of their behavior: (1) Both are nonlinear systems; (2) under appropriate conditions, both can undergo self-sustaining oscillations; (3) both are excitable in the sense that an adequate stimulus can bring the system to its threshold for initiation of nondecremental wave propagation; (4) once activated, both systems undergo a refractory period during which no new activity may be initiated; and (5) similar laws of diffusion apply in both for the propagation of information from one region to another: In the case of the heart, electrochemical gradients provide the driving force for the depolarization wave to move from one cell to its neighbors; in the B-Z reaction, the exchange involves concentration gradients established between regions in which certain molecules have recently been synthesized and neighboring regions in which synthesis has not yet occurred.

The difference, however, is that unlike the B-Z reaction, the heart is a highly inhomogeneous and discontinuous anisotropic medium. Nevertheless, the behavioral similarities of the two systems are so pervasive that they have prompted a number of investigators to use the B-Z reaction as a basis for developing numerical and analytic models to make predictions about dynamics of wave propagation in 2D and

3D cardiac muscle.[8,30] The most remarkable of such predictions is that normal cardiac muscle can indeed sustain spiral wave activity.

The theory of spiral waves has significantly improved our understanding of functionally determined reentry in the heart. Here we discuss the influence of curvature on the dynamics and characteristics of spiral waves in the heart.

What is a Spiral Wave?

We may define spiral wave as a rotating "wavebreak" (see Figure 7). A wavebreak is a discontinuous wave whose depolarizing front and repolarizing tail touch each other at a specific point (q).[8] At the very tip of the spiral wave (Q), the curvature reaches a maximum value. Beyond this point, the wave fails to activate the tissue ahead and, instead, forces the entire wave front to rotate around a small region of unexcited tissue (ie, the core; circle with radius r_q). Note that even though cells in the core area may be excitable throughout the period of rotation, they remain unexcited as a result of the pronounced curvature of the tip of the rotating wave front. Thus, the wavebreak acts effectively as the pivoting point that forces the wave to rotate around the core.

A wavebreak need not develop into a spiral wave. As shown originally in the B-Z reaction[31,32] and more recently in computer simulations and cardiac tissue[14] (see Figure 6), wavebreaks are susceptible to lateral instabilities, and small changes in the excitability of the medium may dramatically alter their dynamics. At relatively low levels of excitability, a wavebreak is unable to rotate and instead travels as a wavelet in a rectilinear direction. At even lower levels of excitability, a wavebreak may contract gradually, undergo decremental conduction, and eventually disappear.[23]

The essential step in the initiation of reentrant activity in 2D or 3D media is the formation of a wavebreak. Wavebreaks may occur as a result of the interaction of the wave front with an anatomic (Figure 6) or a functional obstacle. This is not much different from what was originally proposed as the mechanism for initiation of reentrant activity. A new concept for the initiation of reentry, however, is the notion that reentry may be initiated in totally (anatomically and functionally) homogeneous media. In fact, if properly timed S1-S2 stimulation is applied from different sites (ie, cross-field stimulation), reentry can be predictably initiated, as demonstrated in computer simulations as well as in experimental models.[33,34] Cross-field stimulation consists of the following: Basic and premature plane waves are initiated from linear orthogonally located stimulators; a properly timed premature wave

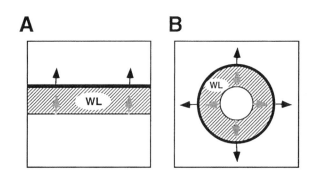

Figure 7. Schematic of planar, circular, and spiral wave in a homogeneous excitable medium. Thick and thin borders represent activation wave front and its repolarizing tail, respectively. Straight arrows at front and tail indicate normal propagation direction. Dashed curved arrows in C are lines of current and indicate future position of specific points on wave front. WL indicates wave length; q, wavebreak in which wave front and wave tail touch each other. This point separates regions with positive and negative dV/dt; Q, point of maximum curvature or critical curvature for propagation (v_k). Segment Q-q of wave front is composed of cells passively depolarized (ie, no active propagation is possible as a result of pronounced curvature at Q). Dashed and dotted circles with radii r_q and r_Q represent trajectories of points q and Q, respectively.

(S2) collides with the repolarizing tail of the basic wave (S1). As a result, the S2 wave front breaks at the point of collision and begins to curl to initiate a rotor (see Reference 26 for full description). With cross-field stimulation, both the location of the rotor and the type of rotation can be controlled by the parameters of stimulation.[35]

Curvature and Core Size

As shown in Figure 6 above, at relatively low levels of excitability, the trajectory of the wavebreak tends to open. In the case of a rotating wavebreak (ie, spiral wave), a decrease in excitability will be reflected as changes in the size of the core. We tested these predictions in our experimental model. Figure 8A shows a snapshot of a stationary counterclockwise rotating spiral obtained in a thin slice of sheep epicardial muscle. Gray levels indicate the instantaneous position of the rotating wave during the entire cycle of the spiral. The outlined area in the center represents the core size (1.49×2.35 mm). In panel B, during tetrodotoxin (15 μmol/L) superfusion, the excitability was reduced, the core became more rounded, and the size increased to 3.73×1.71 mm (6.4 mm^2).

Curvature and Rotation Period

According to the classic description of functionally determined reentry in the heart (ie, leading-circle model), the wave front rotates at the maximum possible speed allowed by its own repolarizing tail.[36–38] Thus, a relatively small change in the duration of the action potential should substantially alter the rotation period. According to the theory of spiral waves, such a situation may indeed occur in cases in which the excitability of the tissue is very high.[8] Thus, prolongation of the action potential duration will be followed by enlargement of the core size and slowing of the activity. Eventually, there will be interruption of the activity. However, if a fully excitable gap is present, changes in action potential duration may have no significant effects on the rotation period. Instead, changes in excitability may lead to pronounced modifications of both the core size and the rotation period. As shown in Figure 8, decreases in excitability lead to enlargement of the size of the core. Hence, there is an increase in the distance traveled by the wavebreak that leads to an increase of the rotation period. In addition, conduction velocity of the propagating wave is significantly decreased. This is illustrated in panel B by the grouping of the 16-ms isochrones compared with panel A.

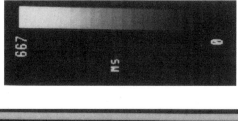

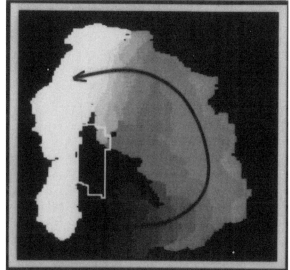

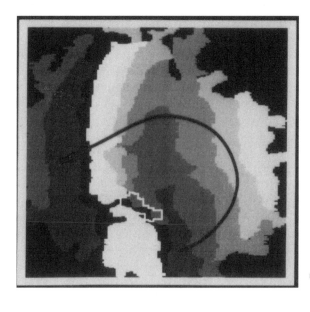

Figure 8. Effect of tetrodotoxin on size of core of a spiral wave activity initiated in isolated cardiac muscle. Gray coded regions represent position of wave front at different times during spiral cycle as indicated by scale. Core area is outlined in white. A, Control; B, during perfusion of 15 μmol/L tetrodotoxin.

Curvature and the Excitable Gap

For many years, cardiac electrophysiologists have argued about the existence as well as the mechanism of the so-called "excitable gap" (ie, period of time of full excitability) in functionally determined reentry.[36,38] Although the excitable gap during reentry in ventricular muscle has been attributed to the presence of anisotropy,[39] this mechanism has been shown to be unlikely, at least in computer simulations,[34] in which neither the period of rotation nor the refractory period changes when the anisotropic ratio is increased by as much as four times. The only effect of anisotropy is that of changing the shape of the spiral from circular to elliptical. Accordingly, the spatial distribution of excited tissue in a given instant in time is different from that of the isotropic medium. The concept of curvature seems to be more important in the understanding of the excitable gap. Clearly, a very steep positive (ie, convex) curvature occurs near the tip of the spiral wave front.[8,33] As a result, both local current density and safety factor for excitation of tissue ahead of the tip are greatly reduced, and thus, conduction velocity of the impulse is also reduced. A curved wave front is never able to achieve full velocity regardless of how excitable the tissue ahead is. Because of the presence of curvature in the front of a spiral wave, such activity will necessarily have an excitable gap. The existence of excitable gap is proved by the ability of externally induced propagating waves with lower curvature to invade the core region during spiral wave activity.[40]

Curvature and Drifting Spiral

Because the core may remain excitable during spiral wave activity, it is not surprising that small changes in the properties of the spiral wave front may lead to the activation of the core area. In fact, numerical simulations have shown that relatively minor changes in the curvature of the spiral tip may allow the wave front to short-circuit the core.[33,34] Under such conditions, the tip may loose its cyclic trajectory (either circular or elliptical) and develop a cycloid motion within an enclosed area (meandering spirals) or it may follow a rather linear pathway (drifting spiral).

Interaction Between Two or More Waves

Curvature and the Common Pathway in Figure-8 Reentry

Figure-8 reentry has been recognized as an important pattern of reentry in the late stages of myocardial infarction.[41] In most cases, two counterrotating waves coexist at a relatively short distance from each other. As described for the case of single reentrant circuits, each wave of the figure-8 reentry circulates around a "line of block." The region separating the lines of block is called the "common pathway." A detailed description of the common pathway is of great practical importance as a strategic region for surgical or catheter ablation in this type of reentry.[42] Figure-8 reentry is equivalent to two counterrotating spirals separated by a relatively small distance. In the case of pairs of counterrotating spirals, the common pathway is a region in which the propagation pattern is largely dependent on the interaction between the wave fronts arising from each spiral. Thus, the common pathway may show varying propagation patterns and velocities depending on the curvature of the resultant wave fronts. We have used both numerical and biological experiments to analyze the characteristics of propagation through the common pathway.

Computer simulations were conducted in a homogeneous matrix of FitzHugh-Nagumo cells in which stable pairs of spirals were initiated on the basis of the concept of the "pinwheel experiment."[40] In brief, a premature stimulus was delivered through a relatively large circular electrode to intersect the repolarizing tail of a planar wave. As a result, two wavebreaks occurred on the premature wave front at the points of intersection with the repolarizing tail of the planar wave. The distance between the cores of the resulting spirals was determined by the size of the electrode used to deliver the premature stimulus. As shown in Figure 9A, appreciable interaction between two curved wave fronts takes place at the common pathway. First, as the two spiral tips continue their rotating course, there is a region in which the wave fronts collide and fuse (frame 1). Immediately after that fusion (frame 2), propagation is interrupted in the direction normal to the collision line. However, propagation of the two fused wave fronts (F) continues toward the ends of the collision line (frames 2 and 3). Conduction velocity in the orthodromic (upward) and antidromic (downward) directions is accelerated by the presence of a negative curvature at each fusion line. A slightly different situation is shown in the example in Figure 9B. In this case, the distance between the two cores is shorter than that shown in panel A. As a result, although the antidromic (downward) wave front still shows a negative curvature (frame 1), the orthodromic wave front (upward) develops a positive curvature that leads to a decrease in conduction velocity (frame 3).

We have measured conduction velocity in the region of the common pathway during both reentry and planar wave activity in three optical mapping experiments using thin slices of epicardial muscle. Figure-8 reentry was initiated in all cases by stimulation applied during single spiral-wave activity. Conduction velocity at the common path-

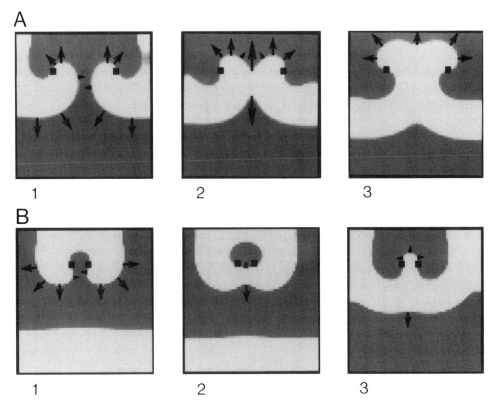

Figure 9. Propagation pattern in common pathway of figure-8 reentry in a computer simulation. A, Relatively long intercore distance. Frame 1, Common pathway is invaded by two curved wave fronts. Frames 2 and 3, Collision of wave fronts leads to formation of two new wave fronts with negative curvature. As a result of negative curvature, propagation in both orthodromic (upward) and antidromic (downward) directions is faster than normal. B, Relatively short intercore distance. Frame 1, Common pathway is invaded by two curved wave fronts. Frames 2 and 3, Collision of wave fronts generates two new wave fronts. In antidromic direction, new wave front has negative curvature, so that conduction velocity is faster than normal. In orthodromic direction, however, curvature of new wave front is positive, and as a result, propagation is slower than normal. Reprinted with permission from Reference 16.

way was faster during reentrant activity than the conduction velocity of planar waves at the same locations. Figure 10 shows one example. Panel A shows a snapshot obtained during figure-8 reentry. As indicated by the arrows, the spiral on the right rotates in the clockwise direction, while the spiral on the left rotates in the counterclockwise direction. Panel B shows the action potentials recorded from selected points over the common pathway as indicated by the numbers in panel

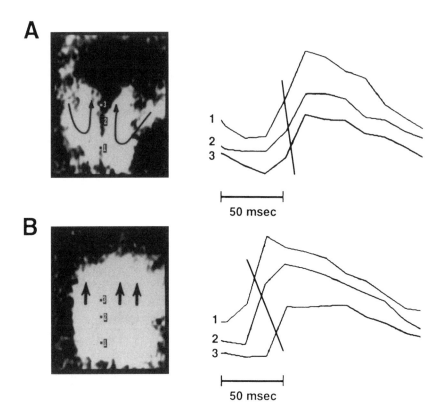

Figure 10. Propagation pattern in common pathway of figure-8 reentry in sheep epicardial muscle. Numbered squares indicate sites of recordings shown in B. A, Snapshot obtained during sustained figure-8 reentry. B, Action potential recordings obtained during same episode. Complete activation of common pathway occurs within 16 ms. Reprinted with permission from Reference 16.

A. Conduction velocity over the common pathway (measured by use of all recording points over the common pathway) was extremely fast (157 cm/s). Note that in this example, only the orthodromic (upward) propagation is visible, because the lower region of the preparation was outside the recording area. Panel B shows a snapshot obtained during the propagation of a planar wave initiated from the bottom border of the same preparation a few seconds before the initiation of the reentrant activity. As illustrated by the action potentials recorded from the same points as shown in panel B, conduction velocity during planar wave was slower (45 cm/s) than that during reentrant activity.

It is important to note that in clinical cases of reentrant tachycardia, conduction velocity of the common pathway may be affected by preexisting local abnormalities of the tissue. However, our results demonstrate that even in completely homogeneous systems, conduction velocity is greatly influenced by the interaction of two curved wave fronts. Thus, conduction velocity during figure-8 reentry may be expected to be faster than that during the propagation of a planar wave.

Conclusions

We have discussed the characteristics of propagation in two-dimensional cardiac tissue. The overall results indicate that the curvature of the wave front plays an important role in determining the success or failure of propagation as well as the velocity of propagation in the following conditions: (1) initiation of a propagating wave from a small source, (2) propagation through a narrow isthmus, (3) propagation of a wave front around an anatomic obstacle with sharp borders, (4) the wave front of rotating spiral waves, and (5) interaction between two or more waves.

References

1. Rushton WAH. Initiation of the propagated disturbance. *Proc R Soc Lond [Biol]*. 1937;124:210–243.
2. Fozzard HA, Schoenberg M. Strength-duration curves in cardiac Purkinje fibres: effects of liminal length and charge distribution. *J Physiol (Lond)*. 1972;226:593–618.
3. Noble D. The relation of Rushton's 'liminal length' for excitation to the resting and active conductances of excitable cells. *J Physiol (Lond)*. 1972;226: 573–591.
4. Zipes DP, Mendez C, Moe Gk. Evidence of summation and voltage dependency in rabbit atrioventricular nodal fibers. *Circ Res*. 1973;32:170–177.
5. Cranefield PF, Hoffman BF. Conduction of the cardiac impulse, II: summation and inhibition. *Circ Res*. 1971;28:220–233.
6. Spach MS, Miller WT III, Dolber PC, Kootsey JM, Sommer JR, Mosher CE Jr. The functional role of structural complexities in the propagation of depolarization in the atrium of the dog: cardiac conduction disturbances due to discontinuities of effective axial resistivity. *Circ Res*. 1982;50:175–191.
7. Spach MS, Miller WT III, Geselowitz DB, Barr RC, Kootsey JM, Johnson EA. The discontinuous nature of propagation in normal canine cardiac muscle: evidence of recurrent discontinuities of intracellular resistance that affect the membrane currents. *Circ Res*. 1981;48:9–54.
8. Zykov VS. *Simulation of Wave Processes in Excitable Media*. Manchester, UK: Manchester University Press; 1987.
9. Zykov VS. Analytical evaluation of the dependence of the speed of an excitation wave in a two-dimensional excitable medium on the curvature of its front. *Biofizica*. 1980;25:888–892.
10. Keener JP, Tyson JJ. Spiral waves in the Belousov-Zhabotinskii reaction. *Physica D*. 1986;21:307–324.

11. Tyson JJ, Keener JP. Singular perturbation theory of travelling waves in excitable media (a review). *Physica D.* 1988;32:327–361.
12. Foerster P, Muller SC, Hess B. Curvature and propagation velocity of chemical waves. *Science.* 1988;241:685–687.
13. Foerster P, Muller SC, Hess B. Critical size and curvature of wave formation in an excitable medium. *Proc Natl Acad Sci U S A* 1989;86:6831–6834.
14. Cabo C, Pertsov AM, Baxter WT, Davidenko JM, Gray RA, Jalife J. Wave front curvature as a cause of slow conduction and block in isolated cardiac muscle. *Circ Res.* 1994;75:1014–1028.
15. Cabo C, Pertsov AM, Baxter WT, Davidenko JM, Jalife J. Measurements of curvature in an ionic model of cardiac tissue. *Chaos Solitons Fractals.* 1995; 5:481–489.
16. Davidenko JM. Spiral waves in the heart: experimental demonstration of a theory. In: Zipes DP, Jalife J, eds. *Cardiac Electrophysiology: From Cell to Bedside.* Philadelphia, Pa: WB Saunders Co; 1995:478–488.
17. Barr RC, Plonsey R. Propagation of excitation in idealized anisotropic two-dimensional tissue. *Biophys J.* 1984;45:1191–1202.
18. Plonsey R, Barr RC. Current flow patterns in two-dimensional anisotropic bisyncytia with normal and extreme conductivities. *Biophys J.* 1984;45:557–571.
19. Pertsov AM, Ermakova EA, Shnol EE. On the diffraction of autowaves. *Physica D.* 1990;44:178–190.
20. Luo C-H, Rudy Y. A model of ventricular cardiac action potential: depolarization, repolarization, and their interaction. *Circ Res.* 1991;68:1501–1526.
21. de la Fuente D, Sasyniuk B, Moe GK. Conduction through a narrow isthmus in isolated canine atrial tissue: a model of the W-P-W syndrome. *Circulation.* 1971;44:803–809.
22. Fast VG, Kléber AG. Tissue geometry as a determinant of unidirectional conduction block: assessment of microscopic excitation spread by optical mapping in patterned myocyte cultures. *Circulation.* 1993;88(Suppl I):I-623. Abstract.
23. Cabo C, Pertsov AM, Davidenko JM, Baxter WT, Gray RA, Jalife J. Vortex shedding as a precursor of turbulent electrical activity in cardiac muscle. *Biophys J.* 1996;70:1105–1111.
24. Suzuki R. Electrochemical neural model. *Adv Biophys.* 1976;9:115–156.
25. Winfree AT. *The Geometry of Biological Time.* New York, NY: 1980. Springer-Verlag.
26. Müller SC, Plesser T, Hess B. The structure of the core of the spiral wave in the Belousov-Zhabotinsky reagent. *Science.* 1985;230:661–663.
27. Gerish G. Stadienspezifische Aggregationsmuster bei *Dictyostelium discoideum. Wilhelm Roux Archiv Entwick Org.* 1965;156:127–144.
28. Goldbeter A. Mechanism for oscillatory synthesis of cAMP in *Dictyostelium discoideum. Nature.* 1975;253:540–542.
29. Gorelova NA, Bures J. Spiral waves of spreading depression in the isolated chicken retina. *Neurobiology.* 1983;14:353–363.
30. Winfree AT. Spiral waves of chemical activity. *Science.* 1972;175:634–636.
31. Pertsov AM, Panfilov AV, Medvedeva FU. Instability of autowaves in excitable media associated with the phenomenon of critical curvature. *Biofizica.* 1983;28:1000–102.
32. Nay-Ungvarai A, Pertsov AM, Hess B, Muller SC. Lateral instabilities of a wave front in the Ce-catalyzed Belousov-Zhabotinsky reaction. *Physica D.* 1992;61:205–212.

33. Davidenko JM, Pertsov AM, Salomonsz R, Baxter W, Jalife J. Stationary and drifting spiral waves of excitation in isolated cardiac muscle. *Nature.* 1992;355:349–351.
34. Pertsov AM, Davidenko JM, Salomonsz R, Baxter WT, Jalife J. Spiral waves of excitation underlie reentrant activity in isolated cardiac muscle. *Circ Res.* 1993;72:631–650.
35. Frazier DW, Wolf PD, Wharton JM, Tabg ASL, Smith WM, Ideker RE. Stimulus-induced critical point: Mechanism for the electrical initiation of reentry in normal canine myocardium. *J Clin Invest.* 1989;83:1039–1052.
36. Allessie MA, Bonke FIM, Schopman FJC. Circus movement in rabbit atrial muscle as a mechanism of tachycardia. *Circ Res.* 1973;33:54–62.
37. Allessie MA, Bonke FIM, Schopman FJC. Circus movement in rabbit atrial muscle as a mechanism of tachycardia, II: the role of nonuniform recovery of excitability in the occurrence of unidirectional block as studied with multiple microelectrodes. *Circ Res.* 1976;39:168–177.
38. Allessie MA, Bonke FIM, Schopman FJC. Circus movement in rabbit atrial muscle as a mechanism of tachycardia, III: the "leading circle" concept: a new model of circus movement in cardiac tissue without the involvement of an anatomical obstacle. *Circ Res.* 1977;41:9–18.
39. Dillon SM, Allessie MA, Ursell PC, Wit AL. Influence of anisotropic tissue structure on reentrant circuit in the epicardial border zone of subacute canine infarcts. *Circ Res.* 1988;63:182–206.
40. Winfree AT. Electrical instability in cardiac muscle: phase singularities and rotors. *J Theor Biol.* 1989;183:353.
41. El-Sherif N, Smith A, Evans K. Canine ventricular arrhythmias in the late myocardial infarction period, 8: epicardial mapping of reentrant circuits. *Circ Res.* 1981;49:25.
42. El-Sherif N, Mehra R, Gough WB, et al. Reentrant ventricular arrhythmias in the late myocardial infarction period: interruption of reentrant circuits by cryothermal techniques. *Circulation.* 1983;68:644.

Chapter 14

Antiarrhythmic and Proarrhythmic Mechanisms in Cardiac Tissue:
Linking Spiral Waves, Reentrant Arrhythmias, and Electrocardiographic Patterns

C. Frank Starmer, PhD, and Josef Starobin, PhD

Although reentrant arrhythmias have been the focus of intense experimental and theoretical study for almost 100 years,[1–3] we are just now gaining insight into the detailed mechanisms responsible for their initiation and maintenance. Much recent progress is based on combined theoretical, numerical, and experimental studies that jointly consider membrane properties and the discontinuous nature of cell-to-cell propagation. Arising from these studies is an increased awareness of the critical importance of the coupling of currents arising from membrane ion channels (as a source of charge) to adjoining cells by gap junctions (supporting the load).[4] These new results not only improve our understanding of normal electrophysiology but also provide important insights into arrhythmogenesis.

Propagation is a complex process involving (1) formation of an impulse (an excited region) and (2) subsequent expansion of this impulse away from the stimulus site. When a region of adjoining cells is excited by a suprathreshold current, an impulse is formed, and depending on the size of the impulse and the load presented by surrounding

Supported in part by a grant, HL32994, from the National Heart, Lung, and Blood Institute, NIH.

From: Spooner PM, Joyner RW, Jalife J (eds). *Discontinuous Conduction in the Heart.* Armonk, NY: Futura Publishing Company, Inc.; © 1997.

cells, the boundary of the impulse (wave front) will propagate either decrementally away from the stimulus site (impulse size<liminal size) and eventually die (conduction velocity = 0) or will propagate incrementally away from the stimulus site (impulse size>liminal size) and eventually achieve a stable conduction velocity. Typically, the wave front is continuous, that is, one can trace the wave front in either a clockwise or counterclockwise manner and return to the starting point. Normal coordination of cardiac excitation is maintained by the propagation of a continuous wave front.

Arrhythmogenic processes (spiral-wave reentry) often arise from formation of discontinuous wave fronts. A major factor for successful propagation and maintenance of continuity of the wave front is the relationship between the charge available within the propagating wave front and the charge requirements for excitation of adjoining cells. If the charge available within the wave front is altered (eg, reduced with sodium channel blockade) or the load is altered (eg, by alteration of the distribution of side-to-side gap junctions as seen in hypertrophy or aging[5]), the wave front may become fractionated because of localized block that occurs when the local charge requirements are not fulfilled. Reentrant arrhythmias can result from discontinuous wave fronts arising from either abnormal or incomplete impulse formation (unidirectional block) secondary to premature stimulation or from a wave fragment created from local block associated with either increased load or spatial dispersed refractory properties.

Features of a propagating wave front that are important to consider when exploring initiation of reentry are (1) the initial size of the impulse; (2) the gradient of potential associated with the leading edge of the impulse (which provides the source charge); (3) the spatial action potential wavelength (which influences the reentrant path); and (4) the distribution of cellular gap junctions (which couple charge that can flow between a source cell and adjacent load cells). Propagation of a wave front is a complex process that involves the transfer of charge residing within the leading edge of the impulse through gap junctions to adjacent cells. By careful analysis of simple models of the flow of charge from the propagating wavefront to the load presented by adjacent cells, it is possible to identify some basic arrhythmogenic properties associated with abnormal wave-front formation[6-8] and with alterations in the distribution of gap junctions connecting source and load cells.[4]

The complexity of cardiac tissue cannot be overemphasized. Only recently have numerical models come close to approximating the cellular complexity and connectivity of myocardium.[4] Analytic models are far behind. However, because impulse formation and propagation are essentially generic properties of any excitable medium and depend on only a single inward excitatory current (that exhibits a negative resistance region) and an outward repolarizing current, membrane models of reduced complexity have yielded a number of surprisingly useful insights. Because of the inherent complexity of cardiac cells and myocardial propagation, we believe that it is essential to first understand the generic mechanisms of impulse formation and propagation on the basis of properties of minimally complex excitable membranes before the impact of cellular and structural complexities associated with physiological cells can be fully appreciated. From this basis, we can explore whether complexities associated with cardiac cells attenuate or amplify the generic underlying antiarrhythmic or proarrhythmic properties.

To understand some of the physical mechanisms behind reentrant arrhythmias and the related QRS morphologies observed in the electrocardiogram (ECG), we start with a review of the basic concepts of an excitable membrane, impulse formation and propagation in a homogeneous medium. With these basic concepts, we will illustrate that reentry is the result of a wavebreak or discontinuity in a propagating wave front. Discontinuities can be caused by sudden changes in the electrical load encountered by a propagating front, by regional variations in the membrane refractory period, or by transient gradients of excitability that exist in the wake of a propagating wave (the vulnerable period). We will illustrate how drugs targeted at suppression of premature ventricular contractions (PVCs) via sodium channel blockade can simultaneously increase the period of vulnerability. Next, we will explore the nature of reentrant activation once it has been initiated. Here we will show how prolongation of the action potential wavelength can destabilize reentry once it is initiated and with sufficient prolongation can lead to an ECG characterized by polymorphic QRS Complexes. Finally, we will explore models that contain simple discontinuities. To analyze wave-front propagation in the presence of simple discontinuities (obstacles), we will introduce the concept of the balance between the charge available in the wave front (source) and the charge required to excite adjacent medium (sink). We will demonstrate that alterations in some medium parameters (eg, g_{Na}) can lead to wave-front–obstacle separation, which is a major proarrhythmic mechanism.

The theoretical basis from which these results are derived is a result of analyses of nonlinear reaction-diffusion equations in a homogeneous medium.[9] These analyses have revealed that several types of arrhythmogenic behavior are generic and a property of any excitable medium. We have observed in our studies that media properties associated with "health" (ie, rapid propagation and uniform anisotropy) make it difficult to meet the requirements for successful initiation of arrhythmic activity. With "disease," however, slowed conduction secondary to a depolarized rest potential and nonuniform anisotropic cellular coupling amplifies latent arrhythmogenic processes,[4,5,10] thus increasing the likelihood of initiating serious atrial and ventricular reentrant arrhythmias. The majority of the analyses presented here are based on a very simple, two-current (an inward, noninactivating excitation current and an outward repolarizing current) model of an excitable cell linked together in either 1D or 2D arrays of identical cells. Such simple models reveal that much of the complexity of membrane ionic currents (eg, inactivation, pumps, etc) is not essential for understanding several basic arrhythmogenic mechanisms and that control of arrhythmogenesis by pharmacological alteration of membrane ion channels can be inherently proarrhythmic.[6,7] Studies of simple discontinuities embedded in a homogeneous medium confirm experimental studies[4,5,10] that wave-front propagation through a region of discontinuities of electrical load is a major factor in reentrant arrhythmogenesis.[8]

Background: Cellular Electrophysiology, Ion Channel Blockade, and Propagation

Cardiac cells are classified as excitable because the transmembrane potential in an isolated cell can be switched between two states: a resting, polarized state and an excited, depolarized state by injection of a small, depolarizing pulse of current. Faced with cells of extraordinary complexity, the cardiac electrophysiologist must somehow decide what is essential for describing normal and pathological cellular responses and how to identify the mechanisms behind these responses. Mathematical models have provided the electrophysiologist with a useful tool for such explorations, and when these are combined with cellular and tissue studies, the electrophysiologist has been able to make great progress in understanding the basic nature of cellular electrical stability and propagation. With simplified physical models, the investigator has a measuring stick with which he or she can decide which of the cellular mechanisms are essential for certain responses. These physical and mathematical models provide a tool for identifying the minimal complexity of a cell and then asking whether additional complexity amplifies or attenuates responses that are associated with the minimally complex model. With such tools, the actual "cause" of a complex arrhythmogenic process can be isolated and identified.

The Hodgkin-Huxley (H-H) model[11] was the first model of an excitable cell and was composed of several novel features that provided a physical foundation for contemporary electrophysiology. In exploring the electrical properties of the squid giant axon, Hodgkin and Huxley observed that an ion transport process with voltage-sensitive and ion-selective permeability was essential. They proposed the concept of a "channel," a passive, transmembrane conduit, whose permeability was controlled by voltage-sensitive and time-dependent gates.

For simplicity, the mechanism for controlling ionic fluxes was visualized as an alteration in the channel conformation that followed simple, first-order transitions between open and closed conformations. They proposed a sodium channel whose conductance was modulated by a rapid activation process, m, a slower inactivation process, h, and a potassium channel whose conductance was modulated by a slow activation process, n, described by

$$\underset{[(1-m),(1-h),(1-n)]}{\text{Closed}} \quad \overset{\alpha}{\underset{\beta}{\longleftrightarrow}} \quad \underset{[m,h,n]}{\text{Open}}$$

where m, n, and h are the fraction of open channel "gates" and α and β are voltage-dependent rate constants. Considering the dynamics of the "m" process, the rate of transition from the closed conformation to the open conformation is proportional to the fraction of closed gates, $1-m$, while the rate of transition from the open to closed conformation is proportional to the fraction of open gates, m. The coefficients α and β then represent the proportionality constants, and the time-dependent fraction of channel gates in the open conformation is characterized by

$$\frac{dm}{dt} = \alpha(1-m) - \beta m \tag{1}$$

The advent of single-channel recordings has provided opportunities to directly observe the dynamics of the openings and closings of cardiac channels.[12] These measurements have confirmed the validity of assuming that channels follow simple first-order kinetics. This is readily seen by recognizing that at the single-channel level, the probability that a closed channel opens during the interval Δt is $\alpha \Delta t$ and the probability that an open channel closes during the interval Δt is $\beta \Delta t$. The exponential solution to Equation 1 for macroscopic currents is equivalent to a single-channel characterization of channel opening,[12] which displays similar exponential behavior.

This gating model led to a general characterization of the time- and voltage-dependent properties of the inward, sodium excitation current, and the outward, repolarizing potassium current by use of Ohm's law:

$$I_{Na} = g_{Na} \, m^3 h \, (V - V_{Na}) \tag{2}$$

$$I_K = g_K n^4 \, (V - V_K) \tag{3}$$

and

$$I_{leak} = g_l \, (V - V_l) \tag{4}$$

where V is the transmembrane potential, g_{Na}, g_K, and g_l are the maxi-

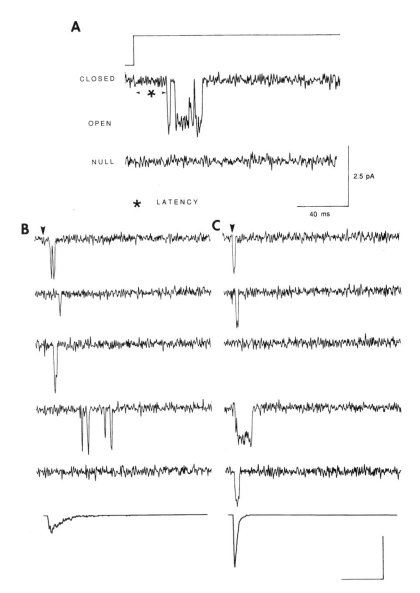

Figure 1. Single cardiac sodium channel currents. Multiple single sodium channels contribute to macroscopic sodium current that is essential for excitation and propagation. A, Rapid opening and closure (inactivation) of a single channel in response to depolarizing step in membrane potential. After change in membrane potential, there is a brief latency (*) before channel opens and conducts sodium ions. This initial opening is followed by several brief closures,

mum macroscopic conductances of the sodium, potassium, and leakage currents, V_{Na}, V_K, and V_l are the reversal potentials, and m^3h and n^4 represent the fraction of channels in the open configuration.

The currents described by these equations represent the sum of all single-channel events for each type of current (Figure 1). The macroscopic conductance is related to the single-channel conductance by $g_{Na} = N_{Na} \times g_{single}(Na)$, where N_{Na} is the number of individual sodium channels and $g_{single}(Na)$ is the single sodium channel conductance (≈ 20 pS). Hodgkin and Huxley[11] used the functions m and h to describe the time-dependent probability of a channel being in the excited (m^3) and noninactivated (h) state as modeled by the hypothesized chemical model. The product of these two probabilities, m^3h, provides the probability of the channel being open and thus models the time- and voltage-dependent properties of the macroscopic conductance.

It is interesting to note that the exponents of m and n were empirically determined by Hodgkin and Huxley[11] to improve the agreement between the time-dependent currents as predicted by the gating models and the currents observed during voltage-clamp experiments. They observed that when the membrane potential was switched from a polarized potential to a depolarized potential, the membrane current initially increased at a slow rate, ie, $dI/dt \approx 0$. The observation that the initial slope of I_{Na} and I_K as a function of time was small (or zero) was not compatible with a channel having a single gating particle as predicted by the solutions to Equation 1 $\{I(t) = I_{max}[1 - e^{-(\alpha + \beta)t}]\}$. The assumption of four "gating particles" produced much better agreement between the observed and predicted time dependence of the ionic currents. The remarkable feature of the H-H analysis is that molecular studies of the sodium and potassium channel sequences indicate that both channels consist of four membrane-spanning subunits. Sodium channels are composed of four homologous protein domains, whereas potassium channels have been shown to be composed of four identical subunits.[13]

---

then channel remains closed for remainder of depolarizing potential (probably, channel has switched to inactivated state). Voltage dependence of channel openings and latencies are shown in B and C. B, Membrane potential is stepped to -60 mV, slightly positive to threshold of Na channel activation. Under this condition, there is an extended latency before opening followed by rapid inactivation, resulting in a short open time. C, Membrane potential is stepped to a more positive potential, -40 mV, where channel responds with a shorter latency before opening and a longer open time. Bottom trace in each panel shows cumulative current obtained by adding open events observed in 100 consecutive steps. Note that summed current appears similar to that measured in traditional whole-cell voltage clamp studies and can be accurately characterized with Hodgkin-Huxley model of a voltage-sensitive ion channel.

It is indeed remarkable that the insights derived from the H-H curve-fitting exercises were the results of mathematical analyses carried out with their mental imagery and desk-top calculators!

Noting that the cell membrane is basically an insulator penetrated by channels, Hodgkin and Huxley modeled the membrane as a capacitor (capacitive current, $I = C_m \, dV/dt$) in parallel with membrane ionic channels, which schematically appears as

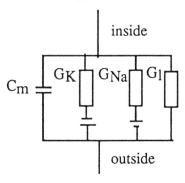

The total membrane current is composed of the capacitive and channel currents:

$$I_m = C_m \frac{\partial V}{\partial t} + I_{Na} + I_K + I_l \tag{5}$$

From Ohm's law, the axial current flowing down the length of the axon, which is available for extending the wave front, can be expressed as

$$I_a = \frac{1}{r_a} \frac{\partial V}{\partial x} \tag{6}$$

where r_a is the axial resistance. Since conservation of charge requires that the change in axial current, $\partial I_a / \partial x$, must equal the membrane current, one can "discover" the telegraph equation developed to describe the current flow in a leaky telegraph wire by Lord Kelvin[14]:

$$\frac{\partial I_a}{\partial x} = \frac{\partial}{\partial x}\left(\frac{1}{r_a}\frac{\partial V}{\partial x}\right) = I_m = C_m \frac{\partial V}{\partial t} + I_{Na} + I_K + I_l \tag{7}$$

Since Hodgkin and Huxley[11] were studying long segments of axon in which the axial resistance, r_a, was essentially constant down the length of the axon, the cable equation can be simplified to

$$\frac{\partial^2 V}{\partial x^2} = r_a C_m \frac{\partial V}{\partial t} + I_{Na} + I_K + I_l \tag{8}$$

To summarize, the left side of Equation 8 represents the current that flows along the long axis of the cell to extend the wave front, whereas the right side of Equation 8 represents the current that flows across the membrane (inward during wave-front formation and outward during recovery). Later, we will explore arrhythmogenic processes, whereby we will focus on the wave-front extension process, and we will consider only the region of large spatial gradients in potential, ie, the wave-front thickness, L_f. Because wave-front extension is limited to behavior within L_f, it will be possible to use very simple models to understand several arrhythmogenic mechanisms, eg, unidirectional block and reentry.

Under voltage-clamp conditions, $\partial V/\partial x = 0$, ie, there is no axial current, and consequently, no propagation, so

$$C_m \frac{\partial V}{\partial t} = -(I_{Na} + I_K + I_l) \qquad (9)$$

which expresses the relationship between membrane ion channels and the potential of a patch of membrane. For squid giant axon, the membrane is forced to be equipotential ($\partial V/\partial x = 0$, voltage clamping) by insertion of a low-resistance wire parallel to the internal longitudinal axis of the axon. If a single microelectrode is used with cardiac cells, the equipotential condition is approximated only when the cell is small (<10 μm in diameter).

Beeler and Reuter[15] adapted the H-H model to cardiac ventricular tissue by altering the kinetics of the sodium and delayed rectifier (I_x) currents and adding a calcium and inward rectifying potassium current. The resulting equations provided a description of the ventricular action potential (Figure 2) that for the first time permitted studies of both patches and propagating ventricular action potentials as well as the possibility to explore the role of ion channel blockade on propagating action potentials.[16,17]

Clinical Links

Remembering that the sodium current activates rapidly relative to the potassium and calcium currents (Figure 2), then according to Equation 9, the maximum of $\partial V/\partial t$ will coincide with the maximum inward sodium current ($-I_{Na}$). For this reason, many early studies, before the advent of cell isolation techniques, used dV/dt_{max} as an indicator of the amplitude of the fast inward sodium current. There is a rich literature concerning the limitations of this approximation; however, cardiac electrophysiology would have made little progress if one had had to wait for the availability of reliable whole-cell isolation techniques and patch-clamp amplifiers.[18–20] Particularly with reference to early studies of ion channel blockade, use of dV/dt_{max} served to indicate

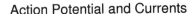

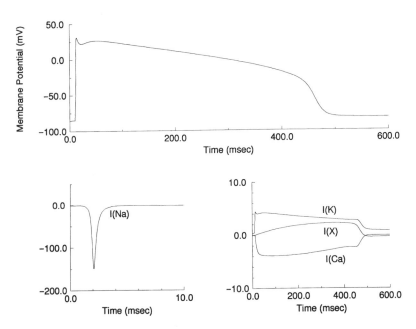

Figure 2. Computed action potential and membrane currents. Action potential computed from Beeler-Reuter[15] model of a ventricular cell. For sodium, calcium, and delayed rectifier currents, Beeler-Reuter model uses Hodgkin-Huxley gating model with voltage-dependent rate constants extracted from studies of cardiac muscle cells. Macroscopic sodium, I(Na), calcium, I(Ca), time-dependent delayed rectifier, I(X), and time-independent inward rectifier, I(K), membrane currents are shown in lower panels. Note that sodium current (lower right) activates very rapidly and produces initial upstroke of action potential. In addition, it is completely inactivated within 2 ms. In this model, membrane repolarization is due to excess of outward currents [from I(K) and I(X)] relative to more slowly activating I(Ca). Delayed rectifier potassium current [lower right, I(X)] activates very slowly and reaches equilibrium only after 400 ms. Note small amplitude of potassium and calcium currents relative to sodium current.

the directional changes of I_{Na} and provided a rich literature that was very effective in characterizing the antiarrhythmic properties of various ion channel blocking agents.

Of course, the most important use of dV/dt_{max} is in the study of events in tissue, in which isolation of loading effects of neighboring cells is impossible.[4,5,10,21–24] Here, derivatives of the membrane potential have provided a basis for understanding many basic events associated with discontinuous propagation as well as how ion channel blockade alters propagation.

Background: Ion Channel Blockade

The finding that drugs could alter the membrane electrical properties was recognized in early studies by Weidman[21] and Johnson and McKinnon.[22] Weidman[21] first showed that addition of cocaine to the bath containing a Purkinje fiber resulted in "stabilization" of the excitable membrane. In the presence of cocaine, quinidine, procainamide hydrochloride, and diphenylhydramine hydrochloride, stronger currents were required for stimulation, spontaneous oscillation of the membrane potential was slowed or terminated, and conduction of an action potential could be blocked. Using dV/dt_{max} as a measure of the sodium current, Weidmann showed that sodium channel availability in the presence of these agents was attenuated and shifted in the hyperpolarized direction; therefore, these agents were considered to be stabilizers of membrane electrical properties because they reduced cellular excitability.

If, as suggested by Weidmann, cocaine, quinidine, and these other agents altered the sodium-carrying mechanism, Johnson and McKinnon[22] reasoned that the depression in sodium-carrying ability, as indicated by dV/dt_{max}, should be sensitive to the frequency of stimulation. Increasing the stimulation rate of guinea pig ventricular fibers from 0.1 to 8 per second reduced the steady-state value of dV/dt_{max}, indicating that the capacity of the sodium-carrying mechanism was progressively decreased by repetitive stimulation. Their specific interpretation was that quinidine slowed the rate of production of active sodium-carrying units, which is consistent with today's view that blocked channels become available only after a slow unbinding process occurs.

These studies were followed by the ingenious studies by Heistracher,[23,24] who first demonstrated the use-dependent nature of what we now refer to as a drug–ion channel interaction. Using Purkinje fibers exposed to quinidine (as well as procainamide and ajmaline), Heistracher and coworkers measured dV/dt_{max} as a function of time after initial exposure of the fiber to the drug. In one preparation, they stimulated continuously, whereas in a separate preparation, they did not stimulate during the first 30 minutes of exposure. They observed that the absence of stimulation resulted in a dV/dt_{max} for the first stimulus that was equivalent to that of control values before drug exposure (Figure 4 in Reference 24). Then, by altering the rate of stimulation, they observed the frequency-dependent nature of use-dependent drug-channel interactions, ie, that dV/dt_{max} was a function of both the number of prior stimuli and the interval between stimuli.

Armstrong's[25,26] studies provided the first detailed hypothesis of the possible microscopic mechanism of the drug-channel interaction. In studies of tetraethylammonium (TEA) interaction with potassium

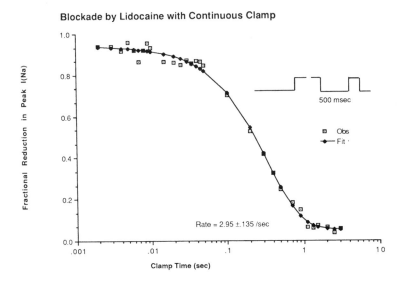

Blockade by Lidocaine with Continuous Clamp

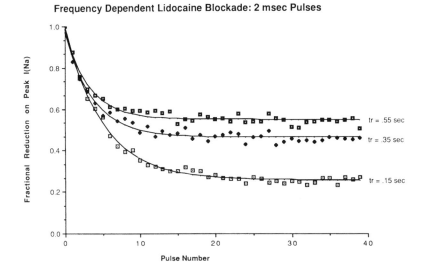

Frequency Dependent Lidocaine Blockade: 2 msec Pulses

Figure 3. Most ligand-receptor reactions occur as if binding site is continuously accessible. Many drugs that block ion channels deviate from this model and bind in a manner consistent with binding to a site that is not continuously

channels in squid giant axon, Armstrong[25,26] observed that the alteration of potassium current was dependent on the length of time the axon was depolarized. On the basis of his observations, he proposed a simple kinetic scheme of TEA interaction with open potassium channels:

$$C \underset{\beta}{\overset{\alpha}{\longleftrightarrow}} O \underset{\ell}{\overset{kD}{\longleftrightarrow}} B \qquad (10)$$

where C represents a closed channel, O represents an open channel, and B represents a blocked channel. From this model, use- and frequency-dependent drug-channel interactions can be readily understood.[27,28] At a polarized resting potential, most of the channels will reside in the C state, and the drug binding site will be "hidden" or guarded. When the membrane potential is switched to a depolarized value, the channel will switch to the O state. While it is in the O state, the binding site is unguarded, and drug can interact with the accessible binding sites. When the membrane is repolarized, recovery of blocked channels will occur at a rate, ℓ, that typically is very small compared with the channel gate transition rates. Consequently, with repetitive stimulation, a progressively larger fraction of channels will reside in the B state, because of incomplete recovery (ie, interstimulus interval $<4/\ell$).

Studies of lidocaine (42 μmol/L) block of Purkinje fibers and atrial

---

accessible, ie, these drugs appear to bind only to specific channel conformations such as open, inactivated, or rest conformation.[27,28] With rapid excitation of a cell, the fraction of drug-complexed channels will increase with each successive stimulus until a steady state is reached that is dependent on frequency of stimulation.[23–26] Dependence of drug-channel interaction with a guarded receptor can be readily demonstrated. Top, Relative magnitude of peak sodium current measured in isolated rabbit atrial cells exposed to lidocaine by a test pulse introduced 500 ms after a single conditioning depolarizing step from a holding potential of -130 to -20 mV of increasing duration (2 ms to 3 seconds). As the duration of the conditioning pulse is increased, peak sodium current follows an exponential function of conditioning pulse duration. Solid line represents least-squares fit of an exponential to observed data. That current continues to be reduced in step with the duration of depolarizing step indicates that drug binds to a channel conformation coupled to the inactivation process. To illustrate drug binding to an openlike conformation, the same cell was stimulated with trains of 2-ms pulses of different frequencies. Shown in lower panel is peak sodium current measured during 2-ms pulses to -20 mV. Peak current decreases with each additional pulse, revealing use- and frequency-dependent blockade of a transiently accessible (guarded) binding site. Note that as the frequency of stimulation increases (recovery interval is reduced from 0.55 to 0.15 second), steady-state current is also reduced, indicating that recovery from blockade is incomplete during the interstimulus interval.

cells[29,30] demonstrated that lidocaine block was dependent on both the duration of a depolarizing pulse and the frequency of a stimulating pulse train (Figure 3). Shown in the top panel is the fractional reduction in peak sodium current in rabbit atrial cells as a function of the duration of a depolarizing pulse. The continuation of blockade after the first few milliseconds of depolarization (ie, after the channel open event is complete) suggests that the bindable substrate is associated with channel inactivation. The data were well described by a first-order (exponential) binding model similar to that used by Armstrong to describe tetraethylammonium block of potassium channels. The data are displayed on a logarithmic time scale to accommodate a 1000-fold range in pulse duration.

The lower panel reveals frequency-dependent reduction in peak sodium current associated with very short depolarizing pulses (2 ms) and demonstrates that lidocaine is also able to bind to a substrate linked to the open state or the opening process. Both modes of blockade can be described by the following scheme:

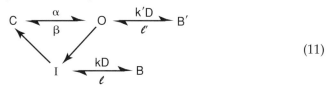

$$\tag{11}$$

where C is a closed sodium channel, O is an open sodium channel, I is an inactivated sodium channel, and B and B' are blocked states. To simplify understanding, we can assume that the open channel component associated with the first pulse is small and limit our attention to block of inactivated channels during long depolarizing pulses. Thus, the above model is simplified to

$$C \underset{\beta}{\overset{\alpha}{\rightleftharpoons}} I \underset{\ell}{\overset{kD}{\rightleftharpoons}} B$$

$$\frac{dc}{dt} = -\alpha c + \beta i \tag{12}$$

$$\frac{db}{dt} = kDi - \ell b$$

$$c + i + b = 1$$

We can assume that the channel gate transition rates are rapid compared with rates of drug binding and unbinding. Under this assumption, we can assume rapid equilibration between channel states C and I so that $dc/dt = 0$ or $c = (\beta/\alpha)i$. From conservation of channel states, $c + i + b = 1$ or $(\beta/\alpha)i + i + b = 1$. Consequently,

$$i = \frac{1-b}{1+\dfrac{\beta}{\alpha}} = \frac{\alpha}{\alpha+\beta}(1-b) \tag{13}$$

In the absence of drug, $\alpha/(\alpha+\beta)$ is the fraction of inactivated channels, $1-h$, so that the equation of block can be rewritten as

$$\frac{db}{dt} = \frac{\alpha}{\alpha+\beta}\, kD(1-b) - \ell b \qquad \text{or}$$

$$\frac{db}{dt} = [(1-h)k]D(1-b) - \ell b \tag{14}$$

Here, the role of channel gating in modulating the rate of drug binding can be readily seen. The apparent rate of blockade is $k(1-h)$, which reveals how the inactivation process acts to guard the binding site from ready access by a drug molecule, thereby imparting an "apparent" voltage dependence to the drug binding mechanism.

There is an interesting ambiguity in Equation 14 relative to interpreting the apparent rate constant. Note that the rate of blocking is a multiplicative term: $(1-h)kD(1-b)$. If we consider $k^* = (1-h)k$ as the apparent binding rate, then we may infer that k^* is voltage dependent, where the voltage modulates the affinity of the binding site. However, if we link $(1-h)$ with the substrate as $(1-h)(1-b)$, we may infer that the substrate availability is modulated by the membrane potential. This latter interpretation is more natural and does not imply any special properties of the drug-channel reaction.

From this model, we can derive several important equations that predict the voltage sensitivity of blockade and alteration of the sodium channel availability curve (h-curve). Assume that after depolarization, the rate of inactivation is rapid relative to binding of drug to inactivated channels; then the unbound channel states can be represented as a single unbound, U, state:

$$U \underset{1}{\overset{(1-h)kD}{\rightleftharpoons}} B$$

which is described by

$$\frac{db}{dt} = (1-h)kD(1-b) - \ell b \tag{15}$$

where U is an unblocked channel and B is a blocked channel. From the H-H[11] formula, the parameter h is the measure of noninactivated channels, where $h=1$ at hyperpolarized potentials (all channels in the rest state) and $h=0$ at depolarized channels (all channels in the inactivated state). To avoid confusion, we will use the term "channel avail-

A

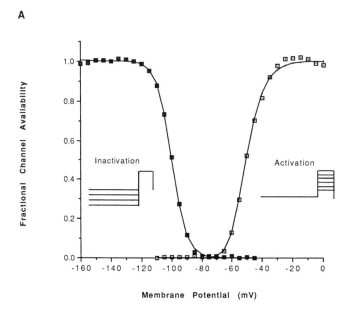

B

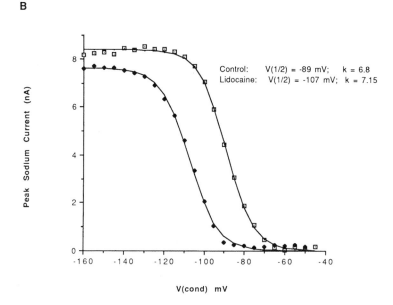

Figure 4. Voltage dependence of activation, m, and inactivation, h, of sodium channels can be readily demonstrated with voltage-clamp studies of single cells. A, Stimulation protocol used to assess sodium channel availability (equivalent to inactivation in absence of drug). Membrane potential was held at − 130 mV, where all channels reside in "rest" state, and was stepped to progressively more depolarized conditioning potentials for 200 ms followed by a test pulse

ability" to describe the fraction of channels that are available to conduct if depolarized. In the absence of drug, h is the fraction of available channels. However, in the presence of drug, channels may be unavailable for conduction as a result of either inactivation or blockade. This is readily illustrated in Figure 4.

In rabbit atrial cells, we determined the fraction of available channels by subjecting the cell to different conditioning potentials followed by a test pulse. Shown in Figure 4A is the fraction of channels available (h) and the fraction of conducting channels (m^3h by the H-H formula) in the absence of drug. In the presence of 80 μmol/L lidocaine (Figure 4B), sodium channel current was reduced during each conditioning potential as a result of the combined effects of channel inactivation and channel blockade. Note that there is a shift in the availability curve in the hyperpolarized direction. The shift in the availability curve is often incorrectly referred to as "shifted inactivation," and this interpretation has led to unnecessarily complex models of ion channel blockade predicated on modified inactivation gating in drug-complexed channels.[31,32]

The shift in availability due to channel blockade can be understood from analysis of equation 15. At equilibrium, the fraction of available channels is described by

$$b = \frac{1}{1 + \frac{\ell}{(1-h)kD}} \tag{16}$$

and the voltage dependence of the H-H inactivation parameter, h, is described as a Boltzmann function:

----

to -30 mV (left inset). Peak current measured during test pulse was measured and normalized by maximum available current (measured at a conditioning potential of -130 mV) and plotted as fraction of available channels. As conditioning potential is progressively depolarized, more channels enter inactivated state, as shown by data points. Solid line is least-squares fit of Boltzmann function: $1/(1 + \exp[(V - V_h)/k_h]$. Voltage dependence of activation, m, was estimated from peak currents divided by driving potential ($V - V_{Na}$) measured during steps from a holding potential (-130 mV) to progressively more depolarized test potentials (right inset). For this cell, threshold of activation was ≈ -70 mV. Solid line is least-squares fit of $1/(1 + \exp[(V_m - V)/V_m]$. B, Sodium channel availability measured as a function of conditioning potential under control conditions (open squares) and in presence of lidocaine (solid diamonds). In absence of drug, reduction in channel availability was due to channel inactivation. In presence of lidocaine, peak current was reduced by both inactivation and drug-complexed channels. Reduced currents observed at very hyperpolarized potentials (sometimes referred to as tonic block) represent mass action associated with blockade of a very small fraction of inactivated channels (see Reference 33 for a detailed discussion of apparent tonic block). Shift in midpoint of availability is compatible with a model of drug binding to inactivated conformation.

$$h = \frac{1}{1 + e^{(V - V_h)/k_h}} \tag{17}$$

At equilibrium, the fraction of available channels is $h^* = h(1 - b)$, which reflects the loss of channels due to both inactivation and blockade. Substituting Equations 16 and 17 into $h^* = h(1 - b)$, the fraction of available channels in the presence of drug can be described by

$$h^* = h(1 - b) = \frac{1}{1 + \left(1 + \dfrac{kD}{\ell}\right)e^{(V - V_h)/k_h}} \tag{18}$$

$$= \frac{1}{1 + e^{[V - V_h + k_h \ln(1 + kD/\ell)]/k_h}}$$

This equation reveals how control of binding site access by the inactivation process shifts channel availability in the presence of drug. The midpoint of the availability curve will be shifted in the hyperpolarized direction by an amount $\Delta V = k_h \ln(1 + kD/\ell)$, which was demonstrated in studies of lidocaine interactions with myocardial cells.[29,30] That shifts in channel availability due to the interaction of the drug with the inactivated conformation of the channel can be accounted for by the Armstrong-like model challenges the utility of more complex models, such as the modulated receptor hypothesis.[31,32]

The mechanism of use- and frequency-dependent blockade can also be readily understood by analysis of Equation 15. The time-dependent characterization of the fraction of blocked channels, $b(t)$, obeys the standard first-order kinetic mechanism:

$$\frac{db}{dt} = (1 - h)kD \, (1 - b) - \ell b \tag{19}$$

The solution is an exponential of the form

$$b(t) = b_\infty + (b_0 - b_\infty)e^{-[(1-h)kD + \ell]t} \tag{20}$$

where

$$b_\infty = \frac{1}{1 + \dfrac{\ell}{(1 - h)kD}}$$

and b_0 is the block at $t = 0$.

The time constant for block is $[(1 - h)kD + \ell]^{-1}$. For a rest potential where $h = 1$, the time constant reflects the unbinding rate, whereas for a test potential where $h = 0$, the time constant reflects the binding rate, kD. Intermediate rates of blockade will depend on the voltage dependence of $h(V)$. For lidocaine at 15°C, $k = 658/(\text{mol/L})/s$ and $\ell = 0.322/s$ at -130 mV, while at -20 mV, $k = 3.59 \times 10^4/(\text{mol/L})/s$ and $\ell = 0.666/s$.

With 80 μmol/L lidocaine, the resulting blockade time constant at -20 mV is 290 ms, whereas at -130 mV, the unblocking time constant is 2.67 seconds.[33] Consequently, with pulse-train stimulation, drug will bind with a time constant of 290 ms during the depolarized segment of the pulse and will unbind with a 2.67-second time constant at the holding potential of -130 mV. When the interstimulus interval is >10 seconds (four time constants), there will be no use-dependent blockade, ie, all the drug that has bound during the action potential duration will unbind during the recovery interval. However, if the interstimulus interval is <10 seconds, then unblocking will be incomplete by the time of the next stimulus such that block will accumulate from pulse to pulse. The pulse-to-pulse reduction in I_{Na} is exponential (Figure 3B). Based on the guarded-receptor model, the frequency- and use-dependent reduction in membrane current was shown to be piecewise exponential.[27,28] The frequency-dependent fraction of blocked channels associated with the nth pulse is

$$b_n = b_{ss} + (b_0 - b_\infty)\, e^{-(\lambda_a t_a + \lambda_r t_r)n} \tag{21}$$

where

$$b(r)_{ss} = b_\infty(a) + \gamma\, [b_\infty(r) - b_\infty(a)]$$

and

$$\gamma = \frac{1 - e^{-\lambda_r t_r}}{1 - e^{-(\lambda_a t_a + \lambda_r t_r)n}}$$

and where b_{ss} is the steady-state fraction of blocked channels, $b(a)$ is block after the depolarizing pulse, and $b(r)$ is the fraction of blocked channels at the end of the recovery interval, λ_r and λ_a are the kinetic rates associated with binding during the recovery and activated phases of the stimulation pulse protocol, and t_r and t_a are the recovery and the activated intervals. Thus, the exponential patterns of peak sodium current (or dV/dt_{max}) observed with repeated stimulation of cardiac tissue in the presence of a use-dependent drug is the result of an underlying piecewise exponential pattern of binding and unbinding, all derived from a standard first-order chemical model of drug-channel interactions with voltage-dependent access to the binding site.[27,28]

Background: Properties of a Minimally Complex Excitable Cell

Even though the H-H equations are relatively simple (three ordinary differential equations to describe channel gating and one partial differential equation to describe the conservation of ionic current), their analytical solution has defied frontal assault. Exploring simpler formulations of an excitable cell, FitzHugh[34] and Nagumo et al[35] found that the major properties of the H-H model could be captured with a two-current model in which one current displayed the "N"-shaped current/voltage (I/V) relationship embedded in the H-H sodium channel (see Reference 36 for a review).

The lingering question, remained however, as to how much useful information could be gleaned from this and other simple models. This question was addressed by early studies by Krinsky and Kokoz[37] and Rinzel.[38] These investigators observed that the H-H model[11] was composed of dynamic events that took place over two basic time scales: a fast sodium activation process and much slower potassium activation and sodium inactivation processes. Defining two variables, a fast and a slow variable, these investigators reduced the four-equation H-H model to a two-equation model that was very similar to the FitzHugh-Nagumo (FHN) model. Scott[36] later showed that the essential features of the sodium negative resistance region in the H-H model was captured with a cubic equation. Thus, with the FHN model, it became possible to explore the basic nature of excitability, impulse formation, and propagation with confidence that these results would also apply qualitatively to more complex models. Moreover, these theoretical studies provided electrophysiology a strong foundation to address "generic" properties of excitable media, ie, what antiarrhythmic and proarrhythmic mechanisms exist in the simplest realization of an excitable cell?

The reduction of the complex H-H model (and even more complex cardiac models) to two state variables (a fast variable and a slow variable) makes it possible to study these simple nonlinear models (and excitable cells) in terms of the phase plane (Figure 5). For illustrative purposes, we will consider the FHN model:

$$\frac{\partial V}{\partial t} = f(V) - W + I_{stim} + D\frac{\partial^2 V}{\partial x^2}$$

$$\frac{\partial W}{\partial t} = \epsilon(\gamma V - W)$$

(22)

where D is the diffusion constant that determines the passive spread of current, f(V) represents the I/V relationship (including a negative resistance region) of the fast inward current, W is the slow outward current, ϵ is a small parameter (similar to the membrane capacitance), I_{stim} is the stimulation current, and γ represents the voltage sensitivity of the outward repolarizing current.

For a single cell, the diffusion term, $\partial^2 V/\partial x^2$, is zero. From these

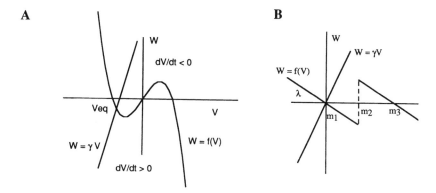

Figure 5. Primary features of impulse formation, liminal length, vulnerability, and propagation observed in cardiac tissue are generic features of any excitable medium. Therefore, it is possible to explore these essential properties in models of reduced complexity. FitzHugh-Nagumo model is a model of excitable unit based on a single excitation current [f(V), similar to fast sodium current] and a single repolarizing current (W, similar to slow potassium current). Current-voltage (I/V) relationship of these two currents is shown in A [for a cubic model of fast sodium current, f(V)] and B (for a piecewise linear model of I/V of fast sodium current), and this graph can be used to estimate qualitative responses of an excitable cell to stimulation. Nullcline equations, W = f(V) and W = γV, obtained from Equation 22 by imposing equilibrium conditions (∂V/∂t = ∂W/∂t = 0) divide phase plane into regions of positive and negative time derivatives, ∂V/∂t and ∂W/∂t. A, "fast" nullcline, f(V), separates phase plane into two regions: above curve, ∂V/∂t<0 (repolarizing) and below curve, ∂V/∂t>0 (depolarizing). Similarly, curve W = γV represents voltage dependence of slow conductance and divides phase plane into two regions where ∂W/∂t<0 (left of line) and ∂W/∂t>0 (right of line). Intersection of W = f(V) and W = γV is equilibrium point and establishes equilibrium rest potential, V_{eq}. B, Piecewise linear approximation of cubic nullcline displayed in A, which is used for analytic convenience.

equations, we can first ask, what happens at equilibrium, ie, when ∂V/∂t = ∂W/∂t = 0 (Figure 5A). Under these conditions, each of the Equations 22 reduces to algebraic equations: W = f(V), the fast nullcline, and W = γV, the slow nullcline. The point at which these two curves intersect is where the two currents are equal, thus defining the equilibrium potential, V_{eq}. These two curves also divide the phase plane (the V-W plane) into two regions: the curve W = f(V) separates the plane such that all points above the line have ∂V/∂t < 0 and all points below the line have ∂V/∂t>0, while the curve is defined by ∂V/∂t=0. Similarly, the curve W = γV separates the phase plane into two regions: to the right of the curve, ∂W/∂t>0, and to the left of the curve, ∂W/∂t<0. For analytical convenience, the cubic equation is often simplified to a piecewise linear function, shown in Figure 5B.

From the phase plane portrait (Figure 6), one can estimate the stability of the equilibrium point, V_{eq}. In panel A, small depolarizations in membrane potential, V, will move the phase point to the right and into the region where $\partial V/\partial t < 0$. Consequently, removing the stimulus will result in the membrane potential decaying back to the equilibrium rest potential. Similarly, hyperpolarizing stimuli will move the phase point to the left and into the region where $\partial V/\partial t > 0$. Removing this stimulus will result in a decay of membrane potential back to V_{eq}.

Applying a depolarizing stimulus with an intensity sufficient to move the phase point from V_{eq} into the region where $\partial V/\partial t > 0$ (threshold) will produce an action potential as illustrated in Figure 6A. Once the phase point is moved past the threshold, A, the membrane potential rapidly increases (the action potential upstroke, $\partial V/\partial t > 0$) until the phase point encounters the other limb of the fast nullcline, B, which separates the region where $\partial V/\partial t > 0$ from the region where $\partial V/\partial t < 0$. At point B, the membrane potential stops increasing, and because the parameter ϵ is small, the slow variable (W) changes at a small rate so that the phase point slowly moves along the fast nullcline from point B to C, defining the action potential plateau. As the slow variable current, W, increases beyond C, the phase point rapidly switches to D, and the membrane potential hyperpolarizes, followed by a gradual decay to the rest potential.

If the intersection of the slow and fast nullclines occurs within the negative resistance region (Figure 6B), then the equilibrium is unstable and the membrane potential oscillates like a pacemaker cell. This property can be readily visualized by analysis of the phase portrait. A small depolarizing stimulus will move the phase point to the right and into the region where $\partial V/\partial t > 0$, and the membrane will continue to depolarize. Similarly, a hyperpolarizing stimulus will move the phase point to the left and into the region where $\partial V/\partial t < 0$. Consequently, the membrane potential will continue to hyperpolarize. Since small variations in membrane potential result in phase point movement away from the nullcline intersection, it is called an unstable equilibrium.

Clinical Links

In cardiac cells, there are two quasi-equilibrium potentials at which cellular electrical stability is of interest: the rest potential and the action potential plateau. At the rest potential, the fast nullcline is defined by the I/V curve of the fast sodium current, whereas during the action potential plateau, the fast nullcline is defined by the calcium I/V curve and the background sodium current. The electrical stability is determined by the nullcline intersections with $i = 0$ and can be altered by

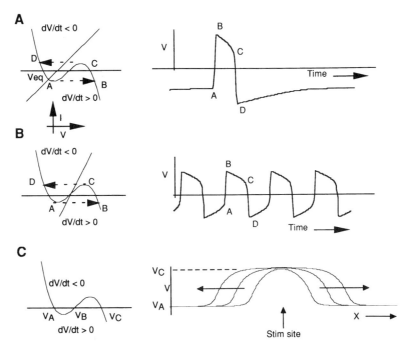

Figure 6. Phase plane portraits and membrane responses. Intersection of fast and slow nullclines determines equilibrium points of electrical properties of cell. A, Equilibrium is stable, and action potential is produced only when cell is stimulated. Cell usually remains at equilibrium potential, Veq, until stimulated. If stimulus is of sufficient strength to move membrane potential into region where dV/dt>0 (threshold, to right of point A), then potential will switch to V_B, slowly decrease (generating action potential plateau) to V_C, and then rapidly switch to V_D and slowly return to equilibrium potential. B, Spontaneous oscillation that results from shifting equilibrium to negative resistance region in middle of fast nullcline (by altering intercept of slow nullcline: $W = \gamma V + \beta$. In this case, membrane potential spontaneously oscillates. C, Propagating trigger wave derived from FitzHugh-Nagumo model, in which slow current is maintained at a constant value, $\partial W/\partial t = 0$; $W(t=0) = W_0$. Left, Plot of a propagating wave front traveling away from center (stimulation point). By varying value of repolarizing current, W_0, one can explore influence of membrane refractoriness on propagation. For $0<W_0<W_{crit}$, trigger wave will incrementally propagate away from stimulus site. For $W_0>W_{crit}$, only decremental propagation is observed.

changes in the permeability of ionic currents at the rest potential or by alterations in the availability of currents active during the action potential plateau. Such alterations are associated with hypokalemia, potassium channel blockade, or augmented g_{Ca}, all of which may shift the equilibrium point of a cell from a stable point to an unstable point, resulting in spontaneous oscillation (at the rest potential) or early afterdepolarizations (at the plateau potential).[39,40] Both calcium[41] and the background sodium currents[42,43] can supply the inward current for this oscillatory behavior.

Background: Properties of a Linear Array of Cells, ie, an Excitable Cable

If one constantly subjects a region of excitable cable to a subthreshold current, then the spatial distribution of current and voltage will reflect the "passive" properties of the cable. Although we now know that the cardiac cell at rest is not passive, this term has been used to represent cable responses to stimulus amplitudes below the threshold necessary for triggering an action potential (ie, limiting the excitation amplitude such that the resultant phase point remains in the $\partial V/\partial t < 0$ region of the phase plane).

With a constant subthreshold stimulus, after a short period of time the membrane potential will stabilize and $\partial V/\partial t = 0$. Under these conditions, the FHN model can be written as

$$D \frac{\partial^2 V}{\partial x^2} = -[f(V) - W + I_{stim}] = -[f(V) - \gamma V + I_{stim}] \tag{23}$$

By realizing that $f(V)$ can be approximated by a straight line for small subthreshold currents, this equation can be approximated by

$$\frac{d^2 V}{dx^2} = -\frac{\alpha V}{D}, \tag{24}$$

where

$$V(0) = \frac{I_{stim}}{r_m}$$

and

$$V(x) = V(0) \, e^{-(\alpha x^2/D)^{1/2}} = V(0) \, e^{-x/\lambda}, \, x > 0 \tag{25}$$

The parameter $\lambda = (D/\alpha)^{1/2}$ is the diffusion length (space constant) and is the distance over which the stimulus voltage is reduced by 63%. Under equilibrium conditions, the membrane potential associated with point excitation decays exponentially as one moves away from the stimulation point (Figure 7A). For cardiac tissue, the space constant is ≈1 mm.[44] Electrodes, however, are not points but rather have a finite length, and because the electrode resistance is minimal, the electrode potential is constant (Figure 7B). Increasing the membrane potential beyond the threshold value results in changes in the membrane resis-

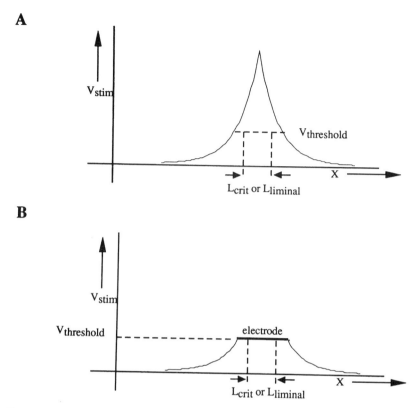

Figure 7. Passive distribution of membrane potential near a stimulating electrode. A, Potential distribution associated with a single point source. Because a critical mass of tissue (liminal length or liminal mass) must be excited to initiate a propagating wave front,[44,45] successful stimulation from "point" electrodes will always exhibit a finite suprathreshold extent that is > liminal region. B, Potential distribution associated with a finite-length electrode. When a finite length electrode is used, its length must be > liminal length to initiate a propagating wave front as first characterized by Rushton.[45]

tance that alter the diffusion length. When the electrode potential is suprathreshold, action potentials will be triggered in cells within the small suprathreshold region, which we call an impulse. An important follow-up question is whether the boundary of this impulse will expand away from the stimulus site, ie, will the wavefront propagate?

When exploring propagation, we must keep in mind that two interacting threshold phenomena are involved: (1) the threshold of stimulation of a single cell as determined by the negative resistance region of the inward, excitatory current and (2) the critical mass of cells (liminal region) that must be excited for the available source current to exceed the requirements for achieving threshold in adjacent cells (load). Abnormal impulse formation usually occurs under conditions different from rest (eg, refractory) so that determination of the liminal region will be quite different from rest conditions. To explore the relationship between source and load under rest and refractory conditions, we use the FHN equation,

$$\frac{\partial V}{\partial t} = f(V) - W + I_{stim} + D \frac{\partial^2 V}{\partial x^2}; \quad \frac{\partial W}{\partial t} = \epsilon\,(\gamma V - W) \tag{26}$$

We first would like to know the relationship between the wave-front velocity, v, and the refractory state as determined by W, the amplitude of the slow, repolarizing current. A large current reflects a highly refractory medium, whereas a small or zero current reflects the rest state. Shown in Figure 6C is a single fast nullcline with equilibria at V_A, V_B, and V_C. After a small pulse of depolarizing current is applied the membrane potential will switch from V_A to V_C in the region of the stimulating electrode. Whether this newly created impulse will propagate away from the stimulation site depends on the magnitude of the repolarizing current, W, and the size of the excited region.

We can explore this question in 1D cable of identical cells by fixing W at a constant value (by requiring $\partial W/\partial t = 0$), creating an impulse by injecting the stimulus current, I_{stim}, in the middle of the cable, and observing the fate of the newly initiated impulse. The action potentials associated with cells (composing the impulse) exposed to suprathreshold excitation will switch from the rest potential (V_A or V_{rest}) to the depolarized potential (V_C or V_{dep}). The leading edges of the impulse define two trigger waves that will propagate either incrementally or decrementally away from the stimulation site, depending on the value of W and the number of excited cells within the impulse (Figure 6C).

Now consider the following experiment. We are able to set the refractory state, W, to any value and then stimulate the medium while observing whether the impulse propagates. We will observe that with $W = 0$, the impulse will propagate away from the stimulation site when the length of excited cells exceeds two thicknesses of the wave front (liminal length). With each increase in refractoriness, $W > 0$; then after stimulation, the trigger wave will propagate at progressively slower velocities depending on the roots of the equation, $f(V) - W = 0$.[9] Eventually a critical value of W, W_{crit}, will be found at which the trigger wave almost fails to propagate (actually, it propagates with a zero velocity), and this value represents the maximal degree of refractoriness at which extension of the leading edges of the impulse (propagation) will succeed.

Rushton[45] was the first to realize that in a rested medium, excitation of a small length of nerve axon may not have enough energy to successfully expand the excited region, ie, initiate a propagating wave front of excitation. To form a propagating wave front in a medium at the rest state, he hypothesized that it would be necessary to inject sufficient stimulus current to exceed the threshold within a critical length ($L_{liminal}$ in Figure 7A) of active membrane so that once a local action potential (established within the bounds of the equipotential region) was initiated, there would be enough additional current flowing away from the active region (source current) into adjoining medium to raise the potential in the "load" region to threshold. The likelihood of actually initiating a propagating wave front is determined by the magnitude of the current flowing from the source region into the adjoining sink regions, which is in turn determined by the difference in membrane potential between the source and sink regions and the resistances of the gap junctions that direct current from the active cell to adjoining "rest" cells. Rushton analyzed the case of a continuous axon and was not concerned with the role of cellular connectivity and its influence on propagation. His analysis resulted in identification of the liminal length of axon that must be excited so that an action potential propagates (nondecrementally) away from the stimulus site into rested medium.

The applicability of the liminal length to cardiac Purkinje fibers was elegantly established by Fozzard and Schoenberg.[44] They realized that if Rushton's liminal length applied to cardiac tissue, then the strength-duration time constants and voltage thresholds for point-stimulated long Purkinje fibers should differ from that of a uniformly charged short fiber. Not only did they confirm this hypothesis, but their studies also revealed that the liminal length in Purkinje fibers was 0.1 to 0.2 λ, where λ is the space constant described above.

The role of two threshold phenomena (voltage threshold and liminal length) in initiating a propagating wave front is illustrated in [Figure 8]. In a 1D cable of FHN cells, we stimulated the center of the cable with a suprathreshold current (10 arbitrary current units applied for 1 time unit) to an electrode of length equal to $3\varDelta x$, which is less than liminal length (panel A) and $5\varDelta x$, which is greater than liminal length (panel B). The potential distribution following stimulation was measured at several points in time (as indicated by the numbers). Panel A shows decremental propagation following the formation of the impulse, and panel B shows incremental propagation of the impulse wave front and eventual splitting of the antegrade and retrograde segments (at $t>10$).

Forming an impulse with subsequent unidirectional propagation in unrested (partially refractory) medium requires addressing a slightly different question. It is well known that reentry can be initiated by premature stimulation within the vulnerable period of a conditioning wave front. Under this condition, the impulse is formed not in rested

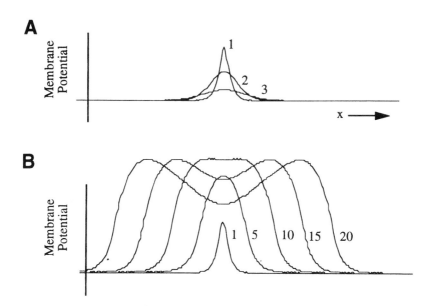

Figure 8. Impulse formation, subsequent propagation, and relationship to liminal length. Propagating wave fronts were computed from FitzHugh-Nagumo cell model (Equation 22) and nullclines illustrated in Figure 5B. Model parameters were $\lambda = 1.0, \gamma = 7.0, \epsilon = 0.01$, and $D = 1$. Zeros of $f(u)$ were $m_1 = 0.0$, $m_2 = 0.85$, and $m_3 = 3.2$. Cable consisted of 401 segments with $\Delta x = 1/8$ and $\Delta t = 1/64$, and Crank-Nicholson semi-implicit method was used to solve discrete representation of Equation 22. A, Fate of an impulse formed by stimulation of an electrode of length $3\Delta x$ (<liminal length) with a current of 10 applied for 1 time unit. Each curve represents potential distribution at $t = 1$, 2, and 3 time units after stimulation and illustrates decremental propagation. Boundary of initial impulse propagates decrementally in both directions away from stimulation site. Slightly increasing electrode length to $5\Delta x$ (>liminal length), larger impulse formed by application of same current for same duration contains enough charge to support incremental propagation of impulse wavefront (B). Curve labeled 1 ($t = 1$) represents potential distribution immediately after application of stimulus current. At later time points, impulse boundaries extend to left and right of stimulus site, and amplitude of action potential increases. For $t > 10$, repolarization process becomes significant, and two wave fronts are seen to begin to split into two individual impulses propagating at a constant velocity.

medium but in a medium that exhibits a gradient of excitability due to nonuniform refractoriness. Whether reentry can be initiated, then, resides with whether the extent of the excited region exceeds that of the liminal length determined for a partially refractory medium. Recently, Starobin et al[7] addressed this issue by asking two essential questions critical for understanding vulnerability: (1) what is the liminal length, L_{crit}, of excitable medium (in a 1D cable) that must be excited to form an impulse whose wave front can propagate in a uniformly refractory medium [$W(x) = W_{crit}$] in both directions at zero velocity and (2) what is the liminal length, L_D, of excitable medium that must be excited to form a wave front that propagates unidirectionally in the wake of the refractory period of a previous wave front, eg, using a spatial approximation of refractoriness where $W(x) = W_{crit} + \sigma(x - x_{stim})$.

Starobin et al[7] derived an equation for the critical liminal length, L_{crit}, when $W(x) = W_{crit}$, eg, when the wave front propagates bidirectionally at zero velocity in a medium with uniform refractoriness. This length was larger than Rushton's liminal length because Rushton's analysis assumed that the impulse was formed in and propagated into a rested medium, a situation that requires less energy. To answer the second question, it was necessary to approximate the nonuniform distribution (gradient) of refractoriness (the residual left by the passage of a conditioning wave front). Assuming a linear variation in refractoriness, they identified a critical liminal length, L_D, that must be excited for a unidirectionally propagating wave front to continue to propagate. For the model parameters they studied, they observed that this critical liminal region was ≈20% of the wave front thickness associated with a stationary propagating wave front (with a velocity of zero) in uniformly refractory medium. That $L_D < L_{crit}$ is readily understood when one realizes that refractoriness becomes less as the wave front propagates in the retrograde direction, so that less charge is required to maintain incremental propagation (because less charge is required to overcome the refractory state at the leading edge of the wave front).

Background: Impulse Formation and Propagation

Without a propagating wave front of excitation, synchronized mechanical contraction of the heart would be impossible. Although excitation of a patch of membrane is the first step in forming a continuous propagating wave front, it represents only part of the process of extending the wave front, eg, the source of current. For impulse formation to succeed and expand (propagate), the source charge available in the leading edge of the impulse must exceed the charge required to excite the surrounding medium (load or sink). This means that a critical mass of medium (liminal length or liminal mass) must be excited for a wave front to propagate away from a stimulus site.[44,45]

The basic processes associated with impulse formation and propagation in a 1D cable can be readily understood from Equation 7. Once the membrane potential in a localized area exceeds the threshold of sodium channel activation, the membrane potential in that region rapidly increases to a potential near the sodium equilibrium potential. This newly created spatial gradient of membrane potential is the wave front and is responsible for the flow of ionic current into adjacent resting cells. Therefore, when exploring propagation, we can restrict our attention to the leading edge of the wave front and its thickness, L_f.

If we remember that the membrane currents described by the right side of Equation 7 supply the axial current responsible for wave front extension, the role of the left side (diffusion current) becomes clear. The diffusive spread of current $[1/r_a\ \partial^2 V/\partial x^2 = \partial/\partial x(1/r_a\ \partial V/\partial x)]$ into the adjacent rested medium begins to depolarize this region. To see the ionic mechanism of wave front extension, we will consider only the role of sodium in the initial moments of impulse formation, since the sodium current activates ≈ 40 to 50 times more rapidly than the potassium currents. For our purposes here, we will ignore channel inactivation and rectification because they do not alter the basic biophysical events associated with propagation.

Consider a cell that is excited by an externally applied stimulus current at $t = 0$. Before stimulation, the cell "rests" at some resting potential, V_{rest}, and the membrane capacitor is charged to that negative potential. Consequently, any attempt to alter the membrane potential must first alter the charge on the cell membrane wall (membrane capacitance). Applying a short pulse of current at $t = 0$ provides positive charge carriers to discharge (or neutralize) some of the negative charge "attached" to the interior side of the cell membrane (capacitor). As the membrane potential slowly depolarizes, the threshold of sodium channel activation is exceeded and a few sodium channels are activated, increasing the inward flow of current, which increases the rate of depolarization, which in turn activates additional sodium channels. The newly accumulated sodium within the cell at the stimulation site displaces internal potassium ions (which have the larger intracellular concentration), which flow away from the stimulation site and through gap junctions to adjacent cells. This local accumulation of positive ions is the "impulse" whose boundaries may or may not expand, depending on the size and amount of "excess" charge that is available in the wave front for discharging adjoining segments of the membrane capacitance. The amount of charge that is available in the membrane can be estimated by the rate of rise of the action potential and the peak action potential amplitude.

When the flow of axial current away from the impulse (impulse size>liminal size) is adequate to discharge the adjacent segments of the membrane capacitance as well as rapidly depolarize this region to the sodium activation threshold, then propagation will succeed. From a qualitative view, the success or failure of propagation and the velocity of propagation are determined by the magnitude of two essential processes: a "source" that feeds sodium ions into the wave front and a "sink" or "load" that receives current necessary for excitation. For our purposes, we include gap junction connections between cells as part of the load, and thus, one can readily see that the availability and the spatial distribution of gap junctions are both critical for multidimensional propagation at the cellular level.

The complexity of conduction in a multidimensional preparation due to the nonuniform distribution of gap junction connections between cells can be readily demonstrated. Simple stimulation along the longitudinal axis, first left to right and then right to left, results in different patterns of activation. This complexity reveals itself in experiments in which one observes dV/dt_{max} at a fixed monitoring site while varying the direction of approach of a wave front. Because the distribution of gap junctions is nonuniform, a left-to-right propagating wave front will encounter different microscopic loads compared with right-to-left propagation, which, in turn, will also differ from top-to-bottom and bottom-to-top propagation.[46] These complexities require new insights into the role played by the distribution of gap junctions and disease-related alterations in gap junction distribution as they control the impulse formation and the flow of excitatory current from one cell to another.[47] Most likely, computational models are the only realistic tools available for dissecting propagation at the cellular and intracellular level.

In an attempt to penetrate the mathematical analysis of propagation in a discontinuous medium, Starobin and coworkers[7,8] developed the concept of charge balance between discrete source and sink regions in a continuous medium and used this idea to explore the detailed extension of a wave front into adjacent excitable medium. As an example, consider a linear wave front of length L_f. Recognizing that successful propagation of the wave front was a function of both the source charge available within the wave front and the sink charge required by adjacent medium to become excited, they developed a simple analytic procedure that could be adapted to wave front propagation in a medium with simple obstacles (discontinuities). Numerical studies revealed that the critical determinant of the source charge was the thickness of the wave front, L_f, which is the distance over which the maximum gradient in membrane potential is developed (phase 0 of the action potential). Therefore, they discretized the medium into squares of size L_f and then computed the charge available within each source square. Similarly, they discretized the sink region into squares of size L_{crit}, because this was the minimal impulse region (liminal region) necessary to propagate at zero velocity.

Figure 9 illustrates their analysis, showing a wave front propagating in the upward direction. The interior squares of the wave front must excite adjoining squares in front of the wave, but the end squares

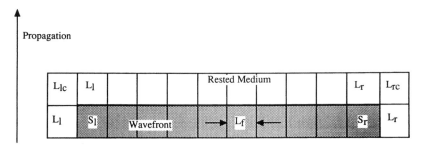

Figure 9. Simplified characterization of a wave front used to visualize safety factor of propagation defined in terms of balance of charge available from leading edge of a wave front and load requirements presented by adjacent medium. Leading edge of an impulse, discretized into squares with each side equal to wave front thickness, L_f, which is the extent of the impulse required for the membrane potential to switch from the rest potential to the maximum depolarized potential. This gradient supplies the driving force for charge transfer into adjoining rested medium. Each interior square of wave front must excite the region directly in front of it. End squares, however, must excite three adjacent squares, representing a larger electrical load than that seen by interior squares of the wave front. Increased load slows extension of end points of the wave front (because of additional time required for the potential in the region adjoining wave-front ends to reach threshold), resulting in wave-front curvature.

must excite not only a region in front but also a region immediately to the left or right of the end points of the wave front. Note that the interior squares must excite only a single square in order to propagate, whereas the left and right end squares must excite three squares. Because the load seen by the end points of the wave front is greater than the load seen by interior source squares, the ends of the wave front propagate more slowly than the interior squares, resulting in curling of the end points, and the initiation of a figure-8 pattern of excitation.

The source and sink properties can be estimated from a discretized variant of Equation 22 in which $dt = \Delta t$ and $dx = L_f$ or L_{crit} (defined in References 7 and 8). The charge, S, available during Δt from a source square characterized by a current-voltage relationship shown in Figure 5B is $S = (m_3 - m_1) \times \Delta t \times L_f \times L_f/2$. The sink requirements are twofold: the charge required to accelerate the three sink squares from a velocity of 0: $L_a = 3 (W_{eq} - W_{crit}) \times \Delta t \times L_{crit} \times L_{crit}$ and the charge that leaks from the two outer edges of the corner square: $L_{leak} = 2(m_3 - m_1) \times \Delta t/L_{crit}$. The wave front will not grow when $S - L_a - L_{leak} = 0$, ie, there is a perfect balance between source and sink charge. When $S < L_a + L_{leak}$, the wave tip retracts (decremental conduction) and eventually dies. When $S > L_a + L_{leak}$, the wave tip will extend itself, and the curvature of the wave front will be determined by the number of squares the source square can activate. Clearly, the greater the wave-front charge, the greater the wave-front charge, the greater the wave-front curvature. This method of analysis can be applied to probing the interaction between a wave front and an obstacle in an otherwise homogeneous medium.

Clinical Links

Let us now consider a basic arrhythmogenic mechanism before returning to more formal analyses of membrane behavior. CAST[48] revealed that survivors of a previous myocardial infarction were approximately three times more likely to die of sudden cardiac death if they were treated with a class I drug compared with untreated patients. The rationale for using class I antiarrhythmic agents was that by blocking sodium channels, one would be able to depress the "excitability" of individual cells, ie, a greater charge would be required to initiate a local action potential because of the loss of available, unblocked sodium channels (the charge source). The underlying assumptions of CAST were that suppression of PVCs would reduce the incidence of sudden cardiac death, and the implied assumption was that unsuppressed PVCs in the presence of drug would be no more malignant than unsuppressed PVCs in the absence of drug with respect to initiating a reentrant arrhythmia. However, it is obvious that reducing the availability of sodium channels will slow propagation by decreasing the charge available within the wave front. Therefore, localized failure of propagation at regions of high electrical load is amplified. In other words, sodium blockade at the cellular level is antiarrhythmic because it depresses excitability, but at the multicellular level, it is proarrhythmic: a result of destabilization of the conditions for maintaining wave-front continuity, either by localized block associated with discontinuous propagation[8] or by unidirectional propagation associated with unsuppressed premature stimuli.[16,49,50]

Background: The Extracellular Potential and ECG

The ECG is a complex electrical signal that is derived from the flow of current between myocardial cells. Development of a detailed model linking the ECG with myocardial potentials has been limited by the complexities introduced by the many different layers of conductive medium between ECG electrode sites and the heart and the irregular geometric shapes of these regions. Despite these difficulties, we can use a simple model assuming a homogeneous conductivity to gain

A

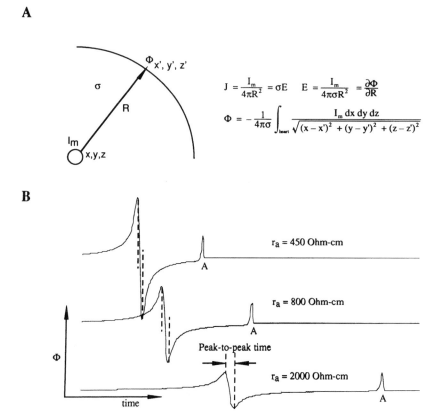

B

Figure 10. Schematic of relationship between surface ECG potential and distribution of charge on myocardial surface. A, Region of charge (cardiac cells) located at x,y,z. Transmembrane current flows into medium surrounding cells and alters potential at site of an electrode (x′, y′, z′). Potential at electrode site is computed by summing (integrating) changes in potential caused by currents flowing from each cell in heart. B, Alterations in electrogram potentials as a function of axial resistance. When axial resistance is small, wave front propagates rapidly, resulting in a large-amplitude, short-duration deflection of electrogram. As axial resistance increases, wave front propagates more slowly, peak-to-peak amplitude is reduced, and duration is increased.

some understanding of the QRS patterns in the ECG. We will assume that the ECG electrodes and heart are immersed in an infinite, homogeneous conducting medium, with the heart located at the center.

Assume that a charge, I_m, is located at x, y, z in an infinite conductive medium (Figure 10A). The potential, Φ, at some distance from the charge source is related to the electrical field, E, associated with the local membrane charge, I_m. The local charge density at the point of measurement of the potential, x', y', z', is distributed over the surface of a sphere of radius r so that $J_{local} = I_m/4\pi R^2$. The local electrical field at the measurement point, E, is the gradient of the potential, Φ, $\Phi = dE/dR$, where R is the vector joining x, y, z with x', y', z' and is related to the current density, J, and conductance, σ, by $J = \sigma E$. Consequently, the potential due to a single membrane charge is

$$E = \frac{d\Phi}{dR} = \frac{1}{\sigma}\frac{I_m}{4\pi R^2} \tag{27}$$

Integrating with respect to R to compute the potential, Φ, yields

$$\Phi = -\frac{1}{4\pi\sigma}\frac{I_m}{R} \tag{28}$$

and the potential due to all the membrane currents is determined by summing the contributions of the local current density:

$$\Phi_{total} = -\frac{1}{4\pi\sigma}\int \frac{I_m}{R}\,dx\,dy\,dz.$$

Since

$$I_m = \frac{\partial}{\partial x}\left(\frac{1}{r_a}\frac{\partial V}{\partial x}\right), \text{ then}$$

$$\Phi_{total} = -\frac{1}{4\pi\sigma}\int \frac{\frac{\partial}{\partial x}\left(\frac{1}{r_a}\frac{\partial V}{\partial x}\right)}{\sqrt{(x-x')^2 + (y-y')^2 + (z-z')^2}}\,dx\,dy\,dz \tag{29}$$

These equations describe a unipolar potential, measured at the location x', y', z', relative to the potential at infinity (which we assume to be 0). From these equations, some general conclusions about the nature of a propagating wave front can be developed. For example, the propagation velocity is a function of both the internal resistance, r_a, and the macroscopic sodium conductance, g_{Na}. When the r_a increases (for instance, in switching from longitudinal to transverse propagation), the amplitude of the numerator is reduced, which reduces the amplitude of the potential, Φ. Similarly, when I_m is reduced, for instance, secondary to sodium channel blockade, then the amplitude of Φ is also reduced.

Clinical Links

The influence of altered conduction velocity is illustrated in Figure 10B, which shows extracellular electrograms computed from a 1D cable for three different values of the internal resistance, r_a. The computations were performed on a uniform cable of 120 segments described by the FHN model.[6] The cable was stimulated at the left end, and the electrogram was monitored by an electrode placed at the middle of the cable (segment 60). The electrogram appears as a biphasic signal, reflecting the passage of the wave front under the monitoring electrode. With slower propagation, the peak-to-peak amplitude was reduced in accordance with the above equations. Similarly, the peak-to-peak duration was prolonged because of the slowed conduction. The top electrogram, computed with $r_a = 450$ $\Omega \cdot cm$, shows a narrow, high-amplitude waveform derived from a rapidly propagating wave front. In contrast, the bottom electrogram, computed with $r_a = 2000$ $\Omega \cdot cm$, reveals a lower-amplitude waveform with a longer peak-to-peak duration. Clearly, careful inspection of unipolar extracellular potentials provides considerable insight into the nature of a propagating wave front. The small, monophasic deflections (labeled A) are artifacts, introduced by collision of the propagating wave front with the end of the cable. The boundary conditions at the cable ends are $dV/dx = 0$, ie, no current flow out of either end of the cable, which could represent a nonconducting object. The electrogram containing this "artifact" derived from the discontinuity in the axial resistance illustrates one aspect of the complexities introduced by resistive discontinuities in a continuous medium.

These concepts can be readily demonstrated in tissue.[51] Figure 11 illustrates the contrast between rapid longitudinal propagation and slower transverse propagation as determined by the sites of stimulation and measurement. Here, three monitoring sites and three stimulation sites were used. When the stimulation and electrogram sites were along the fiber axis, the electrogram was of high amplitude and short duration (Figure 11, panels IA, IIB, IIIC, and IVA, B, and C). However, when the electrogram site was transverse to the axis of propagation, the electrogram amplitude was reduced and exhibited a longer duration (Figure 11, panels IB and C; IIA and C; and IIIA and B).

On the basis of careful observation of extracellular waveforms and their derivatives, Spach and coworkers[51,52] reported that the predictions of continuous theory were inadequate to explain alterations in the cellular action potential when propagation was shifted from longitudinal to transverse. The reader is referred to chapter 1 of this monograph for a detailed discussion of the role of discontinuities in microscopic propagation and the role the distribution of gap junction connections plays in altering the cellular responses to stimulation. Here, we wish simply to illustrate the extraordinary complexities of microscopic propagation introduced by the distribution of gap junctions as revealed by extracellular electrograms (Figure 12).

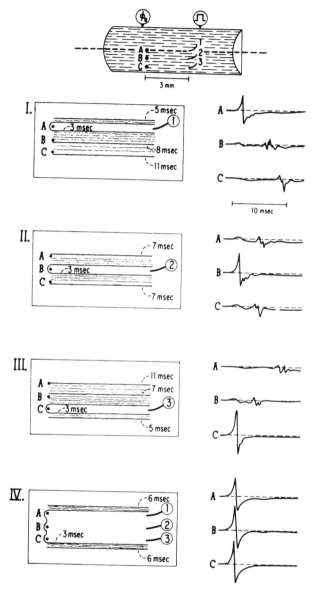

Figure 11. Observed propagation patterns within Bachmann's bundle: dependence on mode of initiation of excitation. Schematic (top) shows location of stimulating electrodes (1–3) and extracellular (ϕ_e) recording electrodes (A-C). Broken line is on crest of bundle. I and III, Activation patterns (left) and extracellular waveforms (right) when excitation was initiated at each stimulus electrode; IV, activation pattern when excitation was initiated at all stimulus electrodes simultaneously. Time of isochrones (in ms) is identified with respect to onset of stimulus. Reprinted with permission from Reference 51.

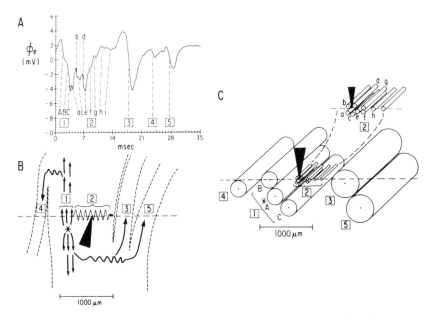

Figure 12. A highly complex polyphasic waveform measured in atrial tissue from a 62-year-old man (A), geometry of underlying structures with pattern of excitation spread (B), and cable model of location of source (C). Numbers in A and B show correspondence between each deflection and structure of origin. A, Letters a through i identify each small deflection produced during transverse propagation in area 2 of major bundle. B, Outline drawing (broken lines) was made from photographs of main bundle and its branches, stimulus site (asterisk), and location of tip of extracellular metal microelectrode (solid triangle). C, Complete geometric configuration of large and small cylinders that produced best theoretical fit of experimental waveform in A along with its first and second derivatives. Reprint with permission from Reference 5.

In studies of propagation in human atrial tissue, Spach and Dolber[5] observed that there was an age-related decrease in the effective transverse propagation velocity, possibly due to the loss of side-to-side gap junction connections between cells. Using the extracellular potential and its derivatives, they found evidence of complex propagation patterns consistent with loss of side-to-side connections between small groups of muscle fibers. With a computer model of a complex arrangement of different-size muscle fibers, they were able to demonstrate many of the extracellular waveforms that were observed experimentally (Figure 12). Here, the unipolar extracellular potential (panel A) shows a complex mixture of small and large-amplitude potentials measured from a preparation from a 62-year-old man. In panel B, the dashed lines highlight the boundaries of the muscle bundles that participated in propagation. Shown is the outline of a main bundle (1 and 2) that was electrically coupled by regions of transverse propagation to bundles 3 and 5 on the right and bundle 4 on the left. The recording electrode is placed in the region of transverse propagation (asterisk). The numbers (1 through 5) shown in panel A are keyed to the regions displayed in panel B, where different modes of propagation are shown by the straight and zigzag arrows. The anatomy was modeled by a group of large and small cylindrical muscle bundles as shown in panel C. From computer simulations, Spach and coworkers were able to determine that the amplitude of the extracellular potentials was dominated by contributions from the "source" membrane ionic currents, whereas the amplitudes of the first and second derivatives of the extracellular potential were primarily a function of the distance between the current source and the recording electrode.

With the basic concepts of a membrane model, propagation in a cable and ion channel blockade, we can now turn our attention to arrhythmogenesis by considering propagation under nonequilibrium conditions in a 1D and 2D medium.

Starting Reentry: Generic Mechanism

When a region of tissue at rest or in equilibrium is excited, under most conditions a small circular or elliptical impulse forms, which in turn expands outward into the adjacent medium. The boundary of the impulse (wave front) is considered continuous because if one walks along the wave front, one eventually returns to the starting point. Although the impulse boundary may be irregular[4] because of variations of propagation velocity associated with variations in the load seen by the advancing wave front, it is still continuous.

A reentrant wave front (spiral wave) is the result of propagation of a discontinuous wave front. As illustrated above (Figure 9), the wave tip at a blocked region will propagate at a slower rate than wave-front segments located some distance from the end points of the wave because of the increased load. A central question in arrhythmogenesis and antiarrhythmic therapy is how to prevent the formation of a discontinuous wave front or, once formed, how to control the resultant discontinuous wave front. Class I and III drugs have been used to try to reduce the likelihood of formation of a discontinuous wave front, and antitachycardia pacing protocols have been used to terminate a reentrant rhythm once initiated. Recently, there has been interest in developing other strategies for control of reentrant activation either by parametric resonance[53–56] or by use of control strategies based on altering the trajectory of the wave front in phase space.[57,58]

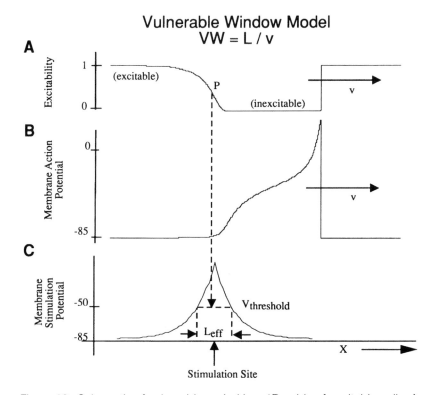

Figure 13. Schematic of vulnerable period in a 1D cable of excitable cells. A, Spatial variation of excitability as approximated by sodium channel inactivation variable (h*j) defined in Luo-Rudy ventricular model.[65] The inactivation variable partitions cable into an excitable region that supports incremental conduction (to left of P) and partially excitable and inexcitable regions that support only decremental conduction. B, Action potential propagating from left to right with velocity v. C, Spatial distribution of membrane potential associated with s2 stimulating electrode. Length of suprathreshold region (where $V_m > -50$ mV) associated with s2 site is indicated by dashed line of length L_{eff}. In the wake of the propagating action potential is a point, P, that separates regions of decremental and incremental conduction. Stimulation of a liminal length (computed for refractory conditions) in the region to left of P (panel A) results in incremental propagation, while stimulation of any length of medium to right of P results in decremental conduction. Time required for P to propagate across suprathreshold region, L_{eff}, defines period of vulnerability. Stimulation before arrival of action potential results in a bidirectionally propagated wave front. If the s2 site is activated while this critical point passes over the suprathreshold region, resultant wave front will propagate incrementally in retrograde direction and decrementally in antegrade direction. If the stimulation site is activated after the critical point passes the suprathreshold region, then propagation in both retrograde and antegrade directions will be incremental. If conduction velocity of initial wave front is v, then period of vulnerability is time required for critical point to propagate across suprathreshold region, L. This time, VW = L/v,

There are three primary mechanisms for creating a discontinuous wave front: (1) premature stimulation when impulse formation in the antegrade direction is inhibited by refractory media[6,7,59,60]; (2) propagation of a wave front into a small region of refractory tissue[61]; and (3) propagation of a wave front into a region of high electrical load leading localized conduction failure.[8,9,62]

After the discontinuity in the wave front has formed, the residual wave fragment (wavelet) may continue to propagate or may fail to propagate depending on its length relative to the cardiac analogue of Rushton's liminal length.[45] If continued propagation is possible, the wave front may fragment again and again, leading to multiple wavelets and fibrillation.[8,63] Thus, we view reentrant arrhythmias, ranging from simple monomorphic tachyarrhythmias to polymorphic tachyarrhythmias to flutter and fibrillation, as different stages of evolution of a discontinuous wave front. By understanding the mechanisms behind incomplete impulse formation, the stability of rotation of a wave-front fragment, and wave-front fractionation, one can explore antiarrhythmic and control strategies within a single conceptual framework.

Starting Reentry: Vulnerability in One Dimension

Although it has long been well known that premature stimulation during the vulnerable period can trigger arrhythmias,[59] it was not until 1946 that the basic mechanism underlying vulnerability was described in analytic terms.[60] Using a finite-state cellular model that assumed that (1) cardiac impulses, once started, would propagate in all directions with a constant velocity; (2) the amplitude of the wave front would be constant and exceed the excitation threshold of adjacent cells; and (3) a cell can reside in either a resting state (from which it can be excited), an active, inexcitable state, or a refractory state of constant duration during which excitability gradually recovered, Wiener and Rosenblueth[60] proposed a model of reentrant arrhythmogenesis for any homogeneous excitable medium. They demonstrated that if one introduced a test stimulus (s2) in a cable of identical cells in the wake of a previously initiated conditioning (s1) wave front, then there was a period of vulnerability, VW, during which test stimuli would initiate a unidirection-

---

is vulnerable period first proposed by Wiener and Rosenblueth.[59] Note that this analysis applies to any "conditioning" wave front. For instance, with multiple premature stimuli (s2, s3 . . .), each successive wave front often propagates with a velocity less than that of its predecessor, thereby extending VW. Thus, it is not surprising that multiple stimuli often can induce reentry more readily than single premature stimuli.

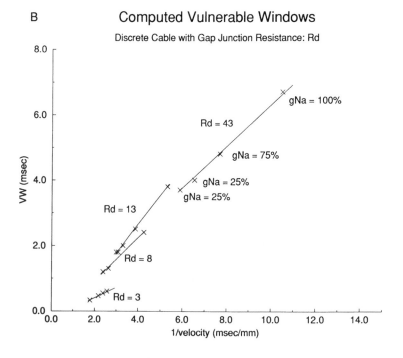

Figure 14. Properties of vulnerable window. A, Two possible hypotheses. Left, Spatial VW that exceeds liminal length; right, spatial VW that is equal to liminal length. Conditioning wave propagated from left to right. Shown are spatial distributions of potential associated with an impulse resulting from stimulation at either left (S_L) or right (S_R) boundary of VW (inner pulse). Propagation is away from stimulation site and is represented by series of curves of potential

ally propagated wave front. The VW was shown to be equal to the length of the suprathreshold stimulus field, L, divided by the conduction velocity of the conditioning wavefront, v: VW = L/v (Figure 13). The role of the s1 conditioning stimulus was to create a propagating wave of excitability. This wave was then "sampled" with s2 stimuli to test for vulnerability (unidirectional propagation).

Vulnerability in a 1D cable can be readily understood by recognizing the existence of a single critical point, P, on the excitability wave that separates the medium capable of supporting incremental propagation (excitable) from the region of the medium that supports only decremental propagation (inexcitable) (Figure 13A). Assume that the conditioning wave propagates from left to right. Then as P propagates from left to right, three conditions arise: (1) if P is to the left of the suprathreshold region of the stimulus field, s2 stimulation results in formation of an impulse that conducts decrementally in both the antegrade and retrograde directions; (2) if P is to the right of the suprathreshold region of the stimulus field, s2 stimulation results in formation of an impulse that conducts incrementally in both the antegrade and retrograde directions; and (3) if P is within the suprathreshold region (as shown in panel C), s2 stimulation results in an impulse that propagates incrementally in the retrograde direction and decrementally in the antegrade direction.

Because a critical mass of excitable medium, L_D or liminal length, must be excited for the impulse boundary resulting from premature stimulation to expand,[7,44,45] the stimulation current must excite a region larger than a single point. Consequently, the vulnerable period cannot be observed when the length of the suprathreshold region, L_{eff}, is less than the liminal length (Figure 13C). For suprathreshold regions>

------

distribution at increasing moments of time. When VW(space)>$L_{liminal}$ (left panel), then stimulation at S_L results in a retrograde decrementally propagating wave, while stimulation at S_R results in an antegrade incrementally propagating wave. Since conditioning wave propagated from left to right, excitability at S_L is greater than excitability at S_R. If this is true, then it is impossible to have a retrograde decrementally propagating wave into medium that is more excitable (at S_L) than an antegrade wave that propagates incrementally into medium of lesser excitability (at S_R). Paradox is only resolved when $S_L - S_R = L_{liminal}$. B, Applicability of VW to a cable of excitable cells (Luo-Rudy model) coupled by gap junctions (discontinuous cable). Shown is a plot of VW observed in numerical experiments (x) as a function of 1/velocity extracted from Table 2 of Reference 64 for four values of gap junction resistance, R_d: 3, 8, 13, and 43 $\Omega \cdot cm^2$. Conduction velocity was altered by reducing maximum sodium conductance, g_{Na}, to values of 100%, 75%, 50%, and 25% for each value of R_d. For each value of gap junction resistance, relationship between VW and 1/velocity was fit by a least-squares procedure (solid lines). Each set of points is well described by a straight line, indicating agreement with VW = L/v.

$L_{liminal}$, the period of vulnerability, VP, is the time required for P to cross this suprathreshold region after compensation for the liminal length: $VP = (L - L_{liminal})/v$, where L is the length of the suprathreshold excitation region and v is the propagation velocity of the conditioning wave front. When the stimulus field is large compared with the liminal length, then the VW can be approximated by L/v. While this equation reveals that in the time domain, the minimum VW is 0 ms, is there a minimum in the spatial domain?

Though often not considered in the context of proarrhythmia, the liminal length plays an essential role in the concept of vulnerability. One might question whether, as we discussed above, the liminal length defines vulnerability or whether there is another "intrinsic" vulnerable period that is determined by the membrane properties. Figure 14A illustrates two possible models of vulnerability: (1) an intrinsic model, in which the vulnerable period (in the spatial domain) is longer than the liminal length, and (2) a liminal length model. Shown are a series of membrane potential distributions as they develop immediately after stimulation and plotted in the spatial domain at successive time intervals. The potential distribution associated with the stimulus current is shown as the innermost impulse. The right and left boundaries of the initial impulse propagate either incrementally or decrementally. The left panel, the intrinsic model, assumes that there is a region of vulnerability that exceeds the liminal length. Assuming that this is correct, then stimulation at the right boundary (S_R) results in a retrograde incrementally propagating wave and an antegrade decrementally propagating wave. Similar events are observed when the medium is stimulated at the left boundary (S_L). Because the conditioning wave front propagates from left to right, the medium at S_L is less refractory than at S_R. This fact creates a paradox: the antegrade wave initiated at S_L propagates decrementally into medium that is more excitable than the incrementally propagating retrograde wave initiated at S_R. The paradox is resolved only when the distance between S_R and S_L is equal to the liminal length (right panel).

Shaw and Rudy[64] extended the analysis of vulnerability to a cable of cells connected by gap junction resistances. Using the Luo-Rudy[65] ventricular model, they explored vulnerability in a cable of 150 cells, each 100 micron in length and connected by gap junction resistances, R_d. In one study, using a stimulation current two times the diastolic threshold and $R_d = 8 \; \Omega \cdot cm^2$, they found that stimulation of the middle third of a single cell (point stimulation) resulted in a VW = 1.2 ms, whereas stimulation of an electrode 21 cells in length resulted in a VW = 5.8 ms, clearly indicating differences in vulnerability. The difference is readily explained in terms of liminal length and examination of the suprathreshold region of the stimulus field (Figure 5 of Reference 64). With point stimulation, the suprathreshold length (approximated by the region in which $V > -50$ mV) was ≈5 cells and larger than $L_{liminal}$. For the finite-length electrode (panels C and D), the suprathreshold region was ≈25 cells. Using the observed conduction velocity of $v = 0.42$ mm/ms, the VW computed from $VW = L/v$, yields a VW (point) $= 0.5/0.42 = 1.2$ ms and a VW(finite) $= 2.5/0.42 = 5.9$ ms. Both values are equivalent to those determined in their numerical experiments, thus confirming the concept of the VW, defined in terms of propagation of a critical point across the suprathreshold region for either a continuous or discontinuous medium.

Further confirmation of this model when applied to a discontinuous cable was provided in Reference 64 by reanalysis of the relationship between VW and conduction velocity as gap junction resistance was varied. According to Wiener and Rosenblueth's model, for each value of gap junction resistance, R_d, the relationship between VW and 1/velocity should be linear. A least-squares fit of a linear model, $VW = L_{eff}/v$, for each set of VW-g_{Na} values in Table 2 of Reference 64 yielded an excellent fit with $r > 0.95$ for each value of R_d, as shown in Figure 14B.

Starting Reentry: Vulnerability in Two Dimensions

The first demonstration of the vulnerable period in a 2D array of excitable cells was by Gul'ko and Petrov,[66] who used a hybrid computer. They first initiated a wave front with a conditioning stimulus, and then, with a test stimulus timed to occur during the refractory wake, they observed the formation of a reentrant wave front (Figure 15). The propagation of the incompletely formed impulse evolved into a spiral wave, perhaps the first computational demonstration of spiral-wave reentry. These computational studies were followed by additional numerical studies of reentry by van Capelle and Durrer.[67] Their studies were the first to reveal the boundaries of the vulnerable period. Both of these studies demonstrated that reentry initiated by premature stimulation was derived from the existence of a functional obstacle around which the wave front evolving from an incompletely formed impulse would rotate. Moreover, in the model studied by van Capelle and Durrer, the region of functional block was observed to drift by some unknown mechanism (Figure 16). This observation is similar to meandering of spiral waves observed in the B-Z chemical medium[68] and later shown to be a mechanism for producing a polymorphic QRS pattern.[17]

Clinical Links

Initiation of reentry is often related to a transient region of block of unknown source and slowed conduction.[1,2,69] Although many clini-

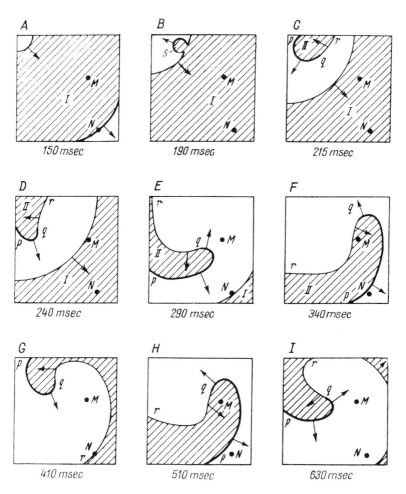

Figure 15. Studies of reentrant wave-front evolution in 2D array of excitable cells. This illustration reveals origin of a closed pathway of conduction of excitation around a functional obstacle in a homogeneous medium after delivery of a test stimulus to the point S at t = 183 ms. A, Conditioning wave front propagating from top left to bottom right. B, Result of premature stimulation: an incompletely formed impulse (discontinuous wave front) at location S. Impulse boundary expands in retrograde direction, curving in response to increased electrical load and eventually forming a spiral wave. Reprinted with permission from Reference 66.

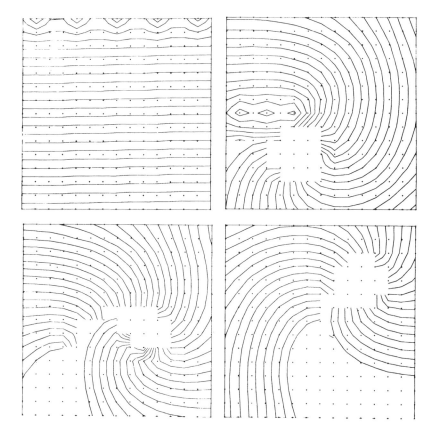

Figure 16. Isochronal lines corresponding to initiation of tachycardia in a 2D model of excitable cells. Distance between lines corresponds to 20 time steps. Top left, Plane wave caused by conditioning stimulus. Top right, Premature beat, which is blocked in antegrade direction, starts a clockwise circus movement around a functionally blocked region. Last isochronal line of this panel corresponds to first one of bottom left. Bottom right, Continuation of bottom left. Isochrones are similar to a spiral and region of block is unstable, drifting from frame to frame. Reprinted with permission from Reference 67.

cians have been acutely aware of the association between slowed conduction and proarrhythmic conditions, we were not aware that slowed conduction also amplified the vulnerable period, thereby increasing the likelihood of initiating reentry with an unsuppressed premature impulse. For this reason, it is helpful to consider reentrant arrhythmias as the result of two distinct processes: (1) an initiating process (incomplete impulse formation or a fractionated wave front) and (2) a maintenance process (reentrant path length that is greater than the refractory wavelength).

Allessie et al[70] demonstrated that the vulnerable period had well-defined and detectable boundaries in their studies of reentry in isolated left atria of rabbit. But what about drug effects on vulnerability? With respect to use-dependent class I antiarrhythmic drugs, it is clear from Wiener and Rosenblueth's model of propagation and vulnerability[60] that although these drugs can suppress early premature excitations by reducing excitability and prolonging the refractory period, the late, unsuppressed premature excitations will be more malignant because of the prolonged period of vulnerability. Demonstrating that the Wiener-Rosenblueth model was directly applicable to a model of cardiac tissue, Starmer and coworkers[16] studied vulnerability in a computer model of identical cells characterized by the Beeler-Reuter model[15] and observed an interesting effect of use-dependent drugs on vulnerability. When sodium channel blockade was modeled as a simple reduction in the maximal sodium conductance, they found that with $g_{Na} = 6$ mS/cm^2, VW = 4 ms, and when g_{Na} was reduced by 50% to 3 mS/cm^2, VW = 8 ms. Propagation failed when g_{Na} was reduced to 2 mS/cm^2.

Class I antiarrhythmic agents are use dependent and bind according to the models described above. When their effect on vulnerability was explored with numerical experiments, it was discovered that prolongation of the VW was much greater than that associated with a constant reduction of g_{Na}.[16] When the drug concentration was held constant, these numerical studies revealed that for rapidly unbinding drugs such as lidocaine, VW = 9 ms, a modest increase of control vulnerability. However, when the unbinding rate was slowed, as with flecainide, the VW was prolonged to 38 mS.

The sensitivity of the vulnerable period to use-dependent sodium channel blockade was first demonstrated[49,50] in studies of flecainide, ethmozin, lidocaine (Figure 17), cocaine, and propoxyphene. In isolated left atria of rabbit, the diastolic interval was scanned with premature stimuli to locate the boundaries of the vulnerable period, VP. Under control conditions, the VP was usually not detectable by use of 1- or 2-ms increments in s1-s2 delay. After exposure to any of the use-dependent class I drugs that were tested, a VP was easily detected and varied in duration from 4 ms for lidocaine to >30 ms for propoxyphene and cocaine.[50] Similar studies were performed in guinea-pig papillary muscle by Nesterenko et al.[49] They observed a well-defined vulnerable period under control conditions that was prolonged with ethmozin, flecainide, and encainide. Application of quinidine reduced the vulnerable period, possibly a response to significant potassium channel blockade.[6]

In light of the dramatic increase in the VP with propoxyphene and cocaine, it is useful to speculate about arrhythmogenesis in the setting of abused substances that block the cardiac sodium channel. Perhaps some of the cardiotoxic effects associated with substances such as co-

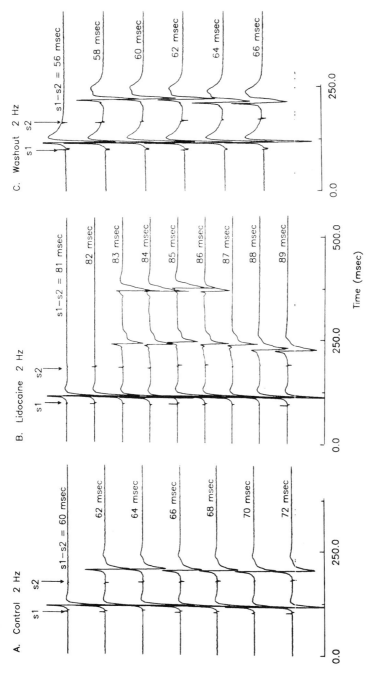

Figure 17. Vulnerability observed in a quasi-2D preparation (isolated rabbit left atrium). Rapidly unbinding lidocaine (42 μmol/L) prolonged duration of vulnerable window. A, Transition between 1:0 (refractory) and 1:1 responses in a typical preparation and absence of VP. After 20 minutes of exposure to lidocaine (B), refractory period was extended by 20 ms, and a 4-ms VP was detected. After 30 minutes of exposure to control solution, VP was no longer detectable at 1-ms precision, and extended refractory period returned to control values. Reprinted with permission from Reference 50.

caine, tricyclic antidepressants, and synthetic opiate derivatives may arise from their ability to block the cardiac sodium channel,[18,71-73] thereby prolonging the VP and amplifying the malignant nature of unsuppressed PVCs. All of these agents have relatively slow unbinding rates, which have been shown to dramatically extend the vulnerable period.[6,7,16] Supporting this hypothesis is the observation that it is possible to reverse some of the ECG alterations associated with drug overdose by competition with a sodium channel blocker that exhibits a rapid unbinding rate.[74,75] In a drug overdose patient, Whitcomb et al[73] were able to reverse the cardiotoxic effects of propoxyphene, a slowly unbinding sodium channel blocker, by competition with lidocaine. The result was a net reduction in the unbinding rate associated with the lidocaine-propoxyphene mixture, which increased the conduction velocity (decreased the QRS duration) and eliminated the recurrence of sustained ventricular tachycardias. Use of magnesium also appears to reduce the cardiotoxic effects of abused substances, perhaps secondary to shifting the sodium channel availability curve to reduce the fraction of drug-complexed inactivated channels.

That the vulnerable period is determined by the propagation velocity of the "conditioning" stimulus provides a simple explanation of why multiple premature stimuli are sometimes more likely to initiate reentry than a single premature stimulus. If a conditioning wave propagates with velocity v_{s1}, then premature stimulation during the refractory period will produce a wave front propagating at a slower velocity, v_{s2}.[10] The vulnerable period associated with the initial, conditioning pulse is then equal to L/v_{s1}. However, if a second test stimulus, s3, is introduced within the wake of the s2 wave front, it will experience a prolonged VP during which it is possible to initiate a unidirectionally propagated wave front: $VP_{s2} < VP_{s3} = L/v_{s2}$. Similarly, additional test stimuli, if placed in the wake of a preceding wave that propagates more slowly than its predecessor wave, will fall with progressively higher probability within the vulnerable period. Consequently, multiple appropriately timed stimuli are more likely to induce reentry than a single test stimulus because of the slowing of each successive conditioning wave responsible for creating the gradient of refractory states.

Starting Reentry: Propagation Into a Region of Refractory Medium

Premature stimulation is not the only way to initiate reentry. Recognizing the importance of creating a discontinuous wave front to initiate reentry (spiral waves), Krinsky[76] proposed that a discontinuity in refractory periods could be used to create conditions leading to wavebreaks, thus providing a plausible mechanism for wave-front fractionation and fibrillation. In fact, there was a very active segment within the Russian (Soviet) school of biophysics that had been actively and intensively studying reentrantlike propagation in an inert chemical reagent discovered by Belousov[77] that exhibited many properties similar to cardiac muscle.

Figure 18 illustrates the Krinsky hypothesis. The medium is characterized by a refractory period of τ_{normal} except for a small region in which the refractory period is $\tau_{long} > \tau_{normal}$. Consider the interval between stimuli as t_s. If the $t_s > \tau_{long}$, then with repetitive stimulation, each successor wave will propagate into fully recovered medium. However, if $t_s < \tau_{long}$, then when a successor wave front encounters the region of prolonged refractoriness, a wavebreak is created. After the area of prolonged refractoriness recovers, then the wave tips of the fractionated wave are able to curl and propagate in the retrograde direction. In other words, after wave front–obstacle collision, the wave tips that form at the discontinuity are required to excite more media than other segments of the wave, leading to slowed conduction (in the region of the tip) and curling. The extension of the wave-front tip continues at a slower rate than the propagation velocity of the incident wave, leading to the development of spiral-wave reentry. Krinsky's model clearly showed the important role of dispersion of cellular refractory properties as a mechanism for creating transient regions of block suitable for initiating reentry.

Starting Reentry: Interaction of a Wave Front With a Structural Discontinuity (Obstacle)

The discontinuity of the wave front created by interaction of a wave front with a transiently refractory region suggests that fractionation of the wave front by nonconducting structural discontinuities may also lead to reentry. Propagation in the presence of recurrent discontinuities is perhaps the least well understood proarrhythmic mechanism, probably because of the inherent complexity associated with the connections between myocardial cells. First recognized by Spach and co-workers,[5,10,51,52] insights into this mechanism require a detailed understanding of the spatial variations in cellular load presented under conditions of uniform and nonuniform anisotropic conditions.

Instead of a creating a wavebreak as a result of a transient obstacle created by a regional dispersion in cellular refractory properties, conduction can be blocked by regional increases in load that lead to the formation of wave fragments. The importance of this mechanism was emphasized by recent studies of arrhythmogenesis in hypertrophic

A

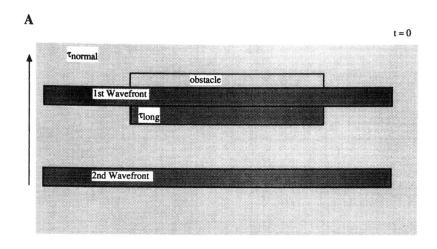

B

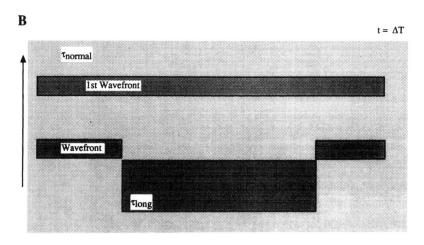

Figure 18. Model of wave-front fractionation in a 2D medium with varied refractory properties. A, Two wave fronts propagating from bottom to top. In middle of medium is a region (obstacle) with a prolonged refractory period. As first wave front propagates through medium, a refractory region remains in its wake. As second wave front encounters region of prolonged refractoriness because interstimulus interval is $< \tau_{long}$ (B), wave front is fractionated and two wave fragments are formed that could curl and evolve to two spiral waves.

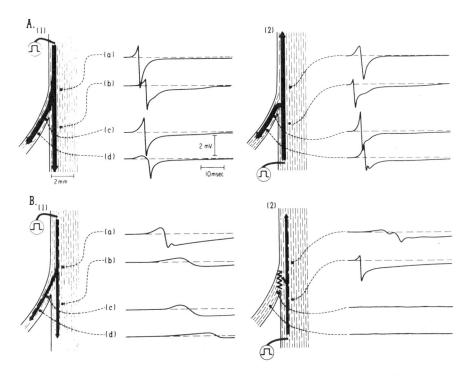

Figure 19. In vitro demonstration of unidirectional block at branch sites. Drawings represent a small branch formed by origin of a pectinate muscle from larger crista terminalis. General direction of fiber orientation (confirmed histologically) is indicated by broken lines. Pattern of propagation is illustrated by solid lines with arrows. Waveforms in A were recorded with extracellular potassium concentration of 4.6 mEq/L, where propagation into branch is successful with both top-to-bottom and bottom-to-top stimulation. Waveforms in B were recorded at an extracellular potassium concentration of 9.0 mEq/L, resulting in a depolarization of resting potential and slowed conduction. Under these conditions, a wavefront initiated from top of preparation successfully propagated into branch, whereas propagation initiated from bottom of preparation failed to propagate into branch because of increased load associated with acute angle of junction. Reprinted with permission from Reference 52.

preparations indicating possible alterations in cellular connectivity associated with the use of ACE inhibitors.[78–80]

    Figure 19 demonstrates the role of alterations in microscopic load leading to propagation failure. In studies of dog atria, Spach and coworkers[51] placed electrodes along the longitudinal axis of a major atrial muscle bundle and an associated branch. When the preparation was bathed with a normal Tyrode's solution ([K] = 4.6 mmol/L), propagation into the branch succeeded when the preparation was stimulated either proximal or distal to the junction of the bundle and its branch. Increasing the bath [K] to 9.0 mmol/L resulted in a depolarization of the resting potential and concomitant reduction in available sodium channels (increased inactivation). Under these conditions, when the preparation was stimulated from a distal site, where the angle between the branch and primary bundle encountered by the incident wave was small, the wave front was able to propagate into the branch. However, when the preparation was stimulated at a site proximal to the branch, the incident wave faced a much greater branch-bundle angle, resulting in an increased load at the branch-bundle junction. Insufficient charge was available within the wave front to excite this additional load, so that propagation into the branch was blocked.

These results display the interaction between the wave front (source of current for supporting propagation) and the load presented by the underlying connectivity between adjacent cells (sink or load). That propagation failed in the above example can be viewed as evidence of the reduction in sodium channel availability due to the depolarized rest potential. Consequently, it would be instructive to explore with theoretical models the critical conditions, eg, sodium channel availability, for initiating reentry as a result of wave front–obstacle collisions.

In addition to alterations in cellular loading associated with the direction of propagation, Spach and Dolber[5] found in histological studies of human atrial tissue that there was an age-related increase in interstitial fibrosis (Figure 20). The loss in side-to-side connections would increase the transverse resistance and alter the properties of transverse propagation leading to alterations in the safety factor of propagation. If the increase in transverse resistance becomes large enough to be considered an obstacle, then wave-front fractionation might arise during transverse propagation. Such alterations, secondary to aging or perhaps hypertension,[5,47] could be considered arrhythmogenic.

The difficulties of studying discontinuous propagation has led to some clever studies that shed new light on the complex role cellular load plays in arrhythmogenic processes. By introducing a simple nonconducting obstacle into an otherwise homogeneous medium, it has been possible to study numerically[8,81] and analytically[8] the results of wave front–obstacle collisions and gain some insight into experimental studies of discontinuous propagation.[52]

Pertsov et al.[81] first explored the outcome of wave front–obstacle collisions with numerical studies of the FHN model by observing the results of a collision between a wave front and an obstacle while varying the amount of wave-front charge (Figure 21). The wave front charge was controlled by the parameter g_f (similar to the maximum sodium

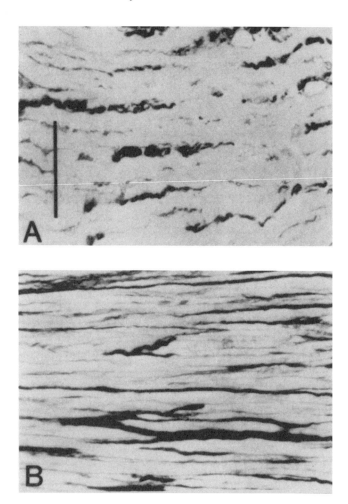

Figure 20. Collagenous septa in atrial tissue at different ages: longitudinal sections of pectinate muscle bundles from 12-year-old (A) and a 62-year-old (B) subjects stained by picrosirius red technique; septa appear dark gray to black. Collagen content is similar in two sections, but septa are generally much longer in B than in A, indicative of loss of side-to-side coupling in adjacent cells. Vertical bar in A = 200 μm; applicable to B as well. Reprinted with permission from Reference 5.

conductance, g_{Na}), which determined the peak-to-peak amplitude of f(V) in the FHN model (Equation 22). After wave front–obstacle collision, they observed two possible outcomes depending on the amplitude of f(V) as determined by the parameter g_f: (1) either the wave front collided with the obstacle and formed fragments that remained attached to the obstacle boundary or (2) the wave front collided with the

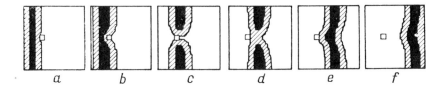

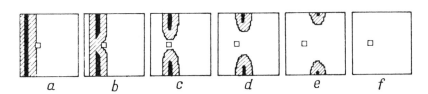

Figure 21. Wave front–obstacle interactions in a 2D array of FitzHugh-Nagumo cells. Top, Propagation of a wave in medium containing a nonexcitable portion (square close to center of medium). Parameter g_f used in these studies altered peak-to-peak amplitude of fast nullcline (sodium current) and is similar to parameter λ in Figure 5B. Stable regime ($g_f = 0.75$) is characterized by maintenance of wave front–obstacle contact after collision. a through c, Formation of break of wave; d through f, its disappearance. Dark regions to value of potential $E > 1.0$; shaded, $1 > E > 0$; and together, dark and light regions approximate spatial extent of wave. Interval in time between individual frames $\Delta t = 16$ (dimensionless units). Bottom, Unstable propagation of wave (gzf = 0.65). In this frame, conduction is slower, as indicated by shorter spatial extent of wave. Reduction in wave-front charge results in insufficient charge to maintain wave front–obstacle attachment so that wave front separates from obstacle. Reprinted with permission from Reference 81.

obstacle and formed fragments that separated from the obstacle. In case 1 (Figure 21, top), $g_f = 0.75$ and the wave fragments recombined after passing the obstacle, thus restoring the original wave front. In case 2 (Figure 21, bottom), $g_f = 0.65$, which reduced the wave-front charge such that the wave fragments were unable to maintain attachment with the obstacle boundary. The factor that separated wave-front attachment from wave-front separation was the peak-to-peak amplitude of the fast FHN nullcline, f(V) (Figure 5B), which is analogous to the sodium conductance in a nerve or cardiac model. Attenuating the peak-to-peak amplitude of f(V) by reducing g_f slowed propagation secondary to the reduction of the wave-front charge. Note the more narrow waves in the lower panels of Figure 21 compared with the waves in the upper panels. When the charge was reduced below a critical value, the tip of the wave fragment was no longer able to maintain contact with the obstacle boundary as the parent wave front continued to propagate. Consequently, the wave front separated from the obstacle.

Starobin et al[8] extended these exploratory studies and found that if the obstacle was sufficiently large, then the separated wave fragment could evolve into a reentrant wave. Moreover, they observed that if the obstacle was asymmetric, then a wave fragment could be pinched off after the mother fragments reattached, thus initiating a spiral wave (Figure 22). These studies[8,81] were the first to explore very primitive discontinuities, approximating those encountered in normal (Figure 19) and diseased tissue (Figure 20), in an otherwise homogeneous medium, and provided a theoretical basis for Spach's model of the arrhythmogenic potential of microscopic discontinuous propagation.[10]

It must be emphasized here that these theoretical and numerical studies were based on very primitive models of discontinuous propaga-

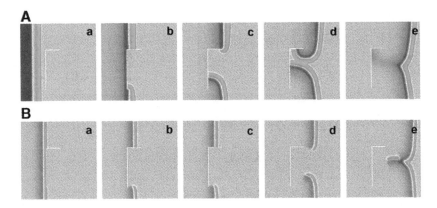

Figure 22. Dynamic studies of wave front–obstacle interactions and subsequent spawning of a wavelet in a 2D array of FitzHugh-Nagumo cells (same parameters as used to generate Figure 8). A and B, L-shaped obstacle and wave propagating from left to right. After wave front collides with obstacle, wave fragments either remain attached to obstacle (A) or separate from obstacle (B), depending on amount of source charge available in tip of wave. Wave-front (source) charge was controlled by slope of fast nullcline, λ (Figure 5B). When $\lambda = 0.9$, there was adequate charge to maintain contact between wave tip and obstacle (A). After collision, two wave fragments rejoined and restored original incident wave. When λ was reduced to 0.7 (similar to sodium channel blockade by a class I antiarrhythmic), charge in wave front was insufficient to maintain contact between wave tip and obstacle, resulting in separation. Right separated wave tip curled in response to increased load, and when two wave fragments collided and recombined, curled tip was "pinched off" and propagated as an independent wave fragment perpendicular to incident velocity vector. Such a mechanism can act as a source of multiple wavelets for atrial or ventricular fibrillation.[8]

tion. From the results of Starobin et al,[8] it became clear that under conditions of normal propagation velocities, the size of an obstacle necessary to initiate reentry almost always exceeded the size of the heart. However, if propagation velocity was impaired secondary to ion channel blockade or altered conduction due to reduced gap junction connectivity, then the size requirements were similarly reduced such that responses to premature stimulation and wave front–obstacle collisions could successfully lead to reentry.

The concept of wave front–obstacle separation represents an important new insight derived from analytic and numerical studies, for it provides an answer to the central question raised in Moe's multiple-wavelet hypothesis of fibrillation[63]: where did the multiple wavelets come from? As discussed above, wave fronts that collided with either a structural or functional (transiently refractory) obstacle either remained attached to or separated from the obstacle. If they remained attached, then the parent wave front was reconstructed as the two fragments recombined. However, if the fragments separated from the obstacle, then new wavelets were formed. Because recovery of excitability in Moe's model was proportional to the interstimulus interval, high-frequency stimulation resulted in reduced conduction velocity. Moe et al[63] found no evidence of arrhythmias with low-frequency stimulation. However, high-frequency stimulation resulted in a fibrillatory arrhythmia, indicating that slowed conduction was an essential element of the process of creating multiple wavelets. As we see in the studies by Pertsov et al[81] and Starobin et al,[8] separation following wave front–obstacle collisions secondary to reduced conduction velocities was an important new insight into arrhythmogenic conditions and provided another hypothesis compatible with the CAST results.[48]

Reentrant Activation and QRS Morphology

Once a wave fragment (discontinuous wave front) is created by blocked conduction, the fragment will curl in response to the local load seen by each point along the wave front. Typically, the ends of the fragment experience a greater load than the interior segments, such that the ends develop greater curvature, forming a figure-8 pattern of reentry. If there is adequate space for the wave front to curl, then reentry will succeed and a spiral wave will be formed (Figure 23).

The tip of the reentrant (spiral) wave is of particular interest. The tip can either rotate about a fixed structural obstacle or a stationary functional obstacle (depolarized region of block) or may drift and meander about the myocardium. When the wave front rotates about a fixed or stationary region (spiral core or region of block) and each

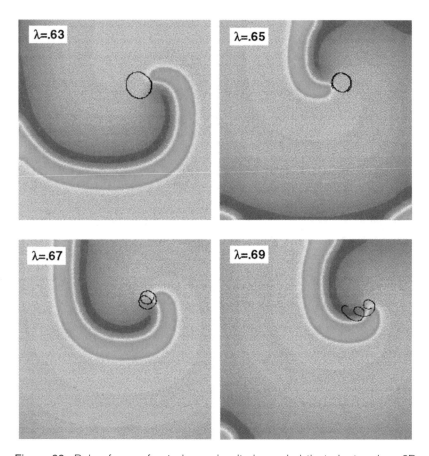

Figure 23. Role of wave-front charge in altering spiral tip trajectory in a 2D array of FitzHugh-Nagumo cells (same parameters as Figures 8 and 21). A through D, Spiral tip trajectory for increasing amounts of wave-front charge as determined by slope of fast nullcline (Figure 5B). When $\lambda = 0.62$, tip traced outline of a circle and produced a monomorphic pattern of QRS complexes seen in Figure 24. As slope was increased (B), Diameter of tip trajectory decreased. When $\lambda = 0.67$, tip diameter was similar to wave-front thickness, and tip departed from circular trajectory as if separating from an obstacle of high curvature. When λ was further increased to 0.69, meandering became more pronounced and ECG pattern became polymorphic as shown in Figure 22.

rotation of the wave front is associated with one rotation about the core, then the activation sequence from one reentrant cycle to the next will remain more or less constant. Such a stationary, repetitive activation sequence will produce the same QRS complex from one reentrant cycle to the next, resulting in a monomorphic pattern as seen on the ECG (Figure 24). However, if the range of tip motion is large and more

A   **Computed EKG**

Effect of gK on Polymorphic Waveforms

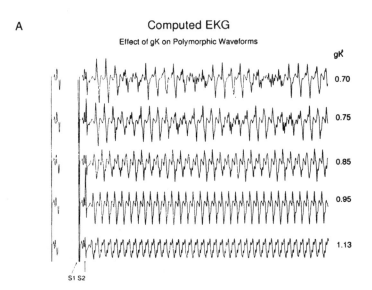

B   **Trajectory of the Spiral Tip**

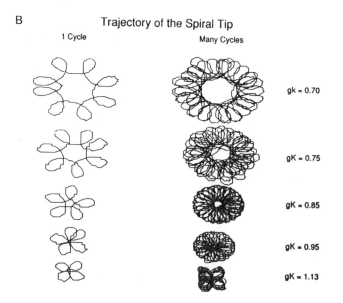

than one reentrant cycle is required for the tip to return to a starting point (as illustrated in Figure 23, lower panels), then the activation sequence will vary considerably from cycle to cycle, producing polymorphic QRS complexes in the ECG.[17,81-84] This complex tip behavior was recognized by Zykov[85] as being due to compound rotation derived from rotation of the tip around one region and the rotation of the spiral around its tip. The compound motion is that of two sinusoidal processes and hence gives a frequency spectrum that consists of two energy peaks, one associated with each rotational process.

Starmer and coworkers[17,82,86] were the first to confirm with numerical studies that increasing the action potential wavelength (by prolonging the action potential duration with potassium channel blockade) resulted in polymorphic QRS complexes during reentry. (Similar results have been obtained with increasing the amplitude of the background sodium current.) As shown in Figure 24, from studies of the FHN and Beeler-Reuter models, they found that either reducing the magnitude of the repolarizing current or increasing the magnitude of the depolarizing current prolonged the action potential duration (similar to that seen in long-QT syndrome [LQTS]) and amplified the range of tip motion. With the medium parameters used in these studies, the tip exhibited a simple meandering pattern characterized by a compound motion: that due to rapid rotation of the spiral wave (at a frequency f_{spiral}) and that due to a slower rotation around a core region (at a frequency f_{tip}). The resultant interaction of these two frequencies produced a Fourier spectrum characterized by sum and difference frequencies (Figure 25). As the magnitude of the repolarizing current was reduced, the action potential duration was prolonged, the size of the meandering pattern increased, and the degree of polymorphism in the ECG was amplified.

The relationship between the range of tip movement and the size of the medium reveals an interesting relationship between QRS morphology and the range of motion of the spiral tip.[86] When the range of motion is less than $\approx 25\%$ of the medium, the ECG will display mono-

---

Figure 24. Role of potassium conductance in destabilizing spiral tip trajectory in a 2D array of FitzHugh-Nagumo cells. Large values of g_K produced a short APD, which led to a small region of meandering of spiral tip. Activation sequence varied only slightly from one reentry cycle to next, producing a monomorphic ECG. A, As potassium conductance was reduced (from 1.13 to 0.7), region of meander was progressively increased, producing great variability in activation sequence, as reflected by increasing degrees of polymorphic QRS complexes in computed ECG. B, Trajectory of spiral tip is shown here as a single rotation of spiral tip around an unstable region of block (left) and multiple rotations (right).

Computed EKG

Monomorphic and Polymorphic EKGs

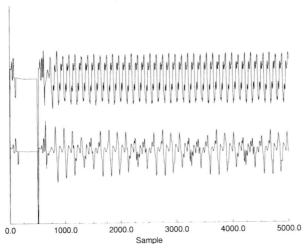

Fourier Spectrum

Monomorphic and Polymorphic EKGs

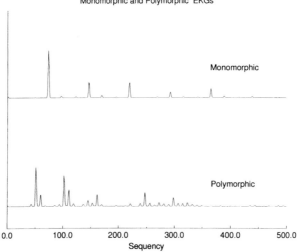

morphic QRS complexes. As the range of spiral tip motion increases, the QRS complexes associated with successive reentrant cycles becomes progressively more polymorphic, as shown in Figure 24. If one continues to increase the range of tip movement, then eventually the spatial requirements for sustaining reentry will be exceeded and the wave will die.

Inoue and colleagues[87] observed this unstable pattern of reactivation in epicardial activation patterns of torsade de pointes in canine myocardium during a period of quinidine-induced long QT (Figure 26). Mapping activation sequences during tachycardia induced by programmed stimulation, they observed that the point of earliest breakthrough varied in proportion to the degree of polymorphism. A monomorphic ECG was associated with a small variation in the points of earliest breakthrough, whereas a polymorphic ECG was associated with much greater variation in the points of earliest breakthrough. In studies of spiral drift in the presence of quinidine, Fast and Pertsov[88] showed that the curvature of the tip trajectory was altered as the tip crossed from a quinidine-free region of tissue to a quinidine-exposed region of tissue. More recently, Gray and colleagues,[89] using optical mapping techniques, observed polymorphic QRS patterns associated with unstationary motion of the spiral tip.

From both experimental and numerical studies of polymorphic tachyarrhythmias, it appears that the spatial duration of the action potential is a critical determinant of the motion of the tip of the wave front. Rapid reentrant tachyarrhythmias that exhibit longer spatial action potential durations are more likely to be polymorphic, and slower reentrant tachyarrhythmias are more likely to be monomorphic. Horowitz et al[90] have observed in patients with polymorphic tachyarrhythmias induced by programmed stimulation that adding a sodium

---

Figure 25. Because reentry is a repetitive process, stability of reentry, as reflected by degree of polymorphic patterns in ECG, can be evaluated with a Fourier transform of ECG. Shown here are computed monomorphic ECG and a polymorphic ECG as generated by different degrees of reduction in repolarizing current. Because monomorphic ECG reflects rotation around a small core region, activation sequence from one reentry cycle to next showed little variation, and Fourier transform revealed a single peak at reentry frequency and a simple pattern of harmonics. When repolarizing current was reduced, core became larger and unstable, producing significant variations in activation sequence between successive reentry cycles. This complex activation pattern was reflected by splitting of primary energy peaks seen in monomorphic spectrum, consistent with a model of two rotating processes: (1) reentrant wave front rotating around tip, and (2) tip rotating around unstable core as described in References 9 and 85.

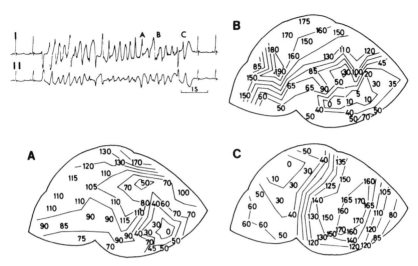

Figure 26. Episode of quinidine-associated torsade de pointes in a dog showing torsion of sharp points in both surface leads. Maps A through C correspond to beats A through C in surface ECG. A, QRS complex deflection was upward in lead I and downward in lead II. Earliest activation site was located in posterior left ventricle, and activation spread radially. B, Transitional QRS morphology. Earliest epicardial activation site had migrated to anterior left ventricle. Although activation spread radially away from point of earliest activation, activation sequence was more complex than observed in A and C. C, QRS complex showed downward deflection in lead I and upward in lead II. Earliest activation site moved far away from posterior left ventricle, where earliest activation site of beat A was located, to base of anterior right ventricle. Migration of points of earliest activation is consistent with that predicted by a meandering spiral wave. Reprinted with permission from Reference 87.

channel blocker (quinidine or procainamide) results in an inability to induce additional runs of polymorphic tachycardia. Rather, only monomorphic tachyarrhythmias were observed, and the rate of the monomorphic arrhythmia was less than that of the associated polymorphic episode (Figure 27). Thus, there is good qualitative agreement between the theoretical insights of spiral tip movement and the morphological variations of the QRS during reentry and observations derived from patient and animal studies.

Clinical Links: Long-QT Syndrome

It is amazing that within the space of 6 years, the links from alterations of a gene to the ECG manifestations of a serious cardiac arrhythmia, LQTS,[17,82,86,91–96] have all been identified. LQTS is an inherited

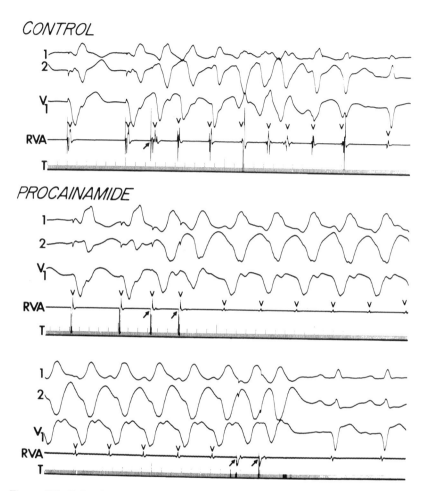

Figure 27. Role of conduction velocity in morphological composition of tachy-arrhythmias. Conversion of torsade de pointes to sustained ventricular tachy-cardia by conduction slowing secondary to procainamide. ECG leads 1, 2, and V_1 are shown, with electrograms recorded in right ventricular apex (RVA) and 10-ms time lines (T). In control panel, a single premature stimulus (arrow) initiated a spontaneously terminating polymorphic paroxysm of torsade de pointes. No other ventricular arrhythmia could be initiated by programmed stimulation (single or double extrastimuli) in control state. After 1500 mg of procainamide, which produced a blood level of 12.8 mg/L, sustained ventricu-lar tachycardia with a uniform, stable morphology was initiated with two prema-ture stimuli (arrows). Ventricular tachycardia was terminated by double extra-stimuli (bottom, arrows). Reprinted with permission from Reference 89.

disorder that is associated with delayed ventricular repolarization and reveals itself in terms of a high incidence of polymorphic ventricular arrhythmias and sudden cardiac death. Torsade de pointes is frequently observed in LQTS patients, and it is perhaps the only disease-related arrhythmia for which there is direct evidence of ion channel dysfunction. The tools to attack LQTS have come from many disciplines: molecular biology, computer science, the physics of excitable media, and cardiac electrophysiology, demonstrating the power of a multidisciplinary approach. Mathematical models of ion channels and excitable cells have provided the final link, showing that altered repolarization will lead to unstable reentrant activation that reveals itself as a polymorphic ECG.[17,82,86]

Genetic linkage studies of families with members exhibiting LQTS revealed alterations of three chromosomes, 3,[91] 7,[92] and 11,[93] and two of these (3 and 7) contain genes (SCN5A and HERG) that code for sodium[94] and potassium channels.[95] The mutant sodium channel exhibited delayed inactivation, whereas the mutant potassium channel exhibited an inactivation mechanism and may be similar to I_{Kr}, the rapidly inactivating delayed rectifier channel. The fact that both mutant sodium and potassium channels delay repolarization by reducing the net repolarizing current established the link between mutant channels and the disease.

Delayed repolarization increases the interval between the Q wave and the T wave under normal sinus conditions. Since different mutant genes code for different channels that can alter repolarizing currents, Moss et al[96] hypothesized that the T-wave morphology might vary, depending on the particular mutation a patient was carrying. With an elegant study, this team found that the ECG obtained from patients exhibiting each class of mutation displayed different T-wave morphologies. Those with alterations in chromosome 3 exhibited prolonged QT with a normal T-wave morphology, whereas those with alterations in chromosome 7 displayed prolonged QT with low-amplitude T wave, and those with alterations in chromosome 11 displayed prolonged QT with early-onset, broad-based T waves.

To complete the path from gene to polymorphic ECGs, one must identify the mechanism that links delayed repolarization to alterations in successive activation sequences during reentry. This question was answered with numerical studies.[17,82] They showed that after reentry initiated by programmed stimulation (simulating an early alterdepolarization), the reentrant wave front rotated around a region of block (core) that was nonstationary. The mobility of the core resulted in drift that altered the activation sequence from one reentrant cycle to the next, which was revealed by changes in the QRS complex between successive reentry cycles. These model studies provided the first direct link between polymorphic ECGs and delayed repolarization, thus completing the chain linking altered chromosomes that code for membrane ion channels with prolonged QT intervals in sinus rhythm ECGs and with polymorphic QRS patterns during reentry. On the basis of these numerical studies and the ECG studies of Moss et al,[96] we would anticipate that the polymorphic patterns observed during reentry in patients with LQTS will display unique patterns that are associated with the particular mutant gene that the patient carries.

Conclusions

What do we know about the link between spiral waves, reentrant arrhythmias, and the ECG? It is clear that physical/mathematical models of membrane ion channels and excitable membrane can be combined to build models of an excitable medium.[7,8,11,15,25,27,34,35,44,60,65] Carefully used, these models have proved to be useful tools for probing the properties of idealized continuous systems[6,7,16,17,66,67] and under some conditions, exploring propagation in the presence of discontinuities.[4,5,8,81]

The processes of impulse formation, liminal length, propagation, and vulnerability are generic properties of an excitable medium.[6–9,36,44,68] Consequently, basic arrhythmic processes that result from abnormal impulse formation, discontinuous propagation, and vulnerability can be explored at a preliminary level by use of a minimal model of an excitable medium, eg, the FHN model.[34,35] The beauty of the FHN model is that it is a minimally complex model consisting of a single, noninactivating inward and a single outward current. Because of its simplicity, proarrhythmic processes associated with alterations in liminal regions, threshold phenomena, and vulnerability can be explored analytically as well as numerically. Any property we find in an array of FHN cells, such as impulse formation, propagation, vulnerability, and meandering and reentrant activation, is highly likely to appear in any more complex system. The importance or significance of each property in arrhythmogenesis, however, may be either attenuated or amplified by the additional complexities that appear in physiological cells. In addition, the FHN model provides a computationally and analytically tractable basis for asking many questions about the generic nature of arrhythmogenesis and links between excitation patterns and QRS morphologies.

We have found that these primitive models accurately predict the existence of the vulnerable period[60] and its prolongation by sodium channel blockade (class I agents).[6,7,16] Similarly, they link a monomorphic ECG with a single reentrant wave front that rotates in a 1:1 manner (ie, one rotation of the tip around a stationary region for each rotation of the excitation wave front) about a small, stable region of block and a polymorphic ECG with a reentrant wave front that rotates in a 1:n manner about an unstable region of block.[17,82–86] These models permit primitive analysis of a medium with simple discontinuities,[8,81] which demonstrates initiation of reentry resulting from a propagating wave front experiencing a localized increase in load, similar to that observed in tissue studies.[5,52] These studies illustrate very clearly that explicit consideration of discontinuities in a conducting medium in theoretical and numerical studies must be aggressively pursued to improve our understanding of arrhythmogenesis associated with disease or aging.

Finally, what about arrhythmia control: should we focus on drugs or devices? The lessons of CAST can be viewed in the following light: Using drugs to alter ion channel properties in patients in whom there was little evidence of diseased-related channel dysfunction but considerable evidence of structural alterations did not succeed (ie, as my wise father told me, "Don't try to fix something that isn't broken"). Ion channel blockers, though, will probably find an increasingly important role in managing arrhythmias in patients with known ion channel dysfunction as seen in LQTS.[91–96] Here, rapidly unbinding drugs that bind to inactivated channels, such as lidocaine and mexiletine, may be particularly appropriate for suppressing early alterdepolarizations in patients with mutant *SVN5A* genes.[97]

With respect to "structural" disease that amplifies the effects of discontinuities in cellular interconnections, there may be a role for therapy that is unrelated to ion channel function.[47] There is considerable evidence of arrhythmias and sudden cardiac death associated with structural alterations in myocardial architecture secondary to myocardial infarction, hypertension, and aging. For hypertension- and age-related structural changes, agents such as ACE inhibitors that can reverse the accumulation of collagen in the interstitial space may turn out to be useful antiarrhythmic tools.[78–80] However, reversal of the proarrhythmic substrate resulting from loss of side-to-side cellular connections is predicated on whether gap junction connections between cells can be reestablished after reduction in interstitial collagen, thereby increasing the degree of uniform anisotropic connectivity.

Devices, starting with pacemakers and more recently with implantable defibrillators and antitachycardia devices, are clearly specific, and their efficacy appears to be high. But what about new devices that might alleviate some of the problems associated with today's implantable defibrillators? Here again, the theory of spiral waves sugggests an approach based on parametric resonance.[53–56] Recently Biktashev and Holden[98] demonstrated in numerical studies of atrial tissue that it was possible to terminate atrial reentry within 10 seconds of initiating a control strategy. Their strategy consisted of applying an external stimulus in synchrony with the frequency of reentry to alter the trajectory of the spiral tip.

Simple and complex models of membrane ionic currents and multicellular preparations are playing an important role both in understanding the detailed nature of cell excitation, impulse formation, and wave-front propagation and in designing arrhythmia control devices. Although continuous models have provided important insights into arrhythmogenic mechanisms, it is clear that for some situations, extending our understanding of conduction from a continuous medium to a discontinuous medium is limited. Thus, models of continuous and discontinuous media will remain important laboratory tools.

We wish to acknowledge the many "running" discussions between Dr. Starmer and Dr. M.S. Spach that brought a new awareness of the link between cellular connections, membrane ionic currents, and propagating wave fronts.

References

1. Mayer AG. The cause of pulsation. *Popular Sci Monthly.* 1908;73:481–487.
2. Mines GR. On dynamic equilibrium in the heart. *J Physiol.* 1913;46:349–383.
3. Garrey WE. The nature of fibrillary contraction of the heart: its relation to tissue mass and form. *Am J Physiol.* 1914;33:397–414.
4. Spach MS, Heidlage JF. The stochastic nature of cardiac propagation at a microscopic level: electrical description of myocardial architecture and its application to conduction. *Circ Res.* 1995;76:366–380.
5. Spach MS, Dolber PC. Relating extracellular potentials and their derivatives to anisotropic propagation at a microscopic level in human cardiac muscle: evidence for electrical uncoupling of side-to-side fiber connections with increasing age. *Circ Res.* 1986;58:356–371.
6. Starmer CF, Biktashev VN, Romashko DN, Stepanov MR, Makarova ON, Krinsky VI. Vulnerability in an excitable medium: analytical and numerical studies of initiating unidirectional propagation. *Biophys J.* 1993;65: 1775–1787.
7. Starobin J, Zilberter YI, Starmer CF. Vulnerability in one-dimensional excitable media. *Physica D.* 1994;72:321–341.
8. Starobin J, Zilberter YI, Rusnak EM, Starmer CF. Wavefront formation in excitable cardiac tissue: the role of wavefront-obstacle interactions in initiating high frequency fibrillatory-like arrhythmias. *Biophys J.* 1996;70:581–584.
9. Mikhailov AS. *Foundations of Synergetics I.* 2nd ed. Heidelberg, Germany: Springer-Verlag; 1994.
10. Spach MS, Dolber PC, Heidlage JF. Influence of the passive anisotropic properties on directional differences in propagation following modification of the sodium conductance in human atrial muscle: a model of reentry based on anisotropic discontinuous propagation. *Circ Res.* 1988;62:811–832.
11. Hodgkin AL, Huxley AF. A quantitative description of the membrane current and its application to conduction and excitation in nerve. *J Physiol (Lond).* 1952;117:500–544.

12. Grant AO, Starmer CF, Strauss HC. Unitary sodium channels in isolated cardiac myocytes of rabbit. *Circ Res.* 1983;53:823–829.
13. Alberts B, Bray D, Lewis J, Raff M, Roberts K, Watson JD. *Molecular Biology of the Cell.* 3rd ed. New York, NY: Garland; 1994:534–535.
14. Thomson W. On the theory of the electric telegraph. [From the *Proc R Soc,* May, 1855.] In: Sir William Thomson (Lord Kelvin). *Mathematical and Physical Papers, Vol. 2.* Cambridge, UK: Cambridge University Press; 1885: 61–76.
15. Beeler GW, Reuter H. Reconstruction of the action potential of ventricular myocardial fibers. *J Physiol (Lond).* 1977;286:177–210.
16. Starmer CF, Lastra AA, Nesterenko VV, Grant AO. Proarrhythmic response to sodium channel blockade: theoretical model and numerical experiments *Circulation.* 1991;84:1364–1377.
17. Starmer CF, Romashko DN, Reddy RS, et al. Proarrhythmic response to potassium channel blockade: numerical studies of polymorphic tachyarrhythmias. *Circulation.* 1995;92:595–605.
18. Cohen IS, Strichartz GR. On the voltage-dependent action of tetrodotoxin. *Biophys J.* 1977;17:275–279.
19. Walton M, Fozzard HA. The relation of V_{max} to I_{Na}, G_{Na} and h_∞ in a model of the cardiac Purkinje fiber. *Biophys J.* 1979;25:407–420.
20. Cohen CJ, Bean BP, Tsien RW. Maximal upstroke velocity as an index of available sodium conductance: comparison of maximal upstroke velocity and voltage clamp measurements of sodium current in rabbit Purkinje fibers. *Circ Res.* 1984;54:636–651.
21. Weidmann S. Effects of calcium ions and local anaesthetics on electrical properties of Purkinje fibers. *J Physiol. (Lond).* 1955;129:568–582.
22. Johnson EA, McKinnon MG. The differential effect of quinidine and pyralamine on the myocardial action potential at various rates of stimulation. *J Pharmacol Exp Ther.* 1957;120:460–468.
23. Heistracher P. Elektrophysiologische Untersuchungen über den Mechanismus der Wirkung eines Antifibrillans auf die Anstiegssteilheit des Aktionspotentials von Purkinje-Fasern. *Pflugers Arch.* 1964;279:305–329.
24. Heistracher P. Mechanism of action of antifibrillatory drugs. *Naunyn Schmiedeberg Arch Pharmacol.* 1971;269:199–212.
25. Armstrong CM. Time course of TEA-induced anomalous rectification in squid giant axons. *J Gen Physiol.* 1966;50:491–502.
26. Armstrong CM. Inactivation of the potassium conductance and related phenomena caused by quaternary ammonium ion injection in squid axons. *J Gen Physiol.* 1969;54:553–575.
27. Starmer CF, Grant AO. Phasic ion channel blockade: a kinetic model and method for parameter estimation. *Mol Pharmacol.* 1985;28:348–356.
28. Starmer CF, Packer DL, Grant AO. Ligand binding to transiently accessible sites: mechanisms for varying apparent binding rates. *J Theor Biol.* 1987; 124:335–341.
29. Bean BP, Cohen CJ, Tsien RW. Lidocaine block of cardiac sodium channels. *J Gen Physiol.* 1983;81:613–642.
30. Gilliam FR, Starmer CF, Grant AO. Blockade of rabbit atrial sodium channels by lidocaine: characterization of continuous and frequency-dependent blocking. *Circ Res.* 1989;65:723–739.
31. Hille B. Local anesthetics: hydrophilic and hydrophobic pathways for the drug-receptor reaction. *J Gen Physiol.* 1977;69:497–515.
32. Hondeghem LM, Katzung BG. Time and voltage-dependent interactions

of antiarrhythmic drugs with cardiac sodium channels. *Biochim Biophys Acta.* 1977;472:373–398.

33. Starmer CF, Nesterenko VV, Undrovinas AI, Grant AO, Rosenshtraukh LV. Lidocaine blockade of continuously and transiently accessible sites in cardiac sodium channels. *J Mol Cell Cardiol.* 1991;23(suppl I):75–83.

34. FitzHugh R. Impulses and physiological states in theoretical models of nerve membrane. *Biophys J.* 1961;1:445–466.

35. Nagumo J, Arimoto S, Yoshizawa S. An active pulse transmission line simulating nerve axon. *Proc IRE.* 1962;50:2061–2070.

36. Scott AC. The electrophysics of a nerve fiber. *Rev Mod Phys.* 1975;47:487–533.

37. Krinsky VI, Kokoz YM. Analysis of equations of excitable membranes, I: reduction of the Hodgkin-Huxley equations to a second order system. *Biofizika.* 1973;18:506–511.

38. Rinzel J. Excitation dynamics: insights from simplified membrane models. *Fed Proc.* 1985;44:2944–2946.

39. Gadsby DC, Cranefield PF. Two levels of resting potential in cardiac Purkinje fibers. *J Gen Physiol.* 1977;70:725–746.

40. Hiraoka M, Sunami A, Fan Z, Sawanobori T. Multiple ionic mechanisms of early afterdepolarization in isolated ventricular myocytes from guinea-pig hearts. *Ann N Y Acad Sci.* 1992;644:33–47.

41. January CT, Riddle JM. Early afterdepolarizations: mechanism of induction and block: a role for L-type Ca^{2+} current. *Circ Res.* 1989;64:977–990.

42. Colatsky TJ. Mechanisms of action of lidocaine and quinidine on action potential duration in rabbit cardiac Purkinje fibers: an effect on steady state sodium current? *Circ Res.* 1982;50:17–27.

43. Zilberter YI, Starmer CF, Starobin J, Grant AO. Late Na channels in cardiac cells: the physiological role of background Na channels. *Biophys J.* 1994;67:153–160.

44. Fozzard HA, Schoenberg M. Strength-duration curves in cardiac Purkinje fibres: effects of liminal length and charge distribution. *J Physiol.* 1972;226:593–618.

45. Rushton WAH. Initiation of the propagated disturbance. *Proc R Soc Lond B.* 1937;124:210–243.

46. Spach MS, Heidlage JF, Darken ER, Hofer E, Raines KH, Starmer CF. Cellular Vmax reflects both membrane properties and the load presented by adjoining cells. *Am J Physiol.* 1992;263:H1855–H1863.

47. Spach MS, Starmer CF. Altering the topology of gap junctions: a major therapeutic target for atrial fibrillation. *Cardiovasc Res.* 1995;30:336–344.

48. The Cardiac Arrhythmia Suppression Trial (CAST) Investigators. Preliminary report: effect of encainide and flecainide on mortality in a randomized trial of arrhythmia suppression after myocardial infarction. *N Engl J Med.* 1989;321:406–412.

49. Nesterenko VV, Lastra AA, Rosenshtraukh LV, Starmer CF. A proarrhythmic response to sodium channel blockade: prolongation of the vulnerable period in guinea-pig ventricular myocardium. *J. Cardiol Pharmacol.* 1992;19:810–820.

50. Starmer CF, Lancaster AR, Lastra AA, Grant AO. Cardiac instability amplified by use-dependent Na channel blockade. *Am J Physiol.* 1992;262:H1305–H1310.

51. Spach MS, Miller WT, Dolber PC, Kootsey JM, Sommer JR, Mosher CE. The functional role of structural complexities in the propagation of depolar-

ization in the atrium of the dog: cardiac conduction disturbances due to discontinuities of effective axial resistivity. *Circ Res.* 1982;50:175–191.

52. Spach MS, Miller WT, Geselowitz DB, Barr RC, Kootsey JM, Johnson EA. The discontinuous nature of propagation in normal canine cardiac muscle: evidence for recurrent discontinuities of intracellular resistance that affect the membrane currents. *Circ Res.* 1981;48:39–54.

53. Grill S, Zykov VS, Muller SC. Feedback-controlled dynamics of meandering spiral waves. *Phys Rev Lett.* 1995;75:3368–3371.

54. Munuzuri AP, Gomez-Gesteira M, Perez-Munuzuri V, Krinsky VI, Perrez-Villar V. Mechanism of the electric-field-induced vortex drift in excitable media. *Phys Rev E.* 1993;48:R3232–R3235.

55. Krinsky VI, Agladze KI. Interaction of rotating waves in an active chemical medium. *Physica D.* 1983;8:50–56.

56. Marcus M, Nagy-Ungvaray Z, Hess B. Phototaxis of spiral waves. *Science.* 1992;257:225–227.

57. Garfinkel A, Spano ML, Ditto WL, Weiss JN. Controlling cardiac chaos. *Science.* 1992;257:1230–1235.

58. Schiff SJ, Jerger K, Duong DH, Chang T, Spano ML, Ditto WL. Controlling chaos in the brain. *Nature.* 1994;370:615–620.

59. Wiggers CJ, Wegria R. Quantitative measurement of the fibrillation thresholds of the mammalian ventricle with observations on the effects of procaine. *Am J Physiol.* 1940;131:296.

60. Wiener N, Rosenblueth A. The mathematical formulation of the problem of conduction of impulses in a network of connected excitable elements, specifically in cardiac muscle. *Arch Inst Cardiol Mex.* 1946;16:205–265.

61. Krinsky VI. Mathematical models of cardiac arrhythmias (spiral waves). *Pharmacol Ther.* 1978;3(pt B):539–555.

62. Joyner RW. Effects of the discrete pattern of electrical coupling on propagation through an electrical syncytium. *Circ Res.* 1982;50:192–200.

63. Moe GK, Reinbolt WC, Abildskov JA. A computer model of atrial fibrillation. *Am Heart J.* 1964;67:338–356.

64. Shaw RM, Rudy Y. The vulnerable window for unidirectional block in cardiac tissue: characterization and dependence on membrane excitability and intercellular coupling. *J Cardiovasc Electrophysiol.* 1995;6:115–131.

65. Luo C, Rudy Y. A dynamic model of the cardiac ventricular action potential, I: simulation of ionic currents and concentration changes. *Circ Res.* 1994;74:1071–1096.

66. Gul'ko FB, Petrov AA. Mechanism of the formation of closed pathways of conduction in excitable media. *Biofizika.* 1972;17:271–282.

67. van Capelle FJL, Durrer D. Computer simulation of arrhythmias in a network of coupled excitable elements. *Circ Res.* 1980;47:454–466.

68. Winfree AT. *When Time Breaks Down.* Princeton, NJ: Princeton University Press: 1987:181–186.

69. Wit AL, Rosen MR, Hoffman BF. Electrophysiology and pharmacology of cardiac arrhythmias, II: relationship of normal and abnormal electrical activity of cardiac fibers to the genesis of arrhythmias, B: reentry. *Am Heart J.* 1974;88:664–670.

70. Allessie RA, Bonke FIM, Schoopman FJG. Circus movement in rabbit atrial muscle as a mechanism of tachycardia, III: the 'leading circle' concept: a new model of circus movement in cardiac tissue without the involvement of an anatomical obstacle. *Circ Res.* 1977;41:9–18.

71. Crumb WB, Clarkson CW. Characterization of cocaine-induced block of cardiac sodium channels. *Biophys J.* 1990;57:589–599.

72. Barber JM, Starmer CF, Grant AO. Blockade of cardiac sodium channels by amitriptyline and diphenylhydantoin: evidence for two use-dependent binding sites. *Circ Res.* 1991;69:677–696.

73. Whitcomb DC, Gilliam FR, Starmer CF, Grant AO. Marked QRS complex abnormalities and sodium channel blockade by propoxyphene reversed with lidocaine. *J Clin Invest.* 1989;84:1629–1636.

74. Clarkson CW, Hondeghem LM. Evidence for a specific receptor site for lidocaine, quinidine, and bupivacaine associated with cardiac sodium channels in guinea pig ventricular myocardium. *Circ Res.* 1985;56:496–506.

75. Starmer CF. Theoretical characterization of ion channel blockade: competitive binding to periodically accessible receptors. *Biophys J.* 1987;52:405–412.

76. Krinsky VI. Spread of excitation in an inhomogeneous medium (state similar to cardiac fibrillation). *Biofizika.* 1966;11:676–683.

77. Belousov BP. A periodic reaction and its mechanism. (From his archives [in Russian], 1951). English translation: In: Field RJ, Berurger M, eds. *Oscillations and Travelling Waves in Chemical Systems.* New York, NY: Wiley;1985: 605–613.

78. Jones JV, James MA. ACE inhibitors and the heart: hypertrophy reversal and antiarrhythmic effects. *J Hum Hypertens.* 1990;4(suppl 4):23–27.

79. Katwa LC, Ratajska A, Cleutjens JPM, et al. Angiotensin converting enzyme and kinase-II-like activities in cultured valvular interstitial cells of the rat heart. *Cardiovasc Res.* 1995;29:57–64.

80. Kohya T, Yokoshiki H, Tohse N, et al. Regression of left ventricular hypertrophy prevents ischemia-induced lethal arrhythmias: beneficial effect of angiotensin II blockade. *Circulation.* 1995;76:892–899.

81. Pertsov AM, Panfilov AV, Medvedeva FU. Instability of autowaves in excitable media associated with the phenomenon of critical curvature. *Biofizika.* 1983;28:103–107.

82. Starmer CF, Reddy MR, Namasivayam A, Singh M. Potassium channel blockade amplifies cardiac instability: numerical studies of torsades de pointes. *Indian J Physiol Pharmacol.* 1994;38:259–266.

83. Gray RA, Jalife J, Panfilov A, et al. Nonstationary vortexlike reentrant activity as a mechanism of polymorphic ventricular tachycardia in the isolated rabbit heart. *Circulation.* 1995;91:2454–2469.

84. Davidenko JM. Spiral wave activity: a possible common mechanism for polymorphic and monomorphic ventricular tachycardias. *J Cardiovasc Electrophysiol.* 1993;4:730–746.

85. Zykov VS. Cycloid circulation of spiral waves in an excitable medium. *Biofizika.* 1986;31:862–865.

86. Starmer CF, Starobin J. Spiral tip movement: the role of the action potential wavelength in polymorphic cardiac arrhythmias. *Int J Chaos Bifurcations.* 1996;6:1909–1923.

87. Inoue H, Murakawa Y, Toda I, et al. Epicardial activation patterns of torsade de pointes in canine hearts with quinidine-induced long QT interval but without myocardial infarction. *Am Heart J.* 1986;111:1080–1087.

88. Fast VG, Pertsov AM. Shift and termination of functional reentry in isolated ventricular preparations with quinidine-induced inhomogeneity in refractory period. *J Cardiovasc Electrophysiol.* 1992;3:255–265.

89. Gray RA, Jalife J, Panfilov AV, et al. Mechanism of cardiac fibrillation. *Science.* 1995;270:1222–1223.

90. Horowitz LN, Greenspan AM, Spielman SR, Josephson ME. Torsade de pointes: electrophysiologic studies in patients without transient pharmacologic or metabolic abnormalities. *Circulation.* 1981;63:1120–1128.

91. Wang Q, Shen J, Splawski I, et al. SCN5A mutations cause an inherited cardiac arrhythmia, long QT syndrome. *Cell.* 1995;80:805–811.
92. Keating M, Atkinson D, Dunn C, Timothy K, Vincent GM, Leppert M. Linkage of cardiac arrhythmia, the long QT syndrome, and the Harvey ras-1 gene. *Science.* 1991;252:704–706.
93. Curran ME, Splawski I, Timothy K, Vincent GM, Green E, Keating MT. A molecular basis for cardiac arrhythmia: HERG mutations cause long QT syndrome. *Cell.* 1995;80:795–803.
94. Bennett PB, Yazawa K, Makita N, George AL. Molecular mechanism for an inherited cardiac arrhythmia. *Nature.* 1995;376:683–685.
95. Trudeau MC, Warmke JW, Ganetky B, Robertson GA. HERG, a human inward rectifier in the voltage-gated potassium channel family. *Science.* 1995;269:92–95.
96. Moss AJ, Zareba W, Benhorin J, et al. ECG T-wave patterns in genetically distinct forms of the hereditary long QT syndrome. *Circulation.* 1995;92: 2929–2934.
97. Schwartz PJ, Priori SG, Locati EH, et al. Long QT syndrome patients with mutations of the *SCN5A* and *HERG* genes have differential responses to Na$^+$ channel blockade and to increases in heart rate: implications for gene-specific therapy. *Circulation.* 1995;92:3381–3386.
98. Biktashev VN, Holden AV. Control of reentrant activity in a model of mammalian atrial tissue. *Proc R Soc Lond B.* 1995;260:211–217.

Section V

Junctional Channels and Molecular Genetics:
Introduction

David C. Spray, PhD

The heart can be viewed as a series of communication compartments in which cells of each compartment are coupled to one another and at compartmental boundaries are coupled to cells that compose other cardiac regions (Figure 1). Fundamental features of cardiac organization include the findings that coupling is stronger in some compartments than in others, that coupling within a compartment may be stronger in one direction than another (anisotropy), and that the different gap junction proteins (connexins) are expressed in the different communication compartments. Because different connexins have different affinities for one another and different physiological properties (see chapters 8 and 15), connexin type may confer selective advantage for conduction speed or ionic selectivity or even to prevent inappropriate connections between compartments (eg, to prevent leakage of current to the underlying myocardium along the length of the conduction system).

Gap junctions are altered in specific disease states and in certain animal models (Table 1). These changes enhance conduction discontinuities, thereby altering conduction velocity, desynchronizing contraction, and exaggerating tissue anisotropy. Because gap junction function is altered under pathological conditions, it is reasonable to ask whether therapeutic strategies might be developed whereby conduction disturbances could be corrected through targeting gap junction function, expression, or distribution. Pharmacological approaches to correction

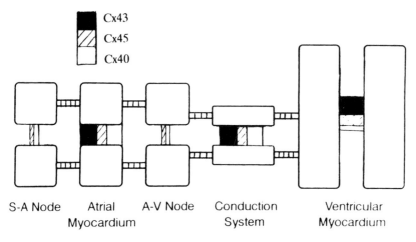

<table>
<tr><td>S-A Node</td><td>Atrial
Myocardium</td><td>A-V Node</td><td>Conduction
System</td><td>Ventricular
Myocardium</td></tr>
</table>

Figure 1. Intercellular communication compartments in the heart and connexins that join them. Cells that compose cardiac tissue include those specialized for pacemaking (sinoatrial [S-A] and atrioventricular [A-V] nodes), contraction (atrial and ventricular myocardium), and conduction (Purkinje system and His bundle). Strength of coupling within and between cardiac cell compartments (indicated diagrammatically by width of parallel lines connecting blocks within compartments) varies from rather weak (nodal tissue) to very strong (conduction system, working myocardium). Type of connexin expressed in each communication compartment also varies, as indicated by relative contribution of symbols for Cx43 (solid box), Cx40 (open box), and Cx45 (hatched box). Coupling at interfaces between compartments (horizontal lines connecting cell types in lower portion of figure) is generally weak, resulting in localized changes in conduction velocity in these regions; connexin types that compose these interfaces are not known, and these connections are symbolized by vertical stripes. Impulse generation and conduction occur from left to right in lower set of compartments.

of gap junction dysfunction need to be more thoroughly explored; this is dealt with in other sections of this volume. The chapters in this section describe the status of knowledge of gene and transcript regulation for the cardiac gap junction proteins and outline various strategies using molecular genetic techniques that are useful in generating experimental models and potentially of therapeutic utility.

Chapter 15 highlights connexin diversity and regional specificity of connexin expression patterns, along with a description of how functional properties may differ and how these channel proteins may be modified posttranslationally by phosphorylation and degraded through the ubiquitin pathway. In addition, this chapter summarizes studies that have been performed in acute or tissue-culture situations using transfection, antisense oligonucleotide, and negative-dominant strategies. Chapter 16 stresses the in vivo approach, emphasizing stud-

Table 1

Alterations in Connexin Expression

Pathological condition	Defect
Chronic *Trypanosoma cruzi* infection	Reduction in Cx43[1]
Acute cardiocyte *T cruzi* infection	Rearrangement of Cx43[2]
Postinfarct myocardium	Reduction and rearrangement of Cx43[3,4]
Stab wound in brain	Reduction in Cx43[5]
Facial nerve lesion	Increase in Cx43[6]
Epileptic cortex	Increase in Cx43[7]
Hypertensive rats	Increase in Cx40, decrease in Cx43[8]
Hypertensive vessels	Abnormal endothelial gap junctions[9]
X-linked Charcot-Marie-Tooth disease	Coding region mutations in Cx32[10]
Heterovisceral atriotaxia	Cx43 phosphorylation site mutations[11]
Transgenic animals	
Cx43 knockout	Ventricular hyperplasia; neonatal lethal[12]
Cx32 knockout	Decreased glucose liver mobilization[13]
Cx46 knockout	Cataracts in lens[14]
Cx37 knockout	Impaired oogenesis[15]
Cx26 knockout	Early embryonic lethal[16]
Cx43 overexpression	Laterality defects[17]
Cx43 underexpression	Embryonic laterality defects[17]
Cx43 negative dominant	Embryonic lethal[18]

ies performed on Cx43 knockout animals, transcriptional control studies in situ, and novel strategies targeting gap junction overexpression or underexpression or connexin swapping in specific cardiac compartments, at specific developmental times, or with promoters that can be turned on and off as needed.

The strategies and concepts represented by these chapters are at the leading edge of the field, pioneering the next phase in our understanding of discontinuous conduction by providing new experimental approaches for testing hypotheses regarding the functions of gap junctions in normal and diseased myocardium. It is a rich and fertile field for physiological, pharmacological, and biochemical studies and will surely result in progress in understanding communication within the heart and the potential benefits for cardiac function of manipulating coupling between different cellular compartments.

References

1. Saez J, Spray DC, Wittner M, et al. Effect of verapamil on cardiac gap junctions in murine Chagas's disease. *Mem Inst Oswaldo Cruz.* 1993;33:64.

2. Campos de Carvalho AC, Tanowitz HB, Wittner M, Dermietzel R, Roy C, Spray DC. Gap junction distribution is altered between cardiac myocytes infected with *Trypanosoma cruzi*. *Circ Res.* 1992;70:733–742.
3. Severs NJ. Pathophysiology of gap junctions in heart disease. *J Cardiovasc Electrophysiol.* 1994;5:461–475. Review.
4. Luke RA, Saffitz JE. Remodeling of ventricular conduction pathways in healed canine infarct border zones. *J Clin Invest.* 1991;87:1594–1602.
5. Muller CM. Gap junction-mediated communication between astrocytes in mammalian cortical slices. In: Spray DC, Dermietzel R, eds. *Gap Junctions in the Nervous System.* RG Austin, TX: Landes; in press.
6. Rohlmann A, Laskawi R, Hofer A, et al. Facial nerve lesions lead to increased immunostaining of the astrocytic gap junction protein (connexin43) in the corresponding facial nucleus of rats. *Neurosci Lett.* 1993;154:206–208.
7. Naus CC, Bechberger JF, Paul DL. Gap junction gene expression in human seizure disorder. *Exp Neurol.* 1991;111:198–203.
8. Bastide B, Neyses L, Ganten D, Paul M, Willecke K, Traub O. Gap junction protein connexin40 is preferentially expressed in vascular endothelium and conductive bundles of rat myocardium and is increased under hypertensive conditions. *Circ Res.* 1993;73:1138–1149.
9. Huttner I, Costabella PM, De Chastonay C, Gabbiani G. Volume, surface, and junctions of rat aortic endothelium during experimental hypertension: a morphometric and freeze fracture study. *Lab Invest.* 1982;46:489–504.
10. Bergoffen J, Scherer SS, Wang S, et al. Connexin mutations in X-linked Charcot-Marie-Tooth disease. *Science.* 1993;262:2039–2042.
11. Britz-Cunninghman, SH, Maithili, MS, Zuppan, CW, Fletcher, WH. Mutations of the connexin43 gap junction gene in patients with heart malformations and defects of laterality. *N Engl J Med.* 1995;332:1323–1329.
12. Reaume, AG, deSousa, PA, Kulkarni, S, et al. Cardiac malformation in neonatal mice lacking connexin43. *Science.* 1995;267:1831–1834.
13. Nelles E, Butzler C, Jung D, et al. Defective propagation of signals generated by sympathetic nerve stimulation in the liver of connexin 32-deficient mice. *Proc Natl Acad Sci USA.* 1996;93:9565–9570.
14. Kumar, N. Gilula NB. Presentation at Keystone Conference, 1996.
15. Simon AM, Goodenough DA, Li E, Paul DL. Female infertility in mice lacking connexin 37. *Nature.* 1997;385:525–529.
16. Willecke K, Winterhager E. Personal communication.
17. Lo CW, Ewart J, Sullivan R. Neural tube defects in transgenic mice with the gain or loss of connexin43 function: relevance to developmental pathologies. 1995 Gap Junction Conference.
18. Paul DL, Yu K, Bruzzone R, Gimlich RL, Goodenough DA. Expression of a dominant negative inhibitor of intercellular communication in the early Xenopus embryo causes delamination and extrusion of cells. *Development.* 1995;121:371–381.

Molecular and Biochemical Regulation of Connexins
Potential Targets for Modulation of Cardiac Intercellular Communication

Eric C. Beyer, MD, PhD,
Jeffrey E. Saffitz, MD, PhD,
Lloyd M. Davis, MBBS, PhD,
James G. Laing, PhD,
Viviana M. Berthoud, PhD,
Peter N. Tadros, MD,
and Richard D. Veenstra, PhD

In the myocardium, gap junction channels facilitate action potential propagation. The microscopic distribution of myocardial gap junctions can have substantial influence on the patterns of electrical conduction in normal cardiac tissues and in regions that have been pathologically disturbed, as by myocardial infarction. It is likely that the molecular composition of cardiac gap junctions may also be an important contributor to cardiac conduction. Many laboratories have contributed to the elucidation of the structure and physiology of cardiac gap junctions. Several years ago, our laboratories began cloning cDNAs and genomic DNA sequences that encode gap junction proteins, especially those expressed in the heart.[1] We have since used those molecular probes to examine the molecular, physiological, cellular, and biochemical regulation of cardiac gap junctions in a variety of tissues.

Supported by NIH grants HL-45466, HL-50598, an American Heart Association Established Investigator Award (to ECB), and a fellowship from the American Heart Association, Missouri Affiliate (to JGL).

From: Spooner PM, Joyner RW, Jalife J (eds). *Discontinuous Conduction in the Heart.* Armonk, NY: Futura Publishing Company, Inc.; © 1997.

To evaluate the role of gap junction pathology in discontinuous cardiac conduction, model systems must be developed with specific perturbations of gap junction expression and distribution. Manipulation of gap junctions may also eventually become a desirable therapeutic intervention, and these studies will be highlighted with our own work in the review that follows.

Gap Junction Structure and Connexin Sequences

Most cardiac gap junctions contain many intercellular channels. Each channel is an oligomeric structure formed of two hemichannels each containing multiple (probably six) subunit proteins called connexins (Cx), which surround a central aqueous pore[2,3] (Figure 1). Molecular cloning studies have demonstrated that there is an extended family of connexin genes; more than a dozen mammalian connexins have been

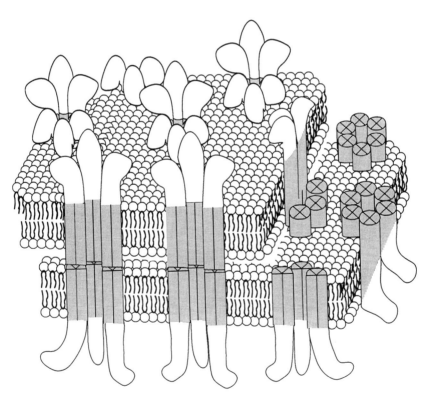

Figure 1. Structural model of a gap junction plaque based on x-ray diffraction and electron microscopy studies of isolated rodent liver gap junctions.

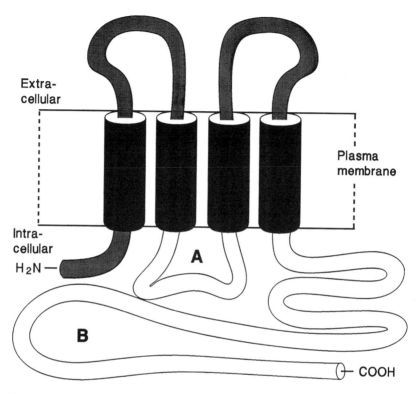

Figure 2. Topological model of connexin orientation within junctional plasma membrane. Shaded regions represent sequences shared among all connexins. Unshaded cytoplasmic domains correspond to unique, connexin-specific regions.

identified thus far. Each connexin contains two regions, each containing ≈100 amino acids, which are highly conserved in all connexins (dark shading in Figures 1 and 2). Hydropathy analyses of the connexin sequences have been used to prepare a topological model of the connexin within the junctional membrane (Figure 2). This model suggests that conserved sequences lie within transmembrane and extracellular regions, whereas connexin-specific sequences are cytoplasmic. This model has been supported by immunocytochemical and proteolysis studies of isolated gap junctions (reviewed in Reference 4).

Connexin Distribution

Different connexins are expressed at different stages of development and within different tissues of the mature organism. Cx43, a major component of ventricular gap junctions, was initially cloned from a cDNA library derived from rat heart, which established its expression in that organ.[1] Many other connexins were cloned from cDNAs from other sources or from genomic DNA. The expression patterns of various connexins have been established by several techniques, including RNA blots of organ homogenates, in situ hybridization, and immunohistochemistry of cells and tissue sections. Cx37, Cx40, Cx43, Cx45, and Cx46 mRNAs have all been detected in heart homogenates.[1,5–10] Immunoreactivity to an MP70 antibody has also been detected in heart.[11] Thus, six (or more) connexins may be expressed in this organ. However, only Cx40, Cx43, and Cx45 have been detected in cardiac myocytes.[7,12] Cx37 mRNA is expressed by cultured endothelial cells derived from bovine aorta and human umbilical vein.[5] The cardiac cells that express the other connexins have not been identified. None of the connexins are "cardiac-specific"; all are also detected in other organs.

Cx40, Cx43, and Cx45 are all expressed in canine ventricular myocytes, as demonstrated by RNA blot analysis and immunofluorescence.[7] Further, these connexins colocalize to identical distributions in the ventricular myocytes, as demonstrated by confocal immunofluorescence microscopy.[12] Double-label immunoelectron microscopy has shown that ultrastructurally identified cardiac myocyte gap junctions contain multiple connexins.[12]

However, despite this colocalization of connexins, the connexins differ in relative amounts within different cardiovascular tissues and regions. Quantitative in situ hybridization and RNA blot analysis demonstrated that Cx40 mRNA is threefold to fivefold more abundant in Purkinje fibers than in ventricular muscle, whereas the abundance of Cx43 mRNA is comparable in the two regions.[13] The connexin phenotypes of selected regions of the canine heart with different conduction properties have been characterized by immunohistochemistry.[14] Junctions in the sinus and atrioventricular nodes and proximal His bundle are virtually devoid of Cx43 but contain both Cx40 and Cx45. Gap junctions in the distal His bundle and the proximal bundle branches stain intensely for Cx40 and Cx43 and to a lesser extent for Cx45. Atrial gap junctions show abundant staining for Cx43, Cx40, and Cx45. Ventricular gap junctions are characterized by abundant staining for Cx43 and Cx45 and much less staining for Cx40. These regions also differ in number and size of gap junctions; for example, gap junctions in the sinus and atrioventricular nodes are small and scarce, whereas those in the Purkinje fibers are large and abundant. These data are summarized in Table 1. The distributions of these connexins in human hearts differ little, except for the presence of low levels of Cx43 in the atrioventricular node.[15] It is reasonable to hypothesize that differences in connexin expression and abundance contribute to the characteristic con-

Table 1

Gap Junction Structure and Connexin Phenotype in Differing Regions of the Canine Heart

Cardiac tissue	Conduction velocity, m/s	Connexin phenotype			Gap junction structure	
		Cx40	Cx43	Cx45	Size of junctions	Number of junctions
Sinus node	0.05	Scant	Absent	Scant	Small	Few
Right atrium	0.3–1	Abundant	Abundant	Moderate	Large	Many
AV node and proximal His bundle	0.1	Scant	Absent	Scant	Small	Few
Distal His bundle and proximal bundle branches	2–4.5	Abundant	Abundant	Moderate	Large	Moderate
Ventricle	0.3–1	Scant	Abundant	Moderate	Moderate	Many

Information on gap junction structure and connexin phenotype is based on the analyses of canine hearts by Kanter et al,[13] Saffitz et al,[16] and Davis et al.[14] Estimates of conduction velocities are based on the literature review of Pressler et al.[89] This table is reprinted with permission and modifications from References 14 and 90.

duction properties of different cardiac tissues. There is also evidence that the anisotropic conduction properties of differing cardiac regions relate to the distributions and orientation of gap junctions connecting myocytes.[16]

Different connexins are also expressed at different stages of development. Beyer[17] has shown that although the chicken heart contains three connexins, Cx42, Cx43, and Cx45, Cx45 mRNA is most abundant in the hearts of 6- to 9-day-old embryos and decreases ≈10-fold by adulthood. Several investigators have shown developmental changes in Cx43 expression within the mammalian heart.[18–21] The patterns of connexin distribution in developing and adult hearts of a number of mammalian organisms have recently been reviewed by van Kempen et al.[22]

The different patterns of connexin expression must represent differential expression of connexin genes. Although the upstream and potential regulatory regions of connexin genes are becoming known,[23–26] important transcriptional regulators remain unknown.

Connexin-Specific Electrophysiological Properties

The multiplicity of connexin sequences can lead to the formation of channels with different inherent gating properties or permeabilities to various molecules and ions. These connexin-specific channel properties have been elucidated by examination of each connexin in the same context, ie, within standardized expression systems. We have used the stable transfection of cells from a single communication-deficient cell line (Neuro 2A) with multiple different connexin DNA sequences. The gap junctional conductances produced by different connexins differ in their gating properties. For example, connexin-specific channel regulation by transjunctional voltage can be described by different parameters from the Boltzmann relation[27] (Table 2).

Each of the connexins also forms channels with differing unitary conductances, from as low as 26 pS for chick Cx45[27,28] to as large as 300 pS for human Cx37[5,29] (Table 2). Many of the connexins exhibit multiple single-channel conductances. Moreno et al[30] suggested that different unitary conductances of Cx43 may derive from different phosphorylated forms of the channel protein. Observations of Cx37 channels have demonstrated that some of these represent subconductance states of the channels.[29] These subconductance states may be favored by different conditions (such as the magnitude of transjunctional potential) and may exhibit permeability properties different from those of the fully open channel.

Differential molecular permeabilities of connexin-specific channels

Table 2

Physiological Properties of Cardiovascular Connexins Expressed in Transfected Cells

Connexin	Source	Transjunctional voltage dependence			Channel conductance, pS
		G_{min}	V_0, mV	z	
Cx37	Human	0.27	28	2.0	295
Cx40	Rat	0.30	50	3	158
Cx42	Mouse	≈0.2	44	4.0	153
	Chicken	0.38	41	2.7	236
Cx43	Human	≈0.4–0.5	60	2	99, 63
	Chicken	0.53	77	1.6	166
	Rat				57
Cx45	Mouse	≈0.24	73	3.7	60
	Chicken	0.09	39	1.4	26

Parameters are derived from a mathematical fit of the normalized steady-state junctional conductance (G_{ss}) vs transjunctional voltage (V_j) relation averaged over several experiments. The two-state Boltzmann equation states $G_{ss} = (1-G_{min})/\{1 + \exp[A(V_j-V_0)]\}$, where G_{min} is the voltage-insensitive component of G_{ss}, V_0 is the half-inactivation voltage for the voltage-sensitive component of G_{ss}, and A is the slope factor expressing the charge sensitivity of the transition between the high- and low-conductance states. A equals zq/kT, where z is the number of equivalent electrons q, k is Boltzmann's constant, and T is absolute temperature. Channel conductances represent the largest observed unitary channel conductances. Data regarding chick Cx42, Cx43, and Cx45, human Cx37, and rat Cx40 and Cx43 are based on experiments performed in stably transfected N2A cells using a pipette solution containing 110 mmol/L potassium glutamate and 15 mmol/L NaCl for chick Cx42 and Cx45 and 120 mmol/L potassium glutamate for chick Cx43, rat Cx43 and Cx40, and human Cx37.[5,27–29,32,33,91] Examinations of human Cx43 were performed in transfected SKHep1 cells with 135 mmol/L CsCl.[92,93] Determinations of properties of mouse Cx40 and Cx43 gap junction channels were performed in Hela cells.[94]

were suggested by observations in two rat osteoblastic cell lines.[31] Intercellular passage of microinjected Lucifer yellow (a fluorescent dye) was abundant in a Cx43-expressing cell line but was very limited in cells that expressed predominantly Cx45. Dye transfer in the poorly dye-coupled cells was increased by transfection with Cx43 DNA, but not Cx45, suggesting that only Cx43 channels are permeable to Lucifer yellow. Veenstra et al[28] found that chicken Cx45 channels expressed in N2A cells were permeable to 2′, 7′-dichlorofluorescein but did not pass 6-carboxyfluorescein. These two molecules have similar charges and molecular masses but differing surface charge distributions.[32] Interestingly, Cx37, which forms large conductance channels, showed only limited permeability to both dyes.[29]

Recently, Veenstra and colleagues[28,29,32,33] used ion substitution experiments in the double whole-cell patch-clamp recordings of transfected N2A cells to examine ionic selectivities of expressed gap junction channels. These studies demonstrate that whereas some connexin channels (including Cx43) exhibit little selectivity between anions and cations, others (including Cx37, Cx40, and Cx45) are preferentially permeable to cations. Permeability and selectivity characteristics of channels expressed from cloned cardiovascular connexins are summarized in Table 3.

Mixing of Connexins

The expression of multiple connexins within an organism and within a single tissue or cell implies that gap junctional plaques may not all be composed of only a homogeneous population of channels containing a single connexin. Rather, connexins may potentially intermingle or mix with each other. Such mixing of connexins has been examined by both morphological and physiological approaches. There are now many examples of coexpression of two connexins within the same cell. This was first documented for Cx26 and Cx32 in hepatocytes.[34] In many cases, immunocytochemistry experiments show colocalization to the same gap junction plaques, as we have seen in canine ventricular myocytes, neonatal rat ventricular myocytes, and the cell line BWEM.[12,35,36] The simplest model consistent with these observations has two populations of channels, each formed of only a single connexin contained within the same plaque. Although confocal immunofluorescence studies suggest that the distributions of two connexins within individual plaques are essentially indistinguishable, Sosinsky[37] recently used scanning transmission electron microscopy to suggest that liver gap junctions may contain discrete domains of Cx32 and Cx26 channels. A few electrophysiological experiments have shown

Table 3
Permeability Properties of Cardiovascular Connexins Expressed in Transfected Cells

| Connexin | Source | Permeability to fluorescent dyes | | Relative anion:cation selectivity (R_p) |
		6-Carboxyfluorescein	Dichlorofluorescein	
Cx37	Human	±	±	0.10
Cx40	Rat	±	±	0.22
Cx43	Chicken	±	+	0.32
	Rat	+	+	0.77
Cx45	Chicken	−	+	0.29

Permeability to fluorescent dyes was estimated by including the fluorescent dye in one pipette of a double whole-cell patch-clamp experiment and scoring for transfer at the conclusion of the recording interval.[28,29,32,33,91] Unitary channel conductances were experimentally determined in KCl and potassium-glutamate pipette solutions, and the relative anion:cation selectivity ratios (R_p) were calculated with a modified Goldman-Hodgkin-Katz current equation divided into separate cationic and anionic components, where R_p is expressed as a scaling factor applied to the anionic term (for details see References 32 and 95).

the presence of multiple discrete channel sizes in a cell that expresses multiple connexins. As examples, A7r5 cells express Cx40 and Cx43,[6,38] and Cx43- or Cx32-transfected SKHep 1 cells contain channels derived from the introduced connexin as well as 30-pS channels, which are likely due to endogenous Cx45.[39–41]

If two cells expressed different connexins, they would have the potential to form heterotypic gap junction channels. The formation of heterotypic channels in vitro has been extensively examined by the pairing of *Xenopus* oocytes injected with RNAs encoding two different connexins.[42,43] The two connexins may sometimes form heterotypic channels with complicated, novel gating properties.[44,45] Not all connexins are compatible partners for the formation of heterotypic channels[42,43,46]; the second extracellular loop in the connexin molecules may contribute to the specificity of these interactions.[47] Heterotypic gap junctions might allow for the interaction of different cells or tissues in vivo and might contribute to the formation of communication compartments with borders determined by the expression of incompatible connexins. Among the cardiac connexins, Cx43 and Cx40 appear to be unable to form heterotypic channels.[36,48] However, except for a single article analyzing hepatocyte gap junctions,[49] heterotypic gap junctions have not yet been definitively demonstrated in vivo.

Finally, coexpression of multiple connexins might allow mixing within a single hemichannel, the formation of heteromeric hemichannels. The potentially large number of different heteromeric mixtures might lead to a large variety of channels. Immunocytochemistry experiments do not have the resolution to detect heteromeric channels. Rigorous biochemical analyses with cross-linking and coimmunoprecipitation or definitive electrophysiological documentation of hybrid channels will be required.

Connexin Protein Modification

Most of the connexins (except Cx26) are phosphoproteins.[35,50–58] In many cases, phosphorylation results in altered electrophoretic mobility of the connexin compared with the unmodified protein; thus, connexin phosphorylation has often been followed according to the electrophoretic variants detected on immunoblots. Of the connexins present in cardiac myocytes, Cx43 and Cx45 are phosphorylated[36,55,59]; Cx40 has not been studied but does contain consensus phosphorylation sites.[6,9,60] Connexin phosphorylation has been implicated in many processes, largely on the basis of studies of cells that express Cx43. Such processes include insertion of connexins into the plasma membrane, assembly of gap junctions, protection from (in the case of Cx32) or increased susceptibility to degradation, and gating of the gap junction channels. All of these possible roles for phosphorylation can lead to changes in intercellular communication, with the most rapid effects due to altered channel gating.

Many different treatments that activate protein kinase pathways lead to changes in intercellular communication, although the effects are connexin and cell-type specific (for a more comprehensive review see Reference 61). Several studies have associated differential phosphorylation of Cx43 with decreased intercellular communication after activation of protein kinase C or tyrosine kinase pathways. In some cases, these functional changes have been associated with increased phosphorylation of serine or tyrosine residues, respectively.

Because several different connexins are expressed in cardiac myocytes and all may be phosphoproteins, it is possible that cardiac gap junctions may be differentially regulated by cellular kinases. Modulation of cellular kinase pathways can alter gating or conductance of cardiac gap junction channels and the abundance of connexins in cardiac myocytes.[62–64] Evidence for differential regulation of two connexins in the same cell type has been provided in other systems. As examples, treatment with the protein kinase activator 12-O-tetradecanoylphorbol ester (TPA) differentially affects the mRNAs for Cx26 and Cx43 in mouse keratinocytes[65] and in human mammary tumor cell lines.[66] In clone 9 cells, a rat liver epithelial cell line that expresses both Cx26 and Cx43, TPA induces a reduction in intercellular communication that recovers spontaneously; these changes are associated with loss of both connexins from the plasma membrane and subsequent reappearance at appositional membranes of only Cx43 at the time of recovery.[66] In BWEM cells, a cardiac-derived cell line, TPA reduced cellular coupling in association with reduced Cx43 electrophoretic mobility and decreased synthesis and phosphorylation of Cx45.[35]

The degradation and remodeling of cardiac intercellular connections at gap junctions may be important in the development of altered conduction after myocardial injury.[67] Turnover studies have demonstrated that connexins are quite dynamic compared with other integral membrane proteins. Their half-lives range from 1.5 to 4 hours in cultured cells[36,55,68] to ≈5 hours in organs.[68] The mechanisms of gap junction/connexin degradation are not fully understood. Electron microscopy studies have suggested that gap junctions may be internalized by endocytosis. Vesicular structures containing morphologically identifiable gap junctions, called annular gap junctions, have been observed in several different systems. These structures have been suggested to be clathrin-coated endosomes,[70,71] phagolysosomes,[72] or multivesicular complex structures.[73] Treatments that lead to a loss of morphologically identifiable gap junctions, such as dissociation of adult hearts to isolate individual cardiac myocytes[73,74] or hepatic ischemia or anoxia, increase the abundance of annular gap junctions.[75] Laing and Beyer[76] recently demonstrated that ubiquitin-mediated proteasomal degradation plays an important role in the degradation of Cx43 in E36 Chinese hamster ovary cells and BWEM cells. The abundance and half-life of Cx43 were only modestly affected by the lysosomotropic amine primaquine, whereas treatment with the proteasomal inhibitor N-acetyl-L-leucyl-L-leucinyl-norleucinal led to a sixfold accumulation of Cx43 and increased its half-life to ≈9 hours. Cx43 degradation was slowed in an E36-derived mutant, ts20, containing a thermolabile ubiquitin-activating enzyme, E1, when grown at the restrictive temperature. Moreover, polyubiquitinated forms of Cx43 were isolated from these cells.

Our understanding of the biochemical and cellular regulation of connexins and gap junctions is still primitive enough that it is difficult to propose specific biochemical or pharmacological strategies to mediate cardiac intercellular communication. Thus far, most of the kinase-activating treatments shown to affect aspects of gap junction function or regulation have used relatively nonselective agents (such as phorbol esters or membrane-permeant cyclic nucleotide analogues). But as specific kinases and their targets within the connexins are identified, it may be possible to modulate connexin phosphorylation selectivity as a means to modulate myocardial intercellular coupling. Additionally, determination of conditions or modifications that target connexins for proteolysis may lead to novel strategies to modulate intercellular coupling.

Molecular Biology–Based Interventions to Perturb Gap Junctional Communication

The successes of investigations that used transfection of cells to overexpress connexins have suggested that it may be possible to use molecular genetic strategies to manipulate connexin expression and intercellular coupling in other systems. Although none of the approaches have yet been applied to manipulations in cardiac myocytes, various studies have been used for both gain and loss of function, largely by manipulation in cultured cells (see Table 4). It is likely that application to expression in the heart will require use of more sophisticated DNA delivery techniques, such as viral vectors (see chapter 16).

The greatest successes in molecular genetic manipulation of gap junction–mediated intercellular communication have come through the overexpression of connexin sequences by the stable transfection of various immortalized cell lines. Increased intercellular coupling has been successfully achieved through this strategy in many different cell

Table 4
Molecular Genetic Strategies to Alter Connexin Expression and Gap Junction-Mediated Intercellular Communication

1. Overexpression
2. Antisense
3. "Dominant-negative"
4. Homologous recombination/knockout

types, including hepatocytes,[77] neuroblastoma cells,[27] glial cells,[78] osteoblasts,[31] insulinoma cells,[79] HeLa cells,[48] and fibroblasts.[80] All of these studies used cells that were poorly coupled or "communication deficient," and the effects of such a strategy in "well-coupled" cells are uncertain.

Intercellular coupling has been reduced by several molecular approaches. Antisense strategies have been used most extensively and successfully in expression experiments in *Xenopus* oocytes. Injection of large amounts of antisense oligonucleotides directed against endogenous *Xenopus* Cx38 eliminates basal coupling due to this connexin but still permits detection of coupling induced by introduction of cRNAs encoding various mammalian connexins.[44] However, the application of antisense strategies to junctional coupling in mammalian cell systems has produced results that are somewhat less impressive and less readily interpretable. Bevilacqua and colleagues[81] found that introduction of antisense RNA to Cx32 led to impairments of cellular coupling and developmental defects in early mouse embryos; however, the direct effectiveness of this treatment on the various connexins present in these embryos is unclear. Moore and Burt[82] found that addition of antisense oligonucleotides to Cx40 or Cx43 selectively reduced the abundance of different-size channels in A7r5 cells. Goldberg et al[81a] showed that stable transfection with an antisense Cx43 construct led to reduced steady-state levels of Cx43 mRNA and protein, reduced cellular coupling, and reduced suppression of foci formation by transformed cells. Davis et al[80] showed that stable transfection with an antisense Cx43 construct led to reductions of Cx43 protein (but not mRNA) and intercellular dye transfer in BHK cells. In both of the latter two studies, effects were variable in different clones, and the antisense transfections never led to complete elimination of Cx43 protein production or cellular coupling.[80,81] Indeed, Davis et al suggested that this strategy was effective only at reducing intercellular communication in poorly coupled cells, because no significant effects could be demonstrated with antisense transfections of well-coupled BWEM cells.

The "dominant-negative" approach has been successfully used to disrupt various cellular processes, especially when introduction of a mutated or truncated protein can impair the oligomerization necessary for normal function. Unfortunately, current knowledge of connexin protein structure and interactions is relatively limited; therefore, application of such strategies to gap junctions has been largely empirical. The most rigorously controlled and analyzed studies were conducted by Paul et al.[83] Injection of a connexin RNA encoding a chimeric Cx32/Cx43 protein into early *Xenopus* embryos led to impaired cellular coupling, delamination and extrusion of cells, and developmental defects. A series of careful controls demonstrated the specificity of this effect in these embryos, but the applicability of this construct to mammalian systems is uncertain. Sullivan and Lo[84] found that transfection of 3T3 fibroblasts with a construct containing Cx43 fused to β-galactosidase partially reduced dye transfer. Koval et al[85] found that transfection of a rat osteoblastic cell line with chicken Cx45 reduced intercellular passage of some but not all fluorescent tracers. Neither of these mammalian cell transfection studies completely eliminated cellular coupling.

Recently, Reaume et al[86] used homologous recombination to generate a Cx43-deficient mouse. In the embryonic stem cells derived by this strategy, intercellular transfer of microinjected Lucifer yellow is dramatically reduced. Although the animals die soon after birth (apparently of right ventricular outflow tract obstruction), hearts from these animals exhibit coordinated contractions before death. This finding and preliminary analyses of isolated hearts or myocyte pairs from these animals[87,88] suggest the presence of electrical conduction mediated by other cardiac connexins.

Summary

The gap junction channels that link cardiac myocytes are formed by several different connexin proteins. Several consequences of the multiplicity of connexins have emerged: (1) Different connexins are expressed in differing distributions within the mature and developing organism. Differences in connexin distribution within specialized cardiac tissues may contribute to differences in cardiac conduction. Because of overlapping expression patterns, multiple connexins can potentially mix within a single cell or even within a single channel. (2) Individual connexins form channels that differ in regulatory, conductance, and permeability properties. (3) Connexins differ in their posttranslational modifications, including phosphorylation by protein kinases. These protein modifications may regulate channel assembly, gating, and degradation. Cardiac coupling might potentially be altered by modulating expression of these connexin genes or by differential modification of the connexin proteins.

References

1. Beyer EC, Paul DL, Goodenough DA. Connexin43: a protein from rat heart homologous to a gap junction protein from liver. *J Cell Biol.* 1987;105: 2621–2629.
2. Makowski L, Caspar DLD, Phillips WC, Goodenough DA. Gap junction structures, II: analysis of the x-ray diffraction data. *J Cell Biol.* 1976;74: 629–645.
3. Unwin PNT, Zampighi G. Structure of the junction between communicating cells. *Nature.* 1980;283:545–549.
4. Beyer EC. Gap junctions. *Int Rev Cytol.* 1993;137C:1–37.
5. Reed KE, Westphale EM, Larson DM, Wang HZ, Veenstra RD, Beyer EC. Molecular cloning and functional expression of human connexin37, an endothelial cell gap junction protein. *J Clin Invest.* 1993;91:997–1004.
6. Beyer EC, Reed KE, Westphale EM, Kanter HL, Larson DM. Molecular cloning and expression of rat connexin40, a gap junction protein expressed in vascular smooth muscle. *J Membr Biol.* 1992;127:69–76.
7. Kanter HL, Saffitz JE, Beyer EC. Cardiac myocytes express multiple gap junction proteins. *Circ Res.* 1992;70:438–444.
8. Paul DL, Ebihara L, Takemoto LJ, Swenson KI, Goodenough DA. Connexin46, a novel lens gap junction protein, induces voltage-gated currents in nonjunctional plasma membrane of Xenopus oocytes. *J Cell Biol.* 1991; 115:1077–1089.
9. Haefliger JA, Bruzzone R, Jenkins NA, Gilbert DJ, Copeland NG, Paul DL. Four novel members of the connexin family of gap junction proteins: molecular cloning, expression, and chromosome mapping. *J Biol Chem.* 1992;267:2057–2064.
10. Hennemann H, Schwarz HJ, Willecke K. Characterization of gap junction genes expressed in F9 embryonic carcinoma cells: molecular cloning of mouse connexin31 and −45 cDNAs. *Eur J Cell Biol.* 1992;57:51–58.
11. Gourdie RG, Green CR, Severs NJ, Thompson RP. Immunolabelling patterns of gap junction connexins in the developing and mature rat heart. *Anat Embryol.* 1992;185:363–378.
12. Kanter HL, Laing JG, Beyer EC, Green KG, Saffitz JE. Multiple connexins colocalize in canine ventricular myocyte gap junctions. *Circ Res.* 1993;73: 344–350.
13. Kanter HL, Laing JG, Beau SL, Beyer EC, Saffitz JE. Distinct patterns of connexin expression in canine Purkinje fibers and ventricular muscle. *Circ Res.* 1993;72:1124–1131.
14. Davis LM, Kanter HL, Beyer EC, Saffitz JE. Distinct gap junction phenotypes in cardiac tissues with disparate conduction properties. *J Am Coll Cardiol.* 1994;24:1124–1132.
15. Davis LM, Rodefeld ME, Green K, Beyer EC, Saffitz JE. Gap junction protein phenotypes of the human heart and conduction system. *J Cardiovasc Electrophysiol.* 1995;6:813–822.

16. Saffitz JE, Kanter HL, Green KG, Tolley TK, Beyer EC. Tissue-specific determinants of anisotropic conduction velocity in canine atrial and ventricular myocardium. *Circ Res.* 1994;74:1065–1070.
17. Beyer EC. Molecular cloning and developmental expression of two chick embryo gap junction proteins. *J Biol Chem.* 1990;265:14439–14443.
18. Yancey SB, Biswal S, Revel JP. Spatial and temporal patterns of distribution of the gap junction protein connexin43 during mouse gastrulation and organogenesis. *Development.* 1992;114:203–212.
19. Fromaget C, el Aoumari A, Dupont E, Briand JP, Gros D. Changes in the expression of connexin 43, a cardiac gap junctional protein, during mouse heart development. *J Mol Cell Cardiol.* 1990;22:1245–1258.
20. Fishman GI, Hertzberg EL, Spray DC, Leinwand LA. Expression of connexin43 in the developing rat heart. *Circ Res.* 1991;68:782–787.
21. Ruangvoravat CP, Lo CW. Connexin 43 expression in the mouse embryo: localization of transcripts within developmentally significant domains. *Dev Dyn.* 1992;194:261–281.
22. van Kempen MJA, Ten Velde I, Wessels A, et al. Differential connexin distribution accommodates cardiac function in different species. *Microsc Res Tech.* 1995;31:420–436.
23. Miller T, Dahl G, Werner R. Structure of a gap junction gene: rat connexin-32. *Biosci Rep.* 1988;8:455–464.
24. Sullivan R, Ruangvoravat C, Joo D, et al. Structure, sequence and expression of the mouse Cx43 gene encoding connexin 43. *Gene.* 1993;130:191–199.
25. Yu W, Dahl G, Werner R. The connexin43 gene is responsive to estrogen. *Proc R Soc Lond.* 1994;255:125–132.
26. Chen Z-Q, Lefebvre D, Bai X, Reaume A, Rossant J, Lye SJ. Identification of two regulatory elements within the promoter region of the mouse connexin 43 gene. *J Biol Chem.* 1995;270:3863–3868.
27. Veenstra RD, Wang HZ, Westphale EM, Beyer EC. Multiple connexins confer distinct regulatory and conductance properties of gap junctions in developing heart. *Circ Res.* 1992;71:1277–1283.
28. Veenstra RD, Wang HZ, Beyer EC, Brink PR. Selective dye and ionic permeability of gap junction channels formed by connexin45. *Circ Res.* 1994;75: 483–490.
29. Veenstra RD, Wang HZ, Beyer EC, Ramanan SV, Brink PR. Connexin37 forms high conductance gap junction channels with subconductance state activity and selective dye and ionic permeabilities. *Biophys J.* 1994;66: 1915–1928.
30. Moreno AP, Saez JC, Fishman GI, Spray DC. Human connexin43 gap junction channels: regulation of unitary conductances by phosphorylation. *Circ Res.* 1994;74:1050–1057.
31. Steinberg TH, Civitelli R, Geist ST, et al. Connexin43 and connexin45 form gap junctions with different molecular permeabilities in osteoblastic cells. *EMBO J.* 1994;13:744–750.
32. Veenstra RD, Wang HZ, Beblo DA, et al. Selectivity of connexin-specific gap junctions does not correlate with channel conductance. *Circ Res.* 1995; 77:1156–1165.
33. Beblo DA, Wang HZ, Beyer EC, Westphale EM, Veenstra RD. Unique conductance, gating, and selective permeability properties of gap junction channels formed by connexin40. *Circ Res.* 1995;77:813–822.
34. Traub O, Look J, Dermietzel R, Brummer F, Hulser D, Willecke K. Comparative characterization of the 21-kD and 26-kD gap junction proteins in murine liver and cultured hepatocytes. *J Cell Biol.* 1989;108:1039–1051.

35. Laing JG, Westphale EM, Engelmann GL, Beyer EC. Characterization of the gap junction protein connexin45. *J Membr Biol.* 1994;139:31–40.
36. Darrow BJ, Laing JG, Lampe PD, Saffitz JE, Beyer EC. Expression of multiple connexins in cultured neonatal rat ventricular myocytes. *Circ Res.* 1995; 76:381–387.
37. Sosinsky G. Mixing of connexins in gap junction membrane channels. *Proc Natl Acad Sci U S A.* 1995;92:9210–9214.
38. Moore LK, Beyer EC, Burt JM. Characterization of gap junction channels in A7r5 vascular smooth muscle cells. *Am J Physiol.* 1991;260:C975–C981.
39. Fishman GI, Spray DC, Leinwand LA. Molecular characterization and functional expression of the human cardiac gap junction channel. *J Cell Biol.* 1990;111:589–598.
40. Moreno AP, Eghbali B, Spray DC. Connexin32 gap junction channels in stably transfected cells: unitary conductance. *Biophys J.* 1991;60:1254–1266.
41. Moreno AP, Laing JG, Beyer EC, Spray DC. Properties of gap junction channels formed of connexin45 endogenously expressed in human hepatoma (SKHep1) cells. *Am J Physiol.* 1995;268:C356–C365.
42. Swenson KI, Jordan JR, Beyer EC, Paul DI. Formation of gap junctions by expression of connexins in Xenopus oocyte pairs. *Cell.* 1989;57:145–155.
43. Werner R, Levine E, Rabadan Diehl C, Dahl G. Formation of hybrid cell-cell channels. *Proc Natl Acad Sci U S A.* 1989;86:5380–5384.
44. Barrio LC, Suchyna T, Bargiello T, et al. Gap junctions formed by connexins 26 and 32 alone and in combination are differently affected by applied voltage. *Proc Natl Acad Sci U S A.* 1991;88:8410–8414.
45. Verselis VK, Ginter CS, Bargiello TA. Opposite voltage gating polarities of two closely related connexins. *Nature.* 1994;368:348–351.
46. Bruzzone R, Haefliger JA, Gimlich RL, Paul DL. Connexin40, a component of gap junctions in vascular endothelium, is restricted in its ability to interact with other connexins. *Mol Biol Cell.* 1993;4:7–20.
47. White TW, Bruzzone R, Wolfram S, Paul DL, Goodenough DA. Selective interactions among the multiple connexin proteins expressed in the vertebrate lens: the second extracellular domain is a determinant of compatibility between connexins. *J Cell Biol.* 1994;125:879–892.
48. Elfgang C, Eckert R, Lichtenberg-Frate H, et al. Specific permeability and selective formation of gap junction channels in connexin-transfected HeLa cells. *J Cell Biol.* 1995;129:805–817.
49. Verselis VK, Bargiello TA, Rubin JA, Bennett MVL. Comparison of voltage dependent properties of gap junctions in hepatocytes and in Xenopus oocytes expressing Cx32 and Cx26. In: Hall JE, Zampighi GA, Davis RM, eds. *Gap Junctions: Progress in Cell Research, vol 3.* Amsterdam, Netherlands: Elsevier; 1993:105–112.
50. Saez JC, Spray DC, Nairn AC, Hertzberg E, Greengard P, Bennett MV. cAMP increases junctional conductance and stimulates phosphorylation of the 27-kDa principal gap junction polypeptide. *Proc Natl Acad Sci U S A.* 1986;83:2473–2477.
51. Traub O, Look J, Paul D, Willecke K. Cyclic adenosine monophosphate stimulates biosynthesis and phosphorylation of the 26 kDa gap junction protein in cultured mouse hepatocytes. *Eur J Cell Biol.* 1987;43:48–54.
52. Takeda A, Saheki S, Shimazu T, Takeuchi N. Phosphorylation of the 27-kDa gap junction protein by protein kinase C in vitro and in rat hepatocytes. *J Biochem (Tokyo).* 1989;106:723–727.
53. Crow DS, Beyer EC, Paul DL, Kobe SS, Lau AF. Phosphorylation of con-

nexin43 gap junction protein in uninfected and Rous sarcoma virus-transformed mammalian fibroblasts. *Mol Cell Biol.* 1990;10:1754–1763.

54. Filson AJ, Azarnia R, Beyer EC, Loewenstein WR, Brugge JS. Tyrosine phosphorylation of a gap junction protein correlates with inhibition of cell-to-cell communication. *Cell Growth Differ.* 1990;1:661–668.

55. Laird DW, Puranam KL, Revel JP. Turnover and phosphorylation dynamics of connexin43 gap junction protein in cultured cardiac myocytes. *Biochem J.* 1991;273:67–72.

56. Berthoud VM, Ledbetter MLS, Hertzberg EL, Saez JC. Connexin43 in MDCK cells: regulation by a tumor-promoting phorbol ester and Ca^{2+}. *Eur J Cell Biol.* 1992;57:40–50.

57. Jiang JX, Paul DL, Goodenough DA. Posttranslational phosphorylation of lens fiber connexin46: a slow occurrence. *Invest Ophthalmol Vis Sci.* 1993; 34:3558–3565.

58. Berthoud VM, Cook AJ, Beyer EC. Characterization of the gap junction protein connexin56 in the chicken lens by immunofluorescence and immunoblotting. *Invest Ophthalmol Vis Sci.* 1994;35:4109–4117.

59. Lau AF, Hatch Pigott V, Crow DS. Evidence that heart connexin43 is a phosphoprotein. *J Mol Cell Cardiol.* 1991;23:659–663.

60. Hennemann H, Suchyna T, Lichtenberg Frate H, et al. Molecular cloning and functional expression of mouse connexin40, a second gap junction gene preferentially expressed in lung. *J Cell Biol.* 1992;117:1299–1310.

61. Saez JC, Berthoud VM, Moreno AP, Spray DC. Gap junctions: multiplicity of controls in differentiated and undifferentiated cells and possible functional implications. In: Shenolikar S, Nairn AC, eds. *Advances in Second Messenger and Phosphoprotein Research Vol. 27.* New York, NY: Raven Press, Ltd; 1993:163–198.

62. Takens Kwak BR, Jongsma HJ. Cardiac gap junctions: three distinct single channel conductances and their modulation by phosphorylating treatments. *Pflugers Arch.* 1992;422:198–200.

63. Darrow BJ, Laing JG, Saffitz JE, Beyer EC. Differential regulation of connexin expression in cultured neonatal rat ventricular myocytes. *Circulation.* 1993;88(suppl I):I–174. Abstract.

64. Moreno AP, Saez JC, Fishman GI, Spray DC. Human connexin43 gap junction channels: regulation of unitary conductances by phosphorylation. *Circ Res.* 1994;74:1050–1057.

65. Brissette JL, Kumar NM, Gilula NB, Dotto GP. The tumor promoter 12-O-tetradecanoylphorbol-13-acetate and the *ras* oncogene modulate expression and phosphorylation of gap junction proteins. *Mol Cell Biol.* 1991;11: 5364–5371.

66. Lee SW, Tomasetto C, Paul D, Keyomarsi K, Sager R. Transcriptional downregulation of gap-junction proteins blocks junctional communication in human mammary tumor cell lines. *J Cell Biol.* 1992;118:1213–1221.

67. Luke RA, Saffitz JE. Remodeling of ventricular conduction pathways in healed canine infarct border zones. *J Clin Invest.* 1991;87:1594–1602.

68. Musil LS, Beyer EC, Goodenough DA. Expression of the gap junction protein connexin43 in embryonic chick lens: molecular cloning, ultrastructural localization, and post-translational phosphorylation. *J Membr Biol.* 1990; 116:163–175.

69. Fallon RF, Goodenough DA. Five-hour half-life of mouse liver gap-junction protein. *J Cell Biol.* 1981;90:521–526.

70. Larsen WJ, Tung HN. Origin and fate of cytoplasmic gap junctional vesicles in rabbit granulosa cells. *Tissue Cell.* 1978;10:585–598.

71. Larsen WJ, Tung HN, Murray SA, Swenson CA. Evidence for the participation of actin microfilaments in the internalization of gap junction membrane. *J Cell Biol.* 1979;83:576–587.
72. Ginzberg RD, Gilula NB. Modulation of cell junctions during differentiation of the chicken otocyst sensory epithelium. *Dev Biol.* 1979;68:110–129.
73. Severs NJ, Shovel KS, Slade AM, Powell T, Twist VW, Green CR. Fate of gap junctions in isolated adult mammalian cardiomyocytes. *Circ Res.* 1989; 65:22–42.
74. Mazet F, Wittenberg BA, Spray DC. Fate of intercellular junctions in isolated adult rat cardiac cells. *Circ Res.* 1985;56:195–204.
75. Traub O, Druge PM, Willecke K. Degradation and resynthesis of gap junction protein in plasma membranes of regenerating liver after partial hepatectomy or cholestasis. *Proc Natl Acad Sci U S A.* 1983;80:755–759.
76. Laing JG, Beyer EC. The gap junction protein connexin43 is degraded via the ubiquitin proteasome pathway. *J Biol Chem.* 1995;270:26399–26403.
77. Eghbali B, Kessler JA, Spray DC. Expression of gap junction channels in communication-incompetent cells after stable transfection with cDNA encoding connexin 32. *Proc Natl Acad Sci U S A.* 1990;87:1328–1331.
78. Zhu D, Caveney S, Kidder GM, Naus CC. Transfection of C6 glioma cells with connexin 43 cDNA: analysis of expression, intercellular coupling, and cell proliferation. *Proc Natl Acad Sci U S A.* 1991;88:1883–1887.
79. Beyer EC, Veenstra RD. Molecular biology and electrophysiology of cardiac gap junctions. In: Peracchia C, ed. *Handbook of Molecular and Cellular Physiology of Membrane Channels.* San Diego, Calif: Academic Press; 1994:379–401.
80. Davis LM, Saffitz JE, Beyer EC. Modulation of connexin43 expression: effects on cellular coupling. *J Cardiovasc Electrophysiol.* 1995;6:103–114.
81. Bevilacqua A, Loch Caruso R, Erickson RP. Abnormal development and dye coupling produced by antisense RNA to gap junction protein in mouse preimplantation embryos. *Proc Natl Acad Sci U S A.* 1989;86:5444–5448.
81a. Goldberg GS, Martyn KD, Lau AF. A connexin43 antisense vector reduces the ability of normal cells to inhibit the foci formation of transformed cells. *Mol Carcinog.* 1994;11:106–114.
82. Moore LK, Burt JM. Selective block of gap junction channel expression with connexin-specific antisense oligodeoxynucleotides. *Am J Physiol.* 1994;267: C1371–C1380.
83. Paul DL, Yu K, Bruzzone R, Gimlich RL, Goodenough DA. Expression of a dominant negative inhibitor of intercellular communication in the early Xenopus embryo causes delamination and extrusion of cells. *Development.* 1995;121:371–381.
84. Sullivan R, Lo CW. Expression of a connexin 43/β-galactosidase fusion protein inhibits gap junctional communication in NIH3T3 cells. *J Cell Biol.* 1995;130:419–429.
85. Koval M, Geist ST, Kemendy AE, et al. Transfected connexin45 alters gap junction permeability in cells expressing endogenous connexin43. *J Cell Biol.* 1995;130:987–995.
86. Reaume AG, Desousa PA, Kulkarni S, et al. Cardiac malformation in neonatal mice lacking connexin43. *Science.* 1995;267:1831–1834.
87. Guerrero PA, Schuessler RB, Davis LM, Beyer EC, Saffitz JE. Characterization of left ventricular conduction in hearts of fetal mice. *Circulation.* 1995; 92(suppl I):I–41. Abstract.
88. Vink MJ, Fishman GI, Vieira D, Spray DC. Properties of gap junction channels in neonatal cardiac myocytes from wild type and connexin43 (Cx43) knockout (KO) mice. *Circulation.* 1995;92(suppl I):I–41. Abstract.

89. Pressler ML, Munster PN, Huang X-d. Gap junction distribution in the heart: functional relevance. In: Zipes DP, Jalife J, eds. *Cardiac Electrophysiology: From Cell to Bedside.* Philadelphia, Pa: WB Saunders Co; 1995:144–151.
90. Beyer EC, Davis LM, Saffitz JE, Veenstra RD. Cardiac intercellular communication: consequences of connexin distribution and diversity. *Brazilian J Med Biol Res.* 1995;28:415–425.
91. Beblo DA, Wang HZ, Beyer EC, Westphale EM, Veenstra RD. Unique conductance, gating, and selective permeability properties of gap junction channels formed by connexin40. *Circulation.* 1994;90(suppl I):I–359. Abstract.
92. Fishman GI, Moreno AP, Spray DC, Leinwand LA. Functional analysis of human cardiac gap junction channel mutants. *Proc Natl Acad Sci U S A.* 1991;88:3525–3529.
93. Spray DC, Moreno AP, Eghbali B, Chanson M, Fishman GI. Gating of gap junction channels as revealed in cells stably transfected with wild type and mutant connexin cDNAs. *Biophys J.* 1992;62:48–50.
94. Traub O, Eckert R, Lichtenberg-Frate H, et al. Immunochemical and electrophysiological characterization of murine connexin40 and -43 in mouse tissue and transfected human cells. *Eur J Cell Biol.* 1994;64:101–112.
95. Veenstra RD. Size and selectivity of gap junction channels formed from different connexins. *J Bioenerg Biomembr.* 1996;28:317–337.

Chapter 16

Can We Learn About Conduction by Use of Genetic Approaches?

Glenn I. Fishman, MD, Monique J. Vink, MD, and David C. Spray, PhD

Contemporary views of cardiac conduction suggest that impulse propagation at the microscopic level is discontinuous, resulting from irregularities in cell structure.[1] Furthermore, it has been proposed that alterations in the arrangement of gap junctional channels within the heart may strongly influence the propensity for cardiac arrhythmogenesis by modifying the extent of discontinuous propagation.[2] To date, however, evidence to support the view that rhythm disturbances can involve gap junction dysfunction is largely circumstantial. Gene targeting methodologies, in which gap junction channel expression is specifically modified in vivo, provides a powerful strategy for directly testing this hypothesis.[3,4] Such an approach permits one to manipulate conduction at the molecular level, potentially highlighting the stochastic nature of discontinuous propagation and providing novel insights into arrhythmogenic mechanisms. In this chapter, we briefly review the molecular genetics of the connexins, focusing on those specific isoforms expressed in the heart. Recent studies of human gap junction channel diseases as well as animal model systems resulting in connexin overexpression or loss of function are also described, and potentially useful strategies still under development are also considered. These newer genetic approaches should more firmly establish the extent to which gap junction channel dysfunction contributes to cardiac arrhythmogenesis.

Dr. Fishman is an Established Investigator of the American Heart Association.

From: Spooner PM, Joyner RW, Jalife J (eds). *Discontinuous Conduction in the Heart.* Armonk, NY: Futura Publishing Company, Inc.; © 1997.

Connexin Multigene Family

Gap junction channels are formed by the association of membrane-spanning protein subunits called connexins.[5,6] The connexins are encoded by a multigene family, and individual isoforms are expressed with distinct but sometimes overlapping developmental and spatial profiles.[7-9] The first transcript encoding a gap junction channel protein was isolated from liver, in which antibodies generated against the junctional channel proteins were used to screen complementary DNA expression libraries, resulting in the isolation of Cx32.[10] Subsequently, clones encoding a somewhat larger gap junction channel protein, Cx43, were identified by screening a cardiac cDNA library with the liver isoform at reduced stringency.[11] These initial studies led to a virtual explosion in the cloning of connexin cDNA and genomic sequences.[12] To date, there are 59 entries in Genbank for connexin sequences isolated from a wide variety of species and tissues; 13 distinct connexins have been detected in rodents, all of which presumably have human homologues.

Connexin genes have maintained both highly conserved nucleic acid and amino acid sequences and genomic organization, suggesting important constraints on the functional integrity of the various proteins as well as their transcriptional regulation.[13,14] In all cases examined thus far, a small, noncoding first exon is widely separated from a second exon within which is located the protein-coding region in a single uninterrupted stretch (Figure 1A). This uniformity of structure suggests that a single precursor gene encoding an intercellular channel protein subunit may have undergone repeated duplications and subsequent mutations, leading to the formation of a multigene family. As described elsewhere in this monograph, all connexins are predicted to have four membrane-spanning domains (M1 through M4), amino- and carboxyl-termini oriented within the cytoplasmic compartment, two extracellular loops connecting M1 with M2 and M3 with M4, and a cytoplasmic hinge region linking M2 with M3 (Figure 1B). Variations in the length of the hinge region divide the various connexins into the group 1 (β) and group 2 (α) subfamilies.

Connexin Gene Expression in the Heart

Among the connexin multigene family, only a subset of isoforms, Cx40, Cx43, and Cx45, are expressed within the heart. Interestingly, these cardiac isoforms are all members of the group 2 subfamily. These three genes are expressed with unique developmental and spatial profiles, and this genetic diversity is hypothesized to be important for

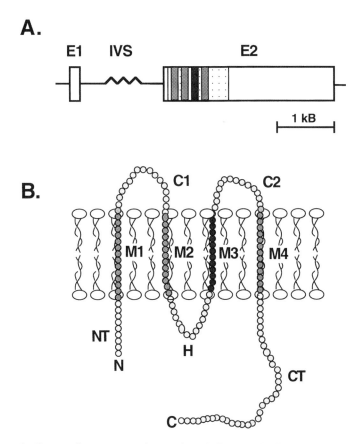

Figure 1. **Connexin genes and proteins.** A, Prototypical connexin gene consists of two widely separated exons (E1 and E2). Entire protein codingregion is located within exon 2. Intron, or intervening sequence (IVS), is of variable length and not drawn to scale. B, Connexin monomers span membrane four times (M1 through M4). Third transmembrane domain is amphipathic and may contribute to the pore. Amino (NT) and carboxyl (CT) termini and cytoplasmic loop or hinge (H) are cytoplasmic, and two extracellular loops (C1 and C2) sit within extracellular gap.

proper heart development as well as for impulse generation and propagation.[15] Cx43 is the most abundant gap junction channel gene expressed in the heart. Studies in rodents have identified Cx43 as early as 10 days after coitum, in the trabeculae and subendocardial layers of the developing ventricles, the outflow tract, the interventricular septum, and the epicardial free wall.[16,17] Transcript levels, at least in rodents, increase substantially between midgestation and early neonatal stages[18,19] and appear to decline modestly in older animals. In the adult heart, Cx43 is abundantly expressed in the working myocardium and within the atrium but in some species is relatively sparse in specialized conduction tissue, including nodal and His-Purkinje cells. In addition to the heart proper, Cx43 is also prominently expressed in the smooth muscle of the vascular wall, where intercellular coupling may play an important role in regulating vasomotor tone.

In addition to Cx43, two additional connexin transcripts (Cx45 and Cx40) have been detected in the mammalian heart, each with a distinct temporal and spatial pattern of expression.[20,21] Cx45 appears to colocalize with Cx43 throughout most regions of the heart. Although no truly quantitative studies have been reported, the contribution of Cx45 to the total junctional protein content within the myocardium appears to be substantially lower than that from Cx43. In the embryonic heart, Cx40 is widely expressed but becomes restricted to the atria and in some species is also localized to the specialized conduction system in the mature heart.[22,23] Cx40 is also observed in the endothelium of both muscular and elastic arteries.[24,25] Transcripts encoding additional isoforms, such as Cx37 and Cx46, have also been detected in the hearts of mammalian species. Although Cx37 protein is readily detected in blood vessel endothelium, transcript accumulation in the heart does not appear to be associated with any significant amount of the encoded protein.[26,27] Unfortunately, the great interspecies variability in the distribution of connexin isoforms, particularly in the heart, greatly complicates efforts to identify functional correlates of this diversity. As alluded to elsewhere, one explanation for connexin diversity may be to facilitate communication compartmentalization; nevertheless, despite the increasingly complete cataloguing of connexin expression in mammalian cardiovascular systems, especially in heart, functional relationships between isoform diversity and conduction patterns remain incompletely explained.

In view of several reports demonstrating alterations in connexin expression in various cardiomyopathies, the regulation of connexin expression within the heart and elsewhere is becoming the focus of important investigation. We have begun to examine the transcriptional control of Cx43 expression in the heart by use of genomic clones encompassing putative 5'-flanking regulatory sequences. Fusion of these sequences to reporter genes, such as the firefly luciferase enzyme, has permitted detection of transcriptional activity both in cultured neonatal cardiac myocytes and when assayed in vivo after direct transfer by intracardiac injection of DNA.[28] In both cell culture and in vivo systems, substantial expression of heterologous reporter genes is obtained by including as few as 175 base pairs of human Cx43 5'-flanking sequence. Inclusion of larger genomic elements results in even greater transcriptional activity, but only in the in vivo gene transfer system. These results suggest that upstream elements between -175 and -2400 are uniquely responsive to hemodynamic or neurohormonal effects. They are also tantalizing in view of the observed downregulation of Cx43 transcript levels in at least two rodent models of hypertension. Very recently, additional studies of human Cx43 transcriptional control in other cell systems have identified *cis*-acting elements that are implicated in the hormonal responsiveness of this gap junction channel gene.[29]

Interestingly, the Cx32 gene, which is expressed in a variety of cell types, including hepatocytes, oligodendrocytes, and Schwann cells, appears to utilize alternative promoters depending on the site of expression.[30] Within cells of the nervous system, a second promoter has been uncovered within the intron. This transcription unit results in the same protein as the originally described mRNA but allows for cell-type–specific transcriptional regulation of a single connexin gene. Whether this phenomenon is also observed in other connexins, such as those expressed within the heart, is currently unexplored. As additional data are forthcoming, one would predict that specific factors that regulate expression of selected connexin genes will be identified and eventually exploited to regulate conduction within the myopathic heart.

Functional Properties of Cardiovascular Gap Junction Channels

The biophysical properties of gap junction channels have been determined by studies of both endogenous channels expressed in various primary and established cell lines and, more recently, by expression in exogenous systems using cloned connexin sequences.[31,32] These approaches are complementary in nature. For example, recordings from primary cells may more faithfully model the behavior of channels in situ, especially where cell-specific posttranslational effects are prominent. However, such studies are complicated by potential expression of numerous connexin isoforms within the same cell, a problem that can be mitigated by exogenous expression of individual connexins in communication-deficient cell lines. Applications of these various approaches are discussed more fully in this monograph and elsewhere.[33]

Connexins and Human Diseases

To date, several human diseases have been attributed to mutations in connexin genes. The X-linked form of Charcot-Marie-Tooth disease (CMTX), a disorder characterized by peripheral neuropathy resulting primarily in lower-extremity weakness, appears to result from mutations in connexin32.[34] The underlying defect in communication is apparently in reflexive junctions located between cytoplasmic processes of myelinating Schwann cells, although details of this function in normal nerve are not entirely clear. Mutations have been detected both within the protein coding region, and in noncoding sequences, suggesting that expression of mutant protein as well as alterations in the levels of wild-type Cx32 may result in pathological states.

Recently, Britz-Cummingham et al[35] presented their findings of mutations in the carboxyl-terminal portion of the Cx43 protein-coding region in six patients with visceroatrial heterotaxia, a congenital abnormality characterized by laterality defects, including complex cardiovascular malformations.

Intriguingly, four of these mutations involved substitutions of phosphorylatable serine residues. In contrast, Gebbia et al[35a] examined a total of 38 additional patients with apparently similar phenotypes and have failed to uncover any mutations within the carboxyl-tail of Cx43. Thus, although Fletcher[35b] argues that the patient samples in reference 35 are from a subset characterized by polysplenia, an association between Cx43 missense mutations and disorders of laterality remains unconfirmed.

Very recently, a pedigree with cases of autosomal dominant deafness was examined and a missense mutation in the Cx26 gene was identified.[35c] Additional mutations resulting in premature stop codons were also found in three pedigrees with autosomal recessive non-syndromic sensorineuronal deafness that had been genetically linked to chromosome 13q11-12, where the Cx26 gene is localized.

Finally, it should be noted that a genetic cardiomyopathy with atrioventricular conduction block mapped to chromosome 1 near the Cx40 locus, prompting speculation as to its candidacy; however, this gap junction channel gene has been excluded as the culprit gene.[36]

In summary, the evidence to date identifying diseases that arise from specific mutations within the connexin family of genes is limited to CMTX, nonsyndromic sensorineuronal deafness and perhaps visceroatrial heterotaxia. These observations prompt speculation as to whether additional genetic diseases will be uncovered as a result of mutations in other isoforms. The answer is almost certainly yes. Mutations with clinically significant but viable phenotypes, such as CMTX, are typically the first to be discovered, because the most deleterious mutations are embryonic-lethal and the more subtle mutations are difficult to discern.

Experimental Studies In Vivo

The most straightforward approach toward understanding the functional role of individual types of gap junction channels in the intact organism is to perturb the normal patterns of expression and examine the animal for phenotypic sequelae. To date, very few studies of dysregulated connexin expression in vivo have been reported. In one of the earliest attempts to modify gap junction channel function in the intact organism, Warner and colleagues[37,38] examined *Xenopus* embryos injected with antisera prepared against the liver gap junction channel protein Cx32. These embryos developed significant developmental defects in neural derivatives,[37] but no evidence for alterations in muscle gene expression were seen.[38] Thus, maintenance of normal intercellular communication was important for at least some facets of embryogenesis. Using a more genetic approach, Lo and colleagues[39] used both the widely expressed human cytomegalovirus promoter and the elongation factor 1 alpha promoter to overexpress either wild-type Cx43 or a Cx43-β-galactosidase fusion protein in transgenic mice. This latter construct has been reported to exhibit dominant-negative effects on intercellular coupling in tissue culture experiments. Their preliminary data describe neural tube defects in these transgenic mice, again supporting the importance of maintaining appropriate levels of intercellular communication during embryogenesis. Moreover, in concert with Warner's studies, these results suggest a particular susceptibility of neural derivatives to perturbations of junctional coupling during embryogenesis. Our laboratory is currently examining transgenic mice in which Cx43 is specifically targeted to cardiac myocytes, using cardiac-restricted transcriptional regulatory elements, such as the α-myosin heavy chain promoter.[40] These studies should help establish whether manipulation of Cx43 expression during early embryogenesis is sufficient to disrupt normal cardiac morphogenesis. In addition, we have also generated a replication-incompetent adenovirus that expresses epitope-tagged Cx43. In vivo experiments using virus-mediated gene transfer technology will address whether enhancement of Cx43-mediated intercellular coupling exerts a protective effect against the development of cardiac arrhythmias.

Several laboratories using homologous recombination and embryonic stem cell methodology have made substantial progress in generating null alleles in several connexin loci. To date, however, the only cardiac connexin knockout that has progressed through the germline stage and yielded homozygous null mice is Cx43, as recently reported by Reaume and colleagues.[41] Given the widespread expression of Cx43 during embryogenesis, it is somewhat surprising that the major abnormality associated with Cx43 deficiency is a localized obstruction of the right ventricular outflow tract. The resulting pulmonary oligemia appears to be the proximate cause of death in these mice shortly after birth. From a pragmatic point of view, the failure of these mice to mature beyond the perinatal period confounds efforts to examine their propensity for cardiac arrythmogenesis. Nonetheless, as described below, our examination of cardiac myocytes derived from these neonatal Cx43 knockout mice establishes that loss of Cx43 is associated with significant functional deficiencies and may provide some explanation for the oberved developmental defect.

The phenotype of Cx32 null mice might be predicted to mimic the findings in patients with CMTX, at least in those human patients with loss-of-function mutations. In fact, in older mice, preliminary studies suggest histological abnormalities in the peripheral nervous system. In addition, defects in mobilization of liver glycogen have been observed, consistent with previous suggestions implicating gap junction channels in metabolic control and homeostasis. Interestingly, transport of Cx26 to the membrane junctional plaques appears to be reduced in the Cx32 knockout mice, suggesting a linkage between the two liver isoforms.[42] Cx26-deficient mice die quite early during embryogenesis, at the trophoblast stage; although the precise defect resulting in this outcome is uncertain, lack of implantation may underscore the importance of this connexin in formation of functional maternofetal exchange within the placenta. Finally, deficiency of Cx46 in the mouse leads to no overt abnormalities, although regeneration of peripheral nerves, in which Cx46 is believed to couple proliferating Schwann cells, has not yet been examined.

Thus, genetic ablation of individual connexin genes may result in exceedingly diverse phenotypes. A simple explanation would be that gap junction channels formed from individual connexins possess both unique and redundant properties, so that deficiencies may be better compensated in some tissues than in others by additional connexins whose expression is either induced by the knockout or constitutive. This conclusion would be consistent with the known differences in gating properties of channels composed of distinct connexin isoforms. However, an alternative hypothesis, which has not been disproved, is that channels formed from different connexins are functionally interchangeable in vivo but that the critical factors in organogenesis and function are spatial and temporal patterns of connexin expression.

Functional Studies of Cx43-Deficient Cardiac Myocytes

Consistent with the belief that Cx43 plays an important roles in cardiac function, deletion of this gene through homologous recombination is lethal. Although this lethality results from a defect in cardiac development, we have investigated consequences of Cx43 deletion on cardiac conduction in cultured myocytes obtained from these animals at birth. Despite the altered morphology of the hearts of the homozygous null animal, they contract rhythmically, implying that other gap junction proteins are either compensatorily or constitutively expressed in adequate abundance to preserve this basic function. Immunostaining with antibodies specific for Cx40 and Cx45 indicates that compensatory upregulation of these isoforms does not occur to any great extent in ventricular myocytes from homozygous Cx43 null ($-/-$) animals. Interestingly, levels of Cx43 in heterozygotes are similar to those in wild-type littermates. Consistent with this lack of compensatory expression, junctional conductances of ventricular myocytes from ($-/-$) animals were significantly lower than in wild-type ($+/+$) mouse heart cells (10.7 ± 1.6 versus 4.6 ± 0.9 nS; $P<.05$). However, Lucifer yellow dye transfer in ($-/-$) cardiocytes was reduced to barely detectable levels, in contrast to the robust dye transfer in ($+/+$) myocytes to multiple contiguous and second-order cells. Also consistent with reduced junctional conductance between these cells, transfer of slow Ca^{2+} waves between ($-/-$) cardiocytes was less extensive and slower than in cardiocytes from ($+/+$) littermates, the average latency for Ca^{2+} transfer from the stimulated cell to its neighbor cells being four times slower for ($-/-$) than for ($+/+$) cells. The average interbeat intervals of ($-/-$) cells were twice as long as the interbeat intervals for ($+/+$) cells, and the ($-/-$) cells showed more dispersion, as reflected in greater variability in interbeat intervals. Thus, although ($-/-$) cardiocytes were able to beat and were electrically coupled, synchrony was clearly impaired.

Single-channel studies on these cell pairs reveal that the channels mediating the coupling are different in ($+/+$) and ($-/-$) animals. Unitary conductances of junctional channels in Cx43 ($-/-$) cardiocytes are shifted toward higher and lower values, whereas the most frequent channel conductances in ($+/+$) cardiocytes are described by a gaussian curve with a peak at 95 ± 0.9 pS, presumably reflecting abundant Cx43; Cx43 ($-/-$) cell pairs display channels with unitary conductances of 57 ± 0.7 and 160 ± 1.2 pS, consistent with the main-state and substate conductances of Cx40 channels. Interestingly, these recordings indicate that channels of the sizes expected for Cx45 contribute a neglible extent to the coupling between ($+/+$) and ($-/-$) myocytes.

To summarize these studies, coupling and conduction between ($-$/$-$) cardiocytes are substantially reduced, although perhaps not to as great an extent as predicted from estimates of the relative levels of other connexins in rodent ventricular myocytes. However, the cells show profound deficiency in Lucifer yellow dye transfer, presumably due to the low relative anion permeability of Cx40 (and Cx45) channels compared with Cx43. This relative impermeability for negatively charged ions might be implicated in the observed developmental defects by restricting diffusion of necessary morphogen(s) at developmentally critical times. Conceivably, disturbances in the patterns of cardiac contraction might also contribute to the observed malformation by changing the load imposed on regions of the developing heart and influencing the process of remodeling that occurs during normal cardiac growth.

Newer Genetic Strategies

The studies of cardiac myocytes from Cx43 knockout mice demonstrate both the power and pitfalls of traditional gene targeting approaches. Rossant's elegant experiments[41] reveal that perturbations of gap junction expression in the heart are associated with severe developmental consequences, i.e., morphogenetic abnormalities that are incompatible with postnatal life. This result is of great interest to developmental biologists, but for the electrophysiologist, these mice fail to establish whether altered cellular connectivity is associated with altered susceptibility to cardiac arrhythmogenesis. To circumvent these confounding developmental issues, novel gene targeting strategies have recently emerged.

Inducible Knockouts

A theoretically straightforward strategy to avoid deleterious knockout phenotypes during early developmental stages would be to delay gene inactivation until the organism has matured beyond the stage when this inactivation is lethal. Taking advantage of various recombinases from bacteriophage or yeast, such an elegant approach has recently been demonstrated in mice.[43] As shown in Figure 2, homologous recombination in embryonic stem cells is first used to introduce site-specific recombination targets, such as the *loxP* target sequences from bacteriophage *Cre* recombinase, into the genomic locus of interest. Mice carrying these modified, fully functional loci are generated by standard techniques and bred to homozygosity. These targeted mice

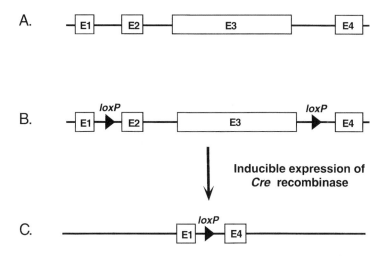

Figure 2. **Inducible gene targeting.** A, Prototypical wild-type allele consisting of four exons. B, Homologous recombination is used to introduce two *loxP* sites into nonprotein codingregions of wild-type allele. Modified allele is fully functional. C, Mice carrying modified allele are crossed with a second strain harboring an inducible *Cre* recombinase transgene; induction of *Cre* expression results in site-specific recombination between two *loxP* sites and gene inactivation.

are then bred with a second transgenic strain, in which *Cre* recombinase is under the regulatory control of an inducible promoter, such as the interferon-inducible *Mx* 1 promoter. Binary transgenic mice carrying both the *loxP* targeted loci and the *Cre* transgene are subsequently identified, and upon induction of the *Mx* 1 promoter with interferon, recombination between the two *loxP* sites can be effected. This paradigm is currently being pursued in our laboratory in an effort to more fully define the functional role of Cx43 in the adult heart.

Conditional Transgene Expression

As described above, constitutive overexpression of Cx43 in the developing mouse may be accompanied by developmental abnormalities, such as neural tube defects. Conditional transgene expression is a useful alternative when traditional gain-of-function approaches lead to such unwanted phenotypes. We have been exploring the potential utility of a tetracycline-regulated transgenic system to regulate cardiac gene expression.[44,45] This approach allows us to repress expression of target genes throughout gestation and subsequently induce them up

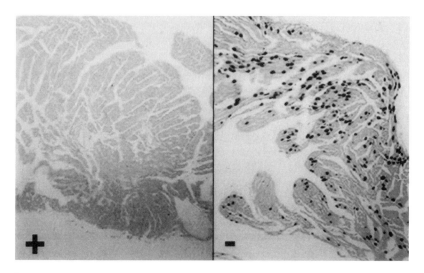

Figure 3. **Conditional expression of transgenes in heart.** Heart sections were prepared from binary transgenic mice harboring an α-myosin heavy chain tetracycline-controlled transactivator (tTA) construct and a tTA-dependent β-galactosidase reporter gene. Mice were treated with either tetracycline (+) or vehicle alone (−). Expression of the nuclear-localized β-galactosidase protein is observed only in the absence of antibiotic.

to 300-fold. As shown in Figure 3, expression of target genes within the heart can be extremely tightly regulated, but induction is heterogeneous. Thus, use of this system to express channels exogenously may be a useful way to exaggerate discontinuities in cardiac conduction and evaluate effects on impulse propagation.

Knock-ins

An extremely elegant approach to examine the nature of connexin isoform diversity is through an approach known as the knock-in, in which gene targeting technology is used to introduce functional mutations into endogenous genetic loci.[46] In this scheme, as illustrated in Figure 4, the coding region for the Cx43 gene can be replaced with another isoform. Expression of the exchanged isoform is predicted to mimic that of Cx43 both temporally and spatially, because it is under the transcriptional control of the endogenous Cx43 locus. If there truly is functional redundancy among the connexins in vivo and diversity is established by differences in patterns of gene expression, then mice harboring the modified allele should be indistinguishable from wild-type mice. However, if gating properties or connexin affinities are criti-

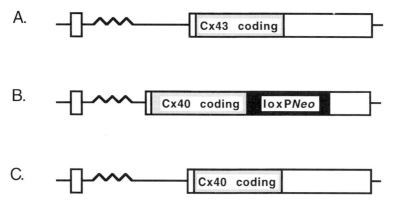

Figure 4. **Genetic knock-ins.** A, Schematic of wild-type Cx43 allele. B, Targeting vector replaces Cx43 protein-coding region with that of Cx40. Neomycin resistance cassette (surrounded by *loxP* sites) is included for positive selection of transfected embryonic stem (ES) cells. ES cell clones that have undergone homologous recombination with the targeting vector are identified by standard techniques. C, Neomyocin resistance cassette can be removed by transient expression of *Cre* recombinase in targeted ES cells. Resulting modified allele expresses Cx40 under regulatory control of the Cx43 locus.

cal variables, then the knock-in should lead to significant phenotypic sequelae. Although such experiments are in their infancy, we anticipate that such an approach will provide important insight into the diversity of gap junction channel isoforms.

Summary

Gap junction channels are essential elements in the ability of the heart to generate and propagate action potentials. However, the structural organization of the heart, including its anatomic complexity and the presence of diverse cell types with distinct patterns of connexin expression, together create discontinuities in impulse propagation at the microscopic level. It is well documented that myopathic states are associated with an increased incidence of cardiac arrhythmias, particularly malignant ventricular tachyarrhythmias. Moreover, experimental evidence is accumulating that alterations in the expression of gap junctions are associated with cardiac myopathies. In several models of heart disease, including hypertensive cardiomyopathy and postinfarct states, specific alterations in the levels of connexin transcripts or encoded proteins are detected.[47] Perhaps more significantly, both in these disease models and in cardiac myocytes acutely infected with *Trypanosoma cruzi*, the causative protozoan parasite in Chagasic cardiomyopathy, changes in the arrangement of gap junctional proteins between neighboring cardiomyocytes have been detected immunologically.[48–50] Unresolved at present, however, is whether or not disturbances in gap junction channel expression in the myopathic heart is a primary cause of these arrhythmias or simply represent a nonspecific or unrelated response of the myopathic heart. Genetic techniques in which modification of connexin expression is the primary perturbation should help resolve this dilemma. Genetic ablation by targeted mutagenesis of Cx43, the major cardiac gap junctional isoform in the mammalian heart, has been achieved. However, the phenotype of perinatal lethality has confounded efforts to establish a cause-and-effect relationship between altered connexin expression and cardiac arrhythmogenesis, at least in intact heart preparations. Newer, more selective genetic approaches through which unwanted developmental sequelae may be avoided promise to circumvent such outcomes and should facilitate more revealing studies of gap junction channel biology and cardiac conduction in vivo.

References

1. Spach MS, Heidlage JF. The stochastic nature of cardiac propagation at a microscopic level: electrical description of myocardial architecture and its application to conduction. *Circ Res.* 1995;76:366–380.
2. Spach MS. Changes in the topology of gap junctions as an adaptive structural response of the myocardium. *Circulation.* 1994;90:1103–1106.
3. Capecchi MR. Targeted gene replacement. *Sci Am.* 1994;270:52–59.
4. Robbins J. Gene targeting: the precise manipulation of the mammalian genome. *Circ Res.* 1993;73:3–9.
5. Beyer EC, Paul DL, Goodenough DA. Connexin family of gap junction proteins. *J Membr Biol.* 1990;116:187–194.
6. Bennett MVL, Barrio LC, Bargiello TA, Spray DC, Hertzberg EL, Saez JC. Gap junctions: new tools, new answers, new questions. *Neuron.* 1991;6: 305–320.
7. Fishman GI, Hertzberg EL, Spray DC, Leinwand LA. Expression of connexin43 in the developing rat heart. *Circ Res.* 1991;68:782–787.
8. Ruangvoravat CP, Lo CW. Connexin43 expression in the mouse embryo: localization of transcripts within developmentally significant domains. *Dev Dyn.* 1992;194:261–281.
9. Dermietzel R, Traub O, Hwang TK, et al. Differential expression of three gap junction proteins in developing and mature brain tissues. *Proc Natl Acad Sci U S A* 1989;86:10148–10152.
10. Paul D. Molecular cloning of cDNA for rat liver gap junction protein. *J Cell Biol.* 1986;103:123–134.
11. Beyer EC, Paul DL, Goodenough DA. Connexin43: a protein from rat heart homologous to a gap junction protein from liver. *J Cell Biol.* 1987;105: 2621–2629.
12. Willecke K, Hennemann H, Dahl E, Jungbluth S, Heynkes R. The diversity of connexin genes encoding gap junction proteins. *Eur J Cell Biol.* 1992;56: 1–7.

13. Fishman GI, Eddy RL, Shows TB, Rosenthal L, Leinwand LA. The human connexin gene family of gap junction proteins: distinct chromosomal locations but similar structures. *Genomics.* 1991;10:250–256.
14. Miller T, Dahl G, Werner R. Structure of a gap junction gene: rat connexin32. *Biosci Rep.* 1988;8:455–464.
15. Spray DC, Fishman GI. Physiological and molecular properties of cardiac gap junctions. In: Morad M, Ebashi S, Trautwein W, Kurachi Y, eds. *Molecular Physiology of Cardiac Ion Channels and Transporters.* Dordrecht, Netherlands: Kluwer Academic Publishers: 1995.
16. Gourde RG, Green CR, Severs NJ, Thompson RP. Immunolabelling patterns of gap junction connexins in the developing and mature rat heart. *Anat Embryol.* 1992;185:363–378.
17. Fromaget C, el Aoumari A, Gros D. Distribution pattern of connexin 43, a gap junctional protein, during the differentiation of mouse heart myocytes. *Differentiation.* 1992;51:9–20.
18. Fishman GI, Hertzberg EL, Spray DC, Leinwand LA. Expression of connexin43 in the developing rat heart. *Circ Res.* 1991;68:782–787.
19. Fromaget C, el Aoumari A, Dupont E, Briand JP, Gros D. Changes in the expression of connexin 43, a cardiac gap junctional protein, during mouse heart development. *J Mol Cell Cardiol.* 1990;22:1245–1258.
20. Kanter HL, Saffitz JE, Beyer EC. Cardiac myocytes express multiple gap junction proteins. *Circ Res.* 1992;70:438–444.
21. Kanter HL, Laing JG, Beau SL, Beyer EC, Saffitz JE. Distinct patterns of connexin expression in canine Purkinje fibers and ventricular muscle. *Circ Res.* 1993;72:1124–1131.
22. Gourdie RG, Severs NJ, Green CR, Rothery S, Germroth P, Thompson RP. The spatial distribution and relative abundance of gap-junctional connexin40 and connexin43 correlate to functional properties of components of the cardiac atrioventricular conduction system. *J Cell Sci.* 1993;105(pt 4): 985–991.
23. Gros D, Jarry-Guichard T, Ten Velde I, et al. Restricted distribution of connexin40, a gap junctional protein, in mammalian heart. *Circ Res.* 1994; 74:839–851.
24. Hennemann H, Suchyna T, Lichtenberg-Frate H, et al. Molecular cloning and functional expression of mouse connexin40, a second gap junction gene preferentially expressed in lung. *J Cell Biol.* 1992;117:1299–1310.
25. Bruzzone R, Haefliger JA, Gimlich RL, Paul DL. Connexin40, a component of gap junctions in vascular endothelium, is restricted in its ability to interact with other connexins. *Mol Biol Cell.* 1993;4:7–20.
26. Reed KE, Westphale EM, Larson DM, Wang HZ, Veenstra RD, Beyer EC. Molecular cloning and functional expression of human connexin37, an endothelial cell gap junction protein. *J Clin Invest.* 1993;91:997–1004.
27. Willecke K, Heynkes R, Dahl E, et al. Mouse connexin37: cloning and functional expression of a gap junction gene highly expressed in lung. *J Cell Biol.* 1991;114:1049–1057.
28. De Leon JR, Buttrick PM, Fishman GI. Functional analysis of the connexin43 gene promoter in vivo and in vitro. *J Mol Cell Cardiol.* 1994;26:379–389.
29. Geimonen E, Etchelsu O, Jiang W, et al. An AP-1 site in the human connexin43 promoter sequence mediates induction of transcription in uterine smooth muscle cells following treatment with phorbol ester. *Biol Chem.* 1996;271(39):23667–23674.
30. Neuhaus IM, Dahl G, Werner R. Use of alternate promoters for tissue-

specific expression of the gene coding for connexin32. *Gene*. 1995;158: 257–262.

31. Dahl G, Miller T, Paul D, Voellmy R, Werner R. Expression of functional cell-cell channels from cloned rat liver gap junction complementary DNA. *Science*. 1987;236:1290–1293.

32. Fishman GI, Spray DC, Leinwand LA. Molecular characterization and functional expression of the human cardiac gap junction channel. *J Cell Biol*. 1990;111:589–598.

33. Spray DC. Physiological and pharmacological regulation of gap junction channels. In: Citi S, ed. *Molecular Mechanisms of Epithelial Cell Junctions: From Development to Disease*. Austin, Tex: Medical Intelligence Unit, RG Landes Co, Biomedical Publishers: 1994:195–215.

34. Bergoffen J, Scherer SS, Wang S, et al. Connexin mutations in X-linked Charcot-Marie-Tooth disease. *Science*. 1993;262:2039–2042.

35. Britz-Cunningham SH, Maithili MS, Zuppan CW, Fletcher WH. Mutations of the connexin43 gap junction gene in patients with heart malformations and defects of laterality. *N Engl J Med*. 1995;332:1323–1329.

35a.Gebbia M, Towbin JA, Casey B. Failure to detect connexin43 mutations in 38 cases of sporadic and familial heterotaxy. *Circulation*. 1996;94(8):1909–12.

35b.Casey B, Ballabio A, Splitt MP, Burn J, Goodship J, Fletcher WH, Britz-Cunningham SH, Zuppan CW. *N Engl J Med*. Connexin43 mutations in sporadic and familial defects of laterality. 1995;333(14):941. Correspondence.

35c.Kelsell DP, Dunlop J, Stevens HP, Lench NJ, Liang JN, Parry G, Mueller RF, Leigh IM. Connexin 26 mutations in hereditary non-syndromic sensorineural deafness. *Nature*. 1997;387:80.

36. Kass S, MacRae C, Graber HL, et al. A gene defect that causes conduction system disease and dilated cardiomyopathy maps to chromosome 1p1-1q1. *Nat Genet*. 1994;7:546–551.

37. Warner AE, Guthrie SC, Gilula NB. Antibodies to gap-junctional protein selectively disrupt junctional communication in the early amphibian embryo. *Nature*. 1984;311:127–131.

38. Warner A, Gurdon JB. Functional gap junctions are not required for muscle gene activation by induction in Xenopus embryos. *J Cell Biol*. 1987;104: 557–564.

39. Lo CW, Ewart J, Sullivan R. Neural tube defects in transgenic mice with the gain or loss of connexin43 function: relevance to developmental pathologies. 1995 Gap Junction Conference.

40. Seiler SH, Fishman GI. Cx43 phosphorylation mutants: effects on gap junction channel activity and cardiac development. Keystone Symposia: *Molecular Biology of the Cardiovascular System*. 1996.

41. Reaume AG, de Sousa PA, Kulkarni S, et al. Cardiac malformation in neonatal mice lacking connexin43. *Science*. 1995;267:1831–1834.

42. Nelles E, Jung D, Gabriel HD, et al. Characterization of connexin32 deficient mice generated by gene targeting. 1995 Gap Junction Conference.

43. Kuhn R, Schwenk F, Aguet M, Rajewsky K. Inducible gene targeting in mice. *Science*. 1995;269:1427–1429.

44. Fishman GI, Kaplan ML, Buttrick PM. Tetracycline-regulated cardiac gene expression in vivo. *J Clin Invest*. 1994;93:1864–1868.

45. Passman R, Fishman GI. Regulated expression of foreign genes in vivo after germline transfer. *J Clin Invest*. 1994;94:2421–2425.

46. Hanks M, Wurst W, Anson-Cartwright L, Auerbach AB, Joyner AL. Rescue

of the En-1 mutant phenotype by replacement of En-1 with En-2 *Science.* 1995;269:679–682.

47. Bastide B, Neyses L, Ganten D, Paul M, Willecke K, Traub O. Gap junction protein connexin40 is preferentially expressed in vascular endothelium and conductive bundles of rat myocardium and is increased under hypertensive conditions. *Circ Res.* 1993;73:1138–1149.

48. Severs NJ. Pathophysiology of gap junctions in heart disease. *J Cardiovasc Electrophysiol.* 1994;5:462–475. Review.

49. Luke RA, Saffitz JE. Remodeling of ventricular conduction pathways in healed canine infarct border zones. *J Clin Invest.* 1991;87:1594–1602.

50. de Carvalho AC, Tanowitz HB, Wittner M, Dermietzel R, Roy C, Spray DC. Gap junction distribution is altered between cardiac myocytes infected with *Trypanosoma cruzi. Circ Res.* 1992;70:733–742.

Section VI

Discontinuous Conduction in Myocardial Ischemia
Introduction

Penelope A. Boyden, PhD

It is rare that troublesome arrhythmias occur in normal cardiac muscle, and it may be even rarer that these arrhythmias are related to the discontinuous nature of conduction of the cardiac impulse. More common, and thus the focus of this section, is the relationship between serious ventricular arrhythmias occurring after myocardial ischemia/infarction (MI) and the occurrence of (either de novo or enhanced) discontinuous cardiac conduction. While admittedly too simple, this discussion of ventricular arrhythmias associated with MI is divided into two sections: arrhythmias (phase 1a and 1b) secondary to acute ischemia (chapter 17) and those occurring in the healing/healed phases after MI (chapter 18). Although in each of these chapters, the relationship between experimentally measured areas of slowed and/or discontinuous conduction and various parameters is discussed, the focus is on the role of cell-to-cell coupling in the manifestation of these critical electrical abnormalities. These chapters then follow from the overall hypothesis that derangements in gap junction function may represent a fundamental mechanism causing electrical discontinuities leading to reentrant arrhythmias in both experimental models of MI (this section) and humans (see chapters 5 and 6).

It is clear that in the setting of MI, we must begin to unravel the mechanism of the observed gap junction dysfunction not only by hypothesizing disease-induced changes in intracellular ions (eg, hydrogen

Supported by NHLBI HL 30557 and HL 34477

ions) but also long-term remodeling of the various connexin proteins in surviving myocytes. This requires our complete knowledge of not only posttranslational modifications (eg, phosphorylation) but also the transcriptional controls of the connexin proteins. In terms of this latter point, it is clear from morphological studies of post-MI hearts in both experimental models and humans (see chapters 4 and 18) that connexin proteins seem to be absent or to redistribute on the cell surface of surviving myocytes. The crucial questions yet to be answered are, of course, how does this redistribution of connexin proteins alter their function on a microscopic level, and/or does it alone account for discontinuities in conduction observed to occur on the macroscopic level? Interestingly, recent data suggest that at least one potassium channel α-subunit protein (Kv1.5), which appears to be localized near connexin proteins at the intercalated disks of normal epicardial cells, also redistributes along myocyte cell surfaces in post-MI epicardial border zone tissue.[1] During this period of time, distinct changes occur in the function and density of the native potassium channels in these surviving border zone myocytes.[2] It is intriguing to postulate that both ion channels (gap junction and Kv1.5 potassium channels) act in a synergistic manner to give rise to discontinuities in cardiac conduction.

Although changes in potassium channel density and function may well help to promote discontinuities in conduction, recent data also suggest that the function of the L-type calcium channel gains significance as cells become relatively uncoupled (see chapter 21). The critical relationship of this finding to discontinuities of conduction in the arrhythmogenic substrates in acute ischemia and during the healing/healed phase post-MI is not clear at this time. However, the rate-dependent manifestation of conduction slowing as described by Gettes et al (chapter 17) and/or the mechanism of conduction in areas of "pseudo-block" during reentrant arrhythmias as described by Wit (chapter 18) may well be critically dependent on the alteration in pattern and extent of gap junction proteins along myocytes, as well as on L-type calcium channel function and its subsequent impact on intracellular calcium handling. In this latter regard, clearly the chronic changes observed to occur in L-type calcium channel function and Ca_i handling in myocytes that survive in the epicardial border[3,4] would only serve to exacerbate the changes in cardiac conduction occurring secondary to gap junction redistribution.

In chapter 19, Rosen and I address the issue of pharmacology of gap junctions. It is certainly clear that this field is rapidly expanding, but we are hesitant to promote excessive therapeutic benefit from "the pharmacological modification of discontinuous conduction." Clearly, reasonable arguments can be made for use of both specific "cell couplers" and specific "cell uncouplers" for treatment of various arrhythmias after MI. The problem here, of course, is that we lack any "specific" agents at this time, making our testing of worthiness of such agents difficult. Furthermore, our knowledge of the pivotal role of intact gap junctions in providing a myocyte-to-myocyte form of cell signaling in health and disease is at this time limited. In particular here, and probably key for myocytes that survive in hearts after MI, is the importance of changes in calcium ions associated with calcium oscillations. These calcium oscillations are initiated at a specific site and spread across adjacent cardiac cells in the form of an intercellular calcium wave. Importantly, pharmacological manipulations to "close" gap junctions appear to block calcium-wave propagation in syncytial myocardium (see chapter 10) and presumably not within a myocyte.

In sum, the nature of discontinuous cardiac conduction is variable, depending on the underlying anatomic and electrical substrates. This is only too well recognized in discussions of the importance of discontinuous conduction in arrhythmias in myocardial ischemia. Therefore, a corollary must be that the pharmacology of discontinuous conduction in this setting (as well as in others) is evolving.

References

1. Tamkun MM, Mays DJ, Boyden PA. Redistribution of the Kv1.5 K channel protien on the surface of myocytes from the epicardial border zone of the infacted canine heart. *CV Pathobiology.* 1997. In press.
2. Lue WM, Boyden PA. Abnormal electrical properties of myocytes from chronically infarcted canine heart: alterations in V_{max} and the transient outward current. *Circulation.* 1992;85:1175–1188.
3. Aggarwal R, Boyden PA. Diminished Ca^{2+} and Ba^{2+} currents in myocytes surviving in the epicardial border zone of the 5 day infarcted canine heart. *Circ Res.* 1995;77:1180–1191.
4. Licata A, Aggarwal R, Robinson R, Boyden PA. Frequency dependent effects on Ca^{2+} transients and cell shortening in myocytes that survive in the infarcted heart. *Cardiovasc Res.* 1997;33:341–350.

Chapter 17

Characteristics and Causes of Conduction Changes Associated with 1a and 1b Arrhythmias in Acute Ischemia

Leonard S. Gettes, MD,
Wayne E. Cascio, MD,
Timothy A. Johnson, PhD,
Barbara Muller-Borer, PhD,
and the Experimental Cardiology Group

In 1979, Kaplinsky et al[1] described two phases of ventricular arrhythmias occurring within 30 minutes of the onset of acute myocardial ischemia. Phase 1a occurred within the first 5 to 10 minutes and was followed by a period of 10 to 15 minutes that was arrhythmia free. This was then followed by the onset of phase 1b arrhythmias, which occurred within 20 to 30 minutes of the onset of acute no-flow ischemia. This chapter discusses the causes of the changes in macroscopic conduction that occur during these phases, addresses the specific role of cell-to-cell electrical uncoupling in the genesis of these conduction changes, and considers whether the changes in macroscopic conduction that contribute to the genesis of arrhythmias during acute ischemia are related to spatial inhomogeneities of impulse propagation.

The speed at which an impulse propagates is determined by both active and passive membrane properties.[2] The most important active membrane property is the rate at which the individual membrane segments depolarize. This is related to the magnitude of the inward cur-

Supported in part by 5-PO1-HL27430, 5-RO1-HL48769, 5-RO1-HL49818, 1-T32-HL07793

From: Spooner PM, Joyner RW, Jalife J (eds). *Discontinuous Conduction in the Heart.* Armonk, NY: Futura Publishing Company, Inc.; © 1997.

rents and is reflected by the maximum rate of rise of the action potential upstroke. Changes in resting membrane potential exert a major effect on this component by virtue of their effect on the inactivation and the recovery from inactivation of the rapid sodium inward current.[3] The passive membrane properties most important to impulse propagation are the external and internal longitudinal resistances (r_o and r_i). r_o refers to the extracellular component of the local membrane circuit, and r_i reflects primarily the resistance at the gap junction, or coupling resistance. The relationship between changes in upstroke velocity of the action potential, changes in coupling resistance, and changes in longitudinal conduction are predicted reasonably well by one-dimensional cable theory, which states that changes in conduction velocity are related directly to the square root of changes of the upstroke of the action potential and inversely to the square root of changes in coupling resistance.[2]

Whether such changes in conduction velocity are continuous or discontinuous is, in part, a matter of definition, and whether such changes will lead to reentry or to the development of reentrant tachyarrhythmias will depend on a variety of factors, some of which are poorly understood. Conduction is discontinuous when impulse propagation is blocked. However, such a discontinuity in conduction may not lead to reentry or to the development of tachyarrhythmias unless the block itself is regional and/or inhomogeneous. On the other hand, slowing of activation may or may not be discontinuous. If such slowing is inhomogeneous, it may promote the development of unidirectional block and lead to the development of reentry and to reentrant tachyarrhythmias.

The delay in ventricular activation that occurs within the center of the ischemic zone after the acute interruption of flow in the left anterior descending coronary artery of the pig is illustrated in Figure 1. Within the first 10 minutes of the onset of no-flow ischemia, which corresponds to the 1a phase of arrhythmias, there is an activation delay of 35 ms. This activation delay is then followed by a period of spontaneous improvement that lasts for ≈10 minutes and is followed by a second phase of activation delay that continues until activation block occurs. This second period of activation delay corresponds to the 1b phase of arrhythmias. The changes in extracellular potassium ($[K^+]_e$) and extracellular pH (pH_e) that occur in the setting of acute ischemia and accompany these changes in activation are shown in Figures 1 and 2.

The changes in $[K^+]_e$, like the changes in activation, are triphasic.[4] There is an initial rise during the first 10 minutes, which is followed by a period during which $[K^+]_e$ changes only slightly, and then, after ≈20 to 30 minutes, a second phase during which $[K^+]_e$ slowly rises.

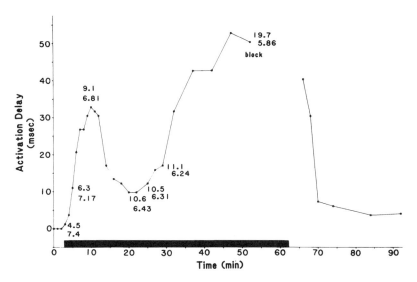

Figure 1. Activation delay recorded in center of ischemic zone by a bipolar electrode referenced to an electrode in nonischemic zone during 60-minute occlusion of left anterior descending coronary artery in situ pig heart. Pairs of numbers at various times represent values of extracellular K^+ (top number) and extracellular pH (bottom number) recorded by ion-selective electrodes positioned at same location.

Extracellular pH falls rapidly in the first 10 minutes. In the period during which activation and $[K^+]_e$ show either a spontaneous improvement or only minimal change, pH_e continues to decrease, albeit at a somewhat slower rate, and eventually plateaus at levels of ≈ 5.5 to 6.0 after 30 minutes of ischemia. The changes in extracellular potassium during these periods are markedly inhomogeneous both in the center and at the margin of the ischemic zone.[5] These inhomogeneities are paralleled by inhomogeneous changes in activation.[6] However, it is important to note that the changes in activation are more pronounced than can be explained solely by the rise in $[K^+]_e$.[4,7]

In our experience, the incidence of ventricular fibrillation during the 1a phase of ventricular arrhythmias, ie, during the first 8 minutes after occlusion of the left anterior descending coronary artery below the first diagonal branch in the anesthetized pig, is $\approx 25\%$.[8] However, we have not been able to identify those animals that fibrillate on the basis of the magnitude or inhomogeneities of the ionic changes or on the basis of the magnitude or inhomogeneities of the changes in activation that occur in the center of the ischemic zone. We have recently shown[8] that if $[K^+]_e$ in the center of the ischemic zone is elevated to 8 mmol/L before complete interruption of left anterior descending coro-

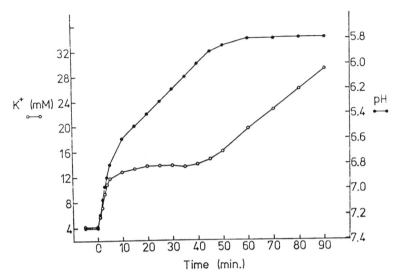

Figure 2. Changes in extracellular K^+ (open circles) and extracellular pH (closed circles) recorded from center of ischemic zone in situ pig heart during 90-minute occlusion of left anterior descending coronary artery. Reprinted with permission from Gettes LS, Cascio WE. Effect of acute ischemia on cardiac electrophysiology. In: Fozzard H, et al, eds. The Heart and Cardiovascular System: *Scientific Foundation.* 2nd ed. New York, NY: Raven Press Ltd; 1992: 2021–2054.

nary flow, then the incidence of ventricular fibrillation rises to ≈80% within 2 minutes of interruption of coronary flow. This high incidence of ventricular fibrillation is associated with a more marked delay in activation than occurs if ischemia is induced without the prior elevation of potassium, an activation delay that corresponds to a slowing of longitudinal conduction to <10 cm/s.[8] In contrast, when ischemia is induced without the prior elevation of $[K^+]_e$, longitudinal conduction slows to no less than 20 cm/s and then blocks (Figure 3). We believe that the marked slowing of conduction to <10 cm/s is due to calcium current– or slow inward sodium current–mediated conduction rather than to the partial inactivation of the rapid sodium current. We believe that inactivation of the rapid inward current is the mechanism responsible for the reduction in conduction velocity to 20 cm/s but that this mechanism is incapable of causing slower conduction velocities. It is our hypothesis that during acute ischemia, reentry occurs at the ischemic margin in areas in which very slow conduction, most likely calcium channel mediated, results from unique changes in $[K^+]_e$ and pH_e. The evidence for this can be found in the work of Pogwizd and Corr[9] and Wilensky et al.[10] Pogwizd and Corr demonstrated the development of reentry at

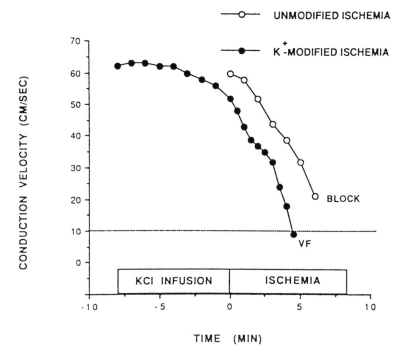

TIME (MIN)

Figure 3. Changes in conduction velocity recorded by a plaque electrode on center of ischemic zone in situ pig heart during unmodified ischemia (open circles), ie, interruption of flow in left anterior descending coronary artery without prior infusion of KCl, and during K^+-modified ischemia (solid circles). See text for discussion. Reprinted with permission from Fleet WF, Johnson TA, Cascio WE, Shen J, Engle CL, Martin DG, Gettes LS. Marked activation delay caused by ischemia initiated after regional K^+ elevation in situ pig hearts. Circulation. 1994;90:3009–3017.

the subendocardial margin of the ischemic zone, where they estimated a slowing of conduction to ≈8 cm/s, consistent with slow channel–mediated conduction. Wilensky et al studied changes in $[K^+]_e$ and pH_e during acute ischemia as a function of distance from the subendocardial ischemic margin and demonstrated a region between 500 and 900 μm, where $[K^+]_e$ increased to between 8 and 10 mmol/L but pH_e had fallen only slightly, thereby predicting that such regions do in fact exist along ischemic margins. We have observed in ongoing studies[11] that ≈25% of pairs of pH and potassium ion–selective electrodes placed across the lateral ischemic margin demonstrate this combination (Figure 4). We also noted that the location of these electrode pairs is not consistent but rather changes as a function of time and distance along the margin.

The very slow conduction that occurs during the 1a phase of ar-

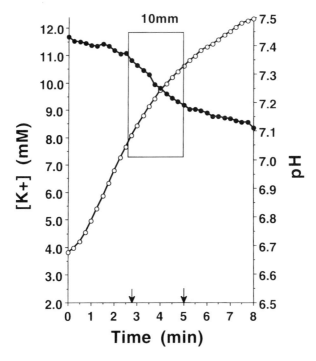

Figure 4. Changes in extracellular K^+ and pH recorded by a pair of ion-selective electrodes placed within 1 mm of each other, 10 mm inside lateral cyanotic border of ischemic zone during occlusion of left anterior descending coronary artery in in situ pig heart. K^+ has risen to >8 mmol/L, but pH has not fallen to <7.2 during interval enclosed in rectangular box and defined by arrows. Discussion in text.

rhythmias is independent of changes in cellular coupling. This conclusion is supported by several studies. Kléber et al[12] showed that in the blood-perfused rabbit papillary muscle, coupling resistance did not increase for ≈10 to 20 minutes after the onset of acute no-flow ischemia, that is, after the time window of the 1a arrhythmias. This result was confirmed by Cascio et al,[13] who showed in the same preparation that the rise in internal longitudinal resistance paralleled the third, or slowly rising, phase of the potassium increase but did not occur during the rise in $[K^+]_e$. This is illustrated in Figure 5, which is based on the data contained in Cascio et al. Recent studies in our laboratories by Smith et al[14] and by Owens et al[15] have extended these observations in the in situ pig heart and in the isolated perfused rabbit heart. Smith et al noted that an increase in whole-tissue resistance, as determined by the four-electrode technique,[16,17] occurred in concert with the third phase of the rise in $[K^+]_e$ ≈20 minutes after the onset of no-flow ischemia in

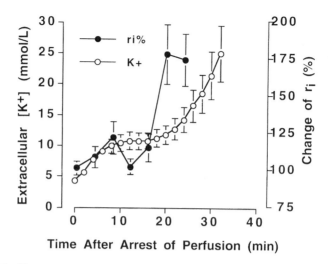

Figure 5. Changes in extracellular K+ and internal longitudinal resistance (r_i) in blood-perfused rabbit papillary muscle during 40 minutes of no-flow ischemia. Note that rise in r_i occurs ≈20 minutes after arrest of perfusion in concert with onset of third or slowly rising phase of K+ change.

the pig. This increase in resistance coincided with the slowing and eventual failure of ventricular conduction and with the onset of the phase 1b arrhythmias.

Owens et al, in association with Dr. Elizabeth Murphy at the National Institute of Environmental Health Sciences,[15] showed a similar relationship in the isolated blood-perfused rabbit heart made globally ischemic by the interruption of the perfusate. They showed that the rise in coupling resistance occurred after intracellular calcium had more than doubled and after intracellular pH had fallen to a level of ≈6.0. It is not clear whether these intracellular ionic changes were the cause of uncoupling or were merely temporally coincident with it. Other factors, such as the long-chain acylcarnitine, lysophosphoglycerides, arachidonic acid, and a decrease in ATP, have also been shown to cause cellular uncoupling and may be equally if not more important than the changes in intracellular pH and calcium.

The results of these studies indicate that the slowing of conduction that occurs 15 to 30 minutes after the onset of ischemia can be attributed not only to changes in active membrane properties, which occur as the rise in $[K^+]_e$ enters its third or slowly rising phase, but also to cellular electrical uncoupling. It is important to note, however, that even with the onset of cellular electrical uncoupling, we have not observed a slowing of conduction velocity to <5 cm/s, nor have we observed the development of fractionated electrograms.

The studies referred to above raised the question of whether discontinuities in conduction during acute ischemia could result from the interaction between the ionic changes and the changes in coupling resistance. To investigate this possibility, Muller-Borer et al[18] recently created a mathematical model to simulate the potassium gradient across the ischemic border and the changes in gap junctional resistance likely to occur during acute ischemia. The model consists of elements, each 10 μm long and 10 μm in diameter, joined to form modeled cells 30 to 130 μm long. The cells are joined in gap junctions to form a 10-mm modeled cardiac fiber. The gap junctional resistance is set at 1275 kΩ. In this model, $[K^+]_e$ concentration is increased in steps of 0.8 mmol/L per 1.0 mm, or 8 mmol/L per centimeter of tissue. Gap junctional resistance is sequentially increased above the control level in each of the regions of increased $[K^+]_e$ and a stimulus introduced from either the high-$[K^+]_e$ end or the low-$[K^+]_e$ end of the fiber. Unidirectional block occurs when the impulse originates from the region of high $[K^+]_e$ when the gap junctional resistance is at least 8 times control, but it does not occur when the impulse originates in the area of low $[K^+]_e$. In this situation, a further increase in gap junctional resistance is required to induce block, and at this level of uncoupling, bidirectional rather than unidirectional block occurs (Figure 6).

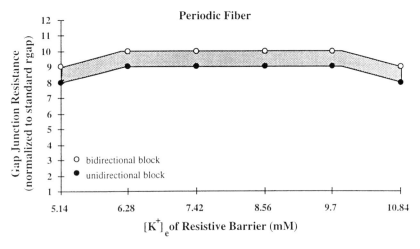

Figure 6. Level of increased gap junctional resistance necessary to produce unidirectional block (solid circles) and bidirectional block (open circles) in nonperiodic fiber model. Unidirectional block occurred when preparation was stimulated from high-K^+ side of resistive barrier. When preparation was stimulated from low-K^+ side of barrier at this level of gap junctional resistance, block did not occur. Bidirectional block indicates that conduction was blocked regardless of stimulation site. Reprinted with permission from Reference 18.

Two other related factors may contribute to macroscopic discontinuities and to the onset of ventricular arrhythmias. The first is that the conduction slowing induced by acute ischemia is rate dependent,[19,20] that is, it becomes more pronounced as the heart rate is increased. The second is that frequently the conduction block that occurs is inhomogeneous. Moreover, the development of complete conduction block is often preceded by a period during which 2:1 conduction block occurs.[8] The inhomogeneous 2:1 behavior, which occurs more commonly at the more rapid rates of stimulation, is a cause of intermittent discontinuous conduction that frequently heralds the onset of ventricular fibrillation. The rate dependency of the conduction slowing is due to a rate-dependent exaggeration of the decrease in V_{max} of the action potential upstroke and to a rate-dependent exaggeration of the rise in coupling resistance.[21] The cause or causes of the rate dependency of these changes in V_{max} and coupling resistance are not obvious. The rise in $[K^+]_e$ during the acute ischemia, while rate dependent in the rabbit, is not rate dependent in the pig, although the rate-dependent changes in conduction during the first 10 minutes of ischemia are very prominent in the pig. Rate-dependent increases in intracellular sodium and intracellular calcium have been proposed as possible mechanisms.[22,23] These changes in intracellular calcium may also contribute to the rate-dependent increase in coupling resistance. However, the possibility of rate-dependent changes in other regulators of gap junctional resistance have not yet been studied.

In conclusion, we believe that during the phase 1a arrhythmias, there are areas of very slow conduction, ie, to <10 cm/s, which are mediated by slow channel–dependent responses and occur in the ab­sence of cellular uncoupling. These areas occur inhomogeneously at regions along the ischemic border where $[K^+]_e$ is >8 and pH_e has not yet fallen to <7.2. These areas of very slow conduction promote the development of spatial inhomogeneities in impulse conduction that permit the creation of reentry pathways and the development of reentrant arrhythmias, including ventricular fibrillation. The conduction slowing that occurs during the phase 1b arrhythmias is associated with cellular uncoupling. This occurs in concert with the slowly rising phase of $[K^+]_e$, a doubling of intracellular calcium, and a fall in intracellular pH to ≈6.0. We believe that the gradual inactivation of the sodium system by the ischemia-induced fall in resting membrane potential is capable of slowing conduction to the range of 20 cm/s but that thereafter, impulse block occurs in an inhomogeneous fashion. Activation of the slow calcium inward current after inactivation of the fast inward sodium current is capable of slowing conduction to the range of 5 to 10 cm/s. However, more marked degrees of conduction slowing due exclusively to changes in active membrane properties have not been recorded. It is likely that conduction slowing to <5 cm/s requires uncoupling of cardiac elements, either by biochemical changes, as occur in the setting of acute myocardial ischemia, or by structural changes that interfere with the integrity of the gap junctions. This mechanism is more likely to occur in the postinfarction period. It is likely that in acute ischemia, the spatial inhomogeneity of conduction is functional, ie, related to the inhomogeneities of metabolic and ionic changes and the location and timing of premature beats. In contrast, macroscopic spatial inhomogeneities of conduction in the postinfarction period on the macroscopic level may be more structural because of fibrosis.

The studies we have reviewed raise many important questions. The cause of the increase in resistance at the gap junction during ischemia, which is rate dependent, is not clearly understood. It appears that the gap junctional resistance is relatively insensitive to changes in both intracellular pH and intracellular calcium if the time-averaged values obtained by nuclear magnetic resonance spectroscopy referred to above provide an accurate representation of the subcellular changes. However, the possibility that inhomogeneous subcellular changes in intracellular calcium and pH may be responsible for cellular uncoupling needs to be addressed. In addition, the role of the other factors referred to above, both in the presence and in the absence of intracellular ionic changes that occur in the setting of acute ischemia, needs to be further defined.

The role of electrical uncoupling and impedance mismatching at the Purkinje ventricular muscle junction in the conduction slowing that occurs during both the 1a and 1b phases of arrhythmias has not been well characterized. In addition, the relationship between the site of origin of premature beats, the changes in active and passive membrane properties, and the creation of spatial inhomogeneities of conduction that lead to reentry and to reentrant tachyarrhythmias in the setting of acute myocardial ischemia requires further investigation. As these issues are addressed and the questions they spawn are answered, our understanding of the characteristics and causes of the conduction changes that occur during acute myocardial ischemia should be significantly broadened and our understanding of the pathogenesis of the phase 1a and 1b arrhythmias made more complete.

References

1. Kaplinsky E, Ogawa S, Balke CW, Dreifus LS. Two periods of early ventricular arrhythmia in the canine acute myocardial infarction model. *Circulation.* 1979;60:397–403.
2. Gettes LS, Buchanan JW Jr, Saito T, Kagiyama Y, Oshita S, Fujino T. Studies concerned with slow conduction. In: Zipes D, Jalife J, eds. *Cardiac Electro-*

physiology and Arrhythmias. New York, NY: Grune & Stratton, Inc (Harcourt Brace Jovanovich, Publishers); 1985:81–87.

3. Gettes LS. Effects of ionic changes on impulse propagation. In: Rosen MR, Janse MJ, Wit AL, eds. *Cardiac Electrophysiology: A Textbook.* Mount Kisco, NY: Futura Publishing Co.; 1990:459–479.

4. Hill JL, Gettes LS. Effect of acute coronary artery occlusion on local myocardial extracellular K^+ activity in swine. *Circulation.* 1980;61:768–778.

5. Johnson TA, Engle CL, Boyd LM, Koch GG, Gwinn M, Gettes LS. Magnitude and time course of extracellular potassium inhomogeneities during acute ischemia in pigs: effect of verapamil. *Circulation.* 1991;83:622–634.

6. Coronel R, Fiolet JWT, Wilms-Schopman FJG, Opthof T, Schaapherder AFM, Janse MJ. Distribution of extracellular potassium and electrophysiologic changes during two-stage coronary ligation in the isolated, perfused canine heart. *Circulation.* 1989;80:165–177.

7. Kléber AG, Janse MJ, Wilms-Schopman FJG, Wilde AAM, Coronel R. Changes in conduction velocity during acute ischemia in ventricular myocardium of the isolated porcine heart. *Circulation.* 1986;73:189–198.

8. Fleet WF, Johnson TA, Cascio WE, et al. Marked activation delay caused by ischemia initiated after regional K^+ elevation in in-situ pig hearts. *Circulation.* 1994;90:3009–3017.

9. Pogwizd SM, Corr PB. Mechanisms underlying the development of ventricular fibrillation during early myocardial ischemia. *Circ Res.* 1990;66: 672–695.

10. Wilenski RL, Tranum-Jensen J, Coronel R, Wilde AAM, Fiolet JWT, Janse MJ. The subendocardial border zone during acute ischemia of the rabbit heart: an electrophysiologic, metabolic and morphologic correlative study. *Circulation.* 1986;74:1137–1146.

11. Fleet WF, Johnson TA, Engle CL, et al. $[K^+]_e$-pH combination at the ischemic margin in the pig. *Circulation.* 1993;88(suppl I):I–7. Abstract.

12. Kléber AG, Riegger CB, Janse MJ. Electrical uncoupling and increase of extracellular resistance after induction of ischemia in isolated, arterially perfused rabbit papillary muscle. *Circ Res.* 1987;61:271–279.

13. Cascio WE, Yan GX, Kléber AG. Passive electrical properties, mechanical activity and extracellular potassium in arterially perfused and ischemic rabbit ventricular muscle: effects of calcium entry blockade or hypocalcemia. *Circ Res.* 1990;66:1461–1473.

14. Smith WT, Fleet WF, Johnson TA, Engle CL, Cascio WE. The Ib phase of ventricular arrhythmias in ischemic in situ porcine heart is related to changes in cell-to-cell electrical coupling. *Circulation.* 1995;92:3051–3060.

15. Owens L, Gettes LS, Cascio WE, Fralix TA, Murphy E. Correlation of extracellular and intracellular events during acute ischemia in the isolated blood perfused rabbit heart. *Circulation.* 1996;94:10–13.

16. Plonsey R, Barr R. The four-electrode resisitivity technique as applied to cardiac muscle. *IEEE Trans Biomed Eng.* 1982;29:541–546.

17. Ellenby MI, Small KW, Wells RM, Hoyt DJ, Lowe JE. On-line detection of reversible myocardial ischemic injury by measurement of myocardial electrical impedance. *Ann Thorac Surg.* 1987;44:587–597.

18. Muller-Borer BJ, Johnson TA, Gettes LS, Cascio WE. Failure of impulse propagation in a mathematically simulated ischemic border zone: influence of direction of propagation and cell-to-cell electrical coupling. *J Cardiovasc Electrophysiol.* 1995;6:1101–1112.

19. Hope RR, Williams DO, El-Sherif N, Lazzara R, Scherlag BJ. The efficacy

of antiarrhythmic agents during acute myocardial ischemia and the role of heart rate. *Circulation.* 1974;50:507–514.

20. Harper JR Jr, Johnson TA, Engle CL, Martin DG, Fleet W, Gettes LS. Effect of rate on changes in conduction velocity and extracellular potassium concentration during acute ischemia in the in situ pig heart. *J Cardiovasc Electrophysiol.* 1993;4:661–671.

21. Hiramatsu Y, Buchannan JW Jr. Kinsley SB, Koch GG, Kropp S, Gettes LS. Influence of rate-dependent cellular uncoupling on conduction change during simulated ischemia in guinea pig papillary muscles: effect of verapamil. *Circ Res.* 1989;65:95–102.

22. Cohen CJ, Fozzard HA, Sheu SS. Increase in intracellular sodium ion activity during stimulation in mammalian cardiac muscle. *Circ Res.* 1982;50: 651–662.

23. Lado MG, Sheu SS, Fozzard HA. Changes in intracellular Ca^{2+} activity with stimulation in sheep cardiac Purkinje strands. *Am J Physiol.* 1982;243: 133–137.

Chapter 18

Discontinuous Conduction in the Epicardial Border Zone of Infarcted Hearts and Its Role in Anisotropic Reentry

Andrew L. Wit, PhD

Reentrant excitation in hearts with myocardial infarction is an important cause of ventricular arrhythmias. The mechanisms causing reentry in this pathological state have been a subject of investigation for a number of years. Many interesting insights into the pathophysiology have been obtained from both clinical investigations and laboratory studies on animal models. One important conclusion from these studies was that mechanisms causing arrhythmias change as infarcts progress from the acute stage through the healing stage to the healed stage.[1]

Our studies have focused on the electrophysiological properties of the arrhythmogenic regions in hearts with healing myocardial infarction during the first week after a coronary artery occlusion. The experimental approach was to map excitation in the epicardial border zone of surviving muscle cells with extracellular electrodes in the in situ canine heart. Using this approach, we have found evidence of "discontinuous conduction" on a macroscopic level rather than on the microscopic level described by others in this monograph. On a macroscopic level, with extracellular electrodes with 3- to 5-mm interelectrode distances, discontinuous conduction appears as a sudden slowing of conduction to the point at which it seems to be almost stationary for a short period of time until it suddenly resumes at its original speed. However, the relationship between this phenomenon and discontin-

Supported by Grants HL-30557 and R32 HL-31393 from the Heart, Lung, and Blood Institute of the National Institutes of Health

From: Spooner PM, Joyner RW, Jalife J (eds). *Discontinuous Conduction in the Heart.* Armonk, NY: Futura Publishing Company, Inc.; © 1997.

uous conduction at a cellular level is uncertain, because the phenomenon of discontinuous conduction at the macroscopic level may actually represent a sudden slowing of conduction without any real discontinuity, that is, without actually stopping and starting again. Therefore, at a level at which conduction is measured with extracellular electrodes, it is more realistic to call it discontinuous activation.

Epicardial Border Zone in Myocardial Infarcts and Anatomic Contribution to Discontinuous Activation

The epicardial border zone is an important site of origin of arrhythmia in healing canine infarcts. Muscle fibers on the epicardial surface of transmural anteroseptal canine infarcts caused by permanent occlusion of the left anterior descending coronary artery (LAD) near its origin survive because they still receive blood flow from epicardial branches of the circumflex artery or from collaterals of the LAD that anastomose with the patent circumflex. A redistribution of coronary blood flow from necrotic endocardial layers to surviving epicardial layers may also maintain their viability.[2]

The microscopic anatomy of the border zone of surviving epicardial muscle in canine infarcts has important influences on the electrophysiological properties of this region that cause arrhythmias. Two aspects of the anatomy influence properties of impulse conduction: thickness of the surviving rim of muscle and orientation of the muscle bundles that form the rim. The border zone of surviving epicardial muscle cells is from one to several hundred cells thick. The number of surviving cell layers is fewest toward the center and increases toward the margin with normal myocardium.[3–5] Very narrow or thin epicardial border zones have properties that favor the occurrence of reentry more than thick ones do, as we describe later.

The surviving epicardial muscle fibers are arranged parallel to one another during the healing phase (during the first 2 weeks) after infarction. The long axis of the muscle fiber bundles is perpendicular to the LAD and extends from the coronary artery toward the lateral left ventricle and apex, the same orientation as epicardial muscle fibers in the noninfarcted anterior left ventricle.[6] The muscle fibers may be either tightly packed together, as they are in the normal subepicardium, or separated by edema, as is commonly seen in a healing infarct. Examples of both kinds of arrangement are shown in Figure 1. Figure 1A shows the muscle fibers widely separated by edema, whereas in 1B they are closely packed together. The parallel orientation forms an anisotropic

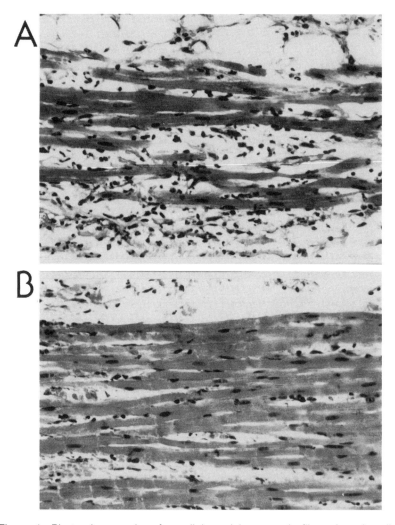

Figure 1. Photomicrographs of parallel surviving muscle fibers in epicardial border zone of healing canine infarct. In some regions (A), muscle fibers are widely separated, while in others (B), they are packed more closely together. In both cases, however, fibers are oriented parallel to each other. Reprinted with permission from Reference 1.

structure that has important influences on conduction properties that may cause reentry in this region.

Conduction in the epicardial border zone of healing canine infarcts is anisotropic, that is, it is markedly influenced by the direction of propagation relative to the orientation of the long axis of the myocardial fibers bundles, which, as mentioned above, are still arranged parallel to one another.[4,7–9] In some infarcts, stimulated wave fronts traveling parallel to the long axis of the muscle fiber bundles in the epicardial border zone may travel at normal conduction velocities of 50 to 60 cm/s in regions in which reentrant circuits were located during periods of tachycardia. Wave fronts traveling transverse to the long axis of the fibers have also been shown to propagate at normal average velocities of 20 to 30 cm/s in some regions,[9] but transverse conduction velocity may be as slow as 5 cm/s in others.[4,9] Regions of the epicardial border zone that have normal conduction velocities during activation parallel to the long axis of myocardial fiber orientation most likely have normal or nearly normal transmembrane resting potentials and action potential upstrokes. Even at rapid rates of stimulation, conduction velocities in these regions slow only slightly, no more than in normal myocardium.[1] Significant rate-dependent slowing of conduction would be expected if the transmembrane potentials were depressed. The same regions are activated slowly by wave fronts propagating transverse to the fiber long axis. The slow activation is a result of the anisotropic properties of the tissue. Where there is very slow activation in the transverse direction, such as those regions with conduction velocities of ≤5 cm/s, the myocardial fiber bundles may be more widely separated by edema or connective tissue, and some of the transverse connections may be disrupted.

We have also found an abnormal distribution of gap junctions in the regions of slow transverse anisotropic conduction.[10] The epicardial border zone overlying 4-day-old infarcts was mapped with a multiple-electrode array and was systematically examined by standard histology and confocal immunolocalization of connexin43 (Cx43), the principal mammalian cardiac gap junctional protein. The surviving myocardium from the interface of surviving border zone muscle fibers with underlying necrotic cells showed a marked disruption of gap junction distribution, with the predominant localization of the Cx43 staining along the lateral surfaces of the cells. Regions occurred in which the disturbances extended throughout the full thickness of the border zone. The location of these regions correlated with the location of the central common pathway in figure-8–type reentrant circuits that could be induced by programmed stimulation.[9] Regions of abnormal gap junction distribution were bounded by the lines of functional block forming the central common pathway. These results suggest that gap-junctional disturbances contribute to very slow transverse conduction that promotes the formation of regions of functional block, thereby contributing to the formation of stable reentrant circuits. Furthermore, the disturbances in gap junction distribution is an early pathophysiological change that is not secondary to fibrotic scarring and distortion that takes place later during healing.

Some of the extracellular electrograms recorded in regions of slow activation in the epicardial border zone in both healing[11] and healed infarcts[12] have a characteristic long duration and fractionated appearance, which is illustrated in Figure 2, top right. The electrogram shown in Figure 2 (right) was recorded from a bipolar electrode (1-mm distance between poles) at the site indicated by the shaded circle on the activation map. Activation of the small region around the electrode (several millimeters) was very slow and required almost 20 ms, causing the long duration of the electrogram compared with electrograms recorded from other regions that were activated more quickly. For example, the electrogram shown at top left was recorded from a region in a healing infarct that was activated in <5 ms. The duration of the electrogram is directly related to the time it takes the propagating wave front to pass beneath the recording electrode, being very long when activation is slow. In addition to the very slow activation causing electrograms with a long duration, it has been shown in these experimental healed infarcts that activation is not homogeneous and that this property causes the fractionated nature of the electrogram.[12] The diagram in Figure 3 offers a simplistic explanation for the relationship of nonhomogeneous, slow activation to the cause of the fractionated electrograms in the epicardial border zone. Three functional bundles of surviving muscle embedded in the infarct scar are shown. Figure 3A shows very few connections between the bundles because of their separation by the connective tissue. Interconnections occur at distant sites not shown in the figure. The larger circles represent the locations of the bipolar electrodes, and the dark arrows show the pattern of impulse propagation between bundles. This model assumes circuitous conduction in the vicinity of the bipolar electrode. Conduction velocity in each of the three functional bundles can be normal because of the normal transmembrane potentials in healed infarcts, but total activation of the region is slow because of the circuitous pathway of propagation made necessary by the lack of interconnections. Isoelectric intervals in the fractionated electrogram at the right (between deflections a, b, and c) occur during the time the impulse is out of the recording field of the bipolar electrode; components of the fractionated electrogram (a, b, and c) occur when the impulse returns in one of the muscle bundles. The model in Figure 3B shows a different possible mechanism for the fractionated electrogram. The arrows again show the propagation pattern in the vicinity of the bipolar recording site indicated by the large circles. This model assumes that are large pauses as excitation passes across connections between adjacent muscle bundles (discontinuous conduction). The pauses might occur if the resistance at intercellular contacts between myocardial fibers is high, causing slow impulse transmission across high-resistance junctions or barriers.[13-15] A high resistance might

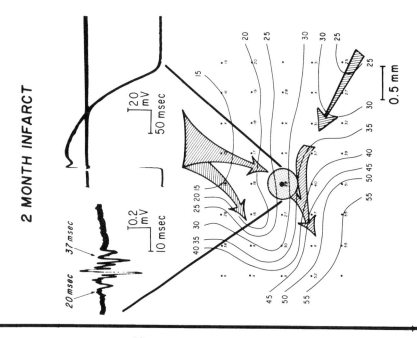

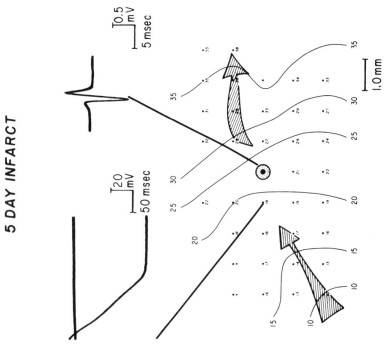

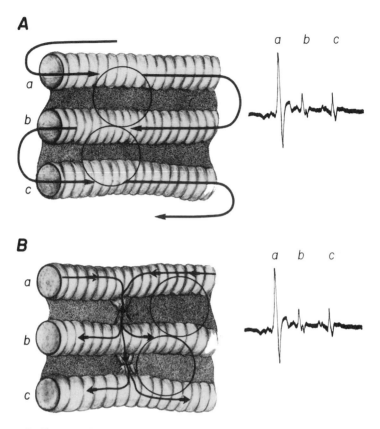

Figure 3. Two models that might explain occurrence of fractionated electrograms. A, Three cardiac fibers or bundles are indicated by cylindrical structures. These fibers are separated by connective tissue and are not interconnected in region shown by diagram. However, interconnections do occur at a distant site. Large circles represent locations of bipolar electrodes; dark arrows show impulse propagation. B, Three cardiac fibers are connected, and impulse propagation occurs in a relatively straight line through these connections, as indicated by arrows. Reprinted with permission from Reference 12.

Figure 2. Activation maps of regions around bipolar electrodes in two different epicardial border zones, one from a 5-day-old infarct (left) and one from a 2-month-old infarct (right). Location and size of electrodes are indicated by stippled circle, and electrograms recorded in each experiment are shown above. Points at which action potentials were recorded are indicated by dots in each panel. Representative action potentials are also shown. Arrows and isochrones show direction of activation. Stimulus sites are not included in maps. Distance scale for each panel is shown below; note that scale is two times larger for 5-day-old infarct preparation than for 2-month-old infarct preparation. Reprinted with permission from Reference 12.

result from the effects of prolonged ischemia on the gap junctions or from a decrease in size or number of intercalated disks because of the increased amount of connective tissue associated with formation of the scar. It also may be related to the altered distribution of Cx43 that we have described.[10] Other possible causes for such exaggerated discontinuous conduction include abrupt changes in cell size or surface-to-volume ratios, marked differences in the number of cells connected across high-resistance barriers, and abrupt cell branching.[14,15] Discontinuities in conduction are often evident by prepotentials or notches on the action potential upstrokes in the healed infarcts in regions in which fractionated electrograms are recorded.[12] Therefore, each component of a fractionated electrogram indicates a functional muscle bundle that is activated out of synchrony with adjacent bundles because of electrophysiological separation either because of abnormal gap junctional properties or by connective-tissue scar during infarct healing. The individual "spikes" of the fractionated electrograms may be rapid because of the fast upstrokes of the underlying action potentials. The amplitude of fractionated electrograms is also much lower than electrograms recorded from normal regions, because of the paucity of muscle fibers in the thin epicardial border zone. Low-amplitude, fractionated electrograms are also routinely recorded in healing or healed human infarcts and may represent discontinuous conduction or activation in these regions.[16–25] Their occurrence in both the experimental canine infarcts and human infarcts suggests a relationship between discontinuous conduction and the occurrence of reentrant arrhythmias.

Electrophysiological Characteristics of Discontinuous Activation During Initiation of Ventricular Tachycardia Caused by Anisotropic Reentry

One of the hallmark features of tachyarrhythmias in hearts with healing or healed infarcts in both canine infarct models and humans is their initiation by programmed premature or overdrive stimulation of the ventricles.[1] Activation maps of the epicardial border zone in the canine model have shown exactly how premature stimuli initiate arrhythmias. An example is shown in Figure 4. Activation times measured simultaneously at 196 sites within a 4×5-cm region went into the construction of these maps. The location and activation times at each of the electrodes is indicated by the numbers. Figure 4, top left, shows that the basic drive stimuli applied on the epicardial surface of the right ventricle adjacent to the LAD (pulse symbol) at a cycle length of 280 ms initiated excitation wave fronts that spread over the epicardial border zone from this margin toward the opposite margin at the apex of the lateral free wall (arrows). The isochrones progress in sequence from 0 to 90 ms. There are no areas of block of the basic drive impulse in this map, although sometimes regions of fixed block occur. Also, there is no evidence of a reentrant circuit in this region, judging by the activation pattern of the basic drive impulses. The prematurely stimulated impulses that initiate arrhythmias have very different activation patterns. Stimulated premature impulses that initiate tachycardias propagate into the epicardial border zone and block.[5,7,9,26,27] The region of conduction block forms a line that extends for several centimeters. Conduction block of a premature impulse with a coupling interval of 150 ms to the last basic drive impulse that resulted in reentry is shown in the activation map in Figure 4, lower left. Activation of the epicardial border zone by this premature impulse occurred from the LAD margin, where it was initiated, to the 60-ms isochrone, about one third of the distance into the border zone before the block occurred. Conduction block is indicated by the thick black line. The line of conduction block sometimes occurs toward the margin of the border zone where there is a transition from the thick normal ventricular wall to the thin layer of surviving epicardial muscle,[5] although it also may occur well into the border zone, as shown in the activation map of Figure 4. As the arc of block is approached, electrogram amplitude diminishes until only very-low-amplitude electrotonic potentials are apparent. The decrease in the electrogram amplitude is caused by the dying out of the premature impulse wave front. At the line of block, the waveform is monophasic, which is characteristic of a waveform that has arrived at the end of its conduction pathway. Reentry occurs when stimulated wave fronts propagate around the extremities of the arc of conduction block and activate myocardium on its distal side after myocardium on the proximal side has recovered excitability. These wave fronts can then reexcite the myocardium on the proximal side. This pattern of activation is shown by the arrows in Figure 4, lower left. The region on the distal side of the line of block was activated at between 150 and 160 ms by wave fronts propagating around both ends of the line of block. Activation on the distal side of the line of block occurred ≈100 ms after block occurred at the proximal side (at 60 ms). This time lapse of 100 ms allowed the proximal side time to recover excitability. The map in Figure 4, lower right, shows the wave front from the distal (asterisks) side of the line of block propagating retrogradely across it to reexcite the proximal side (isochrones 10 to 30). The wave front returned to the LAD margin (40-ms isochrone), where it exited the border zone to excite the ventricles as the first tachycardia impulse (T1). A functional reentrant circuit was therefore formed by

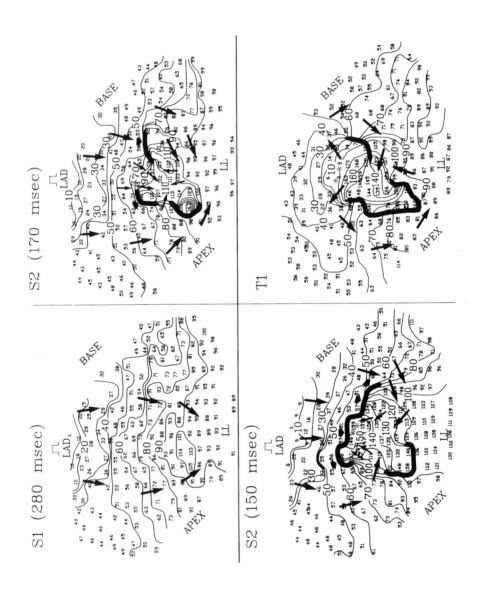

the premature activation. The arc of block, because of its transient nature, acts as an area of unidirectional block that provides the return path for the reentrant impulse; conduction of the premature impulse blocked in the antegrade direction but not in the retrograde direction.

We have found evidence of discontinuous conduction of the premature impulse in the retrograde direction across the line of block, which eventually results in reentry.[28] Electrograms with double potentials can be recorded at the line of block during retrograde propagation. The first deflection indicates the arrival of the premature impulse at the distal side of the line, and the second deflection, occurring after an isoelectric segment of 10 to 50 ms, indicates continuation of retrograde propagation across the line that leads to the first reentrant impulse. The isoelectric segment in the double potential represents the discontinuity in retrograde activation. It may be caused by either a marked and sudden slowing in retrograde conduction or a real stopping and starting of impulse conduction. Whatever the cellular mechanism, it provides a delay in retrograde activation sufficient to allow reentry to occur.[28]

Electrophysiological Characteristics of Discontinuous Activation During Sustained Ventricular Tachycardia

An example of a reentrant circuit in the epicardial border zone of a 4-day-old canine infarct during sustained ventricular tachycardia is

◀───

Figure 4. Activation maps showing initiation of reentrant ventricular tachycardia by a premature stimulus. Ventricles were driven at a regular cycle length (280 ms) by basic drive stimuli (S1) applied through electrodes along LAD margin of epicardial border zone at top of each map. Activation pattern of epicardial border zone during basic drive is shown at top left. Arrows indicate direction of activation. Top right, Activation pattern of a single premature impulse (S2) elicited from same stimulation site at LAD margin at coupling interval of 170 ms. This premature impulse did not initiate reentry, although there were local areas of conduction block, indicated by thick black lines. Bottom left, Activation by another premature impulse elicited with a coupling interval of 150 ms. Conduction of this premature impulse blocked along region indicated by horizontal, thick black line. Conduction around line of block (arrows) initiated reentry. Bottom right, Reentrant excitation pattern of first impulse of tachycardia. Activation in this time window begins at asterisk, point at which activation in previous map and time window (lower left) ended.

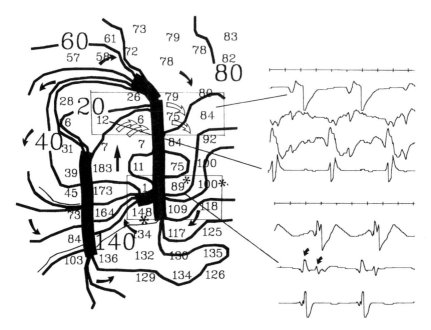

Figure 5. Reentrant excitation in epicardial border zone of 4-day-old canine infarct. Two thick black vertical lines represent interpolated isochrones that form two lines of "apparent" block that bound central common pathway of circuit. Activation times are plotted at each recording site (small numbers). Isochrones drawn every 10 ms are labeled with larger numbers. Reentrant sequence of excitation is shown by black arrows. Open arrows show discontinuous activation across a segment of line of apparent block. Electrograms recorded from selected sites are at right. First four electrograms from top were recorded from sites enclosed within top rectangle. Top electrogram was recorded from site activated at 84 ms; next two electrograms, which are fractionated, were recorded from either side of line of apparent block (activation times, 75 and 6 ms). Fourth electrogram was recorded from site activated at 12 ms. Next three electrograms were recorded from sites within area enclosed by lower rectangle (*). Top electrogram was recorded from site activated at 148 ms; middle electrogram, which has a double component (indicated by arrows), was assigned an activation time of 89 ms (first component); and bottom electrogram had activation time of 100 ms.

shown in Figure 5. Activation begins in the 10-ms isochrone toward the LAD end of the central common pathway. The excitation wave splits into two independent circulating wave fronts, one traveling toward the right and one toward the left. After ≈70 ms, the wave front moving toward the right turns and moves toward the lower margin. The other wave front, moving toward the left, also turns toward the lower margin. After ≈130 ms, the two wave fronts join to form a common wave front that enters the central common pathway between the two parallel lines of block. The joined wave front then moves toward the LAD margin, where it closes the reentrant loop after ≈183 ms.

The two lines of conduction block, indicated by the dark black lines on the map, appear only during reentry. They are established by a large number of interpolated isochrones because of the large activation time differences across distances of ≈6.4 mm. Both of these lines of block are oriented in the direction of the long axis of the myocardial fibers. There are indications that the "lines of block" forming the central common pathway in Figure 5 are not complete block but that activation occurs slowly across them, ie, discontinuous activation transverse to the long axis of the myocardial fibers occurs in some regions. The 80- and 90-ms isochrones adjacent to the right line of block are oriented parallel to it. Regions of similar activation time are located along this line of block within these isochrones. For the isochrones to be oriented as they are, it is likely that this line of block actually permitted very slow conduction (≈6 cm/s) to take place across it (transverse to the long axis of the fiber bundles), as indicated by the open arrows. This slowly conducting transverse excitation wave might have fused with the rapidly moving wave front that propagated around the end of the line of "block," indicated by the black arrows. The electrograms recorded from some regions along the lines of apparent block provide further evidence that there is sometimes slow activation across them transverse to the long axis of the muscle fibers, which may be discontinuous. The electrograms may be fractionated and have long durations. These characteristics are illustrated in Figure 5, right, which shows electrograms recorded from some sites along the right line of apparent block. The first four electrograms (from top to bottom) were recorded from the sites within the upper rectangular box on the activation map. The first (activation time 84) and fourth (activation time 12) electrograms in this group were recorded at a distance from the line of apparent block and have only a single major deflection. However, the two electrograms between them were recorded immediately adjacent to the line of apparent block (at sites 6 and 75) and are characterized by fractionated activity. These characteristics result because there is slowly propagating activity across the line of apparent block in this region, which may be discontinuous. The fractionated components are caused by asynchronous activation of adjacent fiber bundles during transverse propagation in nonuniformly anisotropic tissue (as described previously). The long duration and fractionated characteristics of the electrograms recorded at the lines of apparent block occur only during tachycardia and represent a dramatic change from the characteristics of these electrograms during sinus rhythm or ventricular stimulation.[9] However, there cannot be propagation across the entire line of block because a central obstacle is needed for reentry to occur. The next group of three electrograms in Figure 5, right, were recorded at sites within the lower rectangular box. The top (activation time 148*) and the bottom (activation time 100*) electrograms in this group also have single major components. The middle electrogram recorded at the site with the 89-ms activation time has two distinct components (arrows) coinciding with the deflections at sites on either side of it. This region may be near the fulcrum of the circuit around which the reentrant wave front is revolving, and the two components of the electrogram are coincident with activation on either side of the line of block.[29] This region may be the location of functional block at the center of the circuit (see below).

The characteristics of the reentrant circuits in the epicardial border zone that we just described suggest a model for reentrant tachycardia in healing or healed myocardial infarcts. The cornerstone of the model is that the nonuniform anisotropy is a major cause of slow conduction necessary for reentry and that, therefore, the mechanism is that of anisotropic reentry.[1,9] According to this model, the property of the infarct that enables reentry to occur is the parallel-oriented bundles of surviving muscle fibers, in which there is slow conduction transverse to the fibers and faster conduction parallel to the fibers. In the canine model of LAD occlusion, the parallel bundles are in the epicardial border zone, but in other infarct models or in humans, they may sometimes be located in other regions. Figure 6 illustrates these characteristics. The reentrant circuit is the one described in Figure 5. The large arrows point out the sequence of isochrones moving around the long lines of apparent block. As we pointed out, however, because of the orientation of the isochrones on the distal sides of the lines of apparent block, there is probably slow activation through the block. To indicate this slow activation, the activation map has been redrawn from the one in Figure 5 to show the individual isochrones at the lines of apparent block, which are actually lines of slow activation (Figure 6, right). This is where fractionated electrograms were recorded. In regions of the circuit in which activation is occurring parallel to the fibers, conduction is fast ($\approx$0.5 m/s) and isochrones are widely separated and oriented perpendicular to the long axis of the fibers. In the regions of the circuit in which activation occurs transverse to the long axis, the isochrones are bunched closely together, indicating very slow activation (as slow as 0.05 m/s), and are oriented parallel to the fibers. It is the slow conduction transverse to the long axis of the parallel-oriented muscle bundles that enables reentry to occur in the anisotropic reentry model, not slow conduction caused by severely depressed transmembrane potentials. Therefore, despite the appearance of long lines of apparent block, reentry is actually occurring around a smaller central fulcrum of block.

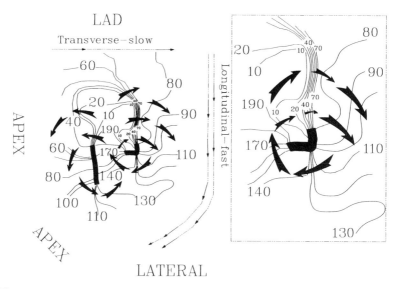

Figure 6. Model of anisotropic reentry in epicardial border zone of canine myocardial infarcts. Reentrant circuit at left is the one described in Figure 5. Right line of apparent block has been redrawn to show individual isochrones resulting from discontinuous and slow propagation transverse to myocardial fiber orientation. Transverse and longitudinal directions relative to long axis of myocardial fibers are indicated. Anisotropic reentrant circuit is enlarged in rectangle at right. Black arrows show activation pattern. Reprinted with permission from Reference 1.

Conclusions

Discontinuous activation, defined as a sudden "bunching" of isochrones in activation maps, followed by a resumption of normal conduction is associated with reentrant ventricular tachycardia in the canine model of myocardial infarct. The cellular basis may be true discontinuous conduction at cell-to-cell junctions, but the exact mechanisms require mapping excitation at a microscopic level.

References

1. Wit AL, Janse MJ. *The Ventricular Arrhythmias of Ischemia and Infarction: Electrophysiological Mechanisms.* Mount Kisco, NY: Futura Publishing Co; 1993.
2. Hirzel HO, Nelson GR, Sonnenblick EH, et al. Redistribution of collateral blood flow from necrotic to surviving myocardium following coronary occlusion in the dog. *Circ Res.* 1976;39:214–222.

3. Wit AL, Allessie MA, Bonke FIM, et al. Electrophysiologic mapping to determine the mechanism of experimental ventricular tachycardia initiated by premature impulses: experimental approach and initial results demonstrating reentrant excitation. *Am J Cardiol.* 1982;49:166–185.
4. Ursell PC, Gardner PI, Albala A, et al. Structural and electrophysiological changes in the epicardial border zone of canine myocardial infarcts during infarct healing. *Circ Res.* 1985;56:436–451.
5. Mehra R, Zeiler RH, Gough WB, et al. Reentrant ventricular arrhythmias in the late myocardial infarction period, 9: electrophysiologic-anatomic correlation of reentrant circuits. *Circulation.* 1983;67:11–24.
6. Roberts DE, Hersh LT, Scher AM. Influence of cardiac fiber orientation on wavefront voltage, conduction velocity and tissue resistivity in the dog. *Circ Res.* 1979;44:701–712.
7. Cardinal R, Vermeulen M, Shenasa M, et al. Anisotropic conduction and functional dissociation of ischemic tissue during reentrant ventricular tachycardia in canine myocardial infarction. *Circulation.* 1988;77:1162–1176.
8. Wit AL, Dillon SM, Coromilas J, et al. Anisotropic reentry in the epicardial border zone of myocardial infarcts. In: Jalife J, ed. *Mathematical Approaches to Cardiac Arrhythmias.* New York, NY: New York Academy of Sciences; 1990;59:86–108.
9. Dillon SM, Allessie MA, Ursell PC, et al. Influence of anisotropic tissue structure on reentrant circuits in the epicardial border zone of subacute canine infarcts. *Circ Res.* 1988;63:182–206.
10. Peters NS, Coromilas J, Severs NJ, Wit AL, et al. Disturbed connexin43 gap junction distribution correlates with the location of reentrant circuits in the epicardial border zone of healing canine infarcts that cause ventricular tachycardia. *Circulation.* 1997;95:988–996.
11. Scheinman MM, Ciaccio EJ, Kassotis J, et al. Use of bipolar electrogram characteristics and activation patterns during sinus rhythm and ventricular pacing to predict the location of ventricular tachycardia reentrant circuits in a canine infarct model. *Circulation.* 1995;92(suppl I):1–257. Abstract.
12. Gardner PI, Ursell PC, Fenoglio JJ Jr, et al. Electrophysiologic and anatomic basis for fractionated electrograms recorded from healed myocardial infarcts. *Circulation.* 1985;72:596–611.
13. Spach MS, Miller WT III, Geselowitz DB, et al. The discontinuous nature of propagation in normal canine cardiac muscle: evidence for recurrent discontinuities of intracellular resistance that affect the membrane currents. *Circ Res.* 1981;48:39–54.
14. Joyner RW, Veenstra R, Rawling D, et al. Propagation through electrically coupled cells: effects of a resistive barrier. *Biophys J.* 1984;45:1017–1025.
15. Joyner RW, Overholt ED, Ramza B, et al. Propagation through electrically coupled cells: two inhomogeneously coupled cardiac tissue layers. *Am J Physiol.* 1984;247:H596–H609.
16. De Bakker JMT, van Capelle FJL, Janse MJ, et al. Reentry as a cause of ventricular tachycardia in patients with chronic ischemic heart disease: electrophysiologic and anatomic correlation. *Circulation.* 1988;77:589–606.
17. Cassidy DM, Vassallo JA, Marchlinski FE, et al. Endocardial mapping in humans in sinus rhythm with normal left ventricles: activation patterns and characteristics of electrograms. *Circulation.* 1984;70:37–42.
18. Vassallo JA, Cassidy DM, Marchlinski FE, et al. Abnormalities of endocardial activation pattern in patients with previous healed myocardial infarction and ventricular tachycardia. *Am J Cardiol.* 1986;58:479–484.

19. Stevenson WG, Weiss JN, Wiener I, et al. Fractionated endocardial electrograms are associated with slow conduction in humans: evidence from pace-mapping. *J Am Coll Cardiol.* 1989;13:369–376.
20. Josephson ME, Simson MB, Harken AH, et al. The incidence and clinical significance of epicardial late potentials in patients with recurrent sustained ventricular tachycardia and coronary artery disease. *Circulation.* 1982;66: 1199–1204.
21. Svenson RH, Littmann L, Gallagher JJ, et al. Termination of ventricular tachycardia with epicardial laser photocoagulation: a clinical comparison with patients undergoing successful endocardial photocoagulation alone. *J Am Coll Cardiol.* 1990;15:163–170.
22. Wiener I, Mindich B, Pitchon R. Determinants of ventricular tachycardia in patients with ventricular aneurysms: results of intraoperative epicardial and endocardial mapping. *Circulation.* 1982;65:856–861.
23. Wiener I, Mindich B, Pitchon R. Fragmented endocardial electrical activity in patients with ventricular tachycardia: a new guide to surgical therapy. *Am Heart J.* 1984;107:86–90.
24. Klein H, Karp RB, Kouchoukos NT, et al. Intraoperative electrophysiologic mapping of the ventricles during sinus rhythm in patients with a previous myocardial infarction: identification of the electrophysiologic substrate of ventricular arrhythmias. *Circulation.* 1982;66:847–853.
25. Kienzle MG, Falcone RA, Kempf FC, et al. Intraoperative endocardial mapping: relation of fractionated electrograms in sinus rhythm to endocardial activation in ventricular tachycardia: surgical implications. *J Am Coll Cardiol.* 1983;1:582. Abstract.
26. El-Sherif N, Smith RA, Evans K. Canine ventricular arrhythmias in the late myocardial infarction period, 8: epicardial mapping of reentrant circuits. *Circ Res.* 1981;49:255–265.
27. El-Sherif N. The figure 8 model of reentrant excitation in the canine postinfarction heart. In: Zipes DP, Jalife J, eds. *Cardiac Electrophysiology and Arrhythmias.* New York, NY: Grune & Stratton; 1985:363–378.
28. Cabo C, Deruyter B, Coromilas J, et al. Mechanisms for absence of inverse relationship between coupling intervals of premature impulses initiating ventricular tachycardia and intervals between premature and first tachycardia impulses. *Circulation.* In press.
29. Restivo M, Gough WB, El-Sherif N. Ventricular arrhythmias in the subacute myocardial infarction period: high-resolution activation and refractory patterns of reentrant rhythms. *Circ Res.* 1990;66:1310–1327.

Chapter 19

Is There a Pharmacology for Discontinuous Conduction?

Michael R. Rosen, MD, and
Penelope A. Boyden, PhD

Discussion of a pharmacological approach specific for any aspect of cardiac rhythm control should meet with skepticism as the result of our experience in the 1990s. This skepticism reflects, in large part, the garden path of expectations that derived from arrhythmia and antiarrhythmic drug research in the 1960s and 1970s, research that culminated in the CAST[1,2] and SWORD[3] trials. These showed conclusively what many had suspected: antiarrhythmic drugs, even when given under careful control in circumstances assumed to be appropriate, have the potential to be lethal. In considering a pharmacology for discontinuous propagation, then, we must first stress the theoretical nature of the argument generated. At the theoretical level, we suppose, one can discuss a pharmacology for almost anything. Beyond this, one must be prepared to demonstrate not only that discontinuous propagation is meaningful as a mechanism for arrhythmias in carefully designed animal, tissue, and computer models but also that it contributes to arrhythmias in human subjects.

If these conditions are satisfied and traditional thinking about antiarrhythmics is applied, then the therapy might be directed at making propagation more discontinuous (ie, inducing conduction block) or less discontinuous (ie, facilitating and/or speeding conduction). In exerting either effect, the agent used might be expected not to interact with structures/channels/receptors in the heart that would exert confounding actions, although interactions that promote the desired effect on discontinuous propagation would, of course, be beneficial.

Some of the studies reported were supported by USPHS-NHLBI grant HL-28958

From: Spooner PM, Joyner RW, Jalife J (eds). *Discontinuous Conduction in the Heart.* Armonk, NY: Futura Publishing Company, Inc.; © 1997.

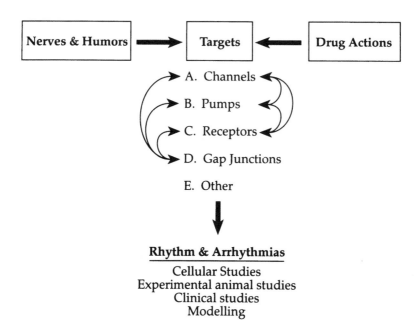

Figure 1. Targets of drug action. There are a variety of targets of drug action, many of which are modified not only by drugs but by other factors, such as neurohumors and peptides. Targets include but are not limited to transmembrane ion channels, ion pumps and exchangers, receptors, and gap junctions. All these targets contribute both to normal cardiac rhythm and to arrhythmias, which can be studied by a number of subcellular, cellular, and other in vitro and in vivo techniques. Reprinted with permission from Reference 4.

A reasonable framework for considering the targeting of such an agent is provided in Figure 1. This is modified from the original Sicilian gambit publication[4] and identifies gap junctions as a target for pharmacological action. Equally important in this figure is the identification of other targets that might modify the conductance of gap junctions. Various receptor-effector coupling systems have additional impact here, as will be detailed.

Does Discontinuous Propagation Contribute to Arrhythmias?

We shall start with the understanding that experimentally, discontinuous propagation can be considered in two ways: (1) by examining discontinuities at the cellular level, which are attributable to cell-to-cell communication via gap junctions, and (2) by considering them at a macroscopic level, deriving from anatomic separation of fiber bundles by various connective-tissue elements. We shall stress the former here. That cell-to-cell uncoupling occurs under a variety of conditions is well documented, whether it is induced by various degrees of myocardial ischemia,[5,6] by other types of tissue injury such as hypoxia or lesioning,[7] or by fiber death in the setting of myocardial infarction.[8] Implicit to the models associated with discontinuous propagation is an understanding that propagation in all directions is discontinuous. This was documented by Spach et al,[9,10] who also showed that the discontinuity that exists in longitudinal conduction is far less than that which occurs transversely. This phenomenon is related, no doubt, to differing densities of gap junctions. The role of discontinuous propagation in the genesis of arrhythmias can be appreciated in the causality of reentry. Rudy and Quan[11] showed that decreased intercellular coupling, by itself, can reduce conduction velocity by up to 20-fold before complete conduction block occurs. The type of slow and decremental conduction seen here is that which in models[11–13] and experimental systems[8,12,14] can induce reentry. The likelihood of unidirectional block and reentry is determined by the degree of cellular uncoupling and by various spatial nonuniformities in uncoupling.

Role of Gap Junctions in Modulating Conduction

As reviewed by Maurer and Weingart,[15] the conduction of the cardiac impulse depends on the summation of local circuit currents, which have four components: excitatory inward current (either Na^+ or Ca^{2+}, depending on the tissue); r_i, the longitudinal intracellular resistance; c_m, the membrane capacitance; and r_o, the longitudinal extracellular resistance. Most research relating to antiarrhythmic drugs that modify conduction has focused on the first of these. However, the role of r_i has been a subject of increasing attention, because it is significantly affected by changes in gap junctional conductance.

Any consideration of the role of gap junctions and their conductance in determining uncoupling depends, in large part, on the distribution of the native population of gap junctions in tissue. Given that connexin43 (Cx43) is the most abundantly expressed gap junctional subunit expressed in heart muscle,[16,17] its density in various tissues should be, and in fact is, reflected in differences in gap junctional density and conduction velocity of the cardiac impulse. Hence, the proportion of Cx43 found to localize at the ends and lateral margins of atrial and ventricular myocytes approximates the 10:1 and 3:1 ratios of longitudinal to transverse conduction velocity that have been measured.[18].

As stated above, the major electrophysiological property that appears to correlate with gap junctional distribution is the internal longitudinal resistance of fibers (r_i), and changes in r_i appear to express themselves in anisotropy of the conduction velocity and susceptibility to block of action potentials.[10,19,20] Ischemia not only increases the likelihood of arrhythmias but concomitantly increases r_i.[6] Similarly, the fatty acids, long-chain acylcarnitines, and lipoxygenase metabolites that accumulate during ischemia uncouple gap junctions.[5,21−23] The fact that remodeling of gap junctions and connexins in the peri-infarction zones occurs in a setting in which lateral connections decrease compared with end-to-end junctions[24,25] could both increase anisotropy and enhance the likelihood of arrhythmias.[18]

A variety of other factors that modify transcription of channel protein or cause posttranslational modification of existing protein can alter gap junctional conductances. These include H^+ and Ca^{2+} ions,[15,26] calmodulin,[27] and cAMP.[28] Neurohumoral interventions have various effects, including upregulation of conductance by β-agonists[28,29] and downregulation by cGMP,[28] angiotensin II,[30] and acetylcholine.[31]

Alteration of Gap Junctional Conductances in Pathological Settings

The gap junctional contribution to anisotropy and reentrant arrhythmias has been the subject of both speculation and experimentation.[9,12] Anisotropic conduction may occur in the setting of ischemia, such that conditions favorable to reentry evolve. Immunohistochemical studies of human myocardium have shown that in the border zones of myocardial infarcts, there is a disorderly arrangement of gap junctions.[24,32] Specifically, the organization of the gap junctions in discrete intercalated disks is disrupted, such that the occurrence of reentry might be facilitated. Chagas disease provides one important example of the devastating effects of gap junctional disruption in pathophysiology.[33]

The case for the involvement of gap junctional conductance changes in pathological settings is strengthened by the demonstration that acute ischemia[6] or hypoxia alone[34] increases r_i. The products of hypoxia, long-chain acylcarnitines and arachidonic acid and its metabolites, decrease gap junctional conductance and are thus proposed to contribute to the ischemia-induced slowing of conduction.[5,22] Similarly, metabolic inhibitors decrease gap potential conductance.[35] Hence, it has been argued that to the extent that one might prevent or reverse the effects of ischemic metabolites to depress gap junctional conductance and/or alter their distribution such that conduction is improved, the propensity to arrhythmias might be reversed. Essential to any therapeutic strategy here would be a precise understanding of the specific transcriptional controls of the connexin proteins.

Phamacological Modification of Gap Junctional Conductances

Modification of gap junctional conductance by pharmacological interventions is a well-studied phenomenon. To the extent that such modulation occurs, it can be expected to either couple or uncouple, and as a result either enhance or depress, conduction. Early studies[36–38] indicated that $[Ca^{2+}]_i$ elevation increases gap junctional resistance, as does increased intracellular acidification.[39–41] Maurer and Weingart[15] studied isolated cell pairs and derived a measure of nexus resistance, r_n, and then determined the effects of elevating $[Ca^{2+}]_i$ via direct elevation of $[Ca^{2+}]_o$, lowering of $[Na^+]_o$, or administration of caffeine or strophanthidin. Elevations of $[Ca^{2+}]_o$ from 0.5 to 10 mmol/L induced no change in r_n in normally coupled cell pairs whose starting r_n was ≈5 MΩ but modestly and reversibly uncoupled those that were slightly uncoupled to start with ($r_n = 50$ MΩ). The high elevations in $[Ca^{2+}]_i$ brought about by removing $[Na^+]_o$ or administering caffeine or strophanthidin were associated with large increases in r_n and cell contracture. It is clear, as well, that the concentrations of the agents administered (caffeine and strophanthidin) were of a level far beyond that which is compatible with life.

More recent evidence produced by techniques to measure Ca_i and pH_i directly has suggested that an increase in intracellular calcium alone does not uncouple adult cell pairs. Rather, it is the level of intracellular H^+ ions that alone[42] and in a complex, synergistic interaction with internal Ca^{2+} ions affects gap junctional conductance.[43] These findings allow us to understand why during each normal Ca^{2+} transient and subsequent tension development, Ca_i-induced cell-to-cell uncoupling does not occur and why under certain conditions, Ca^{2+} ions are the apparent vehicle for gap junction–mediated intercellular communication.[44] Finally, Ca^{2+} ions not only can function as important local cell-to-cell messengers but also can alter their own ability to diffuse through these gap junctions.

Acetylcholine, too, has been shown to decrease gap junctional conductance in rat lacrimal gland cells,[45] as do the phorbol esters PdBu and TPA. These actions have been attributed to a protein kinase C–dependent pathway.[31] Burt and Spray,[28] using carbamylcholine, showed that cholinomimetic interventions also decrease gap junctional conductance in heart. Agents that may act on the cell membrane (eg, altering lipid bilayer mobility) or directly on the gap junctional protein decrease gap junctional conductance: these include the alcohols heptanol[46] and octanol.[25] Other uncoupling agents include Sr^{2+}, Ba^{2+}, Mn^{2+}, Co^{2+}, La^{3+}, metabolic inhibitors, proteolytic enzymes, Ca^{2+} ionophores, hypertonicity, and acidifiers.[35] The role of traditional antiarrhythmic drugs in modifying gap junctional conductance has been the subject of limited study. Whereas lidocaine reportedly has little or no effect on r_i in normal ventricle, acute superfusion with amiodarone appears to alter both active and passive properties of ventricular subepicardial muscle.[47]

Different pharmacological interventions have been shown to improve gap junctional conductance. This phenomenon has been explored particularly with agents that increase intracellular levels of cAMP. In rat hepatocytes plated in culture, there is a rapid loss of gap junctional conductance over 5 to 8 hours, which is attenuated in the presence of a membrane-permeant cAMP analogue.[29] In disaggregated rat cardiac myocytes, β-adrenergic agonists, membrane-permeant analogues of cAMP, and concentrations of isobutyl methylxanthine or caffeine that inhibit phosphodiesterase all increase gap junctional conductance.[28] However, when intracellular levels of Ca^{2+} are high, then the application of cAMP analogues actually decreases gap junctional conductance.[28] In other words, the basal levels and extent of elevation of $[Ca^{2+}]_i$ are critical to the result seen with cAMP elevation. Moreover, in different tissues and under specific circumstances, gap junctional conductance can be increased or decreased by interventions that elevate cAMP.[27] Finally, calmodulin, which is involved in both the synthesis and the breakdown of cAMP, has been shown to decrease gap junctional conductance.[27]

It is as yet uncertain how the various interventions that increase or decrease gap junctional conductance exert their effects. As stated above, alcohols appear to act directly on the gap junctional protein (or on membrane proteins in general). Studies of uncoupling induced by stearic acid[21] have led to the suggestion that these alcohols, and anesthetics like halothane, bind via a carboxyl group to positively charged amino acid residues of the gap junctional proteins, resulting in closure of the channel. Any of the interventions described above might modify conformation of the gap junctional channel proteins. Alternatively, the proteins might themselves function as receptors for other molecules, thereby altering channel configuration and conductance. Finally, these interactions may alter channel phosphorylation as well.

Based on knowledge of the sequence of a number of connexin proteins as well as of the models of their primary structure, recent studies have used molecular approaches to understand mechanisms of transcriptional and posttranslational modification of connexin proteins. For instance, treating cells with antisense oligodeoxynucleotides targeted either toward Cx43 or Cx40 protein synthesis can selectively reduce the frequency of one single gap junction channel with a specific conductance relative to another.[48]

A deletion/mutation approach used by Delmar et al[42] has shown that the addition of a peptide (or particle) designed specifically to interact with the pore region important in pH_i gating of the Cx43 channel protein can alter the well-known effects of pH on gap junctional conductance. Thus, there is now a clear potential that specific peptides could be designed that could protect gap junction channels from closing ("couplers"). Site-directed antibody studies have clearly shown that antibodies to the amino- and carboxy-termini of Cx43 protein are most effective in blocking dye transfer between rat myocytes and that the antibody effects varied depending on external calcium.[49] Yet information is still lacking as to which region of protein precisely controls the permeability of these gap junction proteins.

Is There Potential Therapeutic Benefit of the Pharmacological Modification of Discontinuous Conduction?

In a simplistic sense, one might argue that interventions that improve cell-to-cell coupling and enhance conduction would be antiarrhythmic; and it is this type of argument that historically has led to overly simplistic expectations with respect to antiarrhythmic drug therapy. We tend, in good faith, to set up paradigms for drug-tissue interactions that often have as much of Polyanna as practically in them. Consider the following: in the normal heart, the discontinuities that exist in propagation and the low gap junctional density in specialized tissues such as AV node[50] or at transverse sites of ventricular or atrial myocytes serve the purpose of shaping the directional and temporal characteristics that facilitate orderly propagation of the cardiac impulse and contraction. One need not stretch the imagination a great deal to consider the potentially negative impact of accelerated conduction through the AV node on the contribution of atria and ventricles to systolic and diastolic function in the heart. Similarly, in the setting of ischemia, the alteration of communication between healthy and damaged cells, while potentially arrhythmogenic, serves a positive purpose: it removes, at least in part, a major current sink from the general milieu of the myocardium, and it limits the cell-to-cell spread of metabolites that might otherwise be injurious to healthy cells. Hence, it is not readily apparent that a pharmacological approach to enhancing gap junctional conductance would have a decidedly beneficial effect, nor is it clear that the effect would not be deleterious. In fact, the philosophy of attempting

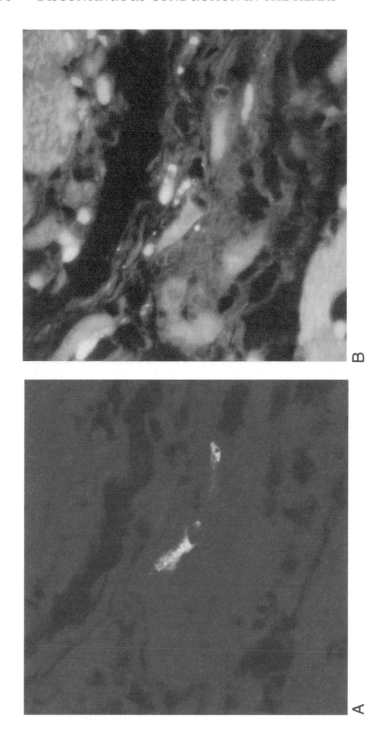

to normalize gap junctional function in an ischemic heart may well be akin to the opening of the portholes in a sinking *Titanic* in an attempt to improve ventilation.

Does this mean that no serious attempts should be made to use the gap junctions in a manner that might be beneficial to cardiac function? Not at all. Recent studies have demonstrated that fetal myocytes implanted into adult heart cells can survive and produce nascent gap junctions with adult cells.[51] Moreover, preliminary data suggest that these junctions are, in fact, functional, in the sense that large molecules can be passed between fetal and adult cells. Specifically, as shown in Figure 2, fetal rat myocytes implanted into adult rat hearts couple with them to the extent that the dye Lucifer yellow is capable of passage from the adult to the fetal cells. Hence, one might think of packaging specific signaling molecules in fetal myocytes and using the gap junctions as a means for providing molecular messages that might be transmitted from cell to cell. These messages might be conceived of as potentially effective modifiers of cellular function.

In sum, we do not foresee the success of a pharmacological approach of the traditional type that gave rise to a generation of antiarrhythmic drugs that have been partially successful and partially dele-

◄───

Figure 2. Evidence of passage of information (in this case, Lucifer yellow dye) between myocytes from fetal and adult hearts via gap junctions. In this experiment, rat cardiocytes were infected with a recombinant adenovirus bearing reporter gene chloramphenicol–acetyl transferase (CAT). Cells were injected into ventricles of adult rats that were killed 1 week later. Strips of left ventricle ≈1 mm in diameter and 5 to 7 mm long that included injection site near one end were placed into a divided tissue chamber perfused with Tyrode's solution. Tissue strips were passed through a small hole in rubber diaphragm that divided chamber. Cut-end method[52] was used, and tissue in side of chamber not containing fetal injection site was perfused with Ca^{2+}-free Tyrode's solution containing 10 μmol/L Lucifer yellow. After 30 minutes of equilibration, perfusion with normal Tyrode's solution was resumed for 6 hours (other end of preparation was perfused with normal Tyrode's solution throughout procedure). Tissue was then removed, fixed in formalin, embedded in paraffin, and cut into 4-μm serial cross sections. These were sequentially incubated with a polyclonal antibody to CAT and a TRITC-labeled anti-rabbit IgG, coverslipped, and examined in an immunofluorescence microscope with excitation and absorption filters of 545 and 610 nm, respectively, for TRITC (red fluorescence) and 405 and 475 nm, respectively, for Lucifer yellow (green fluorescence). Shown here is a preparation stained for CAT (left) and Lucifer yellow (right). Note two fetal cells in center, left, staining positively for CAT in a field of adult cells that stain negatively for CAT. Right, Both fetal and adult cells stain positively for Lucifer yellow, suggesting passage of dye from adult to fetal cells via gap junctions. From a preliminary experiment by A. Kass, L. Leinwand, M. Szabolcs, P. Danilo, R. Robinson, and M. Rosen.

terious in their actions. Rather, we see an approach that uses gap junctions as an internal conduit for passing information that might heal damaged cells and/or modify the machinery of the cells in a fashion that enhances their function.

References

1. The Cardiac Arrhythmias Suppression Trial (CAST) Investigators. Preliminary report of encainide and flecainide on mortality in a randomized trial of arrhythmia suppression after myocardial infarction. *N Engl J Med.* 1989; 321:406–412.
2. Green HL, Roden DM, Kork RJ, et al (CAST Investigators). The Cardiac Arrhythmias Suppression Trial: final CAST...then CAST II. *J Am Coll Cardiol.* 1992;19:894–898.
3. Waldo AL, Camm AJ, deRuyter H, et al (SWORD Investigators). Survival with oral d-sotalol in patients with left ventricular dysfunction after myocardial infarction: rationale, design, and methods (the SWORD trial). *Am J Cardiol.* 1995;75:1023–1027.
4. Task Force of the Working Group on Arrhythmias of the European Society of Cardiology. The Sicilian gambit: a new approach to the classification of antiarrhythmic drugs based on their action on arrhythmogenic mechanisms. *Circulation.* 1991;84:1831–1851.
5. Wu J, McHowat J, Saffitz JE, et al. Inhibition of gap junctional conductance by long-chain acylcarnitines and their preferential accumulation in junctional sarcolemma during hypoxia. *Circ Res.* 1993;72:879–889.
6. Kléber AG, Riegger CB, Janse M. Electrical uncoupling and increase of extracellular resistance after induction of ischemia in isolated, arterially perfused rabbit papillary muscle. *Circ Res.* 1987;61:271–279.
7. De Mello WC. Intercellular communication in cardiac muscle. *Circ Res.* 1982;51:1–9.
8. Janse MJ, Wit AL. Electrophysiologic mechanisms of ventricular arrhythmias resulting from myocardial ischemia and infarction. *Physiol Rev.* 1989; 69:1049–1169.
9. Spach MS, Miller WT III, Geselowitz DB, et al. The discontinuous nature of propagation in normal canine cardiac muscle: evidence for recurrent discontinuities of intracellular resistance that affect the membrane currents. *Circ Res.* 1981;48:39–54.
10. Spach MS, Kootsey JM, Sloan JD. Active modulation of electrical coupling between cardiac cells of the dog: a mechanism for transient and steady state variations in conduction velocity. *Circ Res.* 1982;51:347–362.
11. Quan W, Rudy Y. Unidirectional block and reentry of cardiac excitation: a model study. *Circ Res.* 1990;66:367–382.
12. Rudy Y. Models of continuous and discontinuous propagation in cardiac tissue. In: Zipes DP, Jalife J, eds. *Cardiac Electrophysiology: From Cell to Bedside.* 2nd ed. Philadelphia, Pa: WB Saunders & Co; 1995:326–334.
13. Spach MS. Discontinuous cardiac conduction: its origin in cellular connectivity with long-term adaptive changes that cause arrhythmias. In: Spooner PM, Joyner RW, Jalife J eds. *Discontinuous Conduction in the Heart.* Armonk, NY: Futura Publishing Co., Inc.; 1997;5–51.
14. Rudy Y, Shaw RM. Membrane factors and gap junction factors as determinants of ventricular conduction and reentry. In Spooner PM, Joyner RW,

Jalife J, eds. *Discontinuous Conduction in the Heart.* Armonk, NY: Futura Publishing Co., Inc.; 1997.

15. Maurer P, Weingart R. Cell pairs isolated from adult guinea pig and rat hearts: effects of [Ca²⁺]ᵢ on nexal membrane resistance. *Pflugers Arch.* 1987; 409:394–402.

16. Kanter HL, Saffitz JE, Beyer EC. Cardiac myocytes express multiple gap junction proteins. *Circ Res.* 1992;70:438–444.

17. Kanter HL, Laing JG, Beau SL, et al. Distinct patterns of connexin expression in canine Purkinje fibers and ventricular muscle. *Circ Res.* 1993;72: 1124–1131.

18. Pressler ML, Münster PN, Huang X-D. Gap junction distribution in the heart: functional relevance. In: Zipes DP, Jalife J, eds. *Cardiac Electrophysiology: From Cell to Bedside.* 2nd ed. Philadelphia, Pa: WB Saunders & Co; 1995: 144–151.

19. Clerc L. Directional differences of impulse spread in trabecular muscle from mammalian heart. *J Physiol (Lond).* 1976;255:335–346.

20. Delmar M, Michaels CD. Effects of increasing intercellular resistance on transverse and longitudinal propagation in sheep epicardial muscle. *Circ Res.* 1987;60:780–785.

21. Burt JM. Uncoupling of cardiac cells by doxyl stearic acids: specificity and mechanism of action. *Am J Physiol.* 1989;256:C913–C924.

22. Massey KD, Minnich BN, Burt JM. Arachidonic acid and lipoxygenase metabolites uncouple neonatal rat cardiac myocyte pairs. *Am J Physiol.* 1992; 263:C494–C501.

23. Burt JM, Massey KD, Minnich BN. Uncoupling of cardiac cells by fatty acids: structure-activity relationships. *Am J Physiol.* 1991;260:C439–448.

24. Smith JH, Green CR, Peters NS, et al. Altered patterns of gap junction distribution in ischemic heart disease: an immunohistochemical study of human myocardium using laser scanning confocal microscopy. *Am J Pathol.* 1991;139:801–821.

25. Luke RA, Saffitz JE. Remodeling of ventricular conduction pathways in healed canine infarct border zones. *J Clin Invest.* 1991;87:1594–1602.

26. White RL, Spray DC, Campos de Carvalho AC, et al. Some electrical and pharmacological properties of gap junctions between adult ventricular myocytes. *Am J Physiol.* 1985;249:C447–C455.

27. Peracchia C, Girsch SJ. Functional modulation of cell coupling: evidence for a calmodulin-driven channel gate. *Am J Physiol.* 1985;248:H765–H782.

28. Burt JM, Spray DC. Inotropic agents modulate gap junctional conductance between cardiac myocytes. *Am J Physiol.* 1988;254:H1206–H1210.

29. Sáez JC, Gregory WA, Watanabe T, et al. cAMP delays disappearance of gap junctions between pairs of rat hepatocytes in primary culture. *Am J Physiol.* 1989;257:C1–C11.

30. De Mello WC, Altieri P. Effects of angiotensin II and enalapril on heart cell coupling. *Circulation.* 1992;86(suppl I):1–9. Abstract.

31. Randriamampita C, Giaume C, Neyton J, et al. Acetylcholine-induced closure of gap junction channels in rat lacrimal glands is probably mediated by protein kinase C. Pflugers Arch. 1988;412:462–468.

32. Peters NS, Green CR, Poole-Wilson PA, et al. Reduced content of connexin 43 gap junctions in ventricular myocardium from hypertrophied and ischemic human hearts. *Circulation.* 1993;88:864–875.

33. Campos de Carvalho AC, Masuda MO, Tanowitz HB, et al. Conduction defects and arrhythmias in Chagas' disease: possible role of gap junctions and humoral mechanisms. *J Cardiovasc Electrophysiol.* 1994;5:686–698.

34. Hofmann H. Interaction between a normoxic and hypoxic region of guinea pig and ferret papillary muscles. *Circ Res.* 1985;56:876–883.
35. Peracchia C. Structural correlates of gap junction permeation. *Int Rev Cytol.* 1980;66:81–146.
36. De Mello WC. Effect of intracellular injection of calcium and strontium on cell communication in heart. *J Physiol (Lond).*1975;250:231–245.
37. Dahl G, Isenberg G. Decoupling of heart muscle cells: correlation with increased cytoplasmic calcium activity with changes of nexus ultrastructure. *J Membr Biol.* 1980;53:63–75.
38. Weingart R. The actions of ouabain on intracellular coupling and conduction velocity in mammalian ventricular muscle. *J Physiol (Lond).* 1977;264: 341–365.
39. Reber WR, Weingart R. Ungulate cardiac Purkinje fibres: the influence of intracellular pH on the electrical cell-to-cell coupling. *J Physiol (Lond).* 1982; 328:87–104.
40. Mazet F, Dunia I, Vassort G, et al. Ultrastructural changes in gap junctions associated with CO_2 uncoupling in frog atrial fibers. *J Cell Sci.* 1985;74: 51–63.
41. Noma A, Tsuboi N. Dependence of junctional conductance on protein, calcium and magnesium ions in cardiac paired cells of guinea-pig. *J Physiol.* 1987;382:193–211.
42. Delmar M, Morley GE, Toffet SM. Molecular Analysis of the pH regulation of the cardiac gap junction protein connexin43. In Spooner PM, Joyner RW, Jalife J, eds. *Discontinuous Conduction in the Heart.* Armonk, NY: Futura Publishing Co., Inc.; 1997.
43. White RL, Doeller JE, Verselis VK, et al. Gap junctional conductance between pairs of ventricular myocytes is modulated synergistically by H^+ and Ca^{2+}. *J Gen Physiol.* 1990;95:1061–1075.
44. ter Keurs HEDJ, Zhang YM. Trigger propagated contractions and arrhythmias caused by acute damage to cardiac muscle. In Spooner PM, Joyner RW, Jalife J, eds. *Discontinuous Conduction in the Heart.* Armonk, NY: Futura Publishing Co., Inc.; 1997.
45. Neyton J, Trautmann A. Acetylcholine modulation of the conductance of intercellular junctions between rat lacrimal cells. *J Physiol.* 1986;377: 283–295.
46. Délèze J, Hervé JC. Effect of several uncouplers of cell-to-cell communication on gap junction morphology in mammalian heart. *J Membr Biol.* 1983; 74:203–215.
47. Quinteiro RA, Biagetti MO. Chronic versus acute effects of amiodarone on the $\dot{V}_{max}$-conduction velocity relationship and the space constant in canine myocardium. *J Cardiovasc Pharmacol.* 1994;24:122–132.
48. Moore LK, Burt JM. Selective block of gap junction channel expression with connexin-specific antisense oligodeoxynucleotides. *Am J Physiol.* 1994;267: C1371–C1380.
49. Lak R, Laird DW, Revel J-P. Antibody perturbation analysis of gap-junction permeability in rat cardiac myocytes. *Pflugers Arch.* 1993;422:449–457.
50. Anumonwo JMB, Delmar M. Functional properties of gap junctional currents in adult rabbit atrioventricular (AV) nodal cell pairs. *Circulation.* 1992; 86(suppl I):I–9. Abstract.
51. Soonpaa MH, Koh GY, Klug MG, et al. Formation of nascent intercalated disks between grafted fetal cardiomyocytes and host myocardium. *Science.* 1994;264:98–101.
52. Imanaga I. Cell-to-cell diffusion of procion yellow in sheep and calf Purkinje fibers. *J Membr Biol.* 1974;16:381–388.

Section VII

Contemporary Model Studies of Discontinuous Conduction
Introduction

Ronald W. Joyner, MD, PhD

This section deals with recent efforts to construct and analyze experimental and theoretical models of action potential conduction in cardiac tissue under conditions in which conduction is discontinuous. Action potential conduction in several regions of the heart seems to differ fundamentally from that expected in an electrically well-connected syncytium of cells. In the normal heart, there are directional differences in conduction velocity, corresponding to fiber orientation, as well as specific sites at which conduction delays are normally observed. The difference between continuous and discontinuous conduction needs to be clarified. Conduction in all regions of the heart can be considered to be discontinuous in the sense that the conductance between adjacent cells, facilitated by gap junctions, is localized at the cell boundaries. Some degree of discontinuity has been observed in apparently normal atrial or ventricular muscle, with conduction being less continuous in the direction transverse to the fiber orientation than in a the parallel direction.[1] This phenomenon has been explored in various theoretical studies as well.[2]

Within most of the ventricular and atrial tissue, these studies indicate repeated small delays between adjacent cells or cell bundles that are not easily measured, although the microscopic discontinuities do have effects on the action potential shape during depolarization and repolarization.[3] Other regions of the heart have more macroscopic areas of discontinuous conduction both under normal conditions and, perhaps even more importantly, after the injury of ischemia.

The three chapters in this section illustrate some of the approaches being taken to analyze the mechanisms of the effects of structural irregularities on discontinuous conduction. The primary pathway for electrical conduction between the atria and the ventricles is the AV node, but the AV node often forms a key component in supraventricular arrhythmias and reentrant tachycardias, either with an accessory pathway or with dual pathways within the AV node. Cells within the AV node have been classified into several types based on microelectrode recordings of activation time, action potential shape, and the response to premature atrial stimulation.[4] The characteristic central nodal cells (N cells) have "slow-response" action potential, but cells more closely associated with the atria (AN cells) or His-Purkinje cells (AH cells) have properties intermediate between those of N cells and those of the A or H region. The multidimensional anatomy of the AV node, including the complexity of electrical connections between the atrial tissue and the AV nodal tissue, has not been resolved in terms of the anatomic distribution of cell types and intercellular coupling, although new results with antibodies against nodal cells are making impressive progress.[5] There is abundant evidence from clinical and experimental studies that the AV nodal region demonstrates properties of two somewhat parallel pathways, with an α pathway located inferiorly and posteriorly with slow conduction and a short refractory period and a β pathway, located more anteriorly and superiorly, that has faster conduction but a a longer refractory period.[6] It is not clear how these pathways interconnect with the central node, either as an integral part of the slow pathway or with summation of the pathways proximal to the central region.

Chapter 20 reviews studies on AV nodal conduction, with specific reference to the double potentials observed in mapping studies as a manifestation of the complex, three-dimensional structure of the AV node. The determination of the origin of each component of the double potentials reveals a complex set of pathway that are different for antegrade versus retrograde AV nodal conduction. This approach emphasizes the structural inhomogeneity of the system, with a positive aspect of being conducted on intact cardiac tissue but with the limitation of not fully knowing the membrane properties or the coupling conductance of the cells that constitute the system. There are many examples of cardiac conduction in which the action potential appears to have discrete delays in conduction at specific sites. In normal tissue, the Purkinje–ventricular muscle junction shows this property, whereas in chronic ischemia, there are fractionated electrograms that indicate the occurrence of specific delays.[7,8]

Chapter 21 describes recent work in which we have applied a reductionist approach to the problem of discontinuous conduction by analyzing action potential conduction between cells of a cell pair electrically interconnected by a "coupling clamp" circuit. In this work, the cell pair consists of either two real, isolated cardiac myocytes or one real myocyte coupled to a real-time simulation of a cell model. With this approach, we are able to show that the L-type calcium current begins to play a major role in action potential propagation when the intercellular coupling resistance is high enough to induce a significant conduction delay and that the intercellular coupling resistance plays a major role in enabling both the intrinsic pacing of an ectopic focus and the modulation of surrounding quiescent tissue by such a focus. In this approach, we have the positive aspect of being able to control coupling conductance and to use one or more freshly isolated myocytes as components of the propagating system. The disadvantage of this approach is that we cannot fully represent the complexity of discontinuous conduction with a pair of cells, because in the real tissue, each of these cells would be connected to other cells, which complicates the issues of source current and loading. The use of mathematical simulations to express the characteristics of action potential propagation is common to a number of chapters in this book. This approach summarizes much of what is known about isolated cardiac cells and structure to make predictions about how action potential propagation would occur in real tissue.

Chapter 22 examines the role of membrane properties and gap junction factors in determining propagation of an action potential in a multicellular, one-dimensional model. This model shows the importance of gap junctional uncoupling in supporting very slow conduction, which can lead to reentry, particularly by increasing the vulnerable window in the time domain for induction of unidirectional block.[9] This technique has the particular positive aspect of being able to specify spatial inhomogeneities in membrane properties, which alter refractory period and excitability, and/or the coupling resistance. The disadvantage is that both the specified membrane model and the spatial distribution of resistivity are necessarily models of real cells and real tissues and thus limit the applicability of the results.

The complexity of doing quantitative, mechanistic analyses of discontinuous conduction is well represented by these three chapters. We are still faced with the daunting task of relating the structural complexity of normal and diseased myocardium to the resulting propagational phenomena. Nevertheless, the variety of approaches represented here show great promise and are expected to be instrumental in elucidating the fundamental mechanisms involved.

References

1. Spach MS, Miller WT, Geselewitz DB, Barr RC, Kootsey JM, Johnson EA. The discontinuous nature of propagation in normal canine cardiac muscle. *Circ Res.* 1981;48:39–54.

2. Joyner RW. Effects of the discrete pattern of electrical coupling in propagation through an electrical syncytium. *Circ Res.* 1982;50:192–200.
3. Osaka T, Kodama I, Tsuboi N, Toyama J, Yamada K. Effects of activation sequence and anisotropic cellular geometry on the repolarization phase of action potential of dog ventricular muscles. *Circulation.* 1987;76:226–236.
4. Billette J. Atrioventricular nodal activation during periodic premature stimulation of the atrium. *Am J Physiol.* 1987;252:H163–H177.
5. Oosthoek PW, Viragh S, Mayen AE, van Kempen MJ, Lamers WH, Moorman AF. Immunohistochemical delineation of the conduction system, 1: the sinoatrial node. *Circ Res.* 1993;73:473–481.
6. Iinuma H, Dreifus LS, Mazgaley T. Role of the perinodal region in atrioventricular nodal reentry: evidence in an isolated rabbit heart preparation. *J Am Coll Cardiol.* 1983;2:465–472.
7. Gardner PI, Ursell PC, Fenoglio JJ, Wit AL. Electrophysiologic and anatomic basis for fractionated electrograms recorded from healed myocardial infarcts. *Circulation.* 1985;72:596–611.
8. Veenstra RD, Joyner RW, Rawling DA. Purkinje and ventricular activation sequences of canine papillary muscle: effects of quinidine and calcium on the Purkinje-ventricular conduction delay. *Circ Res.* 1984;54:500–515.
9. Shaw RM, Rudy Y. The vulnerable window for unidirectional block in cardiac tissue: characterization and dependence on membrane excitability and cellular coupling. *J Cardiovasc Electrophysiol.* 1995;6:115–131.

Chapter 20

Discontinuous Conduction in the AV Junctional Area

Jacques M. T. de Bakker, PhD,
and Michiel J. Janse, MD

Structure and Electrophysiology of the AV Node

Transmission of excitation from atrium to ventricle is delayed during passage through the AV junctional area, which comprises, at least in the rabbit heart, transitional cells, midnodal cells, and lower nodal cells[1,2] (Figure 1). The transitional cells, which surround the compact node, contact atrial myocardium. These cells are smaller than atrial cells, are deprived of cross striation, and are separated by numerous strands of connective tissue. Three groups of transitional cells can be distinguished. The posterior group contacts atrial myocardium beneath and behind the coronary sinus. The middle group connects with atrial fibers from the sinus septum (between the ostium of the coronary sinus and the inferior vena cava) and with deeper atrial myocardium on the left side of the interatrial septum, as well as with the myocardium anterior to the coronary sinus. The anterior group of transitional cells passes superficially over the extension of the central fibrous body and overlies the compact node without making contact with the underlying tissue of the node. These overlay cells terminate in the tricuspid valve base. The midnodal cells, together with the circumferential transitional cells, about the bundle of lower nodal cells.

Functionally distinct cell types in the AV junctional area have been subdivided into three major groups, called AN (atrionodal), N (nodal), and NH (nodal-His). These cells have the following characteristics.[3,4]

1. AN cells show fully developed action potentials, the upstroke of which always occurs after the same interval following the atrial com-

From: Spooner PM, Joyner RW, Jalife J (eds). *Discontinuous Conduction in the Heart.* Armonk, NY: Futura Publishing Company, Inc.; © 1997.

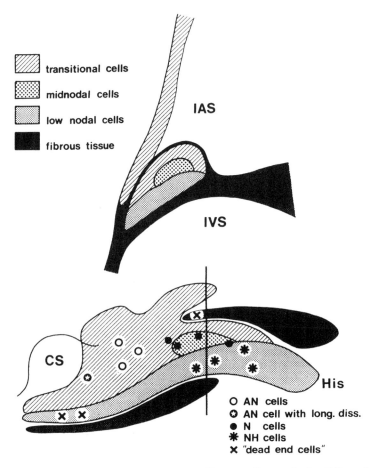

Figure 1. Distribution of morphologically different cell types in the AV junctional area of a rabbit heart. Top, Transverse section showing trilaminar appearance of anterior part of node. Level of sectioning is indicated by bar in lower panel. Bottom, Diagram of AV node indicating location of cells from which typical action potentials were recorded. Reprinted with permission from Janse MJ, et al. In: Wellens et al, eds. *The Conduction System of the Heart.* Leiden, Netherlands: Stenfert Kroese; 1976:296.

plex, regardless of the presence of conduction delay or block farther downstream.

2. N cells have action potentials with slow upstrokes. The action potential configuration changes with each beat of the Wenckebach cycle: the upstroke becomes slower and usually dissociates progressively into two components, while the amplitude becomes smaller, until finally a nonpropagated local response is present.

3. NH cells have generally faster upstrokes than N cells, although the transition is gradual. During the Wenckebach cycle, they are distal to the site at which activation block is produced.

Using microelectrodes containing cobalt chloride for marking cells, Anderson et al[1] showed that action potentials with AN characteristics are recorded from transitional cells. The NH cells were confined to the anterior portion of the bundle of lower nodal cells. Typical N cells were found at the junction of midnodal cells with the circumferential transitional cells but were also found in transitional cells located more posteriorly. Thus, one should realize that N-type action potentials can originate from both transitional cells and midnodal cells.

Mechanisms for Discontinuous Conduction

The exact routes of propagation in the AV junctional area and the mechanism leading to discontinuous conduction curves have not yet been clarified. The structure of the AV junction makes it likely that nodal architecture as well as cellular morphology contributes to nodal electrophysiology. Differences in cell electrophysiology and coupling resistances between cells affect conduction. Gap junctions are thought to be responsible for the electrical coupling of the myocytes. In the heart, connexin43 (Cx43) is an important component of the gap junctions. There are manifest differences in the expression of Cx43 between the AV junction and surrounding myocardium. Cx43 is abundantly present in the atrium and in fibers of the AV bundle but cannot be detected in the myocytes of the AV node.[5] The latter, however, does not mean that this protein is completely absent. Gap junctions have been detected by electron microscopy in the sinus node; compared with atrial myocytes, however, these gap junctions are smaller in size and fewer in number,[6] below the detection level of immunohistochemical staining methods. It is also possible that the gap junctions in the AV node are composed of connexins other than Cx43.[7]

Transitional cells form small strands that are separated by connective tissue; these strands branch frequently. This architecture is ideally suited for activation delay, summation, and longitudinal dissociation, which all affect action potential configuration.[4,8] Activation delay and block occur preferentially at sites at which bundles branch, because of a mismatch between current supply and current demand.[9,10] Double-upstroke action potentials, which are often found in AV junctional area,[11–14] are also recorded at sites at which a mismatch exists between current supply and current demand.[15,16] Conversely, asynchronous arrival of activity in a converging geometry (summation) can also lead to double-component action potentials.[17] A relation between discontinuous AV nodal conduction and any of these factors has never been demonstrated.

Discontinuous Activation in the Presence of Dual Pathways

The demonstration of discontinuous conduction-time curves in human and dog hearts has traditionally been accepted as evidence for the existence of dual-pathway electrophysiology.[18-21] This concept supposes that the anatomic substrate of the AV junctional area consists of two pathways, each with different conduction velocities and refractory periods. The slow pathway has a short refractory period, whereas the refractory period of the fast pathway is long. Differences in the refractory periods of the two pathways have been attributed to intrinsic repolarization differences, which are caused by different kinetics of the ionic channels of the cells in the two pathways. This concept is helpful in explaining the occurrence of echo beats and AV junctional reentrant tachycardia. The existence of dual pathways is supported by radiofrequency catheter ablation for treatment of AV junctional tachycardias. Ablation of one of the two pathways results in conduction via the nonaffected path. Although the traditional two pathways were introduced by Mendez and Moe,[22] evidence for the existence of three or more pathways has been available.[23-25] Despite these observations, there is no evidence that anatomically delineated dual or multiple pathways exist within the AV nodal area. The anatomic studies of Anderson et al[26] and Ho et al[27] showed that the anatomic potentials for multiple, let alone dual, pathways in the junctional area are legion. They showed that the AV nodal region has four atrial inputs. Therefore, it is quite possible that small differences in the time of arrival of atrial impulses over these routes affect AV conduction.

Discontinuous Conduction in the Absence of Dual Pathways

Dual pathways are not a prerequisite for obtaining discontinuous activation and sudden jumps. Jalife[28] showed that in a sucrose gap preparation, heterogeneity in impulse transmission can be induced in a linear Purkinje fiber placed in a three-chamber tissue bath. Under these conditions, a narrow zone of depressed excitability may be created by superfusing the central segment of the fiber with an ion-free sucrose solution. During stimulation of the proximal segment and recording from the distal segment, a discontinuous activation curve was obtained. Premature stimulation at a certain coupling interval resulted in an abrupt delay in activation in the distal segment. Spach and Josephson[29] proposed that the nonuniform anisotropic properties of the AV junctional area could account for discontinuous conduction in the AV node. Spach et al[30] showed that discontinuities in conduction-time curves arise in nonuniform anisotropic myocardial tissue and that the underlying differences in the effective refractory periods of the fast and slow pathways are due to microscopic nonuniformities of electrical load created by the nonuniform anisotropic distribution of the electrical connections between cells. The presence of connective tissue separating bundles of transitional cells[1] suggests that some regions of the AV node have nonuniform anisotropic electrical properties. Fast as well as very slow conduction occurs in the transitional zone of the AV node, along with different shapes and amplitudes of the extracellular waveforms, when activation fronts propagate with a 90° angular difference. Spach and Josephson[29] showed that during stimulation at the anterior extremity of the AV junctional area, conduction was parallel to fiber orientation, with a velocity of 0.39 m/s, and resulted in single large, biphasic electrograms. In contrast, when the stimulation site was just posterior to the posterior zone, conduction was perpendicular to the fiber orientation, was slow (0.07 m/s), and caused low-amplitude, fractionated electrograms. Thus, very slow or fast propagation of the wave front can occur depending on the direction in which the excitatory wave moves with respect to the fiber orientation. According to this concept, the "slow" and "fast" pathways can occupy the same location for different wave fronts. From these data, Spach and Josephson concluded that nonuniform anisotropy provides a major mechanism for dual AV nodal pathway electrophysiology and AV nodal reentry.

Location of the Slow and Fast Pathways

Several mapping studies have demonstrated that the site of earliest atrial excitation during retrograde slow pathway conduction is different from that during fast pathway conduction.[20,31–34] During retrograde fast pathway conduction, the earliest atrial activation is in the anterior zone of the AV junctional area at the apex of Koch's triangle. In contrast, during retrograde slow pathway conduction, the earliest excitation appears to be situated in the posterior approaches to the AV node in the region between the coronary sinus and the tricuspid annulus. These locations have been confirmed by radiofrequency and cryothermal lesions that, when placed at these sites, abolished antegrade slow or fast pathway conduction. A complicating factor is that limited data suggest that antegrade and retrograde pathways are not the same, indicating that multiple fast and slow pathways exist.[35–38]

Are Double Potentials Markers of Slow Pathway Conduction?

Double potentials are extracellular electrograms that show two deflections. It has been suggested that double potentials may help locate the slow pathway, and therefore their location is used as a guide for the delivery of radiofrequency energy in patients with AV nodal reentry tachycardias. At ablation sites at which double potentials are recorded, slow pathway conduction is abolished while fast pathway conduction still persists, suggesting that the double potentials indeed mark the location of the slow pathway. This approach has a success rate of >90%.[39,40]

A similar success rate is obtained with the anatomic approach, in which the ablation catheter is placed posteriorly between the ostium of the coronary sinus and the tricuspid annulus and gradually moved in a more anterior direction if the applied lesion is unsuccessful.[41,42] With this approach, slow pathway ablation can be achieved at sites at which double potentials are absent. Moreover, double potentials may be found at sites distant from the slow pathways and in humans and animals both with and without AV nodal reentrant tachycardias. Such observations bring into question the interpretation of double potentials as a marker for the slow pathway.

Two types of double potentials have been characterized. Jackman et al[39] described a double potential in which a small-amplitude, low-frequency deflection was followed by a large-amplitude, high-frequency component (LH potential, Figure 2). The second type of double potential was first described in a clinical setting by Haissaguerre et al[40] and consists of a high-frequency component followed by a low-frequency component (HL potential, Figure 2). Both types of double potentials can be recorded in humans with and without AV nodal reentrant tachycardias as well as in animals. Because there was some overlap in the regions covered by the two types of double potentials, both types of the low-frequency component could be present in addition to the large high-frequency potential so that the electrogram had three components.

Characteristics and Origin of LH Double Potentials

In human and animal hearts, LH double potentials are found posterior and inferior to the coronary sinus orifice and in the proximal coronary sinus. Studies on isolated, blood-perfused canine hearts showed that rapid atrial pacing had little effect on either component

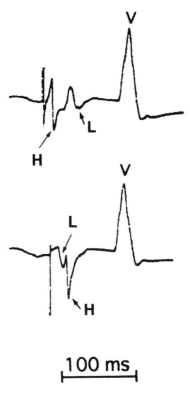

Figure 2. Top, Double potential with HL characteristic recorded in mid nodal area of a dog heart, close to tricuspid valve annulus. Bottom, Double potential with LH characteristic recorded in posterior approach to AV node of a dog heart. Recordings were made during stimulation from high right atrium. Vertical line is stimulus artifact. H indicates high-frequency deflection; L, low-frequency deflection; and V, remote ventricular deflection.

of the LH potential.[43] Timing of the two components was affected by the site of stimulation. Pacing at the site of double potentials even caused reversal of the sequence of the two components so that the high-frequency component preceded the low-frequency deflection.

Combined intracellular and extracellular recordings in the same hearts revealed that LH potentials were caused by asynchronous activation of two muscle bundles separated by the orifice of the coronary sinus. The low-frequency component was a far-field potential caused by activation of the atrial musculature above the mouth of the coronary sinus, whereas the high-frequency component reflected local activity of either atrial or transitional cells in the region between the coronary sinus and the tricuspid valve annulus. Thus, the spatial relation of LH potentials and the slow pathway is merely a fortunate accident.

Characteristics and Origin of HL Double Potentials

HL potentials are found in the posterior approach to the AV node, between the coronary sinus orifice and the tricuspid annulus, in both human and animal hearts.[40,43] The area with HL potentials may extend almost up to the central fibrous body. Characteristics of the slow as well as the fast components in the human hearts did not differ significantly from those in porcine and canine hearts.[44] In virtually all hearts, the low-frequency component showed a gradual transition from a relatively sharp to a slow deflection. The signals exhibiting the sharpest deflections were recorded at sites located posterior to those at which signals had a slow downstroke. The interval between the high- and low-frequency components was also dependent on the recording site, being shortest in the most posterior area (Figure 3).

Premature atrial stimulation and rapid atrial pacing caused little

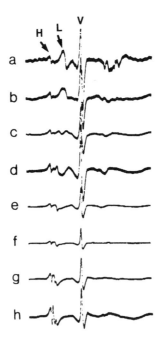

Figure 3. Tracings are extracellular electrograms recorded simultaneously in posterior approach of AV node during sinus rhythm. Recordings were made in a patient with AV nodal reentrant tachycardias. Each tracing comprises HL double potentials followed by a remote ventricular deflection. Note that distance between H and L components decreases from tracing a to h. Recording site of tracing h was located posterior from site a. H indicates high-frequency deflection; L, low-frequency deflection; and V, remote ventricular deflection.

change in the high-frequency component but markedly decreased the amplitude and frequency of the low-frequency component. At rapid rates, the low-frequency component commonly disintegrated, as described by Haissaguerre et al.[40] During ventricular stimulation, the sequence of the two components remains the same, and the low-frequency component occurs only sporadically before the high-frequency deflection.[43,44]

Extracellular mapping of the AV junctional area in patients with AV nodal reentrant tachycardias and in isolated porcine hearts revealed that during sinus rhythm and atrial stimulation, activation generating the high-frequency components spread with a conduction velocity of 0.7 m/s. In contrast, activation causing the low-frequency deflections proceeded with a conduction velocity of only 0.07 m/s. The spread of activation of the two components was usually in opposite directions. During premature atrial stimulation, the activation sequence of the fast components remained similar, but the activation map of the slow component could change markedly.

Simultaneous extracellular and intracellular recordings revealed that HL double potentials are caused by asynchronous depolarization of superficial and deep cell layers near the tricuspid annulus.[43] Both layers were located directly beneath the extracellular recording electrode. The high-frequency component was caused by depolarization of cells in deeper layers. These cells generated triangular action potentials with rapid upstrokes (dV/dt_{max}, 60 to 300 V/s) and high resting membrane potentials (more negative than -75 mV). Rapid pacing caused minor changes in the action potential characteristics. The intrinsic deflection of the slow component in the extracellular electrogram coincided with depolarization of superficial cells. Action potentials from these cells had a low upstroke velocity (dV/dt_{max}, 5 to 25 V/s) and a low resting membrane potential (-65 mV). Extrastimuli and rapid pacing caused marked slowing of the action potential upstroke and amplitude. Notching of the upstroke and Wenckebach-type responses sometimes occurred during rapid pacing. These electrophysiological properties of the action potentials from superficially located cells are characteristic for N cells. It should be noted, however, that they can be recorded many millimeters away from the compact node.

The action potentials with the slowest upstroke velocity were recorded in the superficial layer closest to the tricuspid valve annulus. Cells >15 mm from the tricuspid annulus exhibited action potentials characteristic for atrial cells. Between these two extremes, the superficial cells exhibited a smooth continuum of characteristics. The direction of the gradient of change was perpendicular to the tricuspid annulus. Intracellular mapping showed that the slowest conduction was found in the area in which action potentials had the slowest upstroke velocity, ie, along the annulus.

Histological Characteristics of Superficial and Deeper Layers

The electrophysiological studies suggest the existence of two separate layers in the posterior approach of the AV junctional area. However, action potentials recorded from this area often reveal multiple upstrokes. Microelectrode impalements at the same endocardial location but at several depths showed that activation of superficial cells caused the first upstroke, whereas the second upstroke coincided with the upstroke of the action potential recorded from cells located deeper. This suggests that the two layers are not completely uncoupled (Figure 4). Sections from the sites with double potentials showed that cells in the superficial subendocardial layers had the morphological characteristics of transitional cells. These cells are smaller than those in working atrial myocardium, with less marked striations, and are frequently separated from each other by fine strands of connective tissue. No boundary or morphological characteristic distinguishes the superficial cells with the N-type action potentials from the cells in deeper layers, which causes the high-frequency component.

Slow Components in Double Potentials and Slow Pathway Conduction

The slow components in double potentials arise from activation in cells with N-cell action potential characteristics. These cells are found

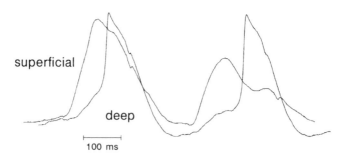

Figure 4. Double-component action potentials recorded from a cell in a superficial and deeper layer in posterior approach to AV node. Two components in both action potentials arise because of a weak coupling between two layers. First component is caused by activation in superficially located cell; second component, by activation in deeper cells. Two components become more pronounced after premature stimulation (second complexes).

in the posterior approach to the AV node, the location of the putative slow pathway. The nodal-type properties of these cells have the characteristics necessary for slow pathway conduction; therefore, they might be the anatomic substrate of the slow pathway. The effects of adenosine on the N-type cells and the slow pathway are the same. The concept that the N cells in the posterior approach to the AV node belong to the slow pathway is supported by observations made in isolated, blood-perfused dog hearts during the induction of ventricular echo beats.[45] In this study, the ventricular extrastimulus that gave rise to an echo beat resulted in a long HA interval, suggesting retrograde slow pathway conduction. A microelectrode impaled at a site along the tricuspid annulus revealed an N-type action potential during retrograde conduction. The upstroke of this action potential was 10 ms before the earliest atrial activation, which had been determined previously with extracellular mapping. The following AH interval was short, suggesting that the antegrade conduction that evoked the echo beat occurred over the fast pathway.

The impaled cell did not participate in antegrade conduction. The short AH interval during antegrade conduction was suggestive of antegrade fast pathway conduction. The action potential upstroke occurred after the His deflection, indicating that during antegrade fast pathway conduction, the impaled cell did not participate in AV conduction but rather was located in a dead-end pathway.

Although these observations are the most direct experimental data that are suggestive of slow pathway conduction, a coincidence cannot be ruled out.

A large number of mechanisms have been proposed for discontinuous conduction in the AV junctional area. However, these mechanisms have usually been proved experimentally in settings other than the AV node. Therefore, it is still questionable whether they indeed participate in discontinuous conduction in the AV junctional area.

References

1. Anderson RH, Janse MJ, van Capelle FJL, et al. A combined morphological and electrophysiological study of the atrioventricular node of the rabbit heart. *Circ Res.* 1974;35:909–922.
2. Becker AE, Anderson RH. Morphology of the human atrioventricular junctional area. In: Wellens HJJ, Lie KI, Janse MJ, eds. *The Conduction System of the Heart: Structure, Function and Clinical Implications.* The Hague, Netherlands: Martinus Nijhoff Medical Division; 1978:263–286.
3. Paes de Carvalho A, De Almeida DF. Spread of activity through the atrioventricular node. Circ Res. 1960;8:801–809.
4. Janse MJ, van Capelle FJL, Anderson A, et al. Electrophysiology and structure of the atrioventricular node of the isolated rabbit heart. In: Wellens

HJJ, Lie KI, Janse MJ, eds. *The Conduction System of the Heart: Structure, Function and Clinical Implications.* The Hague, Netherlands: Martinus Nijhoff Medical Division; 1978:296–316.

5. Oosthoek PW, Virágh S, Lamers WH, et al. Immunohistochemical delineation of the conduction system, II: the atrioventricular node and Purkinje fibers. *Circ Res.* 1993;73:482–491.

6. Sugi Y, Hirakow R. Freeze-fracture studies of the sinoatrial and atrioventricular nodes of the caprine heart, with special reference to the nexus. *Cell Tissue Res.* 1986;245:273–279.

7. Kanter HL, Saffitz JE, Beyer EC. Cardiac myocytes express multiple gap junction proteins. *Circ Res.* 1992;70:438–444.

8. Zipes DP, Mendez C, Moe GK. Evidence of summation and voltage dependency in rabbit atrioventricular nodal fibers. *Circ Res.* 1973;32:170–177.

9. Spach MS, Miller WT Jr, Dolber PC, et al. The functional role of structural complexities in the propagation of depolarization in the atrium of the dog: cardiac conduction disturbances due to discontinuities of effective axial resistivity. *Circ Res.* 1982;50:175–191.

10. Spach MS, Miller WT Jr, Geselowitz DB, et al. The discontinuous nature of propagation in normal canine cardiac muscle: evidence for recurrent discontinuities of intracellular resistance that affect the membrane currents. *Circ Res.* 1981;48:39–54.

11. Mendez C, Moe GK. Some characteristics of transmembrane potentials of AV nodal cells during propagation of premature beats. *Circ Res.* 1966;19:993–1010.

12. Janse MJ. Influence of the direction of the atrial wave front of AV nodal transmission in isolated hearts of rabbits. *Circ Res.* 1969;25:439–449.

13. Sano T, Suzuki F, Takigawa S. The genesis of the step or notch on the upstroke of the action potential obtained from the atrioventricular node. *Jpn J Physiol.* 1964;14:659–668.

14. Watanable Y, Dreifus LS. Second degree atrioventricular block. *Cardiovasc Res.* 1967;1:150–158.

15. Rohr S. Determination of impulse conduction characteristics at a microscopic scale in patterned growth heart cell cultures using multiple site optical recording of transmembrane voltage. *J Cardiovasc Electrophysiol.* 1995;6:551–568.

16. Maglaveras N, de Bakker JMT, van Capelle FJL, et al. Activation delay in healed myocardial infarction: a comparison between model and experiment. *Am J Physiol.* 1995;267(*Heart Circ Physiol* 38):H1441–H1449.

17. van Capelle FJL, Janse MJ. Influence of geometry on the shape of the propagated action potential. In: Wellens HJJ, Lie KI, Janse MJ, eds. *The Conduction System of the Heart: Structure, Function and Clinical Implications.* The Hague, Netherlands: Martinus Nijhoff Medical Division; 1978:316–335.

18. Schuilenburg RM, Durrer D. Atrial echo beats in the human heart elicited by induced atrial premature beats. *Circulation.* 1968;37:680–693.

19. Dennes P, Wu D, Dhingra RC, et al. Demonstration of dual AV nodal pathways in patients with paroxysmal supraventricular tachycardia. *Circulation.* 1973;48:549–555.

20. Sung RJ, Waxman HL, Saksena S, et al. Sequence of retrograde atrial activation in patients with dual atrioventricular nodal pathways. *Circulation.* 1971;64:1059–1067.

21. Moe GK, Preston JB, Burlington HJ. Physiologic evidence for a dual AV transmission system. *Circ Res.* 1956;4:357–375.

22. Mendez C, Moe GK. Demonstration of a dual AV nodal conduction system in the isolated rabbit heart. *Circ Res.* 1966;19:378–393.
23. Kistin AD, Beckley W. Multiple pathways of conduction and reciprocal rhythm with interpolated ventricular premature systoles. *Am Heart J.* 1963; 65:162–179.
24. Gomes JA, Kang PS, Kelen G, et al. Simultaneous anterograde fast-slow atrioventricular nodal pathway conduction after procainamide. *Am J Cardiol.* 1980;46:677–684.
25. Kuck KH, Kuch B, Bleifeld W. Multiple anterograde and retrograde AV nodal pathways: demonstration by multiple discontinuities in the AV nodal conduction curves and echo time intervals. *Pacing Clin Electrophysiol.* 1984; 7:656–662.
26. Anderson RH, Becker AE, Brechenmacher C, et al. The human atrioventricular junctional area: a morphological study of the AV node and bundle. *Eur J Cardiol.* 1975;3:11–25.
27. Ho SY, McComb J, Scott CD, et al. Morphology of the cardiac conduction system in patients with electrophysiologically proven dual atrioventricular nodal pathways. *J Cardiovasc Electrophysiol.* 1993;4:504–512.
28. Jalife J. The sucrose gap preparation as a model of AV nodal transmission: are dual pathways necessary for reciprocation of AV nodal "echoes"? *Pacing Clin Electrophysiol.* 1983;6:1106–1122.
29. Spach MS, Josephson ME. Initiating reentry: the role of nonuniform anisotropy in small circuits. *J Cardiovasc Electrophysiol.* 1994;5:182–209.
30. Spach MS, Dolber PC, Heidlage JF. Influence of the passive anisotropic properties on directional differences in propagation following modification of the sodium conductance in human atrial muscle: a model of reentry based on anisotropic discontinuous propagation. *Circ Res.* 1988;62:811–832.
31. Ross DL, Johnson DC, Denniss AR, et al. Curative surgery for atrioventricular junctional ("AV nodal") reentrant tachycardia. *J Am Coll Cardiol.* 1985; 6:1383–1392.
32. McGuire MA, Johnson DC, Nunn GR, et al. High resolution mapping of the atrial septum in patients with AV junctional ("AV nodal") reentrant tachycardia. *Circulation.* 1992;86(suppl I):I-722. Abstract.
33. Chang BC, Schuessler RB, Stone CM, et al. Computerized activation sequence mapping of the human atrial septum. *Ann Thorac Surg.* 1990;49: 231–241.
34. Lee MA, Morady F, Kadish A, et al. Catheter modification of the atrioventricular junction using radiofrequency energy for control of atrioventricular nodal reentry tachycardia. *Circulation.* 1991;83:827–835.
35. McGuire MA, Lau KC, Johnson DC, et al. Patients with two types of atrioventricular junctional (AV nodal) reentrant tachycardia: evidence that the common pathway of nodal tissue is not present above the reentrant circuit. *Circulation.* 1991;83:1232–1246.
36. Gomes JA, Kang PS, Kelen G, et al. Simultaneous antegrade fast-slow atrioventricular nodal pathway conduction after procainamide. *Am J Cardiol.* 1980;46:677–684.
37. Fujimura O, Guiraudon GM, Yee R, et al. Operative therapy of atrioventricular node reentry and results of an anatomically guided procedure. *Am J Cardiol.* 1989;64:1327–1332.
38. Sethi KK, Jaishankar S, Khalilullah M, et al. Selective blockade of retrograde fast pathway by intravenous disopyramide in paroxysmal supraventricular tachycardia mediated by dual atrioventricular nodal pathways. *Br Heart J.* 1983;49:532–543.

39. Jackman MJ, Beckman KJ, McCelland JH, et al. Treatment of supraventricular tachycardia due to atrioventricular nodal reentry by radiofrequency catheter ablation of slow-pathway conduction. *N Engl J Med.* 1992;327: 313–318.
40. Haissaguerre M, Gaita F, Fischer B, et al. Elimination of atrioventricular nodal reentrant tachycardia using discrete slow potentials to guide application of radiofrequency energy. *Circulation.* 1992;85:2162–2175.
41. Kay GN, Epstein AE, Dailey SM, et al. Selective radiofrequency ablation of the slow pathway for the treatment of atrioventricular nodal reentrant tachycardia: evidence for involvement of perinodal myocardium within the reentrant circuit. *Circulation.* 1992;85:1675–1688.
42. Wu D, Yeh SJ, Wang CC, et al. A simple technique for selective radiofrequency ablation of the slow pathway in atrioventricular node reentrant tachycardia. *J Am Coll Cardiol.* 1993;21:1612–1621.
43. McGuire MA, de Bakker JMT, Vermeulen JT, et al. Origin and significance of double potentials near the atrioventricular node: correlation of extracellular potentials, intracellular potentials, and histology. *Circulation.* 1994;89: 2351–2360.
44. de Bakker JMT, Coronel R, McGuire MA, et al. Slow potentials in the atrioventricular area of patients operated on for atrioventricular node tachycardias and in isolated porcine hearts. *J Am Coll Cardiol.* 1994;23:709–715.
45. McGuire MA, de Bakker JMT, Vermeulen JT, et al. Atrioventricular Junctional Tissue: discrepancy between histological and electrophysiological characteristics. *Circulation.* 1996;94:571–577.

Chapter 21

Experimental Simulations of Variations in Junctional Conductance

Ronald W. Joyner, MD, PhD

Several experimental techniques have been devised to study the interactions among cardiac cells as a function of coupling conductance without the geometric complexity of the multidimensional nature of intact cardiac tissue. Antzelevitch et al[1,2] studied Purkinje strands as one-dimensional systems with the central region of the strand sealed off in a compartment containing sucrose (as an insulator), which was shunted by a variable resistance to provide an effective variable resistance from one region of the strand to another. This technique was also used with sinoatrial node–atrial strips[3] and small papillary muscles.[4] With this technique, the investigators could observe many phenomena related to discontinuous conduction and electrotonic interactions but could not quantitatively determine cellular properties because the tissues on either side of the gap were not isopotential. Studies have also been performed on pairs of heart cells or paired aggregates of heart cells[5–7] in which the coupling conductance is produced by the presence of gap junctions and can be quantitatively measured but poorly modulated or controlled.

Methods

We have developed a technique in which the coupling conductance between a pair of cardiac cells is controlled at some selected value even

Supported by NIH grant HL22562 to Dr. Joyner and by The Children's Heart Center and the Emory Egleston Children's Research Center

From: Spooner PM, Joyner RW, Jalife J (eds). *Discontinuous Conduction in the Heart.* Armonk, NY: Futura Publishing Company, Inc.; © 1997.

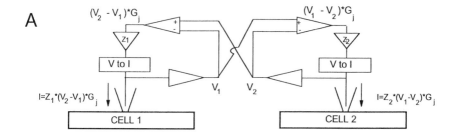

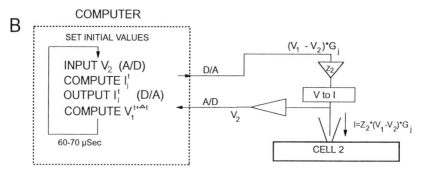

Figure 1. A, Schematic of "coupling-clamp" technique used to supply a coupling conductance, G_c, between two cells recorded simultaneously in "current-clamp" mode. Differential amplifiers at top of diagram continuously produce voltage proportional to difference in potential of two cells, and this difference is used to supply coupling currents to each cell (see Reference 11). B, How this technique can be adapted to couple a real cardiac cell (cell 2) to a real-time simulation of a mathematical model of a cell (cell 1) by use of an A/D and a D/A converter for real-time interactions (see Reference 19).

if the cells are not actually in contact with each other. This "coupling-clamp" technique is illustrated in Figure 1A. For cells 1 and 2, simultaneous recordings are made in "current-clamp" mode, with careful compensation of pipette resistances. If the potentials of cells 1 and 2 are V_1 and V_2, respectively (both functions of time), then the current that would be flowing out of cell 1 and into 2, if the two cells were coupled by a conductance G_c, would be $(V_1 - V_2) \times G_c$. The two amplifiers labeled Z_1 and Z_2 provide an opportunity to vary the effective sizes of cells 1 and 2 by scaling the coupling current applied to cell 1 or to cell 2 such that the effective size of each cell (the inverse of the input resistance) is the real size divided by Z_1 or Z_2, respectively. The resulting "coupling currents" are applied to each cell by the voltage-to-current converter of each channel of the recording amplifier (Axoclamp, Axon Instruments Inc). In this chapter, we describe some of the results obtained with this technique and how they demonstrate fundamental differences in the basic principles and pharmacological modulation of discontinuous compared with continuous cardiac action potential conduction.

Results

In our initial description of the coupling-clamp technique,[8] we documented the technique and showed that coupling an isolated rabbit ventricular cell to a passive resistance-capacitance (RC) circuit representing an inexcitable cell with a normal resting potential produced a progressive shortening of the action potential duration of the ventricular cell as the coupling resistance was decreased with minimal changes in the excitability of the cell. We then studied the effects of "injury current" on an isolated rabbit ventricular cell by performing experiments in which we coupled a ventricular cell to an RC circuit that had a depolarized "resting potential."[9] It had previously been proposed that such an injury current could lead to automatic activity and/or the production of early after depolarizations (EADs) in normal cells coupled to a depolarized region. We found that the effects on APD as we gradually lowered the coupling resistance were biphasic, with decreases in APD while the coupling resistance was quite high and then increases in APD when the coupling resistance was below a critical value. This finding was quite unexpected and may be significant in explaining the wide variability observed in the APD (and refractory period) of cells surrounding an infarct zone. However, we were not able to produce either automaticity or EADs at any value of coupling resistance. We then extended these studies with experiments on guinea pig (GP) ventricular myocytes[10] in which we coupled an isolated cell to a depolarized RC circuit and found that, even though EADs were not produced in normal Tyrode's solution at any value of coupling resistance, we could reproducibly produce EADs in the same cells after we had increased the magnitude of the calcium current with BayK 8644, isoproterenol, forskolin, or intracellular cAMP, or if we used quinidine to partially block potassium current.

We recorded action potentials from two rabbit or GP ventricular cells simultaneously and varied G_c for the cells with our coupling-clamp circuit.[11,12] Figure 2 shows an example of experimental recordings from isolated GP ventricular cells, with a brief stimulus applied to cell 1, at a frequency of 2 Hz and with a G_c of 18.9 nS, close to the critically low G_c for conduction failure. When conduction occurred, cell 2 had a rapid upstroke with a delay from the upstroke of cell 1 of about 16 ms. During the conduction delay, there is a large partial repolariza-

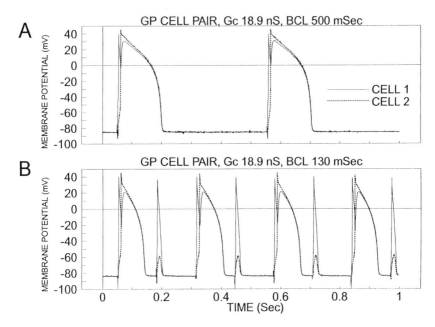

Figure 2. Simultaneous recordings from two isolated GP cells coupled together by "coupling-clamp" circuit with an effective coupling conductance of 18.9 nS. A, Recordings from cell 1 (cell receiving direct stimulus, solid line) and cell 2 (dotted line) at a BCL of 500 ms. B, Results for same two cells, at same coupling conductance, with a BCL of 130 ms. For B, activation of cell 1 occurs with each applied stimulus, but conduction to cell 2 occurs only on alternate activations of cell 1. For activations of cell 1 that do not produce conduction to cell 2, action potential duration of cell 1 is shortened. Modified with permission from Reference 12.

tion of cell 1 due to the electrical load. After activation of cell 2, cell 1 has a recovery of potential up to the normal plateau level, and the subsequent waveforms of potential in cells 1 and 2 were very similar. When we increased the stimulus frequency, we obtained various patterns of success and failure of conduction at cycle lengths <180 ms. Figure 2B shows the potentials of cells 1 and 2 with cell 1 stimulated at a cycle length of 130 ms, with an irregular response of cell 2 after each successful activation of cell 1. Cell 1 has a short action potential duration for each cycle in which cell 2 does not activate. We studied geometric factors responsible for unidirectional block[11] by deliberately choosing cells that were either similar in size or quite different in size (as measured quantitatively by the cell capacitance, the current threshold, and the reciprocal of the input resistance). In cell pairs of asymmetrical size, we showed that bidirectional block occurred at low values of G_c, that bidirectional conduction occurred at higher values of G_c, and that there was a "window" of G_c values over which unidirectional block occurred. Another interesting phenomenon also occurred in these experiments: during the conduction delay between the activation of the stimulated cell (leader cell) and delayed activation of the other cell (follower cell), there was a substantial partial repolarization of the leader cell, which then reversed quickly when the follower cell activated. We also noted that action potential peak amplitude and excitability of the leader cell were not affected by the electrical load that determined conduction failure or success. This suggested that I_{Ca} was much more important in the conduction process than previously considered, at least for cells with discontinuous conduction. We also did experiments[12] in which we coupled pairs of isolated GP ventricular cells over a wide range of G_c and compared the conduction delay and the extent of the partial repolarization of the leader cell in normal Tyrode's solution versus that observed for the same cell pairs with submaximal concentrations of nifedipine. We showed that the critical G_c below which conduction block was produced was increased significantly by nifedipine and that, at a given value of G_c, the conduction delay and the extent of the early repolarization were increased by nifedipine. The extent of the early repolarization in the leader cell also suggested that the actual magnitude of I_{Ca} that flowed during the action potential might be asymmetrical, with more I_{Ca} for the leader than for the follower cell as a result of differences in the early part of the action potential waveform.

We confirmed this prediction[13] by using action potentials recorded from coupled cells (in current-clamp mode) as time-varying command potentials for other cells in voltage-clamp mode. We first simultaneously recorded action potentials from the leader cell (stimulated cell, cell 1) and the follower cell (nonstimulated cell, cell 2) of a cell pair with a fixed G_c between the cells supplied by our coupling circuit. We then applied these recorded action potentials as command potential waveforms for other cells studied in the voltage-clamp mode, for which we used internal and external solutions that isolated I_{Ca}. Figure 3A and 3D are the previously recorded action potentials from a pair of coupled cells (A is from the leader cell, and D is from the follower cell) and are now used as voltage waveforms for voltage clamp. B and E show the currents recorded with the application of waveforms A and D, respectively, with an external solution and an internal (pipette) solution (see "Methods" section), which blocks nearly all ionic currents except I_{Ca}, and we have superimposed on these parts of the figure the results obtained with and without nifedipine in the external solution. Note that nearly all of the inward current is blocked by nifedipine. Figures 3C and 3F show the difference between the results obtained with and without nifedipine and represent the nifedipine-sensitive I_{Ca} for the

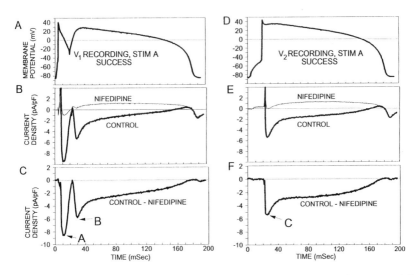

Figure 3. Analysis of L-type calcium current flowing during action potential propagation between two cells of a cell pair. A and D, Action potentials recorded from leader and follower cell, respectively, of a cell pair with coupling conductance slightly above critical value for conduction. B and E, Currents recorded in whole-cell voltage-clamp mode when an isolated GP ventricular myocyte was voltage clamped to the waveforms shown in A and B, respectively, using internal and external solutions that blocked nearly all ionic currents except L-type calcium current. Recordings for B and E are shown before and after addition of 2 μmol/L nifedipine to the external solution to block L-type calcium current. C and F, Differences computed for two traces in B and E, respectively; time course of L-type calcium current in response to waveform of leader and follower cell, respectively. Modified with permission from Reference 13.

waveforms in A and D, respectively. The action potential waveform of the leader cell (A) has a rapid upstroke and then a partial repolarization during the conduction delay before activation of the follower cell. I_{Ca} for the voltage waveform of the leader cell (D) occurred with a large magnitude during the conduction delay, but I_{Ca} for the voltage waveform of the follower cell (F) was nearly zero during the conduction delay. After activation of the follower cell, I_{Ca} was activated for the voltage waveform of the follower cell but not with as large a magnitude as for the voltage waveform of the leader cell. This leads to an asymmetry of I_{Ca} for the two cells, with greater peak I_{Ca} for the leader cell than for the follower cell. When we reversed the direction of conduction by stimulating cell 2, the application of these recorded waveforms for the action potentials for cells 1 and 2 to the voltage-clamped cells also reversed the asymmetry of the magnitude of I_{Ca}. We conclude that discontinuous conduction is associated with a directionally determined asymmetry in I_{Ca}, with the leader cell having a larger I_{Ca} than the follower cell, which may be significant in determining success or failure of conduction.

Many models of the cardiac action potential in single cardiac cells have been published, from the Beeler-Reuter model[14] to the recent Luo and Rudy (LR) model.[15,16] Similarly, numerous models of an SA node action potential have appeared, in particular that of Wilders et al[17] and a similar model by Demir et al.[18] These recent models express multiple ionic currents and electrogenic pumps as well as a quantitative evaluation of the time course of calcium concentration in the cytoplasmic space. The increasing speed of available computers has now made it possible to solve these systems of differential equations in "real time" with a reasonable time step for integration. With an A/D and a D/A converter, the computer can thus produce an "interactive" model in which the solution of the model is coupled in real time by some desired G_c to a real cell from which recordings are being made in the current-clamp mode. The diagram in Figure 1B explains this expansion of our coupling-clamp technique, which is discussed more fully in our recent publication,[19] to include the real-time solution of the LR model (or any other mathematical model of an isolated heart cell) as one of the "cells" to be coupled. We have basically replaced "cell 1" of the cell pair of part A with a computer that, for each time step, samples the voltage present in the real cell (cell 2) via an A/D converter, calculates the value of coupling current for this time step from $I_c = (V_1^t - V_2^t) \times G_c$, sends a voltage proportional to this current to the analog circuit via a D/A converter, and then integrates the LR model for one time step with the coupling current, scaled by Z_1 for an effective change in the area of the computer model, as an additional ionic current to compute $V_1^{t+\Delta t}$. The process is repeated at successive time steps. Using our current hardware (Gateway 120-MHz Pentium processor computer equipped with a Digidata 1200 data acquisition system [Axon Instruments]), we can incorporate this technique with the LR model with a time step of 60 μs. The program also incorporates periodic activation, if desired, of the LR model cell at a variable rate. The computer program also stores as an array the successive samples of V_2 (the potential of the real cell), and with this information, the program can then "replay" the experimental protocol, producing a disk file with a time sequence of the potential of the model cell, the potential of the real cell, the coupling current, and any computed parameters of the model cell (eg, cytoplasmic calcium concentration) as functions of time. In a similar way, we adapted the previously published model of Wilders et al[17] for an SA nodal cell to be coupled in real time to a real cardiac cell. We have done extensive tests of this interactive system, showing that the discrete time step of

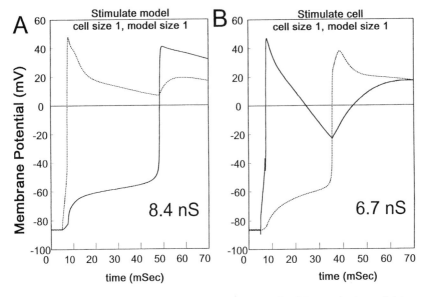

Figure 4. Results obtained by coupling LR model of a GP ventricular cell (dotted line) to a real isolated GP ventricular cell (solid line) using coupling circuit of Figure 3B. Stimulus is applied to LR model cell; B, stimulus is applied to real GP ventricular cell. Reprinted with permission from Reference 19.

60 μs does not seriously distort the computed action potentials or the ionic currents compared with a 1-μs time step.

We show here a few results with this new technique, with more extensive studies presented in our recent publication.[19] When we coupled the LR model cell to a GP ventricular cell, we obtained action potential conduction either from the LR model cell to the real cell or from the real cell to the LR model cell, depending on which cell received direct stimulation and on the G_c. Figure 4 shows results for stimulating the LR model cell (A) or for stimulating the real cell (B) when the two cells were adjusted to be of equal size, based on the recorded current threshold of each cell for a 2-ms current stimulus. For each panel, the potential of the real cell is shown as a solid line and the potential of the LR model cell is shown by a dotted line. These records were selected to represent results obtained near the critical low value of G_c for each direction of conduction (indicated on each panel) for successful conduction. Systematic alteration of G_c and the size of each cell showed the following.[19]

1. When we normalized the real cell size to that of the LR model cell, we found that the required G_c for successful

propagation between a real cell and an LR model cell was greater than that found for successful conduction between two LR model cells (5.4 nS), with a greater disparity (8.27 ± 0.55 nS) when we stimulated the LR model cell than that found (7.02 ± 0.17 nS) when we stimulated the real cell.

2. The extent of electrical loading of the action potentials, as indicated by the extent of the partial repolarization of the leader cell during conduction, was significantly greater for the real cell than for the LR model cell even when the size of the real cell was normalized to that of the LR model cell.

3. When the size of the follower cell was increased by a factor of two, the required G_c for successful conduction was dramatically increased, but this increase was greatest for the condition of conduction from a real cell to an LR model cell, less for conduction from the LR model cell to a real cell, and least for conduction from one LR model cell to another LR model cell. A similar discrepancy occurred when the size of the leader cell was decreased by a factor of 2.

4. For all three conduction conditions (LR model cell to LR model cell, real cell to LR model cell, and LR model cell to real cell), the effects on the required G_c of changes in the ratio of leader size to follower size were greater for changes in the follower size than for changes in the leader size and were also greater for interventions that reduced the ratio of leader size to follower size than for interventions that increased the ratio of leader size to follower size.

5. For all three conduction conditions, the effects on maximal conduction delay were an increase in the maximal conduction delay when the ratio of leader size to follower size was increased and a decrease in the maximal conduction delay when the ratio of leader size to follower size was decreased.

Although in Reference 19 we emphasized the effects of extreme uncoupling of cells, we have also studied the effects of G_c and asymmetry on the size of coupled cells over a wide range of G_c. Figure 5 shows results for stimulating a GP ventricular cell coupled to the LR model while varying G_c but maintaining equal size between the real cell and the model (A) or, for a different cell, maintaining a G_c of 15 nS while varying the LR model cell size with respect to the real cell size (B). In each part, data for the real cell are plotted as solid lines, and data for the LR model cell are plotted as dotted lines. In Figure 5A, the conduction delay progressively increases as G_c is decreased from 50 to 6 nS, with the delay at 50 nS being only 1.0 ms. Note that the early repolariza-

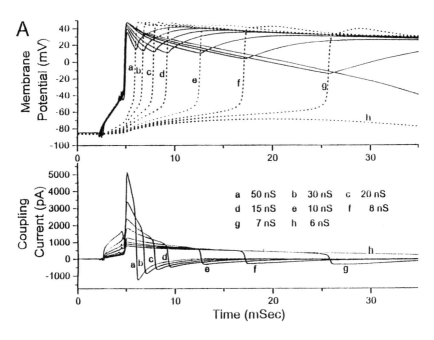

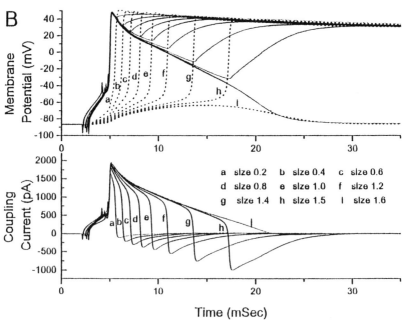

tion of the real cell becomes progressively less steep as G_c is lowered. For values of G_c <7 nS for this cell, there was conduction failure from the real cell to the LR model cell. In B, we show a progressive increase in conduction delay as the relative size of the LR model is increased from 0.2 to 1.6 with a fixed G_c of 15 nS. Note that the early repolarization of the real cell has the same slope for increasing sizes of the LR model cell (compare results in A). The lower panels of A and B show the corresponding coupling currents, with positive current in the direction from the real cell to the model cell.

We have also used pharmacological modulation of the L-type calcium current of one cell of a cell pair in which the leader (stimulated) cell of the cell pair is a GP ventricular cell and the follower cell is the LR model, with the size of the real cell adjusted to have the same current threshold for a 2-ms pulse as the LR model (2.6 nA). Figure 6A is a plot of conduction delay as a function of G_c for a range from 50 nS down to the critical G_c for failure of conduction, which was 7 nS in the control solution (same cell as for Figure 5A) and increased to 9 nS with 1 μmol/L nifedipine. Figure 6B shows action potential recordings of the real cell (solid lines) and the LR model cell (dotted lines) with $G_c = 10$ nS in control (C) and nifedipine (NIF) solution, showing that the delay is clearly increased in the nifedipine solution. At lower values of G_c nifedipine produced a reversible block of conduction for this cell pair. For a different cell pair (again, a real GP ventricular cell coupled to the LR model), Figure 6C shows effects of 20 nmol/L isoproterenol (ISO) at $G_c = 7.3$ nS. In the control solution and after the washout of the isoproterenol, this G_c produced block of conduction. In the ISO solution, conduction became successful. The addition of 20 nmol/L ISO reduced critical G_c from 7.4 to 5.8 nS. We also obtained some exciting results by coupling the Wilders et al[17] sinoatrial node (SAN) model to a GP or a rabbit ventricular cell; some of these results are discussed in a recent manuscript (Kumar et al, submitted). These experiments were not done specifically to ask what would happen if an SAN cell happened to be located within the ventricular wall but rather as a beginning step in understanding how an ectopic focus of depolarized, spontaneously active cells might interact with quiescent but excitable cells of the ventricular or atrial wall. We previously showed with a simulated

Figure 5. Results obtained by coupling LR model (dotted line) to a real GP ventricular cell (solid lines) when real cell receives direct stimuli. A, Size of real cell was adjusted to be equal to that of LR model cell, and multiple traces shown were obtained by varying coupling conductance from 50 nS (trace a) to 6 nS (trace h). B, Coupling conductance was set at 15 nS, and relative size of LR model cell was varied from 0.1 (trace a) to 1.6 (trace i).

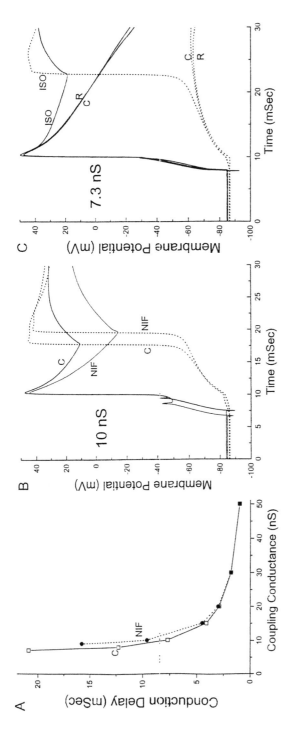

Figure 6. Results obtained by coupling LR model (dotted lines) to a real GP ventricular cell (solid lines) when real cell receives direct stimuli. A, Conduction delay as a function of coupling conductance between real cell and LR model cell under control conditions (C) and with 1 µmol/L nifedipine (NIF). B, Conduction that occurred at 10-nS conductance under control conditions and with 1 µmol/L nifedipine. C, For a different real cell, failure of action potential conduction from real cell to LR model under control conditions, successful conduction with 20 nmol/L isoproterenol (ISO), and failure of conduction again after recovery from isoproterenol solution (R).

pair of cell groups,[20,21] in which one is spontaneously active and the other is excitable but quiescent, that if the size of the group of spontaneously active cells is large enough, then the resulting pattern of activity will progress through three stages as G_c is progressively increased. For the lowest values of G_c, the spontaneous region will pace itself repeatedly but will not drive (activate) the quiescent group.

For an intermediate range of G_c, the spontaneous region will both pace itself and also repeatedly drive the quiescent group. Above a critical value of G_c, the spontaneous group will fail to pace itself (and thus, of course, not be able to drive the quiescent group). We have now documented this phenomenon with our hybrid cell pair system in which one cell is the SAN model and the other is either a GP or a rabbit ventricular cell. Figure 7 shows the results for a rabbit ventricular cell for which coupling at 3 nS (A) or 17 nS (B) was established after the SAN model (size factor of 5) had completed five cycles. After coupling was established, the SAN model continued to pace at a nearly normal cycle length without activating the real ventricular cell ($G_c = 3$ nS, A) or paced at a progressively longer cycle length, with repeated driving of the real ventricular cell, before stopping its automaticity ($G_c = 17$ nS, B). For this cell pair, the critical G_c for the transition from pacing but not driving to pacing and driving was at 7.2 nS. Figure 8 shows results for $G_c = 7$ nS and $G_c = 8$ nS. One very interesting result shown in this figure is that the cycle length is actually shortened by the successful driving of the quiescent cell. This is shown more clearly in Figure 9, in which we show (A) the cycle length as a function of time for this cell pair for values of G_c from 1 to 13 nS, with a size factor of 5 for the SAN model. For all values of G_c for which the SAN model paced itself but did not drive the ventricular cell (shown as solid symbols, $G_c = 1$, 3, 5, and 7 nS), there is a progressive increase in steady-state cycle length for greater values of G_c, but a progressive increase in cycle length with time after coupling is also established. When G_c was then increased to 8 nS (open squares), producing repeated driving of the ventricular cell, the steady-state cycle length then decreased from the value for $G_c = 7$ nS (solid diamonds). As G_c was further increased up to 12 nS, the steady-state cycle length continued to increase, with successful driving of the ventricular cell. In five rabbit ventricular cells for which we used this protocol with an SAN model size factor of 5, the critical G_c for the transition from pacing but not driving to pacing with driving had a mean value of 7.3 ± 0.5 nS and the critical value of G_c for the transition from pacing with driving to not pacing had a mean value of 15.7 ± 0.9 nS. The decrease in cycle length produced by the transition from pacing but not driving to pacing and driving was 66 ± 26 ms. Figure 9B illustrates the results for the same cell pair system for a size factor of 3 for the SAN model cell. Each value of G_c now produces

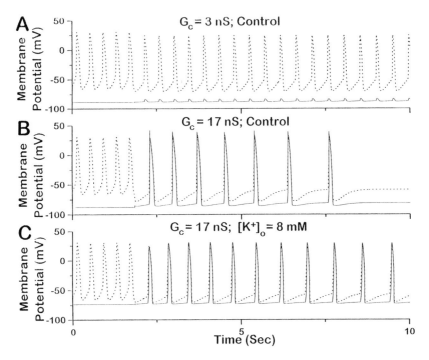

Figure 7. Results obtained by coupling Wilders et al (Reference 17) mathematical model for a sinoatrial node cell (SAN model, dotted line) to a real isolated rabbit ventricular cell (solid line). For A, B, and C, size of SAN model was multiplied by a factor of 5, and we used a protocol of complete uncoupling for the first five cycles of the SAN model and then a coupling conductance as indicated for remainder of trace. A ($G_c = 3$ nS), SAN model paces repeatedly but does not drive (activate) real ventricular cell. B ($G_c = 17$ nS), SAN model does pace and drive for 7 cycles after coupling was established but then becomes quiescent. C (also with $G_c = 17$ nS) was obtained for same real cell after external solution was changed to one containing 8 mmol/L potassium, producing successful pacing and driving of cell pair system.

more slowing of pacing (compared with a size factor of 5, A), and the transition from pacing but not driving to not pacing occurs without any value of G_c that would allow pacing and driving.

As an example of pharmacological modulation of discontinuous conduction, we have done experiments in which we first used a control external solution and located the critical G_c for a cell pair system (SAN model connected to rabbit ventricular cell) for the transition from pacing but not driving to pacing and driving and also the critical G_c for the transition from pacing and driving to not pacing. We then switched the external solution to one with 8 mmol/L K^+ instead of the normal 4 mmol/L K^+ and repeated this protocol. Figures 7C and 8C show data

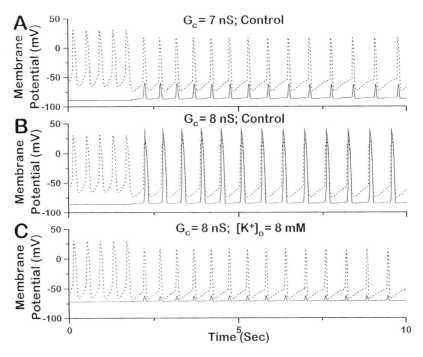

Figure 8. Results obtained by coupling Wilders et al (Reference 17) mathematical model for a sinoatrial node cell (SAN model, dotted line) to a real isolated rabbit ventricular cell (same real cell as Figure 7, solid line). For A, B, and C, size of SAN model was multiplied by a factor of 5, and we used a protocol of complete uncoupling for the first five cycles of the SAN model and then a coupling conductance as indicated for remainder of trace. A ($G_c = 7$ nS), SAN model paces repeatedly but does not drive (activate) real ventricular cell. B ($G_c = 8$ nS) SAN model does pace and drive after coupling was established. C (also with $G_c = 8$ nS) was obtained for same real cell after external solution was changed to one containing 8 mmol/L potassium, producing successful pacing of SAN model cell but not driving of real cell pair system.

from the same cell pair as used for Figures 7 and 8, A and B, for the same G_c values of 17 and 8 nS, respectively, after we switched the bath solution to 8 mmol/L K^+. The depolarization of the ventricular cell (from -87 to -73 mV) produced by the elevated K^+ has reduced the electrotonic load on the SAN model such that a G_c that prevented pacing of the SAN model in control solution (17 nS, Figure 7B) now allows the SAN model to pace and drive the ventricular cell in the 8-mmol/L K^+ solution (Figure 7C). Figure 8C shows the results for a G_c of 8 nS. Figure 8B (8 nS, control solution) demonstrates pacing and driving of the ventricular cell at this G_c, but the switch to 8 mmol/L K^+ (Figure 8C) now produces pacing but not driving of the same cell pair. Note

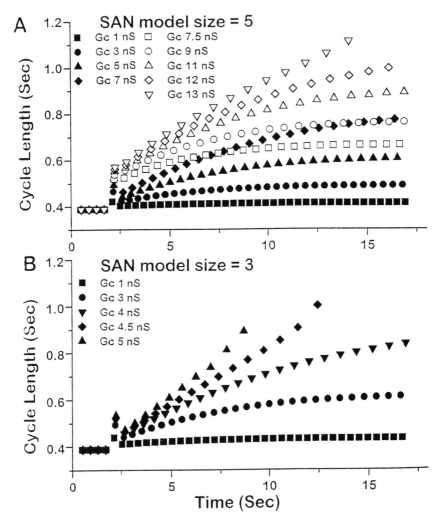

Figure 9. Effects of coupling conductance on cycle length for same hybrid cell pair (SAN model cell connected to real rabbit ventricular cell) as in Figures 7 and 8. A, Cycle length as a function of time with values of G_c ranging from 1 nS (solid squares) to 13 nS (inverted open triangle). For solid symbols, SAN model cell had successful pacing of itself but not driving of real cell. For open symbols, SAN model cell had successful pacing and driving of real cell. B, Same relationships when size of SAN model cell was multiplied by a factor of 3 instead of factor of 5 used for part A.

that the effects of the 8-mmol/L K$^+$ solution on the ability of the SAN model to drive the ventricular cell are opposite for higher values of coupling versus lower values of coupling, with the 8-mmol/L K$^+$ solution raising the upper range of G$_c$ up to which driving of the quiescent cell occurs (from 13 to 20 nS, as illustrated in Figure 7 with G$_c$ = 17 nS) but also raising the lower range over which driving does not occur (from 7.2 to 13 nS, as illustrated in Figure 8 with G$_c$ = 8 nS). All of the effects of the elevated K$^+$ solution were completely reversible upon return to the control solution, with similar effects observed in three additional experiments with elevated K$^+$.

Interactions between the electrotonic loading of the SAN model cell and the periodic direct stimuli of the GP ventricular cell are systematically illustrated in Figures 10 and 11, which are recordings from a single GP ventricular cell (solid lines) that was coupled to the SAN model (dotted lines) at a conductance of 5 nS (Figure 10) or 10 nS (Figure 11). The GP ventricular cell was directly stimulated at a basic cycle length (BCL) as indicated in each part of the two figures, with each occurrence of a direct stimulation of the GP ventricular cell marked by an arrow. Before adjustment of the size of the GP ventricular cell, this cell had a current threshold of 2.8 nA (input resistance, 17.8 MΩ). To normalize the size of this cell, we thus set Z$_2$ to 1.08 (2.8/2.6) (see "Methods"), which made the effective current threshold of this cell 2.6 nA and its input resistance 16.5 MΩ. When uncoupled, the SAN model cell has an intrinsic cycle length of automaticity of 388 ms. For this hybrid cell pair, the critical conductance above which the model cell (size factor of 5) could successfully drive the GP ventricular cell was 7.2 nS. For each part of Figures 10 and 11, we coupled the SAN model cell (size factor of 5) to the GP ventricular cell and allowed the hybrid cell pair to establish a periodic pattern of interactions. For each of parts B through E of Figures 10 and 11, we plotted data from 1.6 seconds before to 1.6 seconds after a direct stimulus to the GP ventricular cell. For Figures 10A and 11A, no direct stimuli were applied to the GP ventricular cell, and the data are plotted for 1.6 seconds before and 1.6 seconds after a spontaneous activation of the SAN model cell. The stable pattern of interaction for Figures 10A and 11A (no direct stimulation) is a periodic automatic pacing of the SAN model, with a resulting cycle length of 396 ms for Figure 10 (G$_c$ = 5 nS) or 743 ms for Figure 11 (G$_c$ = 10 nS), the major difference being that for the higher value of G$_c$ (Figure 11A), the GP ventricular cell is being successfully driven by the SAN model cell and for the lower value of G$_c$ (Figure 10A), the GP ventricular cell has no electrical activity other than the small depolarizations associated with electrotonic current flow from the SAN model cell activations. Every occurrence of successful driving of the GP ventricular cell by activity originating in the SAN model cell is marked by

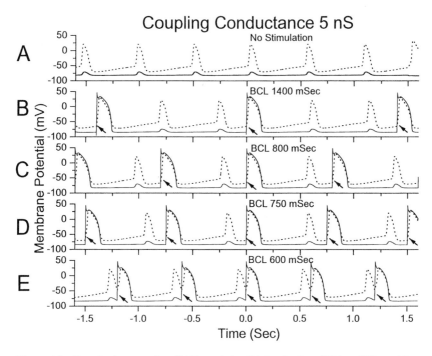

Figure 10. Results for coupling SAN model cell (size factor of 5) to a GP ventricular cell with $G_c = 5$ nS. Results are shown as dotted lines for SAN model cell and as solid lines for the GP ventricular cell. A, No direct stimulation is applied to GP ventricular cell. B through E, Direct stimulation of GP ventricular cell is at a BCL of 1400 ms (B), 800 ms (C), 750 ms (D), or 600 ms (E). Data plotted here are for steady-state condition after coupling was established, with zero time for B through E corresponding to direct stimulation of GP ventricular cell and zero time for A corresponding to spontaneous activation of SAN model cell. B through E, Arrows indicate times of direct stimuli applied to GP ventricular cell. Cell R102495G;5.

an asterisk in each part of Figures 10 and 11. For Figures 10B and 11B, we used direct stimuli to the GP ventricular cell at a BCL of 1400 ms. For both values of G_c, the hybrid cell pair system has established a periodic pattern of interactions. For the lower value of G_c (Figure 10B), the direct activations of the GP ventricular cell propagate to the SAN model, and the SAN model is able to interpolate two cycles of spontaneous activity between each successive direct activation of the GP ventricular cell, but these cycles of spontaneous activity do not propagate to the GP ventricular cell. For the higher value of G_c (Figure 11B), only one spontaneous cycle of the SAN model cell is interpolated between successive direct activations of the GP ventricular cell, and this spontaneous activation of the SAN model cell is able to propagate to the GP

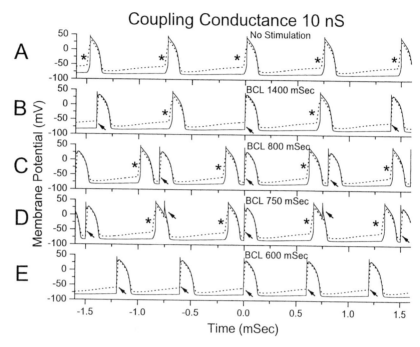

Figure 11. Results for coupling SAN model cell (size factor of 5) to a GP ventricular cell with $G_c = 10$ nS (same cell as for Figure 10). A, No direct stimulation is applied to GP ventricular cell. B through E, Direct stimulation of GP ventricular cell is at a BCL of 1400 ms (B), 800 ms (C), 750 ms (D), or 600 ms (E). Data plotted here are for steady-state condition after coupling was established, with zero time for B through E corresponding to direct stimulation of GP ventricular cell and zero time for A corresponding to spontaneous activation of SAN model cell. For each part of figure, asterisk indicates each occurrence of conduction from SAN model cell to GP ventricular cell, and arrow indicates times of direct stimuli applied to GP ventricular cell. Cell R102495G;5.

ventricular cell (indicated by asterisks). For Figures 10C and 11C, we used direct stimulation of the GP ventricular cell at a BCL of 800 ms. For the lower value of G_c (Figure 10C), each direct activation of the GP ventricular cell produces activation of the SAN model cell, and the SAN model cell is able to interpolate one spontaneous cycle between the direct activations of the GP ventricular cell. For the higher value of G_c (Figure 11C), there is also one interpolated spontaneous cycle of the SAN model cell between successive direct stimuli of the GP ventricular cell, and this spontaneous activation occurs just before each of the direct stimuli of the GP ventricular cell, producing a pattern of activation of the GP ventricular cell of closely coupled activations in which the first activation of each pair originates from the SAN model cell (indicated by asterisks) and the second originates from the direct stimulation of the GP ventricular cell (indicated by arrows). For Figures 10D and 11D, we used direct stimuli to the GP ventricular cell at a BCL of 750 ms. For the lower value of G_c (Figure 10D), the results are very similar to those of Figure 10C, with a resetting of the spontaneous activity of the SAN model cell with each successful propagation from the GP ventricular cell to the SAN model cell, producing a single interpolated spontaneous cycle between successive direct stimuli. For the higher value of G_c (Figure 11D), the slower rate of diastolic depolarization of the SAN model cell, compared with the lower value of G_c (Figure 10D), produces a periodic sequence such that alternate direct stimuli to the GP ventricular cell are occurring during the plateau of the GP ventricular cell action potential that originates from the spontaneous activity of the SAN model cell. The stable pattern of activations of the GP ventricular cell thus alternates between single activations (originating from the SAN model cell, indicated by asterisks) and pairs of closely coupled activations. For Figures 10E and 11E, we used direct stimuli to the GP ventricular cell at a BCL of 600 ms. For the lower value of G_c (Figure 10E), the stable pattern now consists of closely coupled pairs of activations of the SAN model cell, with each direct stimulation of the GP ventricular cell propagating to the SAN model cell and resetting its automaticity. For the higher value of G_c (Figure 11E), the direct stimuli to the GP ventricular cell are now occurring at a BCL that is shorter than the spontaneous cycle length of the SAN model cell with this value of G_c, and thus the direct stimuli now prevent any expression of automaticity from the SAN model cell.

Discussion

In this chapter, we have focused our attention on new techniques that have been developed to understand the basic principles and pharmacological modulation of discontinuous cardiac action potential conduction. It has become clear that cardiac action potential conduction has various degrees of discontinuity in different cardiac regions and with different directions of propagation. It is much less clear in what way the presence of discontinuous conduction leads to the induction and continuation of cardiac arrhythmias. The complex interactions among heart cells with spatial variability in action potential properties and intercellular coupling are poorly understood in the normal heart, and the additional spatial variability induced by ischemia leads to a plethora of proposals for the mechanisms and treatment of cardiac arrhythmias. As recently reviewed by Curtis et al,[22] ischemia induces the accumulation or depletion of a large number of chemical mediators in addition to the loss of oxygen and metabolic substrates. These mediators induce cellular electrophysiological dysfunction (in both the membrane properties of individual cells and the intercellular coupling), which then induces the syncytial electrophysiological dysfunction we call arrhythmias. The cellular electrophysiological dysfunction may lead to conduction slowing and/or block, which can then lead to the development of a reentrant arrhythmic pattern. Alternatively, the cellular electrophysiological dysfunction may lead to one or more localized areas of ectopic spike generation (either as automaticity or as triggered activity) that, if conducted out to the surrounding myocardium, acts as an ectopic focus to generate a nonreentrant arrhythmia. It is important to note that many episodes of acute ischemia are occurring in tissue that is already abnormal in several aspects. Sudden cardiac death is commonly associated with a preexisting "structural abnormality"[23] from prior infarction, hypertrophy, or myopathy that may serve as a substrate from which arrhythmias can arise in the presence of an occurrence or recurrence of electrophysiological dysfunction. The focus of many research efforts is currently either (1) at the level of the isolated cell (or subcellular fraction) to understand the cellular electrophysiological dysfunction or (2) at the level of studying the patterns and modulation of the syncytial electrophysiological dysfunction by mapping the activation sequence of arrhythmias. The effects of discontinuities of conduction may be one of the mechanisms by which cellular electrophysiological dysfunction, in the presence of abnormal spatial distributions of electrical interconnections, produces syncytial electrophysiological dysfunction with respect to ventricular activation.

References

1. Antzelevitch C, Jalife J, Moe GK. Characteristics of reflection as a mechanism of reentrant arrhythmias and its relationship to parasystole. *Circulation.* 1980;61:182–191.
2. Antzelevitch C, Bernstein MJ, Feldman HN, Moe GK. Parasystole, reentry, and tachycardia: a canine preparation of cardiac arrhythmias occurring across inexcitable segments of tissue. *Lab. Invest.* 1983;68:1101–1115.
3. Delmar M, Jalife J, Michaels DC. Effects of changes in excitability and intercellular coupling on synchronization in the rabbit sino-atrial node. *J Physiol.* 1986;370:127–150.
4. Rozanski GK, Jalife J, Moe GK. Determinants of postrepolarization refractoriness in depressed mammalian ventricular muscle. *Circ Res.* 1984;55: 486–496.
5. Veenstra RD, DeHaan RL. Electrotonic interactions between aggregates of chick embryo cardiac pacemaker cells. *Am J Physiol.* 1986;250:H453–H463.
6. Weingart R, Maurer P. Action potential transfer in cell pairs isolated from adult rat and guinea pig ventricles. *Circ Res.* 1988;63:72–80.

7. Burt JM, Spray DC. Inotropic agents modulate gap junctional conductance between cardiac myocytes. *Am J Physiol.* 1988;254:H1206–H1210.
8. Tan RC, Joyner RW. Electrotonic influences on action potentials from isolated ventricular cells. *Circ Res.* 1990;67:1071–1081.
9. Tan RC, Osaka T, Joyner RW. Experimental model of effects on normal tissue of injury current from ischemic region. *Circ Res.* 1991;69:965–974.
10. Kumar R, Joyner RW. An experimental model of the production of early afterdepolarizations by injury current from an ischemic region. *Pflugers Arch.* 1994;428:425–432.
11. Joyner RW, Sugiura H, Tan RC. Unidirectional block between isolated rabbit ventricular cells coupled by a variable resistance. *Biophys J.* 1991;60: 1038–1045.
12. Sugiura H, Joyner RW. Action potential conduction between guinea pig ventricular cells can be modulated by calcium current. *Am J Physiol.* 1992; 263:H1591–H1604.
13. Kumar R, Joyner RW. Calcium currents of ventricular cell pairs during action potential conduction. *Am J Physiol.* 1995;268:H2476–H2486.
14. Beeler GW, Reuter H. Reconstruction of the action potential of ventricular myocardial fibres. *J Physiol.* 1977;268:177–210.
15. Luo CH, Rudy Y. A dynamic model of the cardiac ventricular action potential, 1: simulations of ionic currents and concentration changes. *Circ Res.* 1994;74:1071–1096.
16. Luo CH, Rudy Y. A dynamic model of the cardiac ventricular action potential, 2: afterdepolarizations, triggered activity, and potentiation. *Circ Res.* 1994;74:1097–1113.
17. Wilders R, Jongsma HJ, van Ginneken AC. Pacemaker activity of the rabbit sinoatrial node: a comparison of mathematical models. *Biophys J.* 1991;60: 1202–1216.
18. Demir SS, Clark JW, Murphey CR, Giles WR. A mathematical model of a rabbit sinoatrial node cell. *Am J Physiol.* 1994;266:C832–C852.
19. Wilders R, Kumar R, Joyner RW, et al. Action potential conduction between a ventricular cell model and an isolated ventricular cell. *Biophys J.* 1996;70: 281–295.
20. Joyner RW, Picone J, Rawling D, Veenstra R. Propagation through electrically coupled cells: effects of regional changes in membrane properties. *Circ Res.* 1983;53:526–534.
21. Joyner RW, van Capelle FJL. Propagation through electrically coupled cells: how a small SA node drives a large atrium. *Biophys J.* 1986;50:1157–1164.
22. Curtis MJ, Pugsley MK, Walker MJ. Endogenous chemical mediators of ventricular arrhythmias in ischaemic heart disease. *Cardiovasc Res.* 1993;27: 703–719.
23. Myerburg RJ, Kessler KM, Castellanos A. Interactions between structure and function in sudden cardiac death. In: Akhtar M, Myerburg RJ, Ruskin JN, eds. *Sudden Cardiac Death.* Philadelphia, Pa: Williams & Wilkins; 1994: 32–47.

Chapter 22

Membrane Factors and Gap Junction Factors as Determinants of Ventricular Conduction and Reentry

Yoram Rudy, PhD, and Robin M. Shaw, BS Sc

Propagation of excitation in cardiac tissue is determined by local source-sink relations. For propagation to succeed, the amount of charge supplied by the source must be equal to or exceed the charge required to excite the membrane at the sink location. At the cellular level, this condition is determined by the interplay between the state of membrane excitability and the degree and distribution of intercellular coupling at gap junctions. The state of membrane excitability is determined by the kinetics of membrane ionic currents and has been studied extensively (see Reference 1 for a detailed review of experimental work and References 2 and 3 for theoretical simulations of ionic currents during a ventricular action potential). In a parallel effort, attention has been directed toward the role of the microscopic myocardial architecture in propagation of the action potential.[4] In particular, the role of cell-to-cell coupling at gap junctions has been investigated both experimentally[5-7] and in mathematical models of propagation in cardiac tissue.[8-12]

In this chapter, we use mathematical models to examine the effects of membrane factors and gap junction factors on propagation of the action potential in cardiac tissue. The focus is on changes in membrane excitability and in the degree of cell-to-cell coupling at gap junctions. Altered membrane excitability and reduced cellular coupling are

Preparation of this chapter was supported by National Institutes of Health Grants HL-49054 and HL-33343 (National Heart, Lung, and Blood Institute).

From: Spooner PM, Joyner RW, Jalife J (eds). *Discontinuous Conduction in the Heart.* Armonk, NY: Futura Publishing Company, Inc.; © 1997.

known consequences of various pathological states and can occur together or separately. An example of a pathological state that influences primarily membrane factors is the early stage of acute ischemia.[13,14] Conversely, intercellular decoupling at gap junctions has been demonstrated during the later phases of ischemia[15–17] and in association with various types of injury.[18] An increased degree of separation between fibers has been observed in the setting of infarction.[19] In the studies summarized here, we attempt to provide insights and establish theoretical principles regarding the influence of membrane factors and gap junction factors on propagation of excitation in the heart. We emphasize the roles of these factors in causing slow conduction, decremental conduction, and conduction block. We also investigate their relative effects on the vulnerability of cardiac tissue to the induction of unidirectional block. Since unidirectional block and slow conduction are involved in the development and sustenance of reentry, we evaluate membrane effects and gap junction effects in the context of reentrant activity. This chapter compiles results from several earlier studies; details can be found in previous publications.[20–26]

Theoretical Model

Simulations were conducted in a multicellular one-dimensional model that incorporates membrane ionic processes and intercellular gap junctions.[20] The electrical activity of the membrane is represented, in certain simulations, by the Beeler-Reuter (BR) model.[27] In other simulations, the more recent dynamic Luo-Rudy (LR) model of the ventricular action potential[2,3] is used. This model is based on single-cell and single-channel studies of mammalian ventricle, drawing mainly from studies in the guinea pig. The model incorporates gated ionic channels, ionic pumps, and ionic exchangers. It also accounts for dynamic changes in concentrations of the various ions (importantly, the calcium transient and calcium handling by the sarcoplasmic reticulum and by calcium buffers). The cells in the model are of realistic dimensions (100 μm long) and are connected by gap junctions with 80-Å-long resistive channels (connexons) that provide direct cell-to-cell pathways for current flow. The model permits varying the gap junction conductance over a wide range of values, simulating different degrees of intercellular coupling. A purely resistive representation of the gap junction is adopted. This property is consistent with the behavior of single-channel currents from cardiac gap junctions[28] and with the constancy of the junctional axial resistance over a wide range of voltages.[29]

Properties of Propagation

Membrane Effects on (dV/dt)$_{max}$, Conduction Velocity, and Conduction Block

The effects of reduced membrane excitability on propagation are examined in Figure 1. Membrane excitability is varied by gradually reducing the maximum sodium conductance, $\bar{g}_{Na}$, from 100% (full excitability) to 10%. As excitability is decreased, both (dV/dt)$_{max}$ (the maximum rate of depolarization) and conduction velocity decrease monotonically as a result of decreasing excitatory sodium current, I_{Na}. Over the simulated range of $\bar{g}_{Na}$, (dV/dt)$_{max}$ falls from 240 v/s (at 100% $\bar{g}_{Na}$) to 19 V/s (at 11% $\bar{g}_{Na}$), and the velocity from 54 to 17 cm/s. Further reduction of $\bar{g}_{Na}$ results in insufficient I_{Na} to sustain propagation, and an abrupt conduction block occurs. Note that when membrane excitability is reduced, velocity can be reduced only by a factor of ≈3 before block occurs.

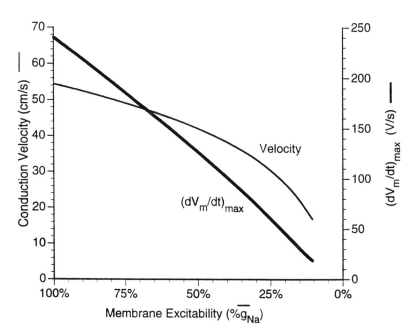

Figure 1. Effects of homogeneous changes in membrane excitability on propagation. Conduction velocity and maximum rate of depolarization, (dV$_m$/dt)$_{max}$, decrease monotonically with decreasing maximum sodium conductance, $\bar{g}_{Na}$.

Gap Junction Effects on $(dV/dt)_{max}$, Conduction Velocity, and Conduction Block

The effects of reduced gap junction coupling on propagation are examined in Figure 2. Conduction velocity and $(dV/dt)_{max}$ are shown as a function of the degree of intercellular coupling for a constant myoplasmic resistivity ($R_{myo} = 150\ \Omega\cdot cm$) and a fully excitable membrane. As cells become progressively less coupled (R_g, the gap junction resistance, increases and G_j, gap junction conductance, decreases), velocity decreases monotonically. In contrast, $(dV/dt)_{max}$ displays a biphasic

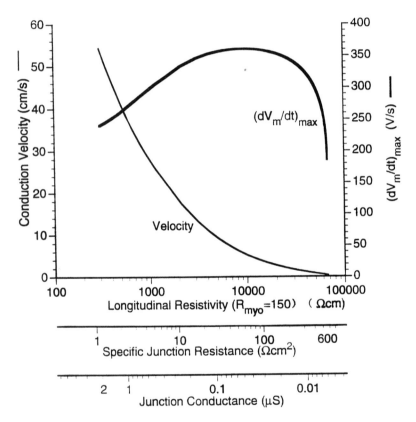

Figure 2. Effects of homogeneous changes in gap junction coupling on propagation. Velocity decreases monotonically, but $(dV_m/dt)_{max}$ displays nonmonotonic behavior as cells become progressively more decoupled. Myoplasmic resistivity, R_{myo}, is held constant at 150 $\Omega\cdot cm$. Abscissa shows (top scale) effective total intracellular resistivity (contribution from both gap junction and myoplasm); (middle scale) specific gap junction resistance; (bottom scale) gap junction conductance.

behavior. In the range of R_g from 1.5 to 100 $\Omega \cdot cm^2$ (G_j from 2.5 to 0.038 μS), $(dV/dt)_{max}$ increases to a maximum value of 360 V/s, reflecting increased confinement of axial current flow in the activated cell. As the cell becomes less coupled to its downstream neighbor, it is subjected to a reduced electrical load, and more current is available for local depolarization. This acts to increase $(dV/dt)_{max}$. At the same time, the reduced coupling creates longer propagation delays in crossing gap junctions, and conduction velocity is reduced. The result is "paradoxical" slow conduction that exhibits normal or even high $(dV/dt)_{max}$ (ie, a highly excitable membrane). Beyond the maximum value, $(dV/dt)_{max}$ decreases with further decrease of intercellular coupling. This is because, for severe uncoupling, the postjunctional charging current becomes very limited, and charging time to threshold (ie, the foot of the action potential) is greatly prolonged. The slow charging process allows for greater inactivation of I_{Na} that is reflected in a reduced $(dV/dt)_{max}$. Note (Figure 2) that very slow conduction (velocity on the order of 1 to 2 cm/s) can be achieved by decoupling of cells at gap junctions.

As cells continue to decouple, a range of severely reduced coupling is reached for which propagation cannot be sustained and conduction block occurs. Figure 3 depicts such an event. The numbers in the body of the figure indicate the cell number relative to the stimulus site. The velocity of propagation decreases progressively with distance from the stimulus site (the velocity could be as slow as 1.5 cm/s). In addition, the action potential duration (APD) and amplitude decrease. Note the spikelike appearance of the action potential, which is consistent with the experimental observations of Sasyniuk and Mendez.[30] Beyond cell 13, complete conduction block occurs. Note that according to continuous-cable theory (in the absence of gap junctions, eg, an axon), conduction block is approached asymptotically as the intracellular resistance becomes infinite. In contrast, in the discontinuous model (cardiac fiber), conduction block occurs for finite values of gap junction resistance. Experimentally, it was observed by Sicouri et al[31] that in the presence of the uncoupler heptanol, "complete blockage was correlated with a fivefold increase in Ri (intracellular resistance), while excitability was unchanged, as demonstrated by the presence of 'nonpropagated' action potentials at the site of intracellular current injection." This experimental finding is consistent with the simulation of Figure 3.

Unidirectional Block

Window of Vulnerability to Unidirectional Block

Unidirectional block is defined as successful propagation in one direction of a cardiac fiber and unsuccessful, or blocked, propagation

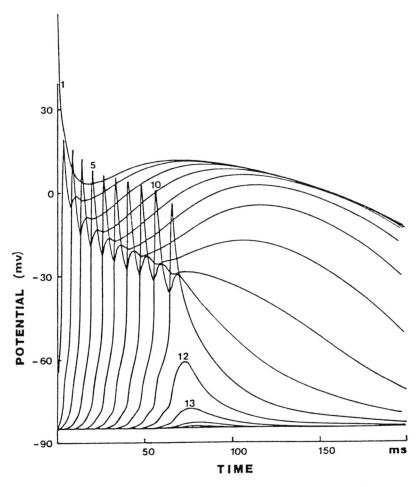

Figure 3. Decremental propagation caused by very high gap junction resistance ($R_g = 380$ $\Omega\cdot cm^2$). Numbers in body of figure indicate cell number relative to stimulus site. Reprinted with permission from Reference 20.

in the other direction. Unidirectional block can occur on the tail of a previous action potential in an otherwise uniform and homogeneous fiber. A directional asymmetry is created by the dispersion of excitability that exists in the wake of the previous action potential. Excitability is regulated by recovery from inactivation of the fast inward sodium channels. During normal sinus rhythm, the duration of the diastolic rest period is sufficient to ensure full recovery from inactivation of the sodium channels. Premature stimuli that occur early in the diastolic period elicit excitatory responses that diminish with increasing degree of prematurity. The development of excitatory responses in both directions, regardless of magnitude, is referred to as bidirectional conduction. If the stimulus is sufficiently premature, then the fiber will be inexcitable in both directions, and bidirectional block will occur.

We define the "vulnerable window" (TW) as the time interval in the refractory period (between plateau and diastole) of a propagating action potential during which unidirectional block and reentry can be induced (Figure 4). The vulnerable window can also be represented as a distance in the space domain (SW) or as a range of membrane potentials in the voltage domain (VW). Outside this window, it is impossible to induce unidirectional block and reentry; an action potential induced by a premature stimulus either propagates or blocks in both directions. When a premature stimulus is applied inside the window, the membrane generates a critical sodium current, giving rise to an action potential that propagates incrementally in the retrograde direction and decrementally in the antegrade direction. This is because in the retrograde direction, the tissue is progressively more recovered as the distance from the window increases in this direction, whereas in the antegrade direction the membrane is progressively less excitable as the distance from the window increases.

Figure 5 demonstrates the relationship between bidirectional conduction, bidirectional block, and unidirectional block. It also serves to

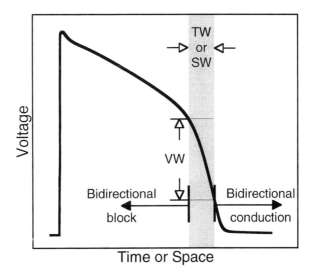

Figure 4. Schematic of vulnerable window during refractory period of propagating action potential. TW, SW, and VW represent the vulnerable window in the time domain, spaced domain, and voltage domain, respectively. Reprinted with permission from Reference 25.

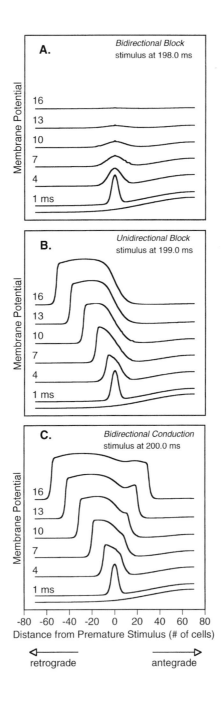

illustrate the concept of the vulnerable window. In this simulation, a multicellular one-dimensional fiber (150 cells connected by gap junctions) is first stimulated at one end to initiate a propagating, conditioning action potential. A second, premature stimulus is applied to cell 80 during the repolarization phase of the conditioning waveform at three different times after the primary stimulus (198, 199, and 200 ms; Figures 5A, 5B, and 5C, respectively).

When the premature stimulus was applied at 198 ms (Figure 5A) after the initial proximal stimulus, conduction block occurred in both the antegrade and retrograde directions. When the premature stimulus was applied 2 ms later at 200 ms (Figure 5C), an excitatory response was achieved in both the antegrade and retrograde directions. At a time between bidirectional block and bidirectional conduction (ie, inside the vulnerable window) at 199 ms (Figure 5B), block occurred in the antegrade direction but excitatory conduction was successful in the retrograde direction (unidirectional block). Note that in the antegrade direction, propagation is decremental, whereas in the retrograde direction, propagation is incremental. This is because in the antegrade direction, the membrane is progressively less excitable (less recovered) as the distance from the window increases (see bottom trace of each panel, which shows the membrane potential due to the conditioning action potential immediately before the premature stimulus). In the retrograde direction, in contrast, the fiber is progressively more recovered with distance from the window, resulting in incremental propagation in this direction.

It is clear from the above discussion that the inducibility of unidirectional block and reentry is related to the spatial inhomogeneity (asymmetry) of excitability at the vulnerable window. Figure 6 shows the distribution of excitability properties in the neighborhood of the vulnerable window. Panel A shows the distribution of the maximum fast sodium channel conductance during the action potential upstroke (g_{Na}) and its spatial gradient, dg_{Na}/dx. Panels B and C display the gating parameters m (activation), h (fast inactivation), and j (slow inactivation) of the sodium current and their spatial gradients at the time of peak g_{Na}. The maximum g_{Na} obtained from an isolated cell stimu-

---

Figure 5. Three types of responses to a premature stimulus. A, Bidirectional block occurred when premature stimulus was applied 198 ms after initiation of conditioning action potential and resulted from inability of premature stimulus to excite fiber in either direction. B, Unidirectional block at 199 ms resulted from successful retrograde but not antegrade excitation. C, Bidirectional conduction at 200 ms when both retrograde and antegrade fibers were excited. Bottom trace in each panel represents membrane potential immediately before stimulus. $R_g = 8 \ \Omega \cdot cm^2$. Reprinted with permission from Reference 23.

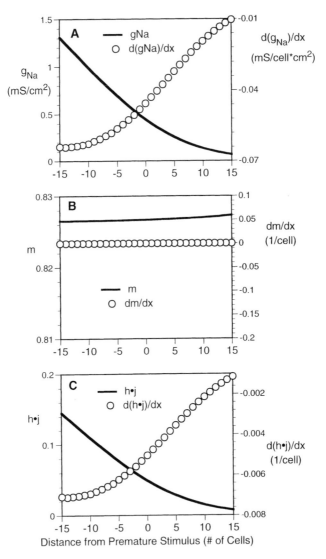

Figure 6. Spatial distribution of excitability, g_{Na}, in vicinity of vulnerable window. Solid curves represent parameters. Circles represent first spatial derivatives. g_{Na} indicates peak sodium conductance; m, activation parameter of I_{NA}; and h and j, fast and slow inactivation parameters of I_{NA}, respectively. Reprinted with permission from Reference 23.

lated at rest with the L-R membrane model is 8.36 mS/cm^2, with values of 0.89, 0.55, and 0.94 for the m, h, and j gates, respectively. The same parameters computed from a cell in the center of the vulnerable window were 0.844 mS/cm^2, 0.88, 0.30, and 0.18 for g_{Na}, m, h, and j, respectively. By separating g_{Na} into its activation (m) and inactivation (h·j) parameters, one observes that the reduction in g_{Na} (89.9%) is determined mostly by unrecovered inactivation (89.6% decrease in h·j). Reduced excitability is therefore not a function of a compromised m gate. The dominance of inactivation on the recovery of excitability is further evidenced by a comparison of the spatial gradient of excitability, dg_{Na}/dx, in Figure 6A with the spatial gradient of activation and inactivation of Figures 6B and 6C. The shape of dg_{Na}/dx follows that of d(h·j)/dx. dm/dx is practically zero (and m is constant) throughout the vulnerable window. Therefore, the spatial functional inhomogeneity of excitability is a reflection of the inhomogeneity of h·j and is not influenced by m. An inhomogeneous recovery from inactivation of I_{Na} creates the conditions for unidirectional block by facilitating excitation from a premature stimulus in the retrograde direction while inhibiting excitation in the antegrade direction. As the local spatial gradient of h·j increases, the spatial functional inhomogeneity of excitability increases, and unidirectional block is more likely to occur.

Gap Junction Effects and Membrane Effects on Vulnerability to Unidirectional Block

The size of the vulnerable window in the time domain (TW) provides a measure of the vulnerability of the tissue to the induction of unidirectional block and reentry. TW is a convenient working expression of the vulnerable window. For a large TW, the time interval during which unidirectional block can be induced is long. Therefore, the probability that a premature stimulus (eg, during clinical electrophysiology study in the catheterization laboratory) will fall inside the window and induce reentry is high. In the following simulation, we examine the effects of cellular decoupling at gap junctions and of membrane excitability on the tissue vulnerability to unidirectional block. Vulnerability (TW) as a function of gap junction resistance is shown in Figure 7 (curve 1). As the gap junction resistance increases, vulnerability increases as well, with an accompanying decrease in propagation velocity (curve 2). For normal cellular coupling ($R_g = 2$ Ω·cm^2), the vulnerability is about 0.5 ms. Very precise timing (TW<0.5 ms) of a premature stimulus is required for induction of unidirectional block and reentry. For a high degree of cellular decoupling ($R_g = 200$ Ω·cm^2), the vulnerability is increased to 30 ms. For such a wide window, unidirectional block

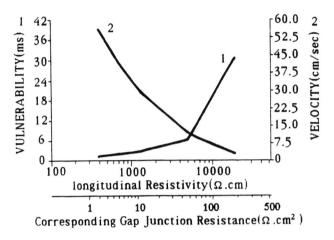

Figure 7. Changes in vulnerability due to changes in gap junction resistance, R_g. Curve 1 shows an increase in vulnerability when R_g increases. Curve 2 shows velocity of propagation as a function of R_g. Reprinted with permission from Reference 24.

can be easily induced. The simulations demonstrate, therefore, that as the degree of cellular decoupling is increased, velocity of propagation decreases (due to long delays at gap junctions) and vulnerability to reentry increases. In the previous section, we showed that the vulnerability is determined by the degree of spatial functional inhomogeneity of excitability at the vulnerable window. As regional propagation delay increases, due to long delays at gap junctions, the degree of spatial functional inhomogeneity in the state of the membrane increases as well. As demonstrated Figure 6, this increased asymmetry at the vulnerable window reflects an increase in the spatial gradient of the sodium inactivation gates h and j.

In contrast to the effect of cellular uncoupling described above, uniform reduction throughout the entire fiber in sodium channel conductance (intrinsic membrane excitability) resulted in slow propagation with decreased vulnerability to the induction of reentry (not shown). This is because a uniform reduction in membrane excitability produces a shift of the vulnerable window to a more recovered portion of the repolarization phase of the action potential (for a less excitable membrane, conditions similar to those under a noncompromised membrane are produced at a more recovered region). This shift to a less steep portion of the action potential brings about reduction in spatial gradients and reduces spatial inhomogeneities in the state of the membrane in the vicinity of the window. The result is lower vulnerability to the induction of unidirectional block and reentry. Quantitatively, the effect is small and operatively negligible; 50% reduction of sodium channel conductance brings about a decrease of the vulnerable window from 0.5 to 0.1 ms. In comparison, a reduction of cellular coupling that causes a similar decrease in conduction velocity is accompanied by a large increase of vulnerability from 0.5 to 30 ms (Figure 7).

It should be emphasized that the slight reduction of vulnerability observed above results from a uniform reduction of excitability along the uniform fiber. Experimentally, increased vulnerability is observed upon administration of drugs that depress membrane excitability (sodium channel blockers). We suspect that the drugs are not distributed uniformly throughout the tissue (drug distribution depends on the spatial organization of vascularization). This nonuniform distribution introduces nonuniformities in the state of the membrane that lead to increased vulnerability to unidirectional block and reentry. Moreover, even if depression of excitability were uniform, it does not occur in a uniform substrate; inhomogeneities in APD, refractoriness, and tissue structure are present in the actual physiological environment. The effects of inhomogeneities in membrane properties and in tissue structure are simulated below in the context of reentry.

Reentry in a Fixed Pathway

To simulate reentry in a closed pathway, the multicellular one-dimensional fiber was formed into a ring that included up to 1500 cells (Figure 8A).[24] In the following studies, we investigate the effects of membrane factors and structural factors on reentrant propagation.

Sustained and Nonsustained Reentry

Reentry induced in the ring could be sustained or nonsustained, depending on the relation between velocity, refractory period, and the length of the reentry pathway. Figure 8 shows an example of nonsustained (8B) and sustained (8C) reentry. The difference between the two simulations is the degree of cellular coupling. In Figure 8B, the gap junction resistance is 2 $\Omega \cdot cm^2$. A primary stimulus is applied at cell 1 of the homogeneous ring model (Figure 8A). A premature stimulus is applied to cell 70. It propagates decrementally in the antegrade direction only for a distance of five cells before it blocks. In the retrograde direction, the premature action potential propagates along the ring fiber, returns to cell 70, reenters, and continues to propagate until it encounters refractoriness and blocks. For a high degree of cellular uncoupling (gap junction resistance of 50 $\Omega \cdot cm^2$), sustained reentry is

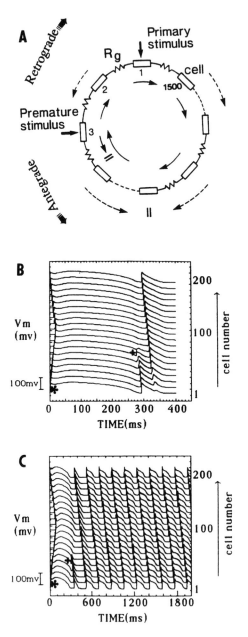

Figure 8. A, Ring-shaped cable model. Ring model consists of up to 1500 cells, each 100 μm in length and 16 μm in diameter. Primary stimulus was applied at top of ring while a premature stimulus was applied at a site in left branch during relative refractory period of propagating action potential initiated by primary stimulus. Solid arrows inside ring represent propagation of prema-

obtained (Figure 8C). The increased uncoupling brings about a fivefold decrease in propagation velocity, and reentry is sustained. The duration of the reentrant action potential is initially very short and then increases during a transient period until stable propagation with a duration of 120 ms (less than half the 270-ms duration of the normal action potential) is obtained. In other simulations (not shown), under conditions of greater head-to-tail interaction of the reentrant action potential, stable beat-to-beat alternans (long-short pattern) of APD are observed.

Effects of Membrane Inhomogeneities and Structural Inhomogeneities on Reentry

In the following simulations, we study the effects of membrane nonuniformities (refractoriness, excitability) and structural nonuniformities (fiber cross section, degree of cellular coupling) on vulnerability to the induction of reentry.

Refractory Period

Inhomogeneity in refractory period was created by reducing the conductance of the slow inward (calcium) channel in the left half (or right half) of the reentry pathway (not shown). A 10% to 15% reduction was used in the simulations. The primary and premature stimuli were both applied at the same location (top cell). For a proper timing of the premature stimulus (during the refractory period), reentry was induced. The size of the vulnerable window is proportional to the difference in refractory periods between the right and left branches of the pathway (ie, the degree of inhomogeneity). Note that with inhomogeneities, reentry could be induced by stimulating from a single site.

Membrane Excitability

Nonuniform distribution of membrane excitability also provides the necessary condition for unidirectional block and reentry. In the

◄——————————————————————————————————

ture (reentrant) action potential. It blocks in antegrade direction (= symbol) and reenters in retrograde direction. Dashed arrows outside ring represent propagation of primary action potential. Due to symmetry, it blocks at bottom (middle) cell of ring. R_g indicates gap junction resistance. B, Nonsustained reentry. Circle length is 2 cm; $R_g = 2$ Ω·cm^2. C, Sustained reentry. Circle length is 2 cm; $R_g = 50$ Ω·cm^2. Location (cell number) and time of application of premature stimuli are depicted by plus sign. Reprinted with permission from Reference 24.

simulation, this inhomogeneity was created by reduction of the conductance of the fast sodium channel, $\bar{g}_{Na}$ (10% to 50% reduction) in the left half of the ring. Both the primary and premature stimuli were applied at the top cell. For a properly timed premature stimulus, reentry was induced (not shown). As in the previous simulation, a window of vulnerability exists at the junction of inhomogeneity. The size of the window is proportional to the difference in the membrane excitability between the left and right branches. In other words, the likelihood of induction of unidirectional block and reentry was proportional to the degree of inhomogeneity in membrane excitability. As in the previous simulation, single-site stimulation was used.

Fiber Cross Section

It is known that sites at which the cross section of interconnected cells suddenly increases may be sites for unidirectional block. An action potential propagating in a strand of small cross section might not supply sufficient current for induction of propagation in the fiber with large cross section. We simulated this situation by introducing nonuniformities in the fiber radius, as shown in Figure 9. There were three fibers with radii of 4, 8, and 16 μm. Unidirectional block could occur at the junction of two fibers with different diameters when propagation traveled from a small-diameter fiber to a large-diameter fiber. For creation of unidirectional block, the ratio of diameters of connected fibers must be sufficiently high. Conduction was not blocked at either the junction between fiber I and fiber II or the junction between fiber II and fiber III, because the ratio of diameters (1:2) of the connected fibers was not high enough. Unidirectional block occurred at the junction between fiber I and fiber III when the impulse propagated from fiber I to fiber III. Note that the ratio of diameters of fibers I and III is 1:4. The stimulus was applied at cell 40. The action potential propagated in both the counterclockwise and clockwise directions. In the clockwise direction, the action potential propagated decrementally (about 20 cells) and completely blocked before it reached the junction between fibers I and III. In the counterclockwise direction, the action potential propagated through all the junctions, returned to the point of initiation, and kept propagating. Sustained reentry was obtained by setting parameters as indicated in Figure 9A. For this type of nonuniform ring, there is a favorable direction of circus movement (counterclockwise).

We noticed that there is a spatial gap on the ring at which a single stimulus could induce reentry. This gap is located close to the unidirectional block site on the small fiber (shown in Figure 9A by a large arrow). The existence of a finite gap results from the requirement that

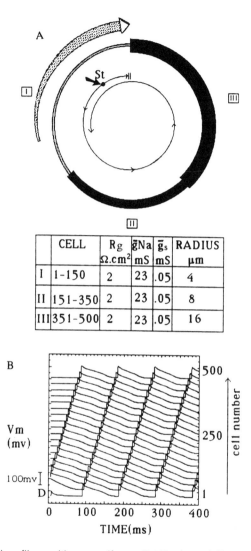

Figure 9. A, Ring fiber with nonuniform distribution of fiber cross sections. Unidirectional block could occur at junction of two fibers with different diameters when propagation is from small-diameter fiber to large-diameter fiber. Sustained circus movement could be induced by a single stimulus (St) applied within gap (large arrow) without need for a premature stimulus. B, Propagating action potentials along ring fiber of panel A. Note decremental propagation in clockwise direction from cell 10 to cell 1 (D). R_g indicates gap junction resistance; $\bar{g}_{Na}$, sodium channel conductance; $\bar{g}_s$, membrane conductance of slow inward channel; and V_m, membrane potential. Reprinted with permission from Reference 24.

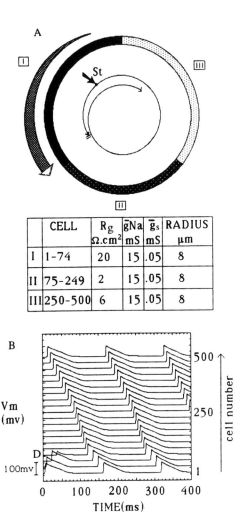

	CELL	R_g $\Omega.cm^2$	$\bar{g}Na$ mS	$\bar{g}_s$ mS	RADIUS μm
I	1-74	20	15	.05	8
II	75-249	2	15	.05	8
III	250-500	6	15	.05	8

Figure 10. A, Ring fiber with nonuniform distribution of gap junction resistances. Unidirectional block could occur at junction of two fibers with different gap junction resistances when propagation is from fiber with higher gap junction resistance to fiber with lower gap junction resistance. Sustained circus movement could be induced by a single stimulus (St) applied within gap (large arrow) without need for a premature stimulus. B, Propagating action potentials along ring fiber of panel A. Note decremental propagation in counterclockwise direction from cell 55 to cell 75 (D). R_g indicates gap junction resistance; $\bar{g}_{Na}$, sodium channel conductance; $\bar{g}_s$, membrane conductance of slow inward current; and V_m, membrane potential. Reprinted with permission from Reference 24.

the tissue be excitable at the time of arrival of the (counterclockwise) reentrant action potential at the I-III junction. The conductance of the slow inward channel, $\bar{g}_s$ (table in Figure 9A), is set to 0.05 (normal, 0.09) for reduction of the APD. However, it is not a necessary condition. If the ring fiber is long enough, reentry can be induced with a normal APD. Figure 9B shows the propagating action potentials along the ring fiber of Figure 9A. Note the decremental propagation (D) in the clockwise direction from cell 10 (stimulus site) to cell 1, where block occurs.

Cellular Coupling

The simulations also predict that nonuniform distribution of gap junction resistance could provide necessary conditions for unidirectional block and reentry that can be induced by a single stimulus without the need for premature stimulation. In Figure 10, there are three segments with gap junction resistances of 20, 2, and 6 $\Omega \cdot cm^2$. Unidirectional block may occur at the junction of two fibers with different gap junction resistances when propagation is from the fiber with higher gap junction resistance to the fiber with lower gap junction resistance.

As in the case of the ring with fibers of nonuniform radii (Figure 9), the ratio of gap junction resistance in adjacent segments is critical for the induction of unidirectional block. Propagation will not block at junctions I-III and III-II because this ratio (10:3 and 3:1, respectively) is not high enough. However, block occurs at junction I-II, at which the ratio of gap junction resistances is 10:1. The stimulus was applied at cell 10. The favorable direction of propagation is clockwise. The gap in which reentry could be induced by a single stimulus is located close to the site of unidirectional block (large arrow in Figure 10A). It should be mentioned that the reduced conductances of the sodium and the slow inward channels ($\bar{g}_{Na}$ and $\bar{g}_s$, Table in Figure 10A) are not necessary for unidirectional block and reentry. These modifications were introduced to decrease conduction velocity and APD so that computing time could be reduced. Figure 10B shows the propagating action potentials along the ring fiber of Figure 10A. Note the decremental propagation (D) in the counterclockwise direction from cell 55 to cell 75, where block occurs.

Conclusions

As stated in the introduction, propagation of excitation in cardiac tissue is determined by the relationship between the availability of depolarizing charge ("source") and the amount of charge required for successful propagation ("sink"). This relationship reflects a complex interaction between the membrane ionic currents that generate the action potential and the microscopic architecture of the tissue that determines the electric load on a depolarizing cell. In particular, the conductance and distribution of gap junctions determines intercellular current flow and conduction. Both membrane factors (eg, excitability in terms of sodium current kinetics) and gap junction factors (eg, conductance and distribution) can be affected by pathological conditions. In this chapter, we use a theoretical model that contains the elementary building block of cardiac tissue (discrete cells connected by gap junctions) to establish certain principles that underlie propagation. In particular, we investigate the roles of membrane excitability and gap junction conductance in determining conduction velocity, conduction block, vulnerability to unidirectional block, and the development of reentry. Conclusions are summarized below.

Properties of Propagation

Reduced membrane excitability reduces both conduction velocity and $(dV/dt)_{max}$. By reducing membrane excitability, velocity can only be reduced by a factor of about 3 (from 54 to 17 cm/s) before block occurs. In comparison, reduced intercellular coupling at gap junctions can support very slow conduction velocities (1 to 2 cm/s). This suggests that cellular decoupling plays an important role in very slow conduction that can be observed during reentry,[32] whereas reduced membrane excitability plays a more important role in the development of conduction block. The ability of reduced gap junction coupling to support very slow conduction is related to the biphasic behavior (increase, then decrease) of $(dV/dt)_{max}$ (Figure 2). This creates conditions for slow conduction with a fully developed rising phase of the action potential. Note that conduction block can result from elevated gap junction resistance, without compromised membrane excitability (Figure 3). However, an extreme degree of uncoupling is necessary for block to occur. We emphasize that to support very slow conduction velocities, gap junction uncoupling must be present. This implies that uncoupling plays an important role in anisotropic reentry, in which extremely slow conduction is observed across a line of apparent block.[33] Uncoupling must also be important to the development of reentry in short pathways ("microreentry"). This is because slow conduction shortens the wavelength of the reentrant action potential (defined as velocity times refractory period) to adapt to the short pathway without an excessive degree of head-to-tail interaction that leads to instabilities and termination of reentry.[25,26,34]

Unidirectional Block

Unidirectional block is a necessary condition for the development of reentry. Therefore, the vulnerability to reentry can be expressed in terms of the vulnerability to the induction of unidirectional block. We have quantified the probability of unidirectional block in terms of the vulnerable window. The vulnerable window is characterized by a spatial asymmetry of excitability, brought about by asymmetry of recovery from inactivation of the excitatory sodium current [ie, $d(h \cdot j)/dx$; see Figure 6 and related text]. Vulnerability to unidirectional block increases with a uniform increase in the degree of cellular decoupling at gap junctions (Figure 7). In contrast, uniform decrease of membrane excitability has a small effect on vulnerability (a slight increase or a slight decrease can be observed, depending on the simulation protocol.[23–25] This last observation seems contradictory to theoretical[35] and clinical[36] observations that vulnerability increases when membrane excitability is depressed by sodium channel blocking agents. A likely explanation of this apparent inconsistency is that in the realistic, physiological environment, the depression of excitability caused by the drug (or by ischemia, for that matter) can never be uniform and never occurs in a completely uniform substrate because inhomogeneities in APD, refractoriness, and tissue structure are present. The inhomogeneities in excitability that are introduced and the reduced excitability on a background of an inhomogeneous substrate enlarge the vulnerable window (see below) and facilitate the induction of unidirectional block.

Reentry and Inhomogeneities

Decreased membrane excitability and decreased intercellular coupling are electrophysiological changes associated with the development of reentry and arrhythmogenesis.[14,15,37] A uniform (or nonuniform) reduction of cellular coupling at gap junctions can transform nonsustained reentry to sustained reentry (Figure 8). As stated above, spatial nonuniformities always exist in the physiological substrate. The importance of inhomogeneities in membrane properties to the formation of unidirectional block and reentry was recognized early.[38] The simulations demonstrate that inhomogeneities both in membrane properties (refractory period, excitability) and in tissue architecture (structural inhomogeneities of fiber cross section or gap junction coupling) create conditions that favor induction of reentry. In fact, vulnerability to reentry is shown to be proportional to the degree of spatial inhomogeneity.

We conclude by noting that in addition to initiation of reentry, membrane factors and gap junction factors influence properties of the reentrant action potential once initiated. In previous simulation studies, we characterized the dynamics of reentry, including alternans and oscillations of APD and of cycle length and the dynamics that lead to termination of reentrant activity. By use of the theoretical model, the underlying mechanisms were analyzed in terms of the kinetics of sodium, potassium, and calcium membrane ionic channels. These studies are beyond the scope of this chapter, and the reader is referred to References 24 through 26 for discussion of these phenomena.

References

1. Spooner PM, Brown AM, eds. *Ion Channels in the Cardiovascular System: Function and Dysfunction.* Armonk, NY: Futura Publishing Co; 1994.
2. Luo C, Rudy Y. A dynamic model of the cardiac ventricular action potential, 1: simulations of ionic currents and concentration changes. *Circ Res.* 1994; 74:1071–1096.
3. Zeng J, Laurita KR, Rosenbaum DS, Rudy Y. Two components of the delayed rectifier K^+ current in ventricular myocytes of the guinea pig type: theoretical formulation and their role in repolarization. *Circ Res.* 1995;77: 1–13.
4. Spach MS, Miller WT, Gezelowitz DB, Barr RC, Kootsey JM, Johnson EA. The discontinuous nature of propagation in normal canine cardiac muscle: evidence for recurrent discontinuities of intracellular resistance that affect the membrane currents. *Circ Res.* 1981;48:39–54.
5. Weingart R, Maurer P. Action potential transfer in cell pairs isolated from adult rat and guinea pig ventricles. *Circ Res.* 1988;63:72–80.
6. Rook MB, Jongsma HJ, van Ginneken ACG. Properties of single gap junctional channels between isolated neonatal rat heart cells. *Am J Physiol.* 1988; 255:H770–H782.
7. Fast V, Kléber A. Microscopic conduction in cultured strands of neonatal rat heart cells measured with voltage-sensitive dyes. *Circ Res.* 1993;73:914–925.
8. Joyner RW. Effects of discrete electrical coupling on propagation through an electrical syncytium. *Circ Res.* 1982;50:192–200.
9. Henriquez CS, Plonsey R. Effects of resistive discontinuities on waveshape and velocity in a single cardiac fibre. *Med Biol Eng Comput.* 1987;25:428–438.
10. Cole WC, Picone JB, Sperelakis N. Gap junction uncoupling and discontinuous propagation in the heart. *Biophys J.* 1988;53:809–818.
11. Spach MS, Heidlage JF. The stochastic nature of cardiac propagation at a microscopic level: electrical description of myocardial architecture and its application to conduction. *Circ Res.* 1995;76:366–380.
12. Leon LJ, Roberge FA. Directional characteristics of action potential propagation in cardiac muscle: a model study. *Circ Res.* 1991;69:378–395.
13. Cascio WE, Johnson TA, Gettes LS. Electrophysiologic changes in ischemic ventricular myocardium, 1: influence of ionic, metabolic, and energetic changes. *J Cardiovasc Electrophysiol.* 1995;6:1039–1062.
14. Wit AL, Janse MJ. *The Ventricular Arrhythmias of Ischemia and Infarction: Electrophysiological Mechanisms.* Armonk, NY: Futura Publishing Co.; 1993.
15. Kléber AG, Riegger CB, Janse MJ. Electrical uncoupling and increase of

extracellular resistance after induction of ischemia in isolated, arterially perfused rabbit papillary muscle. *Circ Res.* 1987;51:271–279.

16. Yan G, Cascio W, Kléber A. Evidence of inhomogeneous cellular uncoupling in ventricular muscle during ischemia. *Circulation.* 1988;78(suppl II): II–639. Abstract.

17. Wu J, McHowat J, Saffitz JE, Yamada KA, Corr PB. Inhibition of gap junctional conductance by long-chain acylcarnitines and their preferential accumulation in junctional sarcolemma during hypoxia. *Circ Res.* 1993;72: 879–889.

18. DeMello WC. Intercellular communication in cardiac muscle. *Circ Res.* 1982; 51:1–9.

19. Janse MJ, Wit AL. Electrophysiological mechanisms of ventricular arrhythmias resulting from myocardial ischemia and infarction. *Physiol Rev.* 1989; 69:1049–1152.

20. Rudy Y, Quan W. A model study of the effects of the discrete cellular structure on electrical propagation in cardiac tissue. *Circ Res.* 1987;61: 815–823.

21. Rudy Y, Quan W. Propagation delays across cardiac gap junctions and their reflection in extracellular potentials: a simulation study. *J Cardiovasc Electrophysiol.* 1991;2:299–315.

22. Rudy Y. Models of continuous and discontinuous propagation in cardiac tissue. In: Zipes DP, Jalife J, eds. *Cardiac Electrophysiology: From Cell to Bedside.* Philadelphia, Pa WB, Saunders Publishers; 1994:326–334.

23. Shaw RM, Rudy Y. The vulnerable window for unidirectional block in cardiac tissue: characterization and dependence on membrane excitability and cellular coupling. *J Cardiovasc Electrophysiol.* 1995;6:115–131.

24. Quan W, Rudy Y. Unidirectional block and reentry of cardiac excitation: a model study. *Circ Res.* 1990;66:367–382.

25. Rudy Y. Reentry: insights from theoretical simulations in a fixed pathway. *J Cardiovasc Electrophysiol.* 1995;6:294–312.

26. Quan W, Rudy Y. Termination of reentrant propagation by a single stimulus: a model study. *Pacing Clin Electrophysiol.* 1991;14:1700–1706.

27. Beeler GW, Reuter H. Reconstruction of the action potential of ventricular myocardial fibers. *J Physiol (Lond).* 1977;286:177–210.

28. Veenstra RD, DeHaan RL. Measurement of single channel currents from cardiac gap junctions. *Science.* 1986;223:972–974.

29. Page E, Shibata Y. Permeable junctions between cardiac cells. *Annu Rev Physiol.* 1981;43:431–441.

30. Sasyniuk BI, Mendez C. A mechanism for re-entry in canine ventricular tissue. *Circ Res.* 1971;28:3–15.

31. Sicouri S, Delmar M, Jalife J. Role of electrical uncoupling on impulse propagation in sheep cardiac Purkinje fibers. *Biophys J.* 1986;49:346a. Abstract.

32. Dillon SM, Allessie MA, Ursell PC, Wit AL. Influence of anisotropic tissue structure on reentrant circuits in the epicardial border zone of subacute canine infarcts. *Circ Res.* 1988;63:182–206.

33. Wit AL, Dillon SM, Coromilas J. Anisotropic reentry as a cause of ventricular tachyarrhythmias in myocardial infarction. In: Zipes DP, Jalife J, eds. *Cardiac Electrophysiology: From Cell to Bedside.* Philadelphia Pa: WB Saunders Publishers; 1994:511–526.

34. Frame LH, Simson MD. Oscillation of conduction, action potential duration and refractoriness: a mechanism for spontaneous termination of reentrant tachycardias. *Circulation* 1988;78:1277–1287.

35. Starmer CF, Lastra AA, Nesterenko VV, et al. Proarrhythmic response to sodium channel blockade: theoretical model and numerical experiments. *Circulation.* 1991;84:1364–1377.
36. The Cardiac Arrhythmia Suppression Trial (CAST) Investigators. Preliminary report: effect of encainide and flecainide on mortality in a randomized trial of arrhythmia suppression after myocardial infarction. *N Engl J Med.* 1989;321:406–412.
37. Nesterenko VV, Lastra AA, Rosenshtraukh LV, et al. A proarrhythmic response to sodium channel blockage: modulation of the vulnerable period in guinea pig ventricular myocardium. *J Cardiovasc Pharmacol.* 1992;19:810–820.
38. Han J, Moe GK. Nonuniform recovery of excitability of ventricular muscle. *Circ Res.* 1974;14:44–60.

Perspectives and Future Directions
Arrhythmias and Discontinuous Conduction

Harold C. Strauss, MD

Cardiac arrhythmias remain a major public health problem despite intensive research on this subject for many years. The relatively limited progress in the clinical sphere reflects our limited understanding of the inordinate complexity of the underlying mechanisms. Specifically, these are related to macroscopic structural and pathological factors as well as to cellular factors such as ion channel function and cell signaling cascades, all of which are intimately involved in the initiation and perpetuation of cardiac arrhythmias.

As stated in the preface to this monograph, one of the considerations of the Hilton Head workshop was to explore different facets of discontinuous conduction, presenting not only perspectives from different laboratories but also the implications for different mechanisms of cardiac arrhythmias. An additional goal was to consider how individual elements of discontinuity, such as gap junctions, might be modulated therapeutically to terminate arrhythmias.

The discovery of the discontinuous nature of conduction at a microscopic level in the heart represented a seminal advance in the field. Recent progress in our understanding of its basis in the heart is elegantly summarized in the preceding chapters in this text. In addition to raising many questions (see below), this work suggests that discontinuous propagation depends on many microscopic and macroscopic factors. Microscopic factors include the properties of different ion and gap junction channels in each cell, the distribution of communication sites and their geometric arrangement at the cellular level, and the different chemical messengers that cells use to communicate with each other. At the macroscopic level, fiber and tissue geometric factors are also potentially important in that they can result in a mismatch of loads that also contribute to arrhythmogenesis. In addition to the factors just described, changes in dynamic variables such as action potential duration and refractoriness also can modulate the degree of discontinuity observed.

There has been particular progress on factors underlying discontinuous conduction, especially in the areas of the functional analysis of different gap junction proteins, the role of spiral waves as generators of experimental cardiac arrhythmias, and new cellular and theoretical models to evaluate the effects of changes in discontinuities on conduction. In addition, promising new gene targeting strategies that have the potential to alter discontinuities in vivo are noted, although at this time their utility seems remote. Other more immediate approaches are also described in an effort to capitalize on the recent progress achieved. Progress in each of these areas has been gleaned from numerous experiments conducted on individual protein molecules and assessment of their integrated function in normal and abnormal systems and in computer simulations of propagation, reentry, and spiral wave generation.

Despite these important advances, numerous issues remain unresolved. Although it is likely that some of the "mechanisms" discussed here may be capable of generating arrhythmias, their relative importance in acquired arrhythmias remains unresolved. The absence of specific diagnostic criteria and selective pharmacological probes precludes a reasonable deductive approach to patients with cardiac arrhythmias that would shed further light on underlying mechanisms. For example, we still do not know whether substantial changes in discontinuities occur before the initiation of an arrhythmic event and under what circumstances they may be detectable in patients. Furthermore, although one may wish to target the gap junction or a specific gap junction protein isoform as a therapeutic modality in patients with certain reentrant arrhythmias, it is still unclear whether one would want to increase or reduce gap junction resistance or alter its properties in other, more subtle ways.

One promising development on which some progress is being made is the area of uniformity of distribution of different connexins and K^+ channels throughout the heart. If the expression of genes for individual connexins and ion channels, or channel gene expression, is not uniform throughout the heart, as it now appears,[1,2] then this may provide insights into underlying principles on which such distributions are based. Elucidation of such principles may be therapeutically important. In this vein, changes in the pattern of channel gene expression that may occur in the border zone surviving an acute myocardial infarction may carry special significance for ischemic arrhythmias.[3,4]

The potential of improved insights into the complexities of discontinuous conduction and, as a result, therapy was the subject of a summary discussion at the Hilton Head workshop. From this meeting, a number of important issues emerged that most if not all of the participants agreed were of importance in furthering our understanding of the mechanisms of cardiac arrhythmias.

One of the foremost issues that emerged at this meeting was the need for developing a full range of models that span the spectrum from the cell at one end, to animal models, to mathematically based theoretical models that can examine discontinuous behavior from different perspectives. It was thought that this broad approach is necessary because the ability to extract information from noninvasive and invasive clinical measurements is quite limited. Given the paucity of relevant clinical information, it is clear that there is a need for clinical studies to identify which of the variables are perturbed and which require modification. Only by exploring a full range of hierarchical models and systems are we likely to identify testable new hypotheses or putative therapeutic strategies of a more sophisticated nature than global depolarization resulting from DC countershock. Given the inordinate complexities underlying cardiac arrhythmias, mathematical models of generic excitable media, which have been useful in the study of the dynamics of a variety of experimental arrhythmias, are likely to be useful for making testable predictions regarding the mechanisms of complex patterns during arrhythmias. In addition, continuation of studies on the dynamics of waves in excitable media and development of computer models that incorporate more biologically relevant factors (eg, discrete structural inhomogeneities and corresponding kinetic and pharmacological channel diversity, as well as diversity of gap junction and channel density) are likely to generate more realistic simulations of electrical activity in the heart. These studies are of equal importance to ongoing work in intact dog models, geometrically defined multicellular systems, and docking incompatibilities between different gap junction proteins.

Another important issue that emerged during the concluding discussions is the need to develop a class of pharmacological agents that selectively modulate gap junction resistance and, as a result, conduction in the heart. The discovery of agents that could predictably modify cell-to-cell communication, especially if they were specific to a particular connexin isoform, could result in novel therapeutic approaches toward preventing or alleviating some arrhythmias. A related approach is to identify specific modulating factors that regulate expression of junctional components. In addition, an approach that selectively modulated expression and translation of cardiac gap junctions, especially if it could be achieved uniquely in different cells or with different connexins, could be very important. Finally, it appears that approaches that advance our understanding of the diversity of ion and gap junction proteins that exist in the heart form an area of unexplored potential.

Extending our knowledge of the genetic basis of arrhythmias resulting from conduction abnormalities is another objective that deserves increased emphasis. Such approaches have recently proved powerful in the discovery of ion channel mutations underlying some types of rare congenital arrhythmias (familial long-QT syndrome).[5,6] This work offers a reasonable template for development of similar approaches to the determinants of cardiac conduction, and in fact, preliminary work on this topic has appeared in the literature.[7]

Given the complexity and diversity of factors that determine the basis of both continuous and discontinuous conduction in the heart, it seems appropriate that a multifaceted approach be pursued to discover fundamental defects responsible for arrhythmias resulting from discontinuous conduction. The work presented here provides important insights into this exciting research field.

Acknowledgments   I am indebted to L.S. Gettes, J. Jalife, R. Joyner, M. Morales, R.L. Rasmusson, P. Spooner, and D. Spray for their critical review of an earlier version of this chapter and to P. Spooner for editorial comments.

References

1. Brahmajothi MV, Morales MJ, Liu SG, Rasmusson RL, Campbell DL, Strauss HC. In situ hybridization reveals extensive diversity of K^+ channel mRNA in isolated ferret cardiac myocytes. *Circ Res.* 1996;78:1083–1089.
2. Brahmajothi MV, Morales MJ, Reimer KA, Strauss HC. Regional localization of *ERG*, the channel protein responsible for the rapid component of the delayed rectifier current (Ikr) in the ferret heart. *Circ Res.* 1997;81:128–135.
3. Peters NS, Coromilas J, Severs NJ, Wit AL. Connexin43 gap junction distribution in the surviving myocytes of the arrhythmogenic border zone of canine four-day-old myocardial infarcts. *Circulation.* 1994;90(Suppl I):I–465. Abstract.
4. Peters NS, Severs NJ, Coromilas J, Wit AL. Disturbed connexin43 gap junction distribution correlates with the location of reentrant circuits in the epicardial border zone of healing canine infarcts that cause ventricular tachycardia. *Circulation.* 1997;95:988–996.
5. Curran ME, Splawski I, Timothy KW, Vincent GM, Green ED, Keating MT. A molecular basis for cardiac arrhythmia: HERG mutations cause long QT syndrome. *Cell.* 1995;80:795–803.
6. Wang Q, Shen J, Splawski I, et al. SCN5A mutations associated with an inherited cardiac arrhythmia, long QT syndrome. *Cell.* 1995;80:805–811.
7. Olson TM, Keating MT. A familial disorder of automaticity and conduction associated with cardiomyopathy maps to chromosome 3p. *Circulation.* 1995; 92(suppl I)I–233. Abstract.

Index

551